EUROPEAN PHARMACOPOEIA - SUPPLEMENT 6.1 TO THE 6th EDITION

published 12 September 2007

The 6th Edition of the European Pharmacopoeia consists of volumes 1 and 2 of the publication 6.0, and Supplement 6.1. These will be complemented by **non-cumulative supplements** that are to be kept for the duration of the 6th Edition. A further supplement will be published in 2007, followed by 3 supplements in each of the years 2008 and 2009. A cumulative list of reagents will be published in supplements 6.4 and 6.7.

If you are using the 6th Edition at any time later than 1 April 2008, make sure that you have all the published supplements and consult the index of the most recent supplement to ensure that you use the latest versions of the monographs and general chapters.

EUROPEAN PHARMACOPOEIA - ELECTRONIC VERSION

The 6th Edition is also available in an electronic format (CD-ROM and online version) containing all of the monographs and general chapters found in the printed version. With the publication of each supplement the electronic version is replaced by a new, fully updated, cumulative version.

In addition to the official English and French online versions, a Spanish online version (5th Edition) is also available for the convenience of users.

PHARMEUROPA

Quarterly Forum Publication

Pharmeuropa contains preliminary drafts of all new and revised monographs proposed for inclusion in the European Pharmacopoeia and gives an opportunity for all interested parties to comment on the specifications before they are finalised. Pharmeuropa also contains information on the work programme and on certificates of suitability to monographs of the European Pharmacopoeia issued by the EDQM, and articles of general interest. Pharmeuropa is available on subscription from the EDQM. The subscription also includes Pharmeuropa Bio and Pharmeuropa Scientific Notes (containing scientific articles on pharmacopoeial matters). Pharmeuropa Online is also available as a complementary service for subscribers to the printed version of Pharmeuropa.

INTERNATIONAL HARMONISATION

See the information given in chapter *5.8. Pharmacopoeial Harmonisation*.

WEBSITE

http://www.edqm.eu
http://www.edqm.eu/store (for prices and orders)

HELPDESK

To send a question or to contact the EDQM, use the HELPDESK, accessible through the EDQM website (visit http://www.edqm.eu/site/page_521.php).

KNOWLEDGE

Consult KNOWLEDGE, the new free database at http://www.edqm.eu to obtain information on the work programme of the European Pharmacopoeia, the volume of Pharmeuropa and of the European Pharmacopoeia in which a text has been published, trade names of the reagents (for example, chromatography columns) that were used at the time of the elaboration of the monographs, the history of the revisions of a text since its publication in the 5th Edition, reference chromatograms, the list of reference standards used, and the list of certificates granted.

COMBISTATS

CombiStats is a computer program for the statistical analysis of data from biological assays in agreement with chapter *5.3* of the 6th Edition of the European Pharmacopoeia. For more information, visit the website (http://www.edqm.eu/combistats).

Members of the European Pharmacopoeia Commission: Austria, Belgium, Bosnia and Herzegovina, Bulgaria, Croatia, Cyprus, Czech Republic, Denmark, Estonia, Finland, France, Germany, Greece, Hungary, Iceland, Ireland, Italy, Latvia, Lithuania, Luxembourg, Malta, Montenegro, Netherlands, Norway, Poland, Portugal, Romania, Serbia, Slovak Republic, Slovenia, Spain, Sweden, Switzerland, 'the former Yugoslav Republic of Macedonia', Turkey, United Kingdom and the European Union.

Observers to the European Pharmacopoeia Commission: Albania, Algeria, Australia, Belarus, Brazil, Canada, China, Georgia, Israel, Madagascar, Malaysia, Morocco, Republic of Kazakhstan, Russian Federation, Senegal, Syria, Tunisia, Ukraine, United States of America and WHO (World Health Organisation).

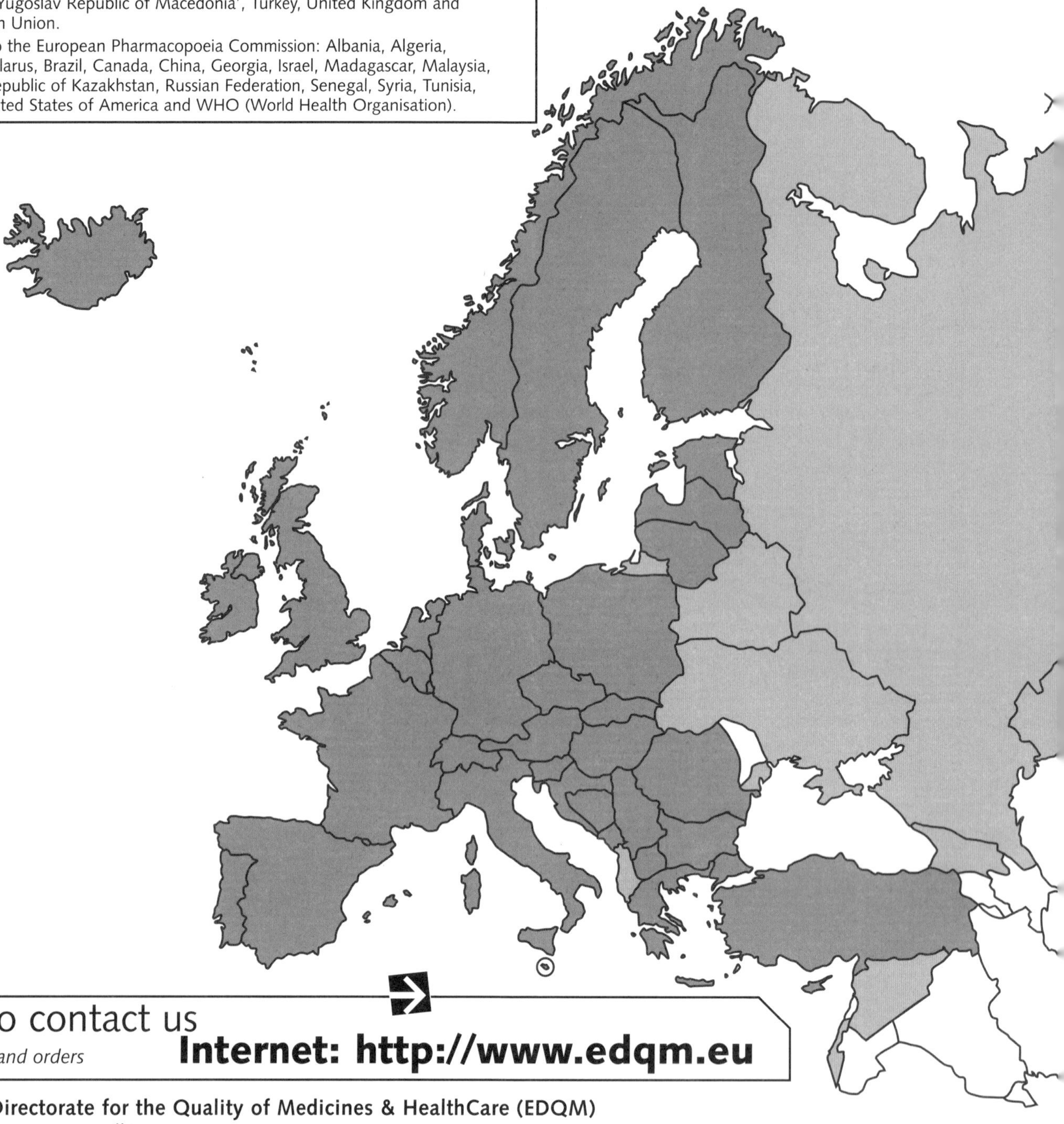

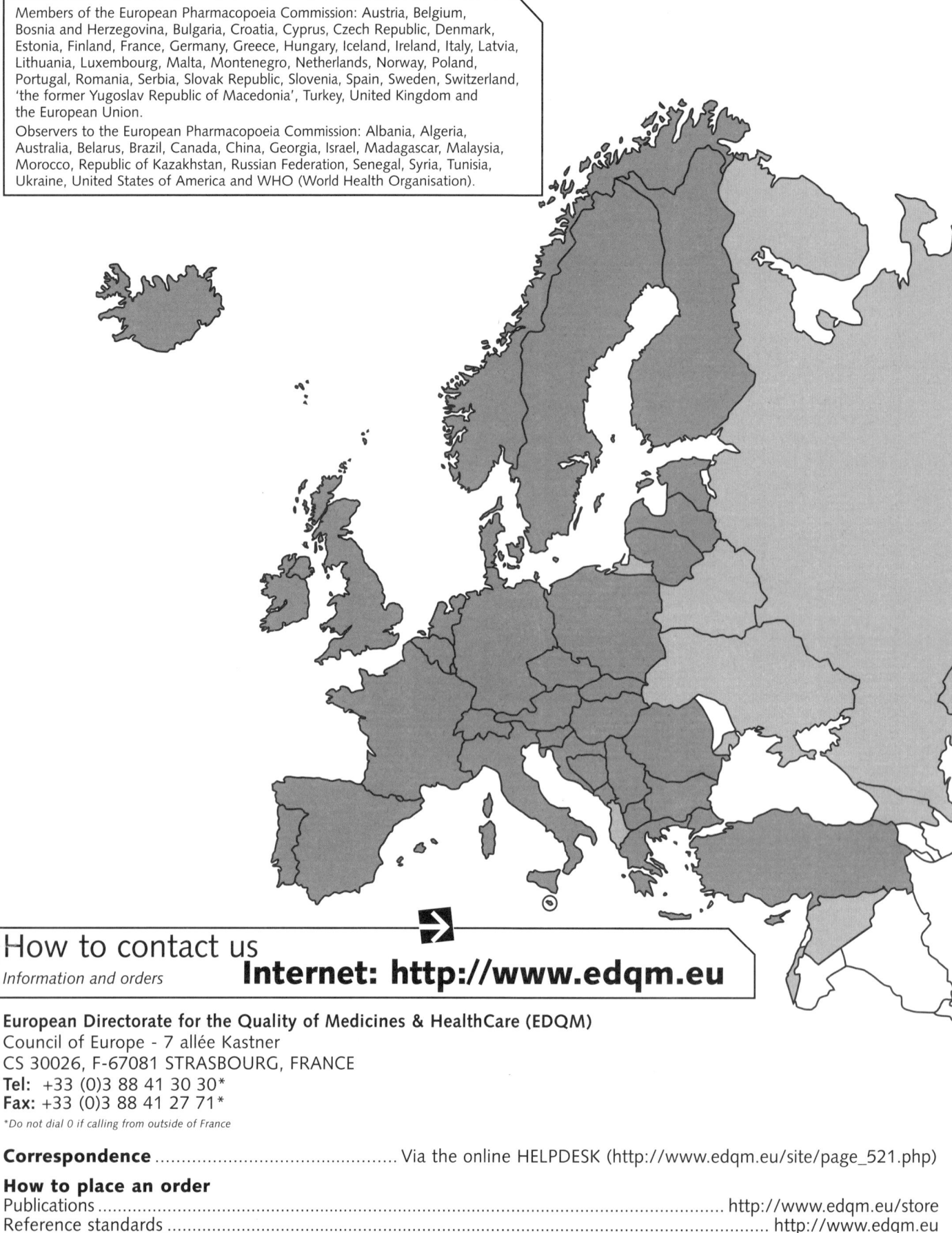

How to contact us

Information and orders **Internet: http://www.edqm.eu**

European Directorate for the Quality of Medicines & HealthCare (EDQM)
Council of Europe - 7 allée Kastner
CS 30026, F-67081 STRASBOURG, FRANCE
Tel: +33 (0)3 88 41 30 30*
Fax: +33 (0)3 88 41 27 71*
**Do not dial 0 if calling from outside of France*

Correspondence .... Via the online HELPDESK (http://www.edqm.eu/site/page_521.php)

How to place an order

Publications .... http://www.edqm.eu/store
Reference standards .... http://www.edqm.eu
Reference standards online order form .... http://www.edqm.eu/site/page_649.php

Further information, including answers to the most frequently asked questions regarding ordering, is available via the HELPDESK.

All other matters ....info@edqm.eu

All reference standards required for application of the monographs are available from the EDQM. A catalogue of reference standards is available on request; the catalogue is included in the Pharmeuropa subscription; it can also be consulted on the EDQM website.

EUROPEAN PHARMACOPOEIA

SIXTH EDITION

Supplement 6.1

EUROPEAN PHARMACOPOEIA

SIXTH EDITION

Supplement 6.1

Published in accordance with the
Convention on the Elaboration of a European Pharmacopoeia
(European Treaty Series No. 50)

European Directorate for the
Quality of Medicines & HealthCare

Council of Europe
Strasbourg

The European Pharmacopoeia is published by the Directorate for the Quality of Medicines & HealthCare of the Council of Europe (EDQM).

ISBN: 978-92-871-6057-7

CONTENTS

CONTENTS OF SUPPLEMENT 6.1	xxxi
GENERAL CHAPTERS	3309
2. Methods of Analysis	3309
2.2. Physical and physicochemical methods	3309
2.2.34. Thermal analysis	3311
2.2.60. Melting point - instrumental method	3313
2.6. Biological tests	3315
2.6.7. Mycoplasmas	3317
2.9. Pharmaceutical technical procedures	3323
2.9.40. Uniformity of dosage units	3325
2.9.43. Apparent dissolution	3327
4. Reagents	3329
4.1.1. Reagents	3331
4.1.3. Buffer solutions	3331
5. General Texts	3333
5.2.7. Evaluation of efficacy of veterinary vaccines and immunosera	3335
5.15. Functionality-related characteristics of excipients	3339
GENERAL MONOGRAPHS	3341
MONOGRAPHS ON VACCINES FOR HUMAN USE	3345
MONOGRAPHS ON VACCINES FOR VETERINARY USE	3369
MONOGRAPHS ON RADIOPHARMACEUTICAL PREPARATIONS	3379
MONOGRAPHS ON HOMOEOPATHIC PREPARATIONS	3383
MONOGRAPHS	3391
INDEX	3571

Note: on the first page of each chapter/section there is a list of contents.

CONTENTS OF SUPPLEMENT 6.1

A vertical line in the margin indicates where part of a text has been revised or corrected. A horizontal line in the margin indicates where part of a text has been deleted. It is to be emphasised that these indications, which are not necessarily exhaustive, are given for information and do not form an official part of the texts. Editorial changes are not indicated.

Individual copies of texts will not be supplied.

NEW TEXTS

GENERAL CHAPTERS

2.2.60. Melting point - instrumental method

5.15. Functionality-related characteristics of excipients

MONOGRAPHS

*The monographs below appear for the first time in the European Pharmacopoeia. They will be implemented on **1 April 2008** at the latest.*

Monographs

Acemetacin (1686)
Bisoprolol fumarate (1710)
Boldo leaf dry extract (1816)
Clopamide (1747)
Desflurane (1666)
Ginkgo dry extract, refined and quantified (1827)
Liquorice dry extract for flavouring purposes (2378)
Magnesium gluconate (2161)
Manganese gluconate (2162)
Marbofloxacin for veterinary use (2233)
Molsidomine (1701)
Niflumic acid (2115)
Pantoprazole sodium sesquihydrate (2296)
Sanguisorba root (2385)
Selamectin for veterinary use (2268)
Sertraline hydrochloride (1705)
Sodium phenylbutyrate (2183)
Sucrose monopalmitate (2319)
Sucrose stearate (2318)
Willow bark dry extract (2312)

REVISED TEXTS

GENERAL CHAPTERS

2.9.40. Uniformity of dosage units

4. Reagents *(new, revised, corrected)*

5.2.7. Evaluation of efficacy of veterinary vaccines and immunosera

MONOGRAPHS

*The monographs below have been technically revised since their last publication. They will be implemented on **1 April 2008**.*

General monographs

Extracts (0765)

Vaccines for human use

Measles, mumps and rubella vaccine (live) (1057)
Measles vaccine (live) (0213)
Mumps vaccine (live) (0538)
Poliomyelitis vaccine (oral) (0215)
Rabies vaccine for human use prepared in cell cultures (0216)
Rubella vaccine (live) (0162)
Smallpox vaccine (live) (0164)
Varicella vaccine (live) (0648)
Yellow fever vaccine (live) (0537)

Vaccines for veterinary use

Avian infectious bronchitis vaccine (live) (0442)
Rabies vaccine (inactivated) for veterinary use (0451)

Monographs

Alfuzosin hydrochloride (1287)
Aluminium hydroxide, hydrated, for adsorption (1664)
Arnica flower (1391)
Atropine (2056)
Atropine sulphate (0068)
Bearberry leaf (1054)
Butcher's broom (1847)
Caffeine (0267)
Carbomers (1299)
Cefadroxil monohydrate (0813)
Cefalexin monohydrate (0708)
Chlorphenamine maleate (0386)
Clotrimazole (0757)
Codeine (0076)
Devil's claw root (1095)
Diethyl phthalate (0897)
Dihydroergotamine mesilate (0551)
Diltiazem hydrochloride (1004)
Disodium phosphate dodecahydrate (0118)
Doxepin hydrochloride (1096)
Estradiol benzoate (0139)
Ethambutol hydrochloride (0553)
Glutathione (1670)
Goldenseal rhizome (1831)
Hamamelis leaf (0909)
Hop strobile (1222)
Hypromellose phthalate (0347)
Ibuprofen (0721)
Lidocaine (0727)
Liothyronine sodium (0728)
Lymecycline (1654)
Morphine hydrochloride (0097)
Morphine sulphate (1244)
Nifuroxazide (1999)
Povidone (0685)
Roselle (1623)

Spiramycin (0293)
Sultamicillin (2211)
Tetracaine hydrochloride (0057)
Triamterene (0058)
Triglycerol diisostearate (2032)
Willow bark (1583)

CORRECTED TEXTS

The texts below have been corrected and are republished in their entirety. These corrections are to be taken into account from the publication date of Supplement 6.1.

GENERAL CHAPTERS

2.2.34. Thermal analysis
2.6.7. Mycoplasmas
2.9.43. Apparent dissolution

MONOGRAPHS

Vaccines for veterinary use

Porcine progressive atrophic rhinitis vaccine (inactivated) (1361)

Radiopharmaceutical preparations

Iobenguane sulphate for radiopharmaceutical preparations (2351)

Homoeopathic preparations

Methods of preparation of homoeopathic stocks and potentisation (2371)

Monographs

Amikacin (1289)
Amikacin sulphate (1290)
Bacampicillin hydrochloride (0808)
Bilberry fruit, fresh (1602)
Cilastatin sodium (1408)
Clemastine fumarate (1190)
Dihydralazine sulphate, hydrated (1310)
Dirithromycin (1313)
Doxylamine hydrogen succinate (1589)
Glyceryl trinitrate solution (1331)
Hypromellose (0348)
Methylcellulose (0345)
Naproxen sodium (1702)
Paclitaxel (1794)
Phenoxymethylpenicillin (0148)
Phenoxymethylpenicillin potassium (0149)
Sertaconazole nitrate (1148)
Sultamicillin tosilate dihydrate (2212)
Terconazole (1270)
Terfenadine (0955)
Xanthan gum (1277)

DELETED TEXTS

*The following texts are deleted as of **1 April 2008**.*

MONOGRAPHS

Vaccines for human use

Pertussis vaccine (0160)

Monographs

Stanozolol (1568)

2.2. PHYSICAL AND PHYSICOCHEMICAL METHODS

01/2008:20234
corrected 6.1

2.2.34. THERMAL ANALYSIS

Thermal analysis is a group of techniques in which the variation of a physical property of a substance is measured as a function of temperature. The most commonly used techniques are those which measure changes of mass or changes in energy of a sample of a substance.

THERMOGRAVIMETRY

Thermogravimetry is a technique in which the mass of a sample of a substance is recorded as a function of temperature according to a controlled temperature programme.

Apparatus. The essential components of a thermobalance are a device for heating or cooling the substance according to a given temperature program, a sample holder in a controlled atmosphere, an electrobalance and a recorder. In some cases the instrument may be coupled to a device permitting the analysis of volatile products.

Temperature verification. Check the temperature scale using a suitable material according to the manufacturer's instructions.

Verification of the electrobalance. Place a suitable quantity of a suitable certified reference material (for example, *calcium oxalate monohydrate CRS*) in the sample holder and record the mass. Set the heating rate according to the manufacturer's instructions and start the temperature increase. Record the thermogravimetric curve as a graph with temperature, or time, on the abscissa, increasing from left to right, and mass on the ordinate, increasing upwards. Stop the temperature increase at about 230 °C. Measure the difference on the graph between the initial and final mass-temperature plateaux, or mass-time plateaux, which corresponds to the loss of mass. The declared loss of mass for the certified reference material is stated on the label.

Method. Apply the same procedure to the substance to be examined, using the conditions prescribed in the monograph. Calculate the loss of mass of the substance to be examined from the difference measured in the graph obtained. Express the loss of mass as per cent $\Delta\ m/m$.

If the apparatus is in frequent use, carry out temperature verification and calibration regularly. Otherwise, carry out such checks before each measurement.

Since the test atmosphere is critical, the following parameters are noted for each measurement: pressure or flow rate, composition of the gas.

DIFFERENTIAL SCANNING CALORIMETRY

Differential Scanning Calorimetry (DSC) is a technique that can be used to demonstrate the energy phenomena produced during heating (or cooling) of a substance (or a mixture of substances) and to determine the changes in enthalpy and specific heat and the temperatures at which these occur.

The technique is used to determine the difference in the flow of heat (with reference to the temperature) evolved or absorbed by the test sample compared with the reference cell, as a function of the temperature. Two types of DSC apparatuses are available, those using power compensation to maintain a null temperature difference between sample and reference and those that apply a constant rate of heating and detect temperature differential as a difference in heat flow between sample and reference.

Apparatus. The apparatus for the power compensation DSC consists of a furnace containing a sample holder with a reference cell and a test cell. The apparatus for the heat flow DSC consists of a furnace containing a single cell with a sample holder for the reference crucible and the test crucible.

A temperature-programming device, thermal detector(s) and a recording system which can be connected to a computer are attached. The measurements are carried out under a controlled atmosphere.

Calibration of the apparatus. Calibrate the apparatus for temperature and enthalpy change, using indium of high purity or any other suitable certified material, according to the manufacturer's instructions. A combination of 2 metals, e.g. indium and zinc may be used to control linearity.

Operating procedure. Weigh in a suitable crucible an appropriate quantity of the substance to be examined; place it in the sample holder. Set the initial and final temperatures, and the heating rate according to the operating conditions prescribed in the monograph.

Begin the analysis and record the differential thermal analysis curve, with the temperature or time on the abscissa (values increasing from left to right) and the energy change on the ordinate (specify whether the change is endothermic or exothermic).

The temperature at which the phenomenon occurs (the onset temperature) corresponds to the intersection (A) of the extension of the baseline with the tangent at the point of greatest slope (inflexion point) of the curve (see Figure 2.2.34.-1). The end of the thermal phenomenon is indicated by the peak of the curve.

The enthalpy of the phenomenon is proportional to the area under the curve limited by the baseline; the proportionality factor is determined from the measurement of the heat of fusion of a known substance (e.g., indium) under the same operating conditions.

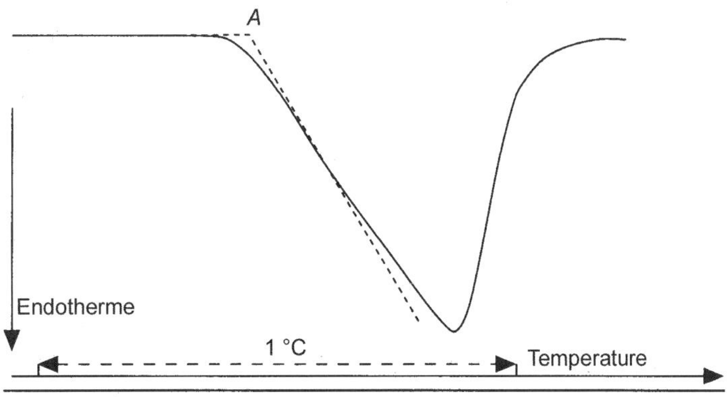

Figure 2.2.34.-1. – *Thermogram*

Each thermogram may be accompanied by the following data: conditions employed, record of last calibration, sample size and identification (including thermal history), container, atmosphere (identity, flow rate, pressure), direction and rate of temperature change, instrument and recorder sensitivity.

Applications

Phase changes. Determination of the temperature, heat capacity change and enthalpy of phase changes undergone by a substance as a function of temperature.

solid - solid transition:	allotropy - polymorphism glass transition desolvation amorphous-crystalline
solid - liquid transition:	melting
solid - gas transition:	sublimation
liquid - solid transition:	freezing recrystallisation
liquid - gas transition:	evaporation

Changes in chemical composition. Measurement of heat and temperatures of reaction under given experimental conditions, so that, for example, the kinetics of decomposition or of desolvation can be determined.

Application to phase diagrams. Establishment of phase diagrams for solid mixtures. The establishment of a phase diagram may be an important step in the preformulation and optimisation of the freeze-drying process.

Determination of purity. The measurement of the heat of fusion and the melting point by DSC enables the impurity content of a substance to be determined from a single thermal diagram, requiring the use of only a few milligrams of sample with no need for repeated accurate measurements of the true temperature.

In theory, the melting of an entirely crystalline, pure substance at constant pressure is characterised by a heat of fusion ΔH_f in an infinitely narrow range, corresponding to the melting point T_0. A broadening of this range is a sensitive indicator of impurities. Hence, samples of the same substance, whose impurity contents vary by a few tenths of a per cent, give thermal diagrams that are visually distinct (see Figure 2.2.34.-2).

The determination of the molar purity by DSC is based on the use of a mathematical approximation of the integrated form of the Van't Hoff equation applied to the concentrations (not the activities) in a binary system [$\ln(1 - x_2) = -x_2$ and $T \times T_0 = T_0^2$]:

$$T = T_0 - \frac{RT_0^2}{\Delta H_f} \times x_2 \qquad (1)$$

x_2 = mole fraction of the impurity i.e. the number of molecules of the impurity divided by the total number of molecules in the liquid phase (or molten phase) at temperature T (expressed in kelvins),

T_0 = melting point of the chemically pure substance, in kelvins,

ΔH_f = molar heat of fusion of the substance, in joules,

R = gas constant for ideal gases, in joules·kelvin^{-1}·mole^{-1}.

Hence, the determination of purity by DSC is limited to the detection of impurities forming a eutectic mixture with the principal compound and present at a mole fraction of less than 2 per cent in the substance to be examined.

This method cannot be applied to:

- amorphous substances,
- solvates or polymorphic compounds that are unstable within the experimental temperature range,
- impurities forming solid solutions with the principal substance,
- impurities that are insoluble in the liquid phase or in the melt of the principal substance.

During the heating of the substance to be examined, the impurity melts completely at the temperature of the eutectic mixture. Above this temperature, the solid phase contains only the pure substance. As the temperature increases progressively from the temperature of the eutectic mixture to the melting point of the pure substance, the mole fraction of impurity in the liquid decreases constantly, since the quantity of liquified pure substance increases constantly. For all temperatures above the eutectic point:

$$x_2 = \frac{1}{F} \times x_2^* \qquad (2)$$

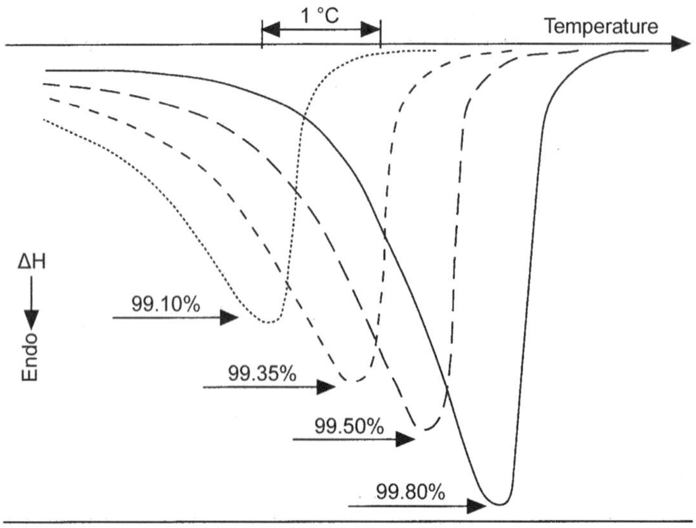

Figure 2.2.34.-2. – *Thermal diagrams according to purity*

F = molten fraction of the analysed sample,

x_2^* = mole fraction of the impurity in the analysed sample.

When the entire sample has melted, $F = 1$ and $x_2 = x_2^*$.

If equation (2) is combined with equation (1), the following equation is obtained:

$$T = T_0 - \frac{x_2^* R T_0^2}{\Delta H_f} \times \frac{1}{F}$$

The value of the heat of fusion is obtained by integrating the melting peak.

The melting point T_0 of the pure substance is extrapolated from the plot of $1/F$ versus the temperature expressed in kelvins. The slope α of the curve, obtained after linearisation, if necessary, corresponding to $RT_0^2 \frac{x_2^*}{\Delta H_f}$ allows x_2^* to be evaluated.

The fraction x_2^*, multiplied by 100 gives the mole fraction in per cent for the total eutectic impurities.

THERMOMICROSCOPY

Phase changes may be visualised by thermomicroscopy, a method which enables a sample subjected to a programmed temperature change to be examined, in polarised light, under a microscope.

The observations made in thermomicroscopy allow the nature of the phenomena detected using thermogravimetry and differential thermal analysis to be clearly identified.

Apparatus. The apparatus consists of a microscope fitted with a light polariser, a hot plate, a temperature and heating rate and/or cooling rate programmer and a recording system for the transition temperatures. A video camera and video recorder may be added.

04/2008:20260

2.2.60. MELTING POINT - INSTRUMENTAL METHOD

This chapter describes the measurement of melting point by the capillary method using an instrumental method of determination.

APPARATUS

There are 2 modes of automatic observation arrangements:

- mode A: by light transmission through the capillary tube loaded with the sample;
- mode B: by light being reflected from the sample in the capillary tube.

In both modes, the capillary tube sits in a hollow of a metal block, which is heated electrically and controlled by a temperature sensor placed in another hollow of the metal block. The heating block is capable of being maintained accurately at a pre-defined temperature (± 0.1 °C) by the heating element, and of being heated at a slow and steady rate of 1 °C/min, after an initial isothermal period.

In mode A, a beam of light shines through a horizontal hollow and crosses the capillary tube. A sensor detects the beam at the end of the cylindrical hole after the capillary tube.

In mode B, a beam of light illuminates the capillary tube from the front and the sensor records the image.

Some apparatuses allow for the visual determination of the melting point.

The temperature at which the sensor signal first leaves its initial value is defined as the beginning of melting, and the temperature at which the sensor signal reaches its final value is defined as the end of melting, or the *melting point*.

Use glass capillary tubes that are open at one end, about 100 mm long, with an external diameter of 1.3-1.5 mm and an internal diameter of 0.8-1.3 mm. The wall thickness of the tube is 0.1-0.3 mm.

Some apparatuses allow for the determination of the melting point on more than 1 capillary tube.

METHOD

Introduce into the capillary tube a sufficient amount of the substance to be examined, previously treated as described in the monograph, to form in each tube a compact column about 4 mm high, and allow the tubes to stand for the appropriate time at the prescribed temperature.

Proceed as follows or according to the manufacturer's instructions. Heat the heating block until the temperature is about 5 °C below the expected melting point.

Place the capillary tube in the heating block with the closed end downwards. Start the temperature programme. When the substance starts melting, it changes its appearance in the capillary tube. As a result, the temperature of the heating block is recorded automatically following the signal changes from the photosensor due to light transmission (mode A, Figure 2.2.60.-1), or following image processing (mode B, Figure 2.2.60.-2).

Carry out the test on 2 other samples and calculate the mean value of the 3 results.

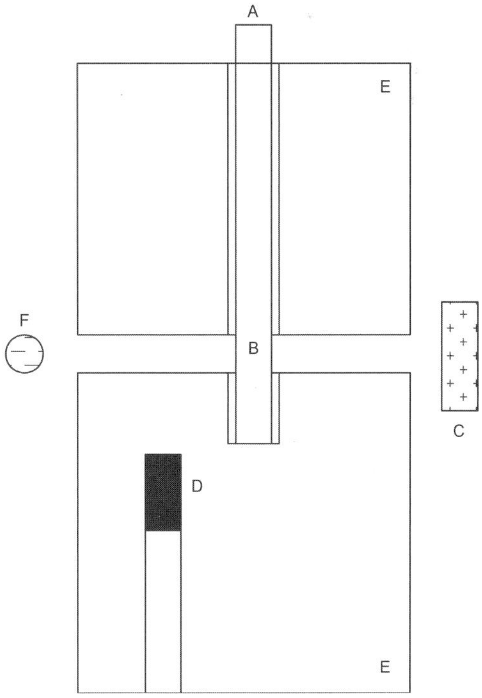

A. glass capillary tube
B. sample
C. photosensor
D. temperature sensor
E. heating block
F. light source

Figure 2.2.60.-1. – *Mode A: transmission*

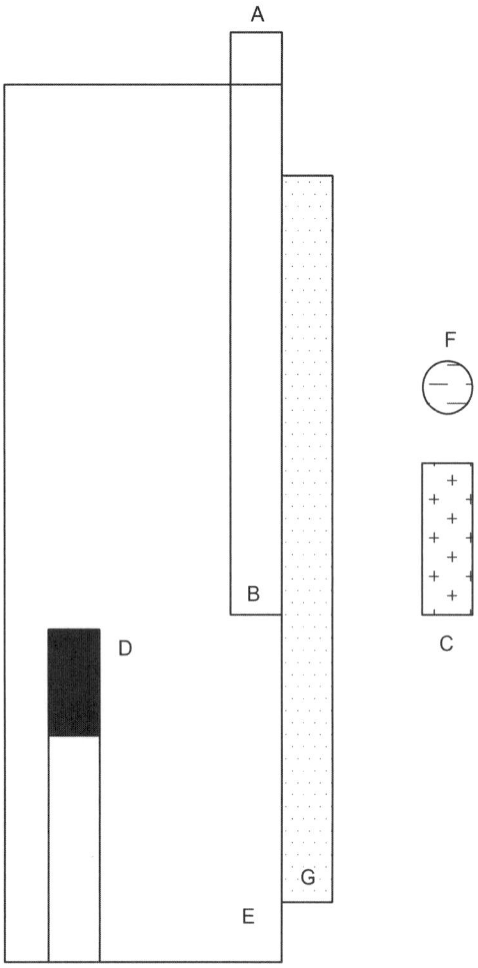

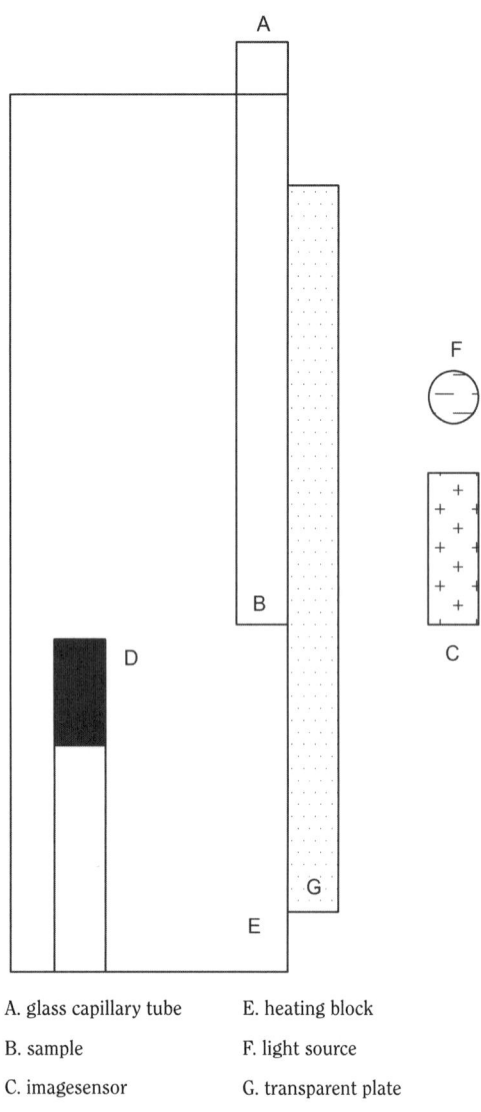

A. glass capillary tube
B. sample
C. imagesensor
D. temperature sensor
E. heating block
F. light source
G. transparent plate

Figure 2.2.60.-2. – *Mode B: reflexion*

CALIBRATION

The temperature scale of the apparatus is checked periodically by measuring the melting point of certified reference materials. Use capillary tubes having the same dimensions as those used for the determination of the melting point (see Apparatus).

Prepare 3 capillary tubes for each of at least 2 certified reference materials. Carry out the test and calculate the mean value of the 3 results for each material.

SYSTEM SUITABILITY

In addition to the calibration, carry out a verification, before the measurements, using a suitable certified reference material whose melting point is close to that expected for the substance to be examined.

Prepare 3 capillary tubes. Carry out the test and calculate the mean value of the 3 results.

The mean value is within the tolerance given on the certificate supplied with the certified reference material.

2.6. BIOLOGICAL TESTS

01/2008:20607
corrected 6.1

2.6.7. MYCOPLASMAS

Where the test for mycoplasmas is prescribed for a master cell bank, for a working cell bank, for a virus seed lot or for control cells, both the culture method and the indicator cell culture method are used. Where the test for mycoplasmas is prescribed for a virus harvest, for a bulk vaccine or for the final lot (batch), the culture method is used. The indicator cell culture method may also be used, where necessary, for screening of media.

Nucleic acid amplification techniques (NAT) may be used as an alternative to one or both of the other methods after suitable validation.

CULTURE METHOD

CHOICE OF CULTURE MEDIA

The test is carried out using a sufficient number of both solid and liquid media to ensure growth in the chosen incubation conditions of small numbers of mycoplasmas that may be present in the product to be examined. Liquid media must contain phenol red. The range of media chosen is shown to have satisfactory nutritive properties for at least the micro-organisms shown below. The nutritive properties of each new batch of medium are verified for the appropriate micro-organisms in the list. When testing for mycoplasmas in the product to be examined, at least 1 of the following species will be included as a positive control:

- *Acholeplasma laidlawii* (vaccines for human and veterinary use where an antibiotic has been used during production);
- *Mycoplasma gallisepticum* (where avian material has been used during production or where the vaccine is intended for use in poultry);
- *Mycoplasma hyorhinis* (non-avian veterinary vaccines);
- *Mycoplasma orale* (vaccines for human and veterinary use);
- *Mycoplasma pneumoniae* (vaccines for human use) or other suitable species of D-glucose fermenter such as *Mycoplasma fermentans*;
- *Mycoplasma synoviae* (where avian material has been used during production or where the vaccine is intended for use in poultry).

The test strains are field isolates having undergone a limited number of subcultures (not more than 15), and are stored frozen or freeze-dried. After cloning, the strains are identified as being of the required species by comparison with type cultures, for example:

A. laidlawii	NCTC 10116	CIP 75.27	ATCC 23206
M. gallisepticum	NCTC 10115	CIP 104967	ATCC 19610
M. fermentans	NCTC 10117	CIP 105680	ATCC 19989
M. hyorhinis	NCTC 10130	CIP 104968	ATCC 17981
M. orale	NCTC 10112	CIP 104969	ATCC 23714
M. pneumoniae	NCTC 10119	CIP 103766	ATCC 15531
M. synoviae	NCTC 10124	CIP 104970	ATCC 25204

Acholeplasma laidlawii BRP, *Mycoplasma fermentans BRP*, *Mycoplasma hyorhinis BRP*, *Mycoplasma orale BRP* and *Mycoplasma synoviae BRP* are suitable for use as low-passage reference strains.

INCUBATION CONDITIONS

Incubate liquid media in tightly stoppered containers at 35-38 °C. Incubate solid media in microaerophilic conditions (nitrogen containing 5-10 per cent of carbon dioxide and sufficient humidity to prevent desiccation of the agar surface) at 35-38 °C.

NUTRITIVE PROPERTIES

Carry out the test for nutritive properties for each new batch of medium. Inoculate the chosen media with the appropriate test micro-organisms; use not more than 100 CFU (colony-forming units) per 60 mm diameter plate containing 9 ml of solid medium and per 100 ml container of liquid medium; use a separate plate and container for each species of micro-organism. Incubate the media and make subcultures from 0.2 ml of liquid medium to solid medium at the specified intervals (see below under Test for mycoplasmas in the product to be examined). The solid medium complies with the test if adequate growth is found for each test micro-organism (growth obtained does not differ by a factor greater than 5 from the value calculated with respect to the inoculum). The liquid medium complies with the test if growth on agar plates subcultured from the broth is found for at least 1 subculture for each test micro-organism.

INHIBITORY SUBSTANCES

The test for inhibitory substances is carried out once for a given product and is repeated whenever there is a change in production method that may affect the detection of mycoplasmas.

To demonstrate absence of inhibitory substances, carry out the test for nutritive properties in the presence and absence of the product to be examined. If growth of a test micro-organism occurs more than 1 subculture sooner in the absence of the product to be examined than in its presence, or if plates directly inoculated with the product to be examined have fewer than 1/5 of the number of colonies of those inoculated without the product to be examined, inhibitory substances are present and they must be neutralised or their effect otherwise countered, for example by passage in substrates not containing inhibitors or dilution in a larger volume of medium before the test. If dilution is used, larger medium volumes may be used or the inoculum volume may be divided among several 100 ml flasks. The effectiveness of the neutralisation or other process is checked by repeating the test for inhibitory substances after neutralisation.

TEST FOR MYCOPLASMAS IN THE PRODUCT TO BE EXAMINED

Inoculate 10 ml of the product to be examined per 100 ml of each liquid medium. If it has been found that a significant pH change occurs upon the addition of the product to be examined, the liquid medium is restored to its original pH value by the addition of a solution of either sodium hydroxide or hydrochloric acid. Inoculate 0.2 ml of the product to be examined on each plate of each solid medium. Incubate liquid media for 20-21 days. Incubate solid media for not less than 14 days, except those corresponding to the 20-21 day subculture, which are incubated for 7 days. At the same time incubate an uninoculated 100 ml portion of each liquid medium and agar plates, as a negative control. On days 2-4 after inoculation, subculture each liquid medium by inoculating 0.2 ml on at least 1 plate of each solid medium. Repeat the procedure between the 6th and 8th days, again between the 13th and 15th days and again between the 19th and 21st days of the test. Observe the liquid media every 2 or 3 days and if a colour change occurs, subculture. If a liquid medium shows bacterial or fungal contamination, the test is invalid. The test is valid if at least 1 plate per medium and per inoculation day can be read. Include in the test positive controls prepared by inoculation of not more than

100 CFU of at least 1 test micro-organism on agar medium or into broth medium. Where the test for mycoplasmas is carried out regularly and where possible, it is recommended to use the test micro-organisms in regular rotation. The test micro-organisms used are those listed under Choice of culture media.

INTERPRETATION OF RESULTS

At the end of the prescribed incubation period, examine all inoculated solid media microscopically for the presence of mycoplasma colonies. The product complies with the test if growth of typical mycoplasma colonies has not occurred. The product does not comply with the test if growth of typical mycoplasma colonies has occurred on any of the solid media. The test is invalid if 1 or more of the positive controls do not show growth of mycoplasmas on at least 1 subculture plate. The test is invalid if 1 or more of the negative controls show growth of mycoplasmas. If suspect colonies are observed, a suitable validated method may be used to determine whether they are due to mycoplasmas.

The following section is published for information.

RECOMMENDED MEDIA FOR THE CULTURE METHOD

The following media are recommended. Other media may be used, provided that their ability to sustain the growth of mycoplasmas has been demonstrated on each batch in the presence and absence of the product to be examined.

HAYFLICK MEDIA (RECOMMENDED FOR THE GENERAL DETECTION OF MYCOPLASMAS)

Liquid medium

Beef heart infusion broth (1)	90.0 ml
Horse serum (unheated)	20.0 ml
Yeast extract (250 g/l)	10.0 ml
Phenol red (0.6 g/l solution)	5.0 ml
Penicillin (20 000 IU/ml)	0.25 ml
Deoxyribonucleic acid (2 g/l solution)	1.2 ml

Adjust to pH 7.8.

Solid medium

Prepare as described above replacing beef heart infusion broth by beef heart infusion agar containing 15 g/l of agar.

FREY MEDIA (RECOMMENDED FOR THE DETECTION OF M. SYNOVIAE)

Liquid medium

Beef heart infusion broth (1)	90.0 ml
Essential vitamins (2)	0.025 ml
Glucose monohydrate (500 g/l solution)	2.0 ml
Swine serum (inactivated at 56 °C for 30 min)	12.0 ml
β-Nicotinamide adenine dinucleotide (10 g/l solution)	1.0 ml
Cysteine hydrochloride (10 g/l solution)	1.0 ml
Phenol red (0.6 g/l solution)	5.0 ml
Penicillin (20 000 IU/ml)	0.25 ml

Mix the solutions of β-nicotinamide adenine dinucleotide and cysteine hydrochloride and after 10 min add to the other ingredients. Adjust to pH 7.8.

Solid medium

Beef heart infusion broth (1)	90.0 ml
Agar, purified (3)	1.4 g

Adjust to pH 7.8, sterilise by autoclaving then add:

Essential vitamins (2)	0.025 ml
Glucose monohydrate (500 g/l solution)	2.0 ml
Swine serum (unheated)	12.0 ml
β-Nicotinamide adenine dinucleotide (10 g/l solution)	1.0 ml
Cysteine hydrochloride (10 g/l solution)	1.0 ml
Phenol red (0.6 g/l solution)	5.0 ml
Penicillin (20 000 IU/ml)	0.25 ml

FRIIS MEDIA (RECOMMENDED FOR THE DETECTION OF NON-AVIAN MYCOPLASMAS)

Liquid medium

Hanks' balanced salt solution (modified) (4)	800 ml
Distilled water	67 ml
Brain heart infusion (5)	135 ml
PPLO Broth (6)	248 ml
Yeast extract (170 g/l)	60 ml
Bacitracin	250 mg
Meticillin	250 mg
Phenol red (5 g/l)	4.5 ml
Horse serum	165 ml
Swine serum	165 ml

Adjust to pH 7.40-7.45.

Solid medium

Hanks' balanced salt solution (modified) (4)	200 ml
DEAE-dextran	200 mg
Agar, purified (3)	15.65 g

Mix well and sterilise by autoclaving. Cool to 100 °C. Add to 1740 ml of liquid medium as described above.

(1) *Beef heart infusion broth*

Beef heart (for preparation of the infusion)	500 g
Peptone	10 g
Sodium chloride	5 g
Distilled water	to 1000 ml

Sterilise by autoclaving.

(2) *Essential vitamins*

Biotin	100 mg
Calcium pantothenate	100 mg
Choline chloride	100 mg
Folic acid	100 mg
i-Inositol	200 mg
Nicotinamide	100 mg
Pyridoxal hydrochloride	100 mg
Riboflavine	10 mg
Thiamine hydrochloride	100 mg
Distilled water	to 1000 ml

(3) *Agar, purified*

A highly refined agar for use in microbiology and immunology, prepared by an ion-exchange procedure that results in a product having superior purity, clarity and gel strength. It contains about:

Water	12.2 per cent
Ash	1.5 per cent
Acid-insoluble ash	0.2 per cent
Chlorine	0
Phosphate (calculated as P_2O_5)	0.3 per cent
Total nitrogen	0.3 per cent
Copper	8 ppm
Iron	170 ppm
Calcium	0.28 per cent
Magnesium	0.32 per cent

(4) *Hanks' balanced salt solution (modified)*

Sodium chloride	6.4 g
Potassium chloride	0.32 g
Magnesium sulphate heptahydrate	0.08 g
Magnesium chloride hexahydrate	0.08 g
Calcium chloride, anhydrous	0.112 g
Disodium hydrogen phosphate dihydrate	0.0596 g
Potassium dihydrogen phosphate, anhydrous	0.048 g
Distilled water	to 800 ml

(5) *Brain heart infusion*

Calf-brain infusion	200 g
Beef-heart infusion	250 g
Proteose peptone	10 g
Glucose monohydrate	2 g
Sodium chloride	5 g
Disodium hydrogen phosphate, anhydrous	2.5 g
Distilled water	to 1000 ml

(6) *PPLO broth*

Beef-heart infusion	50 g
Peptone	10 g
Sodium chloride	5 g
Distilled water	to 1000 ml

INDICATOR CELL CULTURE METHOD

Cell cultures are stained with a fluorescent dye that binds to DNA. Mycoplasmas are detected by their characteristic particulate or filamentous pattern of fluorescence on the cell surface and, if contamination is heavy, in surrounding areas. Mitochondria in the cytoplasm may be stained but are readily distinguished from mycoplasmas.

If for viral suspensions the interpretation of results is affected by marked cytopathic effects, the virus may be neutralised using a specific antiserum that has no inhibitory effects on mycoplasmas or a cell culture substrate that does not allow growth of the virus may be used. To demonstrate the absence of inhibitory effects of serum, carry out the positive control tests in the presence and absence of the antiserum.

VERIFICATION OF THE SUBSTRATE

Use Vero cells or another cell culture (for example, the production cell line) that is equivalent in effectiveness for detecting mycoplasmas. Test the effectiveness of the cells to be used by applying the procedure shown below and inoculating not more than 100 CFU or CFU-like micro-organisms of suitable reference strains of *M. hyorhinis* and *M. orale*. The following strains have been found to be suitable:

M. hyorhinis			ATCC 29052
M. orale	NCTC 10112	CIP 104969	ATCC 23714

The cells are suitable if both reference strains are detected. The indicator cells must be subcultured without an antibiotic before use in the test.

TEST METHOD

1. Seed the indicator cell culture at a suitable density (for example, 2×10^4 to 2×10^5 cells/ml, 4×10^3 to 2.5×10^4 cells/cm^2) that will yield confluence after 3 days of growth. Inoculate 1 ml of the product to be examined into the cell culture vessel and incubate at 35-38 °C.
2. After at least 3 days of incubation, when the cells have grown to confluence, make a subculture on cover slips in suitable containers or on some other surface (for example, chambered slides) suitable for the test procedure. Seed the cells at low density so that they reach 50 per cent confluence after 3-5 days of incubation. Complete confluence impairs visualisation of mycoplasmas after staining and must be avoided.
3. Remove the medium and rinse the indicator cells with *phosphate buffered saline pH 7.4 R*, then add a suitable fixing solution (a freshly prepared mixture of 1 volume of *glacial acetic acid R* and 3 volumes of *methanol R* is suitable when *bisbenzimide R* is used for staining).
4. Remove the fixing solution and wash the cells with sterile *water R*. Dry the slides completely if they are to be stained more than 1 h later (particular care is needed for staining of slides after drying owing to artefacts that may be produced).
5. Add a suitable DNA stain and allow to stand for a suitable time (*bisbenzimide working solution R* and a standing time of 10 min are suitable).
6. Remove the stain and rinse the monolayer with *water R*.
7. Mount each coverslip, where applicable (a mixture of equal volumes of *glycerol R* and *phosphate-citrate buffer solution pH 5.5 R* is suitable for mounting). Examine by fluorescence (for bisbenzimide stain a 330 nm/380 nm excitation filter and an LP 440 nm barrier filter are suitable) at 400 × magnification or greater.
8. Compare the microscopic appearance of the test cultures with that of the negative and positive controls, examining for extranuclear fluorescence. Mycoplasmas produce pinpoints or filaments over the indicator cell cytoplasm. They may also produce pinpoints and filaments in the intercellular spaces. Multiple microscopic fields are examined according to the protocol established during validation.

INTERPRETATION OF RESULTS

The product to be examined complies with the test if fluorescence typical of mycoplasmas is not present. The test is invalid if the positive controls do not show fluorescence typical of mycoplasmas. The test is invalid if the negative controls show fluorescence typical of mycoplasmas.

NUCLEIC ACID AMPLIFICATION TECHNIQUES (NAT)

NAT (*2.6.21*) may be used for detection of mycoplasmas by amplification of nucleic acids extracted from a test sample with specific primers that reveal the presence of the target nucleic acid. NAT indicate the presence of a particular nucleic acid sequence and not necessarily the presence of viable mycoplasmas. A number of different techniques are available. This general chapter does not prescribe a particular method for the test. The procedure applied must be validated as described, taking account of the guidelines presented at the end of this section. Where a commercial kit is used, certain elements of the validation may be carried out by the manufacturer and information provided to the user but it must be remembered that full information on the primers may not be available and that production of the kit may be modified or discontinued.

NAT are applied where prescribed in a monograph. They may also be used instead of the culture method and the indicator cell culture method after suitable validation.

Direct NAT can be applied in the presence of cytotoxic material and where a rapid method is needed.

Cell-culture enrichment followed by NAT: the test sample and a suitable cell substrate (as described under the indicator cell-culture method) are cultured together for a suitable period; the nucleic acids are then extracted from cells and supernatant and used for detection by NAT.

VALIDATION

Reference standards are required at various stages during validation and for use as controls during routine application of the test. The reference standards may be mycoplasmas or nucleic acids.

For validation of the limit of detection, the following species represent an optimal selection in terms of the frequency of occurrence as contaminants and phylogenetic relationships:

- *A. laidlawii*;
- *M. fermentans*;
- *M. hyorhinis* (where cell-culture enrichment is used, a fastidious strain such as ATCC 29052 is included);
- *M. orale*;
- *M. pneumoniae* or *M. gallisepticum*;
- *M. synoviae* (where there is use of or exposure to avian material during production);
- *Mycoplasma arginini;*
- *Spiroplasma citri* (where there is use of or exposure to insect or plant material during production).

Demonstration of specificity requires the use of a suitable range of bacterial species other than mycoplasmas. Bacterial genera with close phylogenetic relation to mycoplasmas are most appropriate for this validation; these include *Clostridium, Lactobacillus* and *Streptococcus.*

Comparability studies for use of NAT as an alternative method. For each mycoplasma test species:

- as an alternative to the culture method: the NAT test system must be shown to detect 10 CFU/ml;
- as an alternative to the indicator cell culture method: the NAT test system must be shown to detect 100 CFU/ml;

or an equivalent limit of detection in terms of the number of copies of mycoplasma nucleic acid in the test sample (using suitable reference standards of mycoplasma nucleic acid).

CONTROLS

Internal controls. Internal controls are necessary for routine verification of absence of inhibition. The internal control may contain the primer binding-site, or some other suitable sequence may be used. It is preferably added to the test material before isolating the nucleic acid and therefore acts as an overall control (extraction, reverse transcription, amplification, detection).

External controls. The external positive control contains a defined number of target-sequence copies or CFUs from 1 or more suitable species of mycoplasma chosen from those used during validation of the test conditions. 1 of the positive controls is set close to the positive cut-off point to demonstrate that the expected sensitivity is achieved. The external negative control contains no target sequence but does not necessarily represent the same matrix as the test article.

INTERPRETATION OF RESULTS

The primers used may also amplify non-mycoplasmal bacterial nucleic acid, leading to false positive results. Procedures are established at the time of validation for dealing with confirmation of positive results, where necessary.

The following section is published for information.

Validation of nucleic acid amplification techniques (NAT) for the detection of mycoplasmas: guidelines

1. *SCOPE*

Nucleic acid amplification techniques (NAT) are either qualitative or quantitative tests for the presence of nucleic acid. For the detection of mycoplasma contamination of various samples such as vaccines and cell substrates, qualitative tests are adequate and may be considered to be limit tests.

These guidelines describe methods to validate qualitative nucleic acid amplification analytical procedures for assessing mycoplasma contamination. They may also be applicable for real-time NAT used as limit tests for the control of contaminants.

The 2 characteristics regarded as the most important for validation of the analytical procedure are the specificity and the detection limit. In addition, the robustness of the analytical procedure should be evaluated.

For the purpose of this document, an analytical procedure is defined as the complete procedure from extraction of nucleic acid to detection of the amplified products.

Where commercial kits are used for part or all of the analytical procedure, documented validation points already covered by the kit manufacturer can replace validation by the user. Nevertheless, the performance of the kit with respect to its intended use has to be demonstrated by the user (e.g. detection limit, robustness, cross-detection of other classes of bacteria).

NAT may be used as:

- a complementary test (for example, for cytotoxic viral suspensions) or for in-process control purposes;
- an alternative method to replace an official method (indicator cell culture method or culture method).

These guidelines will thus separate these 2 objectives by presenting first a guideline for the validation of the NAT themselves, and second, a guideline for a comparability study between NAT and official methods.

2. *GUIDELINE FOR MYCOPLASMA NAT VALIDATION*

3 parameters should be evaluated: specificity, detection limit and robustness.

2-1. **Specificity**. Specificity is the ability to unequivocally assess target nucleic acid in the presence of components that may be expected to be present.

The specificity of NAT is dependent on the choice of primers, the choice of probe (for analysis of the final product) and the stringency of the test conditions (for both the amplification and detection steps).

The ability of the NAT to detect a large panel of mycoplasma species will depend on the choice of primers, probes and method parameters. This ability should be demonstrated using characterised reference panels (e.g. reference strains provided by the EDQM). Since NAT systems are usually based on a mix of primers, the theoretical analysis of primers and probes by comparison with databases is not recommended, because interpretation of the results may be quite complex and may not reflect the experimental results.

Moreover, as it is likely that the primers will detect other bacterial species, the potential cross-detection should be documented in the validation study. Bacterial genera such as gram-positive bacteria with close phylogenetic relation to mycoplasmas are most appropriate for this validation; these include *Clostridium*, *Lactobacillus* and *Streptococcus*. However, this is not an exhaustive list and species to be tested will depend on the theoretical ability (based on primers/probes sequences) of the NAT system to detect such other species.

Based on the results from this validation of the specificity, if a gap in the specificity of the method is identified (such as detection of non-mycoplasmal bacterial nucleic acid), an appropriate strategy must be proposed in the validation study to allow interpretation of positive results on a routine basis. For example, a second test may be performed using an alternative method without this specificity gap or using an official method.

2-2. **Detection limit**. The detection limit of an individual analytical procedure is the lowest amount of target nucleic acid in a sample that can be detected but not necessarily quantitated as an exact value.

For establishment of the detection limit, a positive cut-off point should be determined for the nucleic acid amplification analytical procedure. The positive cut-off point (as defined in general chapter *2.6.21*) is the minimum number of target sequence copies per volume of sample that can be detected in 95 per cent of test runs. This positive cut-off point is influenced by the distribution of mycoplasmal genomes in the individual samples being tested and by factors such as enzyme efficiency, and can result in different 95 per cent cut-off values for individual analytical test runs.

To determine the positive cut-off point, a dilution series of characterised and calibrated (either in CFUs or nucleic acid copies) in-house working strains or EDQM standards should be tested on different days to examine variation between test runs.

For validation of the limit of detection, the following species represent an optimal selection in terms of the frequency of occurrence as contaminants and phylogenetic relationships:

- *A. laidlawii*;
- *M. fermentans*;
- *M. hyorhinis*;
- *M. orale*;
- *M. pneumoniae* or *M. gallisepticum*;
- *M. synoviae* (where there is use of or exposure to avian material during production);
- *M. arginini*;
- *S. citri* (where there is use of or exposure to insect or plant material during production).

For each strain, at least 3 independent 10-fold dilution series should be tested, with a sufficient number of replicates at each dilution to give a total number of 24 test results for each dilution, to enable a statistical analysis of the results.

For example, a laboratory may test 3 dilution series on different days with 8 replicates for each dilution, 4 dilution series on different days with 6 replicates for each dilution, or 6 dilution series on different days with 4 replicates for each dilution. In order to keep the number of dilutions at a manageable level, a preliminary test should be performed to obtain a preliminary value for the positive cut-off point (i.e. the highest dilution giving a positive signal). The range of dilutions can then be chosen around the predetermined preliminary cut-off point. The concentration of mycoplasmas (CFUs or copies) that can be detected in 95 per cent of test runs can then be calculated using an appropriate statistical evaluation.

These results may also serve to evaluate the variability of the analytical procedure.

2-3. **Robustness**. The robustness of an analytical procedure is a measure of its capacity to remain unaffected by small but deliberate variations in method parameters, and provides an indication of its reliability during normal usage.

The evaluation of robustness should be considered during the development phase. It should show the reliability of the analytical procedure with respect to deliberate variations in method parameters. For NAT, small variations in the method parameters can be crucial. However, the robustness of the method can be demonstrated during its development when small variations in the concentrations of reagents (e.g. $MgCl_2$, primers or deoxyribonucleotides) are tested. Modifications of extraction kits or extraction procedures as well as different thermal cycler types may also be evaluated.

Finally, robustness of the method can be evaluated through collaborative studies.

3. *GUIDELINE FOR COMPARABILITY STUDY*

NAT may be used instead of official methods (indicator cell culture method and/or culture method). In this case a comparability study should be carried out. This comparability study should include mainly a comparison of the respective detection limits of the alternative method and official methods. However, specificity (mycoplasma panel detected, putative false positive results) should also be considered.

For the detection limit, acceptability criteria are defined as follows:

- if the alternative method is proposed to replace the culture method, the NAT system must be shown to detect 10 CFU/ml for each mycoplasma test species described in paragraph 2-2;
- if the alternative method is proposed to replace the indicator cell culture method, the NAT system must be shown to detect 100 CFU/ml for each mycoplasma test species described in paragraph 2-2.

For both cases, suitable standards calibrated for the number of nucleic acid copies and the number of CFUs may be used for establishing that these acceptability criteria are reached. The relation between CFUs and nucleic acid copies for the reference preparations should be previously established to compare the performance of the alternative NAT method with the performance of the official methods.

1 of the following 2 strategies can be used to perform this comparability study:

- perform the NAT alternative method in parallel with the official method(s) to evaluate simultaneously the detection limit of both methods using the same samples of calibrated strains;
- compare the performance of the NAT alternative method using previously obtained data from official method validation. In this case, calibration of standards used for both validations as well as their stabilities should be documented carefully.

Comparability study reports should describe all the validation elements described in section 2 (specificity, limit of detection and variability, as well as robustness) in order to assess all the advantages and/or disadvantages of the alternative NAT method compared to official methods.

2.9. PHARMACEUTICAL TECHNICAL PROCEDURES

04/2008:20940

2.9.40. UNIFORMITY OF DOSAGE UNITS

To ensure the consistency of dosage units, each unit in a batch should have an active substance content within a narrow range around the label claim. Dosage units are defined as dosage forms containing a single dose or a part of a dose of an active substance in each dosage unit. Unless otherwise stated, the uniformity of dosage units specification is not intended to apply to suspensions, emulsions or gels in single-dose containers intended for cutaneous administration. The test for content uniformity is not required for multivitamin and trace-element preparations.

The term 'uniformity of dosage unit' is defined as the degree of uniformity in the amount of the active substance among dosage units. Therefore, the requirements of this chapter apply to each active substance being comprised in dosage units containing one or more active substances, unless otherwise specified elsewere in this Pharmacopoeia.

The uniformity of dosage units can be demonstrated by either of 2 methods: content uniformity or mass variation (see Table 2.9.40.-1).

The test for content uniformity of preparations presented in dosage units is based on the assay of the individual contents of active substance(s) of a number of dosage units to determine whether the individual contents are within the limits set. The content uniformity method may be applied in all cases.

The test for mass variation is applicable for the following dosage forms:

(1) solutions enclosed in single-dose containers and in soft capsules;

(2) solids (including powders, granules and sterile solids) that are packaged in single-dose containers and contain no added active or inactive substances;

(3) solids (including sterile solids) that are packaged in single-dose containers, with or without added active or inactive substances, that have been prepared from true solutions and freeze-dried in the final containers and are labelled to indicate this method of preparation;

(4) hard capsules, uncoated tablets, or film-coated tablets, containing 25 mg or more of an active substance comprising 25 per cent or more, by mass, of the dosage unit or, in the case of hard capsules, the capsule contents, except that uniformity of other active substances present in lesser proportions is demonstrated by meeting content uniformity requirements.

The test for content uniformity is required for all dosage forms not meeting the above conditions for the mass variation test. Alternatively, products that do not meet the 25 mg/25 per cent threshold limit may be tested for uniformity of dosage units by mass variation instead of the content uniformity test on the following condition: the concentration Relative Standard Deviation (RSD) of the active substance in the final dosage units is not more than 2 per cent, based on process validation data and development data, and if there has been regulatory approval of such a change. The concentration RSD is the RSD of the concentration per dosage unit (*m/m* or *m/V*), where concentration per dosage unit equals the assay result per dosage unit divided by the individual dosage unit mass. See the RSD formula in Table 2.9.40.-2.

CONTENT UNIFORMITY

Select not less than 30 units, and proceed as follows for the dosage form designated. Where different procedures are used for assay of the preparation and for the content uniformity test, it may be necessary to establish a correction factor to be applied to the results of the latter.

Solid dosage forms. Assay 10 units individually using an appropriate analytical method. Calculate the acceptance value (see Table 2.9.40.-2).

Liquid dosage forms. Assay 10 units individually using an appropriate analytical method. Carry out the assay on the amount of well-mixed material that is removed from an individual container in conditions of normal use. Express the results as delivered dose. Calculate the acceptance value (see Table 2.9.40.-2).

Calculation of Acceptance Value

Calculate the Acceptance Value (*AV*) using the formula:

$$\left|M - \overline{X}\right| + ks$$

for which the terms are as defined in Table 2.9.40.-2.

Table 2.9.40.-1. – *Application of Content Unformity (CU) and Mass Variation (MV) test for dosage forms*

Dosage forms	Type	Sub-Type	Dose and ratio of active substance	
			≥ 25 mg and ≥ 25 per cent	< 25 mg or < 25 per cent
Tablets	uncoated		MV	CU
	coated	film-coated	MV	CU
		others	CU	CU
Capsules	hard		MV	CU
	soft	suspensions, emulsions, gels	CU	CU
		solutions	MV	MV
Solids in single-dose containers	single component		MV	MV
	multiple components	solution freeze-dried in final container	MV	MV
		others	CU	CU
Solutions enclosed in single-dose containers			MV	MV
Others			CU	CU

Table 2.9.40.-2.

Variable	Definition	Conditions	Value
$\overline{X}$	Mean of individual contents (x_1, x_2,..., x_n), expressed as a percentage of the label claim		
$x_1, x_2,..., x_n$	Individual contents of the dosage units tested, expressed as a percentage of the label claim		
n	Sample size (number of dosage units in a sample)		
k	Acceptability constant	If n = 10, then	2.4
		If n = 30, then	2.0
s	Sample standard deviation		$\left[\frac{\sum_{i=1}^{n}(x_i-\overline{X})^2}{n-1}\right]^{1/2}$
RSD	Relative standard deviation		$\frac{100s}{\overline{X}}$
M (case 1) To be applied when $T \le 101.5$	Reference value	If 98.5 per cent $\le \overline{X} \le$ 101.5 per cent, then	$M = \overline{X}$ ($AV = ks$)
		If $\overline{X}$ < 98.5 per cent, then	M = 98.5 per cent ($AV = 98.5 - \overline{X} + ks$)
		If $\overline{X}$ > 101.5 per cent, then	M = 101.5 per cent ($AV = \overline{X} - 101.5 + ks$)
M (case 2) To be applied when T > 101.5	Reference value	If 98.5 per cent $\le \overline{X} \le T$, then	$M = \overline{X}$ ($AV = ks$)
		If $\overline{X}$ < 98.5 per cent, then	M = 98.5 per cent ($AV = 98.5 - \overline{X} + ks$)
		If $\overline{X} > T$, then	$M = T$ per cent ($AV = \overline{X} - T + ks$)
Acceptance value (*AV*)			General formula: $\lvert M - \overline{X}\rvert + ks$ Calculations are specified above for the different cases.
L1	Maximum allowed acceptance value		*L1* = 15.0 unless otherwise specified
L2	Maximum allowed range for deviation of each dosage unit tested from the calculated value of *M*	On the low side, no dosage unit result can be less than 0.75 *M* while on the high side, no dosage unit result can be greater than 1.25 *M* (This is based on *L2* value of 25.0)	*L2* = 25.0 unless otherwise specified
T	Target content per dosage unit at time of manufacture, expressed as a percentage of the label claim. *T* is equal to 100 per cent unless an overage for stability reasons has been approved, in which case it is greater than 100 per cent		

MASS VARIATION

Carry out an assay for the active substance(s) on a representative sample of the batch using an appropriate analytical method. This value is result *A*, expressed as percentage of label claim (see Calculation of Acceptance Value). Assume that the concentration (mass of active substance per mass of dosage unit) is uniform. Select not less than 30 dosage units, and proceed as follows for the dosage form designated.

Uncoated or film-coated tablets. Accurately weigh 10 tablets individually. Calculate the active substance content, expressed as percentage of label claim, of each tablet from the mass of the individual tablets and the result of the assay. Calculate the acceptance value.

Hard capsules. Accurately weigh 10 capsules individually, taking care to preserve the identity of each capsule. Remove the contents of each capsule by suitable means. Accurately weigh the emptied shells individually, and calculate for each capsule the net mass of its contents by subtracting the mass of the shell from the respective gross mass. Calculate the active substance content in each capsule from the mass of product removed from the individual capsules and the result of the assay. Calculate the acceptance value.

Soft capsules. Accurately weigh 10 intact capsules individually to obtain their gross masses, taking care to preserve the identity of each capsule. Then cut open the capsules by means of a suitable clean, dry cutting instrument such as scissors or a sharp open blade, and remove the contents by washing with a suitable solvent. Allow the occluded solvent to evaporate from the shells at room temperature over a period of about 30 min, taking precautions to avoid uptake or loss of moisture. Weigh the individual shells, and calculate the net contents. Calculate the active substance content on each capsule from the mass of product removed from the individual capsules and the result of the assay. Calculate the acceptance value.

Solid dosage forms other than tablets and capsules. Proceed as directed for hard capsules, treating each unit as described therein. Calculate the acceptance value.

Liquid dosage forms. Accurately weigh the amount of liquid that is removed from each of 10 individual containers in conditions of normal use. If necessary, compute the equivalent volume after determining the density. Calculate the active substance content in each container from the mass of product removed from the individual containers and the result of the assay. Calculate the acceptance value.

Calculation of Acceptance Value. Calculate the acceptance value (*AV*) as shown in content uniformity, except that the individual contents of the units are replaced with the individual estimated contents defined below.

$x_1, x_2, ..., x_n$ = individual estimated contents of the dosage units tested;

where

$$x_i = w_i \times \frac{A}{\overline{W}}$$

$w_1, w_2, ..., w_n$ = individual masses of the dosage units tested;

A = content of active substance (percentage of label claim) obtained using an appropriate analytical method (assay);

$\overline{W}$ = mean of individual masses of the units used in the assay.

CRITERIA

Apply the following criteria, unless otherwise specified.

Solid and liquid dosage forms. The requirements for dosage uniformity are met if the acceptance value of the first 10 dosage units is less than or equal to $L1$. If the acceptance value is greater than $L1$, test the next 20 dosage units and calculate the acceptance value. The requirements are met if the final acceptance value of the 30 dosage units is less than or equal to $L1$ and no individual content of the dosage unit is less than $(1 - L2 \times 0.01)M$ or more than $(1 + L2 \times 0.01)M$ in calculation of acceptance value under content uniformity or under mass variation. Unless otherwise specified, $L1$ is 15.0 and $L2$ is 25.0.

01/2008:20943
corrected 6.1

2.9.43. APPARENT DISSOLUTION

This method is mainly used to determine the apparent dissolution rate of pure solid substances. It may also be used for the determination of the apparent dissolution rate of active substances in preparations presented as powders or granules.

APPARATUS

All parts of the apparatus that may come into contact with the sample or the dissolution medium are chemically inert and do not adsorb, react with, or interfere with the test sample. No part of the assembly or its environment contributes significant motion, agitation or vibration beyond that resulting from the flow-through system.

Apparatus that permits observation of the sample is preferable.

The apparatus (see Figure 2.9.43.-1) consists of:

- a reservoir for the dissolution medium;
- a pump that forces the dissolution medium upwards through the flow-through cell;
- a flow-through cell, preferably of transparent material, mounted vertically with a filter system preventing escape of undissolved particles;
- a water-bath that will maintain the dissolution medium at the chosen temperature (generally 37 ± 0.5 °C).

The flow-through cell shown in Figure 2.9.43.-2 consists of 3 parts that fit into each other. The lower part supports a system of grids and filters on which the powder is placed. The middle part, which fits onto the lower part, contains an

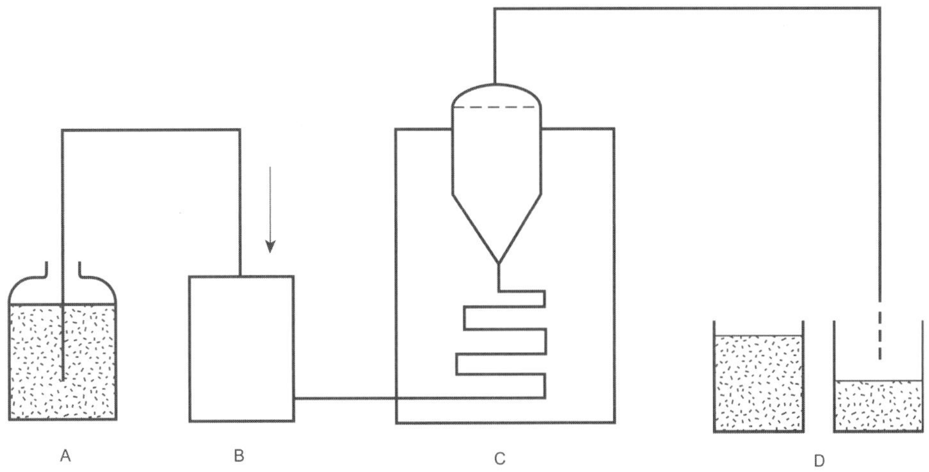

A. reservoir for dissolution medium B. pump C. thermostatically controlled flow-through cell and filter D. collecting vessels for analysis

Figure 2.9.43.-1. – *Flow-through apparatus*

insert that sieves the sample when the dissolution medium flows through the cell. This insert is made up of 2 parts: a conical sieve that is placed on the sample and a clip placed midway down the middle part to hold the sieve in place when the dissolution medium passes through. A 2nd filtration assembly (grid and filter) is placed on top of the middle part before fitting the upper part through which the dissolution medium flows out of the cell.

DISSOLUTION MEDIUM

If the dissolution medium is buffered, adjust its pH to within ± 0.05 units. Remove any dissolved gases from the dissolution medium before the test, since they can cause the formation of bubbles, which significantly affect the results.

METHOD

Place a bead of 5 ± 0.5 mm diameter at the bottom of the cone of the lower part followed by glass beads of suitable size, preferably of 1 ± 0.1 mm diameter. Place a sieve (with 0.2 mm apertures), a suitable filter and a 2nd sieve on top of the lower part. Fit the middle part onto the lower part. Weigh the assembly. Place the sample on the filtration assembly and weigh the sample in the cell. Place the sieve of the insert, cone upwards, on the sample, and position the clip midway down the middle part. Place a sieve (with 0.2 mm apertures) and a suitable filter on top of the middle part. Fit the upper part. Heat the dissolution medium to the chosen temperature. Using a suitable pump, introduce the dissolution medium through the bottom of the cell to obtain a suitable continuous flow through an open or closed circuit at the prescribed rate ± 5 per cent.

SAMPLING

Samples of dissolution medium are collected at the outlet of the cell, irrespective of whether the circuit is opened or closed.

Immediately filter the liquid removed using an inert filter of appropriate pore size that does not cause significant adsorption of the substances from the solution and does not contain substances extractable by the dissolution medium that would interfere with the prescribed analytical method. Proceed with the analysis of the filtrate as prescribed.

ASSESSMENT OF THE RESULTS

When the test is performed for batch release purposes, an adequate number of replicates is carried out.

The results are expressed as:

– the amount of dissolved substance by time unit (if the dissolution is linear);

– the dissolution time of the whole sample and at appropriate intermediate stages.

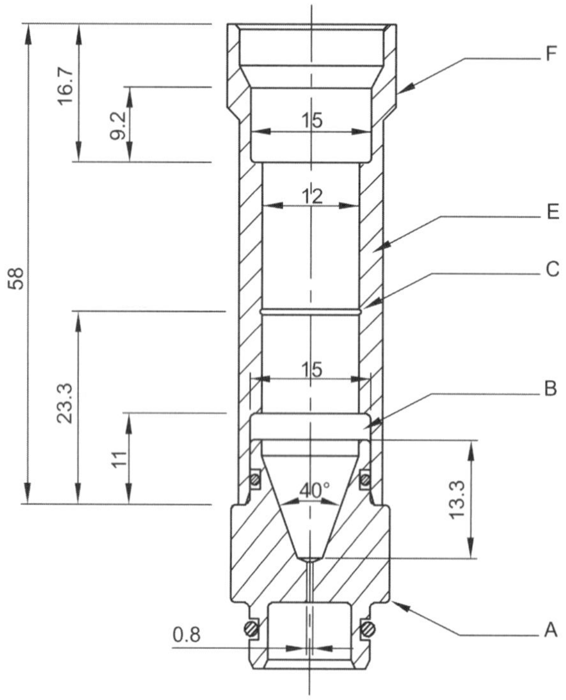

A. lower part C. clip E. middle part

B. sieve D. insert F. upper part

Figure 2.9.43.-2. – *Flow-through cell*

Dimensions in millimetres

4. REAGENTS

04/2008:40101

4.1.1. REAGENTS

3-Benzoylpropionic acid. $C_{10}H_{10}O_3$. (M_r 178.2). *1171000.* [2051-95-8]. 4-Oxo-4-phenylbutanoic acid.

mp: about 118 °C.

Benzyl cyanide. C_8H_7N. (M_r 117.2). *1171100.* [140-29-4]. Phenylacetonitrile.

Content: minimum 95.0 per cent.

Clear, colourless or light yellow liquid.

n_D^{20}: about 1.523.

bp: about 233 °C.

Lavandulyl acetate. $C_{12}H_{20}O_2$. (M_r 196.3). *1114200.* [25905-14-0]. 2-Isopropenyl-5-methylhex-4-en-1-yl acetate.

A colourless liquid with a characteristic odour.

Lavandulyl acetate used in gas chromatography complies with the following additional test.

Assay. Examine by gas chromatography (*2.2.28*) as prescribed in the monograph on *Lavender oil (1338).*

Test solution. The substance to be examined.

The area of the principal peak is not less than 93.0 per cent of the area of all the peaks in the chromatogram obtained.

Linsidomine hydrochloride. $C_6H_{11}ClN_4O_2$. (M_r 206.6). *1171200.* [16142-27-1]. 3-(Morpholin-4-yl)sydnonimine hydrochloride. 3-(Morpholin-4-yl)-1,2,3-oxadiazol-3-ium-5-aminide hydrochloride.

White or almost white powder.

Mandelic acid. $C_8H_8O_3$. (M_r 152.1). *1171300.* [90-64-2]. 2-Hydroxy-2-phenylacetic acid.

White crystalline flakes, soluble in water.

mp: 118 to 121 °C.

(*R*)-(+)-α-Methylbenzyl isocyanate. C_9H_9NO. (M_r 147.2). *1171400.* [33375-06-3]. (+)-(*R*)-α-Methylbenzyl isocyanate. (+)-[(1*R*)-1-Isocyanatoethyl]benzene. (+)-(1*R*)-1-Phenylethyl isocyanate.

Content: minimum 99.0 per cent.

Colourless liquid.

d_{20}^{20}: about 1.045.

n_D^{20}: about 1.513.

bp: 55 °C to 56 °C at 2.5 mm Hg.

Enantiomeric purity: minimum 99.5.

Storage: at a temperature of 2 °C to 8 °C.

Poly(dimethyl)(75)(diphenyl)(25)siloxane. *1171500.*

Stationary phase for chromatography.

Contains 75 per cent of methyl groups and 25 per cent of phenyl groups.

Poly[methyl(trifluoropropylmethyl)siloxane]. *1171600.*

Stationary phase for gas chromatography.

Contains 50 per cent of trifluoropropylmethyl groups and 50 per cent of methyl groups.

2-Pyrrolidone. C_4H_7NO. (M_r 85.1). *1138000.* [616-45-5]. Pyrrolidin-2-one.

Content: minimum 98.0 per cent.

Liquid above 25 °C, miscible with water, with ethanol and with ethyl acetate.

d_4^{25}: 1.116.

Water (*2.5.12*): maximum 0.2 per cent determined on 2.00 g.

Assay. Gas chromatography (*2.2.28*): use the normalisation procedure.

Test solution. Dissolve 1.0 g in *methanol R* and dilute to 10.0 ml with the same solvent.

Column:

– *material*: glass;
– *size*: *l* = 30 m; Ø = 0.53 mm;
– *stationary phase*: *macrogol 20 000 R* (1.0 μm).

Carrier gas: *helium for chromatography R.*

Flow rate: adjusted so that the retention time of 2-pyrrolidone is about 10 min.

Split ratio: 1:20.

Temperature:

	Time (min)	Temperature (°C)
Column	0 - 1	80
	1 - 12	80 → 190
	12 - 32	190
Injection port		200

Detection: flame ionisation.

Injection: 1 μl of the test solution.

Calculate the percentage content of C_4H_7NO.

Silica gel AD for chiral separation. *1171700.*

A very finely divided silica gel for chromatography (5 μm) coated with the following derivative:

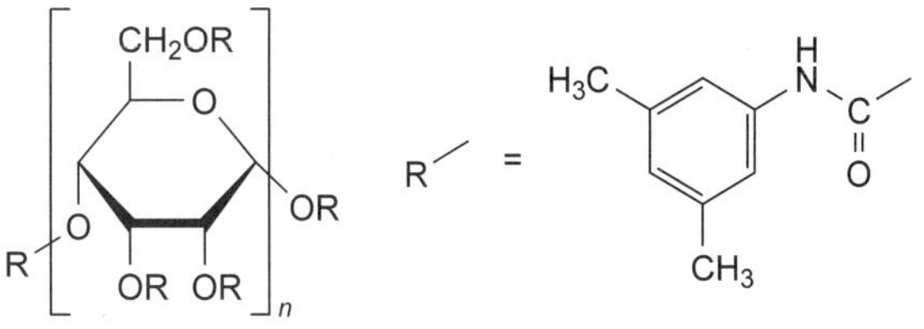

α-Tetralone. $C_{10}H_{10}O$. (M_r 146.2). *1171800.* [529-34-0]. 1-Oxotetraline. 3,4-Dihydronaphthalen-1(2*H*)-one.

bp: about 115 °C.

mp: about 5 °C.

3-Trifluoromethylaniline. $C_7H_6F_3N$. (M_r 161.1). *1171900.* [98-16-8]. 3-(Trifluoromethyl)aniline. α,α,α-Trifluoro-*m*-toluidine. 3-(Trifluoromethyl)benzenamide.

Colourless liquid.

Density: 1.30 g/cm³ (20 °C).

Tropic acid. $C_9H_{10}O_3$. (M_r 166.17). *1172000.* [529-64-6]. (2*RS*)-3-hydroxy-2-phenylpropanoic acid.

04/2008:40103

4.1.3. BUFFER SOLUTIONS

Buffer solution pH 2.2. *4010500.*

Mix 6.7 ml of *phosphoric acid R* with 55.0 ml of a 4 per cent solution of *sodium hydroxide R* and dilute to 1000.0 ml with *water R.*

5.2. GENERAL TEXTS ON BIOLOGICAL PRODUCTS

04/2008:50207

5.2.7. EVALUATION OF EFFICACY OF VETERINARY VACCINES AND IMMUNOSERA

The term 'product' means either a vaccine or an immunoserum throughout the text.

During development of the product, tests are carried out to demonstrate that the product is efficacious when administered by each of the recommended routes and methods of administration and using the recommended schedule to animals of each species and category for which use of the product is to be recommended. The type of efficacy testing to be carried out varies considerably depending on the particular type of product.

As part of tests carried out during development to establish efficacy, the tests described in the Production section of a monograph may be carried out; the following must be taken into account.

The dose to be used is that quantity of the product to be recommended for use and containing the minimum titre or potency expected at the end of the period of validity.

For live vaccines, use vaccine containing virus/bacteria at the most attenuated passage level that will be present in a batch of vaccine.

For immunosera, if appropriate, the dose tested also contains minimum quantities of immunoglobulin or gammaglobulin and/or total protein.

The efficacy evidence must support all the claims being made. For example, claims for protection against respiratory disease must be supported at least by evidence of protection from clinical signs of respiratory disease. Where it is claimed that there is protection from infection this must be demonstrated using re-isolation techniques. If more than one claim is made, supporting evidence for each claim is required.

Vaccines. The influence of passively acquired and maternally derived antibodies on the efficacy of a vaccine is adequately evaluated. Any claims, stated or implied, regarding onset and duration of protection shall be supported by data from trials.

Claims related to duration of immunity are supported by evidence of protection. The test model described under Immunogenicity and/or Potency is not necessarily used to support claims regarding the duration of immunity afforded by a vaccine.

The efficacy of each of the components of multivalent and combined vaccines shall be demonstrated using the combined vaccine.

Immunosera. Particular attention must be paid to providing supporting data for the efficacy of the regime that is to be recommended. For example, if it is recommended that the immunoserum needs only to be administered once to achieve a prophylactic or therapeutic effect then this must be demonstrated. Any claims, stated or implied, regarding onset and duration of protection or therapeutic effect must be supported by data from trials. For example, the duration of the protection afforded by a prophylactic dose of an antiserum must be studied so that appropriate guidance for the user can be given on the label.

Studies of immunological compatibility are undertaken when simultaneous administration is recommended or where it is a part of a usual administration schedule. Wherever a product is recommended as part of an administration scheme, the priming or booster effect or the contribution of the product to the efficacy of the scheme as a whole is demonstrated.

LABORATORY TESTS

In principle, demonstration of efficacy is undertaken under well-controlled laboratory conditions by challenge of the target animal under the recommended conditions of use.

In so far as possible, the conditions under which the challenge is carried out shall mimic the natural conditions for infection, for example with regard to the amount of challenge organism and the route of administration of the challenge.

Vaccines. Unless otherwise justified, challenge is carried out using a strain different from the one used in the production of the vaccine.

If possible, the immune mechanism (cell-mediated/humoral, local/general, classes of immunoglobulin) that is initiated after the administration of the vaccine to target animals shall be determined.

Immunosera. Data are provided from measurements of the antibody levels achieved in the target species after administration of the product, as recommended. Where suitable published data exist, references are provided to relevant published literature on protective antibody levels and challenge studies are avoided.

Where challenges are required, these can be given before or after administration of the product, in accordance with the indications and specific claims to be made.

FIELD TRIALS

In general, results from laboratory tests are supplemented with data from field trials, carried out, unless otherwise justified, with untreated control animals. Provided that laboratory tests have adequately assessed the safety and efficacy of a product under experimental conditions using vaccines of maximum and minimum titre or potency respectively, a single batch of product could be used to assess both safety and efficacy under field conditions. In these cases, a typical routine batch of intermediate titre or potency may be used. Where laboratory trials cannot be supportive of efficacy, the performance of field trials alone may be acceptable.

5.15. FUNCTIONALITY-RELATED CHARACTERISTICS OF EXCIPIENTS

04/2008:51500

5.15. FUNCTIONALITY-RELATED CHARACTERISTICS OF EXCIPIENTS

This chapter and the FRC sections in specific monographs are not mandatory and are published for information and guidance.

PREAMBLE

Excipients that have previously been evaluated for safety are used in the formulation of pharmaceutical preparations to bring functionality to the formulation. The intended function of an excipient is to guarantee the required physical and biopharmaceutical properties of the pharmaceutical preparation.

The functionality of an excipient is determined by its physical and chemical properties and, in some cases, also by its content of by-products or of additives used to improve the intended functionality. In addition, the functionality may depend on complex interactions between the constituents of the formulation and stresses related to the process. Excipient functionality can therefore be evaluated only in the context of a particular formulation and manufacturing process, frequently by the use of a number of analytical methods. Knowledge of excipient functionalities may facilitate the application of Process Analytical Technology (PAT).

Certain excipient properties, such as the particle size of an excipient intended for a solid dosage form or the molecular mass of a polymeric material used as a viscosity-increasing agent, may however relate to functionality in a more general sense. Such functionality-related characteristics (FRCs) can be controlled and may be subject to a product-specific quality specification when the pharmaceutical development work has demonstrated their critical role for the manufacturing process and quality attributes of the medicinal product.

Monographs of the European Pharmacopoeia on excipients are designed to ensure acceptable quality for users. Information on the appearance and characters of the excipient, and requirements concerning identity, chemical and microbiological purity and physical characteristics associated with the chemical structure, such as optical rotation, are given in specific monographs and in the general monograph *Substances for pharmaceutical use (2034)*.

FRCs are included in excipient monographs to aid manufacturers of pharmaceutical products in establishing specifications based on standard analytical methods. They provide manufacturers and users of excipients with a common language to support the supply of excipients with specified properties. FRCs may be labelled (in the certificate of analysis, for example) by the excipient manufacturer with a reference to the Pharmacopoeia monograph, thus indicating the method used to test a particular characteristic. The FRC section in specific monographs contains FRCs that are known to have an impact on the functionality of the excipient for the stated uses. The uses and the FRCs listed are not exhaustive due to the multiple uses of many excipients and the development of new uses.

REGULATORY GUIDANCE

According to current regulatory guidelines, for example ICH Q8 Pharmaceutical Development, the marketing authorisation application should discuss the excipients chosen and their concentration, and demonstrate the characteristics that can influence the medicinal product performance and manufacturability relative to the respective function of each excipient. The ability of excipients to provide their intended functionality throughout the intended period of validity of the formulation should also be demonstrated. The information on excipient performance can be used as appropriate to justify the choice and quality attributes of the excipient.

Excipients are normally produced by batch processes, so there is a possibility of batch-to-batch variation from the same manufacturer. Excipients from different sources may not have identical properties with respect to their use in a specific formulation. The inevitable variation in chemical and physical properties is one of the most important input variables that can impact on a pharmaceutical manufacturing process, since excipients typically make up the major proportion of a medicinal product. Many excipients are of natural origin and composed of a mixture of chemically related compounds. Other excipients are made in chemical plants primarily designed for producing chemicals for industries other than the pharmaceutical industry. The excipient manufacturer's process may therefore be focused on the chemical characteristics and some physical properties addressing the manufacturer's primary market. In many cases, the excipient manufacturer has limited knowledge of the pharmaceutical uses of the product.

The key to a successful, robust formulation is to understand the chemical and physical nature of the active substance(s) and the excipients alone, and how their properties interact with other constituents of the formulation and the manufacturing process. During pharmaceutical development, the ingredient properties that are critical to the manufacturing process and performance of the medicinal product are identified. Having identified the critical properties of the excipients, preferably by a risk-based approach, pharmaceutical development may establish the acceptable range of the critical characteristics including both the physical and chemical property variation. The FRCs concerned may not be properties controlled by the excipient manufacturer and are therefore variable. The design of a robust manufacturing process for the medicinal product that limits the effect of the normal excipient variability is preferable.

PHYSICAL GRADES

Excipients that are particulate solids can be available in a variety of physical grades, for example with regard to particle-size distribution, which is usually controlled by the excipient supplier. However, FRCs for these excipients may concern a wide range of properties, resulting from solid-state properties and properties of the particulate solid, which may not be controlled by the excipient supplier.

Examples of solid-state properties to be considered in the development of solid dosage forms include polymorphism, pseudopolymorphism, crystallinity and density. Complementary techniques to study crystalline forms and solvates are given in the general chapters:

- *5.9. Polymorphism*;
- *2.2.34. Thermal analysis*;
- *2.9.33. Characterisation of crystalline and partially crystalline solids by x-ray powder diffraction (XRPD)*;
- *2.2.42. Density of solids*;
- *2.9.23. Pycnometric density of solids.*

Properties of particulate solids include for example particle-size distribution, specific surface area, bulk density, flowability, wettability and water sorption. Depending on the size range, the particle-size distribution can be determined by sieve analysis (see chapter *2.9.38. Particle-size distribution estimation by analytical sieving*) or instrumental methods, for example, *2.9.31. Particle-size analysis by laser light diffraction*. General method *2.9.26. Specific surface area by gas adsorption* is based on the Brunauer-Emmett-Teller

(BET) technique. Methods to characterise flowability and bulk density of powders are described in chapters *2.9.36. Powder flow* and *2.9.34. Bulk and tapped density*. Solid-state properties may impact on the wettability and water-solid interactions of particulate solids. A range of instrumental methods is available for determining these characteristics, for example, techniques to measure the static and dynamic contact angles and the gravimetric vapour sorption and/or techniques of gravimetric analysis.

CHEMICAL GRADES

Excipients that are available in different chemical grades are of natural, semi-synthetic or synthetic origin. Specific monographs usually control the chemical composition of excipients that are composed of a mixture of related compounds, for example, the composition of fatty acids in vegetable oils or surfactants. There are, however, specific monographs in the Pharmacopoeia each describing a class of polymeric materials that may vary in their composition with regard to the structure of homopolymers, block polymers and copolymers, the degree of polymerisation, and thus the molecular mass and mass distribution, the degree of substitution and in some cases even different substituents on the polymer backbone. This variation may, however, have a profound effect on the functionality of the excipient and should be subject to investigations during the pharmaceutical development, preferably to establish the acceptable range of each characteristic being critical to the manufacturing process and performance of the end-product.

While, in the past, the mandatory part of monographs on polymeric excipients may have contained some tests for physical or chemical characteristics, for example, a test for viscosity including acceptance criteria, such tests will gradually be moved to the non-mandatory FRC section, unless the concerned characteristic is an indispensable part of the identification tests. This development should be seen in light of regulatory guidance on pharmaceutical development and the desired regulatory flexibility based on establishing the acceptable range of material properties within the design space. Thus, evaluation of the chemical grades and, when appropriate, the setting of a specification for the critical characteristics, is a part of the pharmaceutical development irrespective of the non-mandatory character of FRCs.

FUNCTIONALITY-RELATED CHARACTERISTICS SECTION IN MONOGRAPHS

Monographs on excipients may have a section entitled 'Functionality-related characteristics'. This section is included for information for the user and is not a mandatory part of the monograph. The section gives a statement of characteristics that are known to be relevant for certain uses of the excipient. The use for which the characteristic is relevant is stated. For other uses, the characteristic may be irrelevant. For this reason, the section should not be seen simply as a supplement to the monograph. It is the responsibility of the manufacturer of the medicinal product to decide how the information on FRCs will be applied in the manufacturing process in light of the use of the excipient and data from pharmaceutical development.

The information on the functionality-related characteristics may be given in different ways:

- name of the FRC;
- name of the FRC and a recommended method for its determination, referring wherever possible to a general chapter of the Pharmacopoeia;
- name of the FRC with a recommended method for its determination and typical acceptance criteria, which may be in the form of tolerances for the nominal value.

A given characteristic may be the subject of a mandatory requirement in the monograph and may also be mentioned in the FRC section. The degree of polymerisation is used in the mandatory Identification section of the monographs on microcrystalline cellulose and powdered cellulose to distinguish the 2 types. The degree of polymerisation of microcrystalline cellulose is not greater than 350, whereas that of powdered cellulose is 440 to 2250. The actual degree of polymerisation is relevant for certain uses and it is therefore also cited as a relevant FRC that the manufacturer of the medicinal product may choose to specify for the grade used of a particular pharmaceutical preparation.

The section on FRCs is intended to reflect current knowledge related to the major uses of an excipient. In view of the multiple uses of some excipients and the continuous development of new uses, the section may not be complete. In addition, the methods cited for the determination of a particular characteristic are given as recommendations for methods that are known to be satisfactory for the purpose, and the use of other methods is not excluded.

INTERNATIONAL HARMONISATION

A number of excipient monographs are subject to international harmonisation among the European, Japanese and United States Pharmacopoeias (see *5.8. Pharmacopoeial harmonisation*). Introduction of the FRC section in the monographs of the European Pharmacopoeia means that the presentation of harmonised monographs differs. Tests for physical and chemical characteristics regarded as functionality-related in the European Pharmacopoeia are, in the 2 other pharmacopoeias, included in the body of the monograph. The different format has no implications on the specification of excipient characteristics for the manufacturer of the medicinal product. Current regulatory guidance recommends the identification and specification of only such critical properties that impact the manufacturing process and the performance of the end-product. The different legal environments of the 3 pharmacopoeias allow for different formats of the monographs without affecting the international harmonisation status.

GLOSSARY

Critical characteristic: any physical or chemical material characteristic that has been demonstrated to impact significantly on the manufacturability and/or performance of the medicinal product.

Design space: the multidimensional combination and interaction of input variables (e.g. material attributes) and process parameters that have been demonstrated to provide assurance of quality.

Functionality-related characteristic: a controllable physical or chemical characteristic of an excipient that is shown to impact on its functionality.

Functionality testing: the direct testing of the concerned function of an excipient in a particular formulation and manufacturing process to verify that the excipient provides the intended functionality.

Performance tests: analytical tests on the critical properties of a medicinal product.

Process robustness: ability of a process to tolerate variability of materials and changes of the process and equipment without negative impact on quality.

GENERAL MONOGRAPHS

04/2008:0765

EXTRACTS

Extracta

DEFINITION

Extracts are preparations of liquid (liquid extracts and tinctures), semi-solid (soft extracts and oleoresins) or solid (dry extracts) consistency, obtained from herbal drugs or animal matter, which are usually in a dry state.

Where medicinal products are manufactured using extracts of animal origin, the requirements of chapter *5.1.7. Viral safety* apply.

Different types of extract may be distinguished. Standardised extracts are adjusted within an acceptable tolerance to a given content of constituents with known therapeutic activity; standardisation is achieved by adjustment of the extract with inert material or by blending batches of extracts. Quantified extracts are adjusted to a defined range of constituents; adjustments are made by blending batches of extracts. Other extracts are essentially defined by their production process (state of the herbal drug or animal matter to be extracted, solvent, extraction conditions) and their specifications.

PRODUCTION

Extracts are prepared by suitable methods using ethanol or other suitable solvents. Different batches of the herbal drug or animal matter may be blended prior to extraction. The herbal drug or animal matter to be extracted may undergo a preliminary treatment, for example, inactivation of enzymes, grinding or defatting. In addition, unwanted matter may be removed after extraction.

Herbal drugs, animal matter and organic solvents used for the preparation of extracts comply with any relevant monograph of the Pharmacopoeia. For soft and dry extracts where the organic solvent is removed by evaporation, recovered or recycled solvent may be used, provided that the recovery procedures are controlled and monitored to ensure that solvents meet appropriate standards before re-use or admixture with other approved materials. Water used for the preparation of extracts is of a suitable quality. Except for the test for bacterial endotoxins, water complying with the section on Purified water in bulk in the monograph on *Purified water (0008)* is suitable. Potable water may be suitable if it complies with a defined specification that allows the consistent production of a suitable extract.

Where applicable, concentration to the intended consistency is carried out using suitable methods, usually under reduced pressure and at a temperature at which deterioration of the constituents is reduced to a minimum. Essential oils that have been separated during processing may be restored to the extracts at an appropriate stage in the manufacturing process. Suitable excipients may be added at various stages of the manufacturing process, for example to improve technological qualities such as homogeneity or consistency. Suitable stabilisers and antimicrobial preservatives may also be added.

Extraction with a given solvent leads to typical proportions of characterised constituents in the extractable matter; during production of standardised and quantified extracts, purification procedures may be applied that increase these proportions with respect to the expected values; such extracts are referred to as 'refined'.

IDENTIFICATION

Extracts are identified using a suitable method.

TESTS

Where applicable, as a result of analysis of the herbal drug or animal matter used for production and in view of the production process, tests for microbiological quality (*5.1.4*), heavy metals, aflatoxins and pesticide residues (*2.8.13*) in the extracts may be necessary.

ASSAY

Wherever possible, extracts are assayed by a suitable method.

LABELLING

The label states:

- the herbal drug or animal matter used;
- whether the extract is liquid, soft or dry, or whether it is a tincture;
- for standardised extracts, the content of constituents with known therapeutic activity;
- for quantified extracts, the content of constituents (markers) used for quantification;
- the ratio of the starting material to the genuine extract (extract without excipients) (DER);
- the solvent or solvents used for extraction;
- where applicable, that a fresh herbal drug or fresh animal matter has been used;
- where applicable, that the extract is 'refined';
- the name and amount of any excipient used including stabilisers and antimicrobial preservatives;
- where applicable, the percentage of dry residue.

Liquid extracts – extracta fluida

DEFINITION

Liquid extracts are liquid preparations of which, in general, 1 part by mass or volume is equivalent to 1 part by mass of the dried herbal drug or animal matter. These preparations are adjusted, if necessary, so that they satisfy the requirements for content of solvent, and, where applicable, for constituents.

PRODUCTION

Liquid extracts are prepared by using ethanol of a suitable concentration or water to extract the herbal drug or animal matter, or by dissolving a soft or dry extract (which has been produced using the same strength of extraction solvent as is used in preparing the liquid extract by direct extraction) of the herbal drug or animal matter in either ethanol of a suitable concentration or water. Liquid extracts may be filtered, if necessary.

A slight sediment may form on standing, which is acceptable as long as the composition of the liquid extract is not changed significantly.

TESTS

Relative density (*2.2.5*). Where applicable, the liquid extract complies with the limits prescribed in the monograph.

Ethanol (*2.9.10*). For alcoholic liquid extracts, carry out the determination of ethanol content. The ethanol content complies with that prescribed.

Methanol and 2-propanol (*2.9.11*): maximum 0.05 per cent *V/V* of methanol and maximum 0.05 per cent *V/V* of 2-propanol for alcoholic liquid extracts, unless otherwise prescribed.

Dry residue (*2.8.16*). Where applicable, the liquid extract complies with the limits prescribed in the monograph, corrected if necessary, taking into account any excipient used.

General monographs

STORAGE

Protected from light.

LABELLING

The label states in addition to the requirements listed above:

- where applicable, the ethanol content in per cent *V/V* in the final extract.

Tinctures – tincturae

DEFINITION

Tinctures are liquid preparations that are usually obtained using either 1 part of herbal drug or animal matter and 10 parts of extraction solvent, or 1 part of herbal drug or animal matter and 5 parts of extraction solvent.

PRODUCTION

Tinctures are prepared by maceration or percolation (outline methodology is given below) using only ethanol of a suitable concentration for extraction of the herbal drug or animal matter, or by dissolving a soft or dry extract (which has been produced using the same strength of extraction solvent as is used in preparing the tincture by direct extraction) of the herbal drug or animal matter in ethanol of a suitable concentration. Tinctures are filtered, if necessary.

Tinctures are usually clear. A slight sediment may form on standing, which is acceptable as long as the composition of the tincture is not changed significantly.

Production by maceration. Unless otherwise prescribed, reduce the herbal drug or animal matter to be extracted to pieces of suitable size, mix thoroughly with the prescribed extraction solvent and allow to stand in a closed container for an appropriate time. The residue is separated from the extraction solvent and, if necessary, pressed out. In the latter case, the 2 liquids obtained are combined.

Production by percolation. If necessary, reduce the herbal drug or animal matter to be extracted to pieces of suitable size. Mix thoroughly with a portion of the prescribed extraction solvent and allow to stand for an appropriate time. Transfer to a percolator and allow the percolate to flow at room temperature slowly making sure that the herbal drug or animal matter to be extracted is always covered with the remaining extraction solvent. The residue may be pressed out and the expressed liquid combined with the percolate.

TESTS

Relative density (*2.2.5*). Where applicable, the tincture complies with the limits prescribed in the monograph.

Ethanol (*2.9.10*). The ethanol content complies with that prescribed.

Methanol and 2-propanol (*2.9.11*): maximum 0.05 per cent *V/V* of methanol and maximum 0.05 per cent *V/V* of 2-propanol, unless otherwise prescribed.

Dry residue (*2.8.16*). Where applicable, the tincture complies with the limits prescribed in the monograph, corrected if necessary, taking into account any excipient used.

STORAGE

Protected from light.

LABELLING

The label states in addition to the requirements listed above:

- for tinctures other than standardised and quantified tinctures, the ratio of starting material to extraction liquid or of starting material to final tincture;
- the ethanol content in per cent *V/V* in the final tincture.

Soft extracts – extracta spissa

DEFINITION

Soft extracts are semi-solid preparations obtained by evaporation or partial evaporation of the solvent used for extraction.

TESTS

Dry residue (*2.8.16*). The soft extract complies with the limits prescribed in the monograph.

Solvents. Residual solvents are controlled as described in chapter *5.4*, unless otherwise prescribed or justified and authorised.

STORAGE

Protected from light.

Oleoresins – oleoresina

DEFINITION

Oleoresins are semi-solid extracts composed of a resin in solution in an essential and/or fatty oil and are obtained by evaporation of the solvent(s) used for their production.

This monograph applies to oleoresins produced by extraction and not to natural oleoresins.

TESTS

Water (*2.2.13*). The oleoresin complies with the limits prescribed in the monograph.

Solvents. Residual solvents are controlled as described in chapter *5.4*, unless otherwise prescribed or justified and authorised.

STORAGE

In an airtight container, protected from light.

Dry extracts – extracta sicca

DEFINITION

Dry extracts are solid preparations obtained by evaporation of the solvent used for their production. Dry extracts have a loss on drying of not greater than 5 per cent *m/m*, unless a loss on drying with a different limit or a test on water is prescribed in the monograph.

TESTS

Water (*2.2.13*). Where applicable, the dry extract complies with the limits prescribed in the monograph.

Loss on drying (*2.8.17*). Where applicable, the dry extract complies with the limits prescribed in the monograph.

Solvents. Residual solvents are controlled as described in chapter *5.4*, unless otherwise prescribed or justified and authorised.

STORAGE

In an airtight container, protected from light.

VACCINES FOR HUMAN USE

04/2008:1057

MEASLES, MUMPS AND RUBELLA VACCINE (LIVE)

Vaccinum morbillorum, parotitidis et rubellae vivum

DEFINITION

Measles, mumps and rubella vaccine (live) is a freeze-dried preparation of suitable attenuated strains of measles virus, mumps virus and rubella virus.

The vaccine is reconstituted immediately before use, as stated on the label, to give a clear liquid that may be coloured owing to the presence of a pH indicator.

PRODUCTION

The 3 components are prepared as described in the monographs *Measles vaccine (live) (0213)*, *Mumps vaccine (live) (0538)* and *Rubella vaccine (live) (0162)* and comply with the requirements prescribed therein.

The production method is validated to demonstrate that the product, if tested, would comply with the test for abnormal toxicity for immunosera and vaccines for human use (*2.6.9*).

FINAL BULK VACCINE

Virus harvests for each component are pooled and clarified to remove cells. A suitable stabiliser may be added and the pooled harvests diluted as appropriate. Suitable quantities of the pooled harvest for each component are mixed.

Only a final bulk vaccine that complies with the following requirement may be used in the preparation of the final lot.

Bacterial and fungal contamination. Carry out the test for sterility (*2.6.1*), using 10 ml for each medium.

FINAL LOT

For each component, a minimum virus concentration for release of the product is established such as to ensure, in light of stability data, that the minimum concentration stated on the label will be present at the end of the period of validity.

Only a final lot that complies with the requirements for minimum virus concentration of each component for release, with the following requirement for thermal stability and with each of the requirements given below under Identification and Tests may be released for use. Provided that the tests for bovine serum albumin and, where applicable, for ovalbumin have been carried out with satisfactory results on the final bulk vaccine, they may be omitted on the final lot.

Thermal stability. Maintain at least 3 vials of the final lot of freeze-dried vaccine in the dry state at 37 ± 1 °C for 7 days. Determine the virus concentration as described under Assay in parallel for the heated vaccine and for vaccine stored at the temperature recommended for storage. For each component, the virus concentration of the heated vaccine is not more than 1.0 log lower than that of the unheated vaccine.

IDENTIFICATION

When the vaccine reconstituted as stated on the label is mixed with antibodies specific for measles virus, mumps virus and rubella virus, it is no longer able to infect cell cultures susceptible to these viruses. When the vaccine reconstituted as stated on the label is mixed with quantities of specific antibodies sufficient to neutralise any 2 viral components, the 3rd viral component infects susceptible cell cultures.

TESTS

Bacterial and fungal contamination. The reconstituted vaccine complies with the test for sterility (*2.6.1*).

Bovine serum albumin. Not more than 50 ng per single human dose, determined by a suitable immunochemical method (*2.7.1*).

Ovalbumin. If the mumps component is produced in chick embryos, the vaccine contains not more than 1 μg of ovalbumin per single human dose, determined by a suitable immunochemical method (*2.7.1*).

Water (*2.5.12*). Not more than 3.0 per cent, determined by the semi-micro determination of water.

ASSAY

The cell lines and/or neutralising antisera are chosen to ensure that each component is assayed without interference from the other 2 components.

Titrate the vaccine for infective measles, mumps and rubella virus, using at least 3 separate vials of vaccine and inoculating a suitable number of wells for each dilution step. Titrate 1 vial of the appropriate virus reference preparation in triplicate to validate each assay. The virus concentration of the reference preparation is monitored using a control chart and a titre is established on a historical basis by each laboratory. The relation with the appropriate European Pharmacopoeia Biological Reference Preparation is established and monitored at regular intervals if a manufacturer's reference preparation is used. Calculate the individual virus concentration for each vial of vaccine and for each replicate of the reference preparation as well as the corresponding combined virus concentrations, using the usual statistical methods (for example, *5.3*).

The combined estimates of the measles, mumps and rubella virus concentrations for the 3 vials of vaccine are not less than that stated on the label; the minimum measles virus concentration stated on the label is not less than 3.0 log $CCID_{50}$ per single human dose; the minimum mumps virus concentration stated on the label is not less than 3.7 log $CCID_{50}$ per single human dose; the minimum rubella virus concentration stated on the label is not less than 3.0 log $CCID_{50}$ per single human dose.

The assay is not valid if:

- the confidence interval (P = 0.95) of the estimated virus concentration of the reference preparation for the 3 replicates combined is greater than ± 0.3 log $CCID_{50}$;
- the virus concentration of the reference preparation differs by more than 0.5 log $CCID_{50}$ from the established value.

The assay is repeated if the confidence interval (P = 0.95) of the combined virus concentration of the vaccine is greater than ± 0.3 log $CCID_{50}$; data obtained from valid assays only are combined by the usual statistical methods (for example, *5.3*) to calculate the virus concentration of the sample. The confidence interval (P = 0.95) of the combined virus concentration is not greater than ± 0.3 log $CCID_{50}$.

Measles vaccine (live) BRP is suitable for use as a reference preparation.

Mumps vaccine (live) BRP is suitable for use as a reference preparation.

Rubella vaccine (live) BRP is suitable for use as a reference preparation.

Where justified and authorised, different assay designs may be used; this may imply the application of different validity and acceptance criteria. However, the vaccine must comply if tested as described above.

LABELLING

The label states:

- the strains of virus used in the preparation of the vaccine;

- where applicable, that chick embryos have been used for the preparation of the vaccine;
- the type and origin of the cells used for the preparation of the vaccine;
- the minimum virus concentration for each component of the vaccine;
- that contact between the vaccine and disinfectants is to be avoided;
- that the vaccine must not be given to a pregnant woman and that a woman must not become pregnant within 2 months after having the vaccine.

04/2008:0213

MEASLES VACCINE (LIVE)

Vaccinum morbillorum vivum

DEFINITION

Measles vaccine (live) is a freeze-dried preparation of a suitable attenuated strain of measles virus. The vaccine is reconstituted immediately before use, as stated on the label, to give a clear liquid that may be coloured owing to the presence of a pH indicator.

PRODUCTION

The production of vaccine is based on a virus seed-lot system and, if the virus is propagated in human diploid cells, a cell-bank system. The production method shall have been shown to yield consistently live measles vaccines of adequate immunogenicity and safety in man. Unless otherwise justified and authorised, the virus in the final vaccine shall have undergone no more passages from the master seed lot than were used to prepare the vaccine shown in clinical studies to be satisfactory with respect to safety and efficacy; even with authorised exceptions, the number of passages beyond the level used for clinical studies shall not exceed 5.

The potential neurovirulence of the vaccine strain is considered during preclinical development, based on available epidemiological data on neurovirulence and neurotropism, primarily for the wild-type virus. In light of this, a risk analysis is carried out. Where necessary and if available, a test is carried out on the vaccine strain using an animal model that differentiates wild-type and attenuated virus; tests on strains of intermediate attenuation may also be needed.

The production method is validated to demonstrate that the product, if tested, would comply with the test for abnormal toxicity for immunosera and vaccines for human use (*2.6.9*).

SUBSTRATE FOR VIRUS PROPAGATION

The virus is propagated in human diploid cells (*5.2.3*) or in cultures of chick-embryo cells derived from a chicken flock free from specified pathogens (*5.2.2*).

SEED LOT

The strain of measles virus used shall be identified by historical records that include information on the origin of the strain and its subsequent manipulation. Virus seed lots are prepared in large quantities and stored at temperatures below – 20 °C if freeze-dried, or below – 60 °C if not freeze-dried.

Only a seed lot that complies with the following requirements may be used for virus propagation.

Identification. The master and working seed lots are identified as measles virus by serum neutralisation in cell culture, using specific antibodies.

Virus concentration. The virus concentration of the master and working seed lots is determined to monitor consistency of production.

Extraneous agents (*2.6.16*). The working seed lot complies with the requirements for seed lots.

PROPAGATION AND HARVEST

All processing of the cell bank and subsequent cell cultures is done under aseptic conditions in an area where no other cells are handled during production. Suitable animal (but not human) serum may be used in the growth medium, but the final medium for maintaining cells during virus multiplication does not contain animal serum. Serum and trypsin used in the preparation of cell suspensions and culture media are shown to be free from extraneous agents. The cell culture medium may contain a pH indicator such as phenol red and suitable antibiotics at the lowest effective concentration. It is preferable to have a substrate free from antibiotics during production. Not less than 500 ml of the production cell cultures is set aside as uninfected cell cultures (control cells). The viral suspensions are harvested at a time appropriate to the strain of virus being used.

Only a single harvest that complies with the following requirements may be used in the preparation of the final bulk vaccine.

Identification. The single harvest contains virus that is identified as measles virus by serum neutralisation in cell culture, using specific antibodies.

Virus concentration. The virus concentration in the single harvest is determined as prescribed under Assay to monitor consistency of production and to determine the dilution to be used for the final bulk vaccine.

Extraneous agents (*2.6.16*). The single harvest complies with the tests for extraneous agents.

Control cells. If human diploid cells are used for production, the control cells comply with a test for identification. They comply with the tests for extraneous agents (*2.6.16*).

FINAL BULK VACCINE

Virus harvests that comply with the above tests are pooled and clarified to remove cells. A suitable stabiliser may be added and the pooled harvests diluted as appropriate.

Only a final bulk vaccine that complies with the following requirement may be used in the preparation of the final lot.

Bacterial and fungal contamination. The final bulk vaccine complies with the test for sterility (*2.6.1*), carried out using 10 ml for each medium.

FINAL LOT

A minimum virus concentration for release of the product is established such as to ensure, in light of stability data, that the minimum concentration stated on the label will be present at the end of the period of validity.

Only a final lot that complies with the requirements for minimum virus concentration for release, with the following requirement for thermal stability and with each of the requirements given below under Identification and Tests may be released for use. Provided that the test for bovine serum albumin has been carried out with satisfactory results on the final bulk vaccine, it may be omitted on the final lot.

Thermal stability. Maintain at least 3 vials of the final lot of freeze-dried vaccine in the dry state at 37 ± 1 °C for 7 days. Determine the virus concentration as described under Assay in parallel for the heated vaccine and for vaccine stored at the temperature recommended for storage. The virus concentration of the heated vaccine is not more than 1.0 log lower than that of the unheated vaccine.

Vaccines

IDENTIFICATION

When the vaccine reconstituted as stated on the label is mixed with specific measles antibodies, it is no longer able to infect susceptible cell cultures.

TESTS

Bacterial and fungal contamination. The reconstituted vaccine complies with the test for sterility (*2.6.1*).

Bovine serum albumin. Not more than 50 ng per single human dose, determined by a suitable immunochemical method (*2.7.1*).

Water (*2.5.12*). Not more than 3.0 per cent, determined by the semi-micro determination of water.

ASSAY

Titrate the vaccine for infective virus, using at least 3 separate vials of vaccine and inoculating a suitable number of wells for each dilution step. Titrate 1 vial of an appropriate virus reference preparation in triplicate to validate each assay. The virus concentration of the reference preparation is monitored using a control chart and a titre is established on a historical basis by each laboratory. The relation with the appropriate European Pharmacopoeia Biological Reference Preparation is established and monitored at regular intervals if a manufacturer's reference preparation is used. Calculate the individual virus concentration for each vial of vaccine and for each replicate of the reference preparation as well as the corresponding combined virus concentrations, using the usual statistical methods (for example, *5.3*). The combined estimate of the virus concentration for the 3 vials of vaccine is not less than that stated on the label; the minimum virus concentration stated on the label is not less than 3.0 log $CCID_{50}$ per single human dose.

The assay is not valid if:

- the confidence interval (P = 0.95) of the estimated virus concentration of the reference preparation for the 3 replicates combined is greater than ± 0.3 log $CCID_{50}$;
- the virus concentration of the reference preparation differs by more than 0.5 log $CCID_{50}$ from the established value.

The assay is repeated if the confidence interval (P = 0.95) of the combined virus concentration of the vaccine is greater than ± 0.3 log $CCID_{50}$; data obtained from valid assays only are combined by the usual statistical methods (for example, *5.3*) to calculate the virus concentration of the sample. The confidence interval (P = 0.95) of the combined virus concentration is not greater than ± 0.3 log $CCID_{50}$.

Measles vaccine (live) BRP is suitable for use as a reference preparation.

Where justified and authorised, different assay designs may be used; this may imply the application of different validity and acceptance criteria. However, the vaccine must comply if tested as described above.

LABELLING

The label states:

- the strain of virus used for the preparation of the vaccine;
- the type and origin of the cells used for the preparation of the vaccine;
- the minimum virus concentration;
- that contact between the vaccine and disinfectants is to be avoided.

04/2008:0538

MUMPS VACCINE (LIVE)

Vaccinum parotitidis vivum

DEFINITION

Mumps vaccine (live) is a freeze-dried preparation of a suitable attenuated strain of mumps virus. The vaccine is reconstituted immediately before use, as stated on the label, to give a clear liquid that may be coloured owing to the presence of a pH indicator.

PRODUCTION

The production of vaccine is based on a virus seed-lot system and, if the virus is propagated in human diploid cells, a cell-bank system. The production method shall have been shown to yield consistently live mumps vaccines of adequate immunogenicity and safety in man. Unless otherwise justified and authorised, the virus in the final vaccine shall have undergone no more passages from the master seed lot than were used to prepare the vaccine shown in clinical studies to be satisfactory with respect to safety and efficacy.

The potential neurovirulence of the vaccine strain is considered during preclinical development, based on available epidemiological data on neurovirulence and neurotropism, primarily for the wild-type virus. In light of this, a risk analysis is carried out. Where necessary and if available, a test is carried out on the vaccine strain using an animal model that differentiates wild-type and attenuated virus; tests on strains of intermediate attenuation may also be needed.

The production method is validated to demonstrate that the product, if tested, would comply with the test for abnormal toxicity for immunosera and vaccines for human use (*2.6.9*).

SUBSTRATE FOR VIRUS PROPAGATION

The virus is propagated in human diploid cells (*5.2.3*) or in chick-embryo cells or in the amniotic cavity of chick embryos derived from a chicken flock free from specified pathogens (*5.2.2*).

SEED LOT

The strain of mumps virus used shall be identified by historical records that include information on the origin of the strain and its subsequent manipulation. Virus seed lots are prepared in large quantities and stored at temperatures below − 20 °C if freeze-dried, or below − 60 °C if not freeze-dried.

Only a seed lot that complies with the following requirements may be used for virus propagation.

Identification. The master and working seed lots are identified as mumps virus by serum neutralisation in cell culture, using specific antibodies.

Virus concentration. The virus concentration of the master and working seed lots is determined to ensure consistency of production.

Extraneous agents (*2.6.16*). The working seed lot complies with the requirements for seed lots.

PROPAGATION AND HARVEST

All processing of the cell bank and subsequent cell cultures is done under aseptic conditions in an area where no other cells are handled during the production. Suitable animal (but not human) serum may be used in the culture media. Serum and trypsin used in the preparation of cell suspensions and culture media are shown to be free from extraneous agents. The cell culture medium may contain a pH indicator such as

Vaccines

phenol red and suitable antibiotics at the lowest effective concentration. It is preferable to have a substrate free from antibiotics during production. Not less than 500 ml of the production cell cultures is set aside as uninfected cell cultures (control cells). If the virus is propagated in chick embryos, 2 per cent but not less than 20 eggs are set aside as uninfected control eggs. The viral suspensions are harvested at a time appropriate to the strain of virus being used.

Only a single harvest that complies with the following requirements may be used in the preparation of the final bulk vaccine.

Identification. The single harvest contains virus that is identified as mumps virus by serum neutralisation in cell culture, using specific antibodies.

Virus concentration. The virus concentration in the single harvest is determined as prescribed under Assay to monitor consistency of production and to determine the dilution to be used for the final bulk vaccine.

Extraneous agents (*2.6.16*). The single harvest complies with the tests for extraneous agents.

Control cells or eggs. If human diploid cells are used for production, the control cells comply with a test for identification; the control cells and the control eggs comply with the tests for extraneous agents (*2.6.16*).

FINAL BULK VACCINE

Single harvests that comply with the above tests are pooled and clarified to remove cells. A suitable stabiliser may be added and the pooled harvests diluted as appropriate.

Only a final bulk vaccine that complies with the following requirement may be used in the preparation of the final lot.

Bacterial and fungal contamination. The final bulk vaccine complies with the test for sterility (*2.6.1*), carried out using 10 ml for each medium.

FINAL LOT

A minimum virus concentration for release of the product is established such as to ensure, in light of stability data, that the minimum concentration stated on the label will be present at the end of the period of validity.

Only a final lot that complies with the requirements for minimum virus concentration for release, with the following requirement for thermal stability and with each of the requirements given below under Identification and Tests may be released for use. Provided that the tests for bovine serum albumin and, where applicable, for ovalbumin have been carried out with satisfactory results on the final bulk vaccine, they may be omitted on the final lot.

Thermal stability. Maintain at least 3 vials of the final lot of freeze-dried vaccine in the dry state at 37 ± 1 °C for 7 days. Determine the virus concentration as described under Assay in parallel for the heated vaccine and for vaccine stored at the temperature recommended for storage. The virus concentration of the heated vaccine is not more than 1.0 log lower than that of the unheated vaccine.

IDENTIFICATION

When the vaccine reconstituted as stated on the label is mixed with specific mumps antibodies, it is no longer able to infect susceptible cell cultures.

TESTS

Bacterial and fungal contamination. The reconstituted vaccine complies with the test for sterility (*2.6.1*).

Bovine serum albumin. Not more than 50 ng per single human dose, determined by a suitable immunochemical method (*2.7.1*).

Ovalbumin. If the vaccine is produced in chick embryos, it contains not more than 1 µg of ovalbumin per single human dose, determined by a suitable immunochemical method (*2.7.1*).

Water (*2.5.12*). Not more than 3.0 per cent, determined by the semi-micro determination of water.

ASSAY

Titrate the vaccine for infective virus, using at least 3 separate vials of vaccine and inoculating a suitable number of wells for each dilution step. Titrate 1 vial of an appropriate virus reference preparation in triplicate to validate each assay. The virus concentration of the reference preparation is monitored using a control chart and a titre is established on a historical basis by each laboratory. The relation with the appropriate European Pharmacopoeia Biological Reference Preparation is established and monitored at regular intervals if a manufacturer's reference preparation is used. Calculate the individual virus concentration for each vial of vaccine and for each replicate of the reference preparation as well as the corresponding combined virus concentrations, using the usual statistical methods (for example, *5.3*). The combined estimate of the virus concentration for the 3 vials of vaccine is not less than that stated on the label; the minimum virus concentration stated on the label is not less than 3.7 log $CCID_{50}$ per single human dose.

The assay is not valid if:

- the confidence interval (P = 0.95) of the estimated virus concentration of the reference preparation for the 3 replicates combined is greater than ± 0.3 log $CCID_{50}$;
- the virus concentration of the reference preparation differs by more than 0.5 log $CCID_{50}$ from the established value.

The assay is repeated if the confidence interval (P = 0.95) of the combined virus concentration of the vaccine is greater than ± 0.3 log $CCID_{50}$; data obtained from valid assays only are combined by the usual statistical methods (for example, *5.3*) to calculate the virus concentration of the sample. The confidence interval (P = 0.95) of the combined virus concentration is not greater than ± 0.3 log $CCID_{50}$.

Mumps vaccine (live) BRP is suitable for use as a reference preparation.

Where justified and authorised, different assay designs may be used; this may imply the application of different validity and acceptance criteria. However, the vaccine must comply if tested as described above.

LABELLING

The label states:

- the strain of virus used for the preparation of the vaccine;
- that the vaccine has been prepared in chick embryos or the type and origin of cells used for the preparation of the vaccine;
- the minimum virus concentration;
- that contact between the vaccine and disinfectants is to be avoided.

04/2008:0215

POLIOMYELITIS VACCINE (ORAL)

Vaccinum poliomyelitidis perorale

DEFINITION

Oral poliomyelitis vaccine is a preparation of approved strains of live attenuated poliovirus type 1, 2 or 3 grown in *in vitro* cultures of approved cells, containing any one type or any combination of the 3 types of Sabin strains, presented in a form suitable for oral administration.

The vaccine is a clear liquid that may be coloured owing to the presence of a pH indicator.

PRODUCTION

The vaccine strains and the production method shall have been shown to yield consistently vaccines that are both immunogenic and safe in man.

The production of vaccine is based on a virus seed-lot system. Cell lines are used according to a cell-bank system. If primary monkey kidney cell cultures are used, production complies with the requirements indicated below. Unless otherwise justified and authorised, the virus in the final vaccine shall not have undergone more than 2 passages from the master seed lot.

REFERENCE STANDARDS

Poliomyelitis vaccine (oral) types 1, 2, 3 BRP is suitable for use as a virus reference preparation for the assay.

The International Standards for poliovirus type 2 (Sabin) for MAPREC (Mutant Analysis by PCR and Restriction Enzyme Cleavage) assays and poliovirus, type 3 (Sabin) synthetic DNA for MAPREC assays are suitable for use in the tests for genetic markers and the molecular tests for consistency of production.

Reference preparations of each poliovirus type at the Sabin Original + 2 passage level, namely WHO (SO + 2)/I for type 1 virus, WHO (SO + 2)/II for type 2 virus and WHO (SO + 2)/III for type 3 virus are available for comparison of the *in vivo* neurovirulence with that of homotypic vaccines. Requests for the WHO reference preparations for *in vivo* neurovirulence tests are to be directed to WHO, Biologicals, Geneva, Switzerland.

A suitable reference preparation is to be included in each test.

SUBSTRATE FOR VIRUS PROPAGATION

The virus is propagated in human diploid cells (*5.2.3*), in continuous cell lines (*5.2.3*) or in primary monkey kidney cell cultures (including serially passaged cells from primary monkey kidney cells).

Primary monkey kidney cell cultures. *The following special requirements for the substrate for virus propagation apply to primary monkey kidney cell cultures.*

Monkeys used for preparation of primary monkey kidney cell cultures and for testing of virus. If the vaccine is prepared in primary monkey kidney cell cultures, animals of a species approved by the competent authority, in good health, kept in closed or intensively monitored colonies and not previously employed for experimental purposes shall be used.

The monkeys shall be kept in well-constructed and adequately ventilated animal rooms in cages spaced as far apart as possible. Adequate precautions shall be taken to prevent cross-infection between cages. Not more than 2 monkeys shall be housed per cage and cage-mates shall not be interchanged. The monkeys shall be kept in the country of manufacture of the vaccine in quarantine groups for a period of not less than 6 weeks before use. A quarantine group is a colony of selected, healthy monkeys kept in one room, with separate feeding and cleaning facilities, and having no contact with other monkeys during the quarantine period. If at any time during the quarantine period the overall death rate of a shipment consisting of one or more groups reaches 5 per cent (excluding deaths from accidents or where the cause was specifically determined not to be an infectious disease), monkeys from that entire shipment shall continue in quarantine from that time for a minimum of 6 weeks. The groups shall be kept continuously in isolation, as in quarantine, even after completion of the quarantine period, until the monkeys are used. After the last monkey of a group has been taken, the room that housed the group shall be thoroughly cleaned and decontaminated before being used for a fresh group. If kidneys from near-term monkeys are used, the mother is quarantined for the term of pregnancy.

Monkeys from which kidneys are to be removed shall be anaesthetised and thoroughly examined, particularly for evidence of tuberculosis and cercopithecid herpesvirus 1 (B virus) infection.

If a monkey shows any pathological lesion relevant to the use of its kidneys in the preparation of a seed lot or vaccine, it shall not be used, nor shall any of the remaining monkeys of the quarantine group concerned be used unless it is evident that their use will not impair the safety of the product.

All the operations described in this section shall be conducted outside the areas where the vaccine is produced.

The monkeys used shall be shown to be free from antibodies to simian virus 40 (SV40), simian immunodeficiency virus and spumaviruses. The blood sample used in testing for SV40 antibodies must be taken as close as possible to the time of removal of the kidneys. If *Macaca* spp. are used for production, the monkeys shall also be shown to be free from antibodies to cercopithecid herpesvirus 1 (B virus). Human herpesvirus has been used as an indicator for freedom from B virus antibodies on account of the danger of handling cercopithecid herpesvirus 1 (B virus). Monkeys used for the production of new seed lots are shown to be free from antibodies to simian cytomegalovirus (sCMV).

Primary monkey kidney cell cultures for vaccine production. Kidneys that show no pathological signs are used for preparing cell cultures. If the monkeys are from a colony maintained for vaccine production, serially passaged monkey kidney cell cultures from primary monkey kidney cells may be used for virus propagation, otherwise the monkey kidney cells are not propagated in series. Virus for the preparation of vaccine is grown by aseptic methods in such cultures. If animal serum is used in the propagation of the cells, the maintenance medium after virus inoculation shall contain no added serum.

Each group of cell cultures derived from a single monkey or from foetuses from no more than 10 near-term monkeys is prepared and tested as an individual group.

VIRUS SEED LOTS

The strains of poliovirus used shall be identified by historical records that include information on the origin and subsequent manipulation of the strains.

Working seed lots are prepared by a single passage from a master seed lot and at an approved passage level from the original Sabin virus. Virus seed lots are prepared in large quantities and stored at a temperature below − 60 °C.

Only a virus seed lot that complies with the following requirements may be used for virus propagation.

Identification. Each working seed lot is identified as poliovirus of the given type, using specific antibodies.

Virus concentration. Determined by the method described below, the virus concentration is the basis for the quantity of virus used in the neurovirulence test.

Extraneous agents (*2.6.16*). If the working seed lot is produced in human diploid cells or in a continuous cell line, it complies with the requirements for seed lots for virus vaccines. If the working seed lot is produced in primary monkey kidney cell cultures, it complies with the requirements given below under Virus Propagation and Harvest and Monovalent Pooled Harvest and with the tests in adult mice, suckling mice and guinea-pigs given in chapter *2.6.16*.

In addition to the requirements in chapter *2.6.16*, for vaccines produced in cell lines and when the seed lot was produced in primary monkey kidney cell cultures, a validated test for sCMV is performed.

Working seed lots shall be free from detectable DNA sequences from simian virus 40 (SV40).

Neurovirulence. Each master and working seed lot complies with the test for neurovirulence of poliomyelitis vaccine (oral) in monkeys (*2.6.19*). In addition, at least the first 4 consecutive batches of monovalent pooled harvest prepared from these seed lots shall be shown to comply with the test for neurovirulence of poliomyelitis vaccine (oral) in monkeys (*2.6.19*) before the seed lot is deemed suitable for use. Furthermore, the seed lot shall cease to be used in vaccine production if the frequency of failure of the monovalent pooled harvests produced from it is greater than predicted statistically. This statistical prediction is calculated after each test on the basis of all the monovalent pooled harvests tested; it is equal to the probability of false rejection on the occasion of a first test (i.e.1 per cent), the probability of false rejection on retest being negligible. If the test is carried out only by the manufacturer, the test slides are provided to the control authority for assessment.

Genetic markers. Each working seed lot is tested for its replicating properties at temperatures ranging from 36 °C to 40 °C as described under Monovalent pooled harvest. A profile (i.e. percentage of mutant) of the seed virus using the MAPREC assay is prepared. Type 3 virus seed lots comply with the MAPREC assay as described under Monovalent pooled harvest.

VIRUS PROPAGATION AND HARVEST

All processing of the cell banks and subsequent cell cultures is done under aseptic conditions in an area where no other cells are handled during the production. Suitable animal (but not human) serum may be used in the culture media, but the final medium for maintaining cell growth during virus multiplication does not contain animal serum. Serum and trypsin used in the preparation of cell suspensions and media are shown to be free from live extraneous agents. The cell-culture medium may contain a pH indicator such as phenol red and suitable antibiotics at the lowest effective concentration. It is preferable to have a substrate free from antibiotics during production. On the day of inoculation with the virus working seed lot, not less than 5 per cent or 1000 ml, whichever is the less, of the cell cultures employed for vaccine production are set aside as uninfected cell cultures (control cells). Special requirements, given below, apply to control cells when the vaccine is produced in primary monkey kidney cell cultures. The virus suspension is harvested not later than 4 days after virus inoculation. After inoculation of the production cell culture with the virus working seed lot, inoculated cells are maintained at a fixed temperature, shown to be suitable, within the range 33-35 °C; the temperature is maintained constant to ± 0.5 °C; control cell cultures are maintained at 33-35 °C for the relevant incubation periods.

Only a single virus harvest that complies with the following requirements may be used in the preparation of the monovalent pooled harvest.

Virus concentration. The virus concentration of virus harvests is determined as prescribed under Assay to monitor consistency of production and to determine the dilution to be used for the final bulk vaccine.

Molecular tests for consistency of production. The MAPREC assay is performed on each virus harvest. The acceptance/rejection criteria for consistency of production are determined for each manufacturer and for each working seed by agreement with the competent authority. These criteria are periodically reviewed and updated to the satisfaction of the competent authority. An investigation of consistency occurs if a virus harvest gives results that are inconsistent with previous production history.

Control cells. The control cells of the production cell culture from which the virus harvest is derived comply with a test for identity and with the requirements for extraneous agents (*2.6.16*) or, where primary monkey kidney cell cultures are used, as shown below.

Primary monkey kidney cell cultures. *The following special requirements apply to virus propagation and harvest in primary monkey kidney cell cultures.*

Cell cultures. On the day of inoculation with the virus working seed lot, each cell culture is examined for degeneration caused by an infective agent. If, in this examination, evidence is found of the presence in a cell culture of any extraneous agent, the entire group of cultures concerned shall be rejected.

On the day of inoculation with the virus working seed lot, a sample of at least 30 ml of the pooled fluid removed from the cell cultures of the kidneys of each single monkey or from foetuses from not more than 10 near-term monkeys is divided into 2 equal portions. 1 portion of the pooled fluid is tested in monkey kidney cell cultures prepared from the same species, but not the same animal, as that used for vaccine production. The other portion of the pooled fluid is, where necessary, tested in monkey kidney cell cultures from another species so that tests on the pooled fluids are done in cell cultures from at least 1 species known to be sensitive to SV40. The pooled fluid is inoculated into bottles of these cell cultures in such a way that the dilution of the pooled fluid in the nutrient medium does not exceed 1 in 4. The area of the cell sheet is at least 3 cm^2/ml of pooled fluid. At least 1 bottle of each type of cell culture remains uninoculated to serve as a control. If the monkey species used for vaccine production is known to be sensitive to SV40, a test in a 2nd species is not required. Animal serum may be used in the propagation of the cells, provided that it does not contain SV40 antibody, but the maintenance medium after inoculation of test material contains no added serum except as described below.

The cultures are incubated at a temperature of 35-37 °C and are observed for a total period of at least 4 weeks. During this observation period and after not less than 2 weeks' incubation, at least 1 subculture of fluid is made from each of these cultures in the same cell culture system. The subcultures are also observed for at least 2 weeks.

Serum may be added to the original culture at the time of subculturing, provided that the serum does not contain SV40 antibody.

Fluorescent-antibody techniques may be useful for detecting SV40 virus and other viruses in the cells.

A further sample of at least 10 ml of the pooled fluid is tested for cercopithecid herpesvirus 1 (B virus) and other viruses in rabbit kidney cell cultures. Serum used in the nutrient medium of these cultures shall have been shown to be free from inhibitors of B virus. Human herpesvirus has been used as an indicator for freedom from B virus inhibitors on account of the danger of handling cercopithecid herpesvirus 1 (B virus). The sample is inoculated into bottles of these cell cultures in such a way that the dilution of the pooled fluid in the nutrient medium does not exceed 1 in 4. The area of the cell sheet is at least 3 cm^2/ml of pooled fluid. At least 1 bottle of the cell cultures remains uninoculated to serve as a control.

The cultures are incubated at a temperature of 35-37 °C and observed for at least 2 weeks.

A further sample of 10 ml of the pooled fluid removed from the cell cultures on the day of inoculation with the seed lot virus is tested for the presence of extraneous agents by inoculation into human cell cultures sensitive to measles virus.

The tests are not valid if more than 20 per cent of the culture vessels have been discarded for non-specific accidental reasons by the end of the respective test periods.

If, in these tests, evidence is found of the presence of an extraneous agent, the single harvest from the whole group of cell cultures concerned is rejected.

If the presence of cercopithecid herpesvirus 1 (B virus) is demonstrated, the manufacture of oral poliomyelitis vaccine shall be discontinued and the competent authority shall be informed. Manufacturing shall not be resumed until a thorough investigation has been completed and precautions have been taken against any reappearance of the infection, and then only with the approval of the competent authority.

If these tests are not done immediately, the samples of pooled cell-culture fluid shall be kept at a temperature of − 60 °C or below, with the exception of the sample for the test for B virus, which may be held at 4 °C, provided that the test is done not more than 7 days after it has been taken.

Control cell cultures. On the day of inoculation with the virus working seed lot, 25 per cent (but not more than 2.5 litres) of the cell suspension obtained from the kidneys of each single monkey or from not more than 10 near-term monkeys is taken to prepare uninoculated control cell cultures. These control cell cultures are incubated in the same conditions as the inoculated cultures for at least 2 weeks and are examined during this period for evidence of cytopathic changes. The tests are not valid if more than 20 per cent of the control cell cultures have been discarded for non-specific, accidental reasons. At the end of the observation period, the control cell cultures are examined for degeneration caused by an infectious agent. If this examination or any of the tests required in this section shows evidence of the presence in a control culture of any extraneous agent, the poliovirus grown in the corresponding inoculated cultures from the same group shall be rejected.

Tests for haemadsorbing viruses. At the time of harvest or within 4 days of inoculation of the production cultures with the virus working seed lot, a sample of 4 per cent of the control cell cultures is taken and tested for haemadsorbing viruses. At the end of the observation period, the remaining control cell cultures are similarly tested. The tests are carried out as described in chapter *2.6.16*.

Tests for other extraneous agents. At the time of harvest, or within 7 days of the day of inoculation of the production cultures with the working seed lot, a sample of at least 20 ml of the pooled fluid from each group of control cultures is taken and tested in 2 kinds of monkey kidney cell culture, as described above.

At the end of the observation period for the original control cell cultures, similar samples of the pooled fluid are taken and the tests referred to in this section in the 2 kinds of monkey kidney cell culture and in the rabbit cell cultures are repeated, as described above under Cell cultures.

If the presence of cercopithecid herpesvirus 1 (B virus) is demonstrated, the production cell cultures shall not be used and the measures concerning vaccine production described above must be undertaken.

The fluids collected from the control cell cultures at the time of virus harvest and at the end of the observation period may be pooled before testing for extraneous agents. A sample of 2 per cent of the pooled fluid is tested in each of the cell culture systems specified.

Single harvests

Tests for neutralised single harvests in primary monkey kidney cell cultures. A sample of at least 10 ml of each single harvest is neutralised by a type-specific poliomyelitis antiserum prepared in animals other than monkeys. In preparing antisera for this purpose, the immunising antigens used shall be prepared in non-simian cells.

Half of the neutralised suspension (corresponding to at least 5 ml of single harvest) is tested in monkey kidney cell cultures prepared from the same species, but not the same animal, as that used for vaccine production. The other half of the neutralised suspension is tested, if necessary, in monkey kidney cell cultures from another species so that the tests on the neutralised suspension are done in cell cultures from at least 1 species known to be sensitive to SV40.

The neutralised suspensions are inoculated into bottles of these cell cultures in such a way that the dilution of the suspension in the nutrient medium does not exceed 1 in 4. The area of the cell sheet is at least 3 cm^2/ml of neutralised suspension. At least 1 bottle of each type of cell culture remains uninoculated to serve as a control and is maintained by nutrient medium containing the same concentration of the specific antiserum used for neutralisation.

Animal serum may be used in the propagation of the cells, provided that it does not contain SV40 antibody, but the maintenance medium, after the inoculation of the test material, contains no added serum other than the poliovirus neutralising antiserum, except as described below.

The cultures are incubated at a temperature of 35-37 °C and observed for a total period of at least 4 weeks. During this observation period and after not less than 2 weeks' incubation, at least 1 subculture of fluid is made from each of these cultures in the same cell-culture system. The subcultures are also observed for at least 2 weeks.

Serum may be added to the original cultures at the time of subculturing, provided that the serum does not contain SV40 antibody.

Additional tests are made for extraneous agents on a further sample of the neutralised single harvests by inoculation of 10 ml into human cell cultures sensitive to measles virus. This test is also validated for the detection of sCMV.

Fluorescent-antibody techniques may be useful for detecting SV40 virus and other viruses in the cells.

The tests are not valid if more than 20 per cent of the culture vessels have been discarded for non-specific accidental reasons by the end of the respective test periods.

If any cytopathic changes occur in any of the cultures, the causes of these changes are investigated. If the cytopathic changes are shown to be due to unneutralised poliovirus,

Vaccines

the test is repeated. If there is evidence of the presence of SV40 or other extraneous agents attributable to the single harvest, that single harvest is rejected.

MONOVALENT POOLED HARVEST

Monovalent pooled harvests are prepared by pooling a number of satisfactory single harvests of the same virus type. Monovalent pooled harvests from continuous cell lines may be purified. Each monovalent pooled harvest is filtered through a bacteria-retentive filter.

Only a monovalent pooled harvest that complies with the following requirements may be used in the preparation of the final bulk vaccine.

Identification. Each monovalent pooled harvest is identified as poliovirus of the given type, using specific antibodies.

Virus concentration. The virus concentration is determined by the method described below and serves as the basis for calculating the dilutions for preparation of the final bulk, for the quantity of virus used in the neurovirulence test and to establish and monitor production consistency.

Genetic markers. For Sabin poliovirus type 3, a validated MAPREC assay is performed. In this analysis the amount of the mutation at position 472 of the genome (472-C) is estimated and expressed as a ratio relative to the International Standard for MAPREC analysis of poliovirus type 3 (Sabin). A poliovirus type 3 monovalent pooled harvest found to have significantly more 472-C than the International Standard for MAPREC analysis of poliovirus type 3 (Sabin) fails in the MAPREC assay.

The MAPREC analysis of poliovirus type 3 (Sabin) is carried out using a standard operating procedure approved by the competent authority. A suitable procedure (*Mutant analysis by PCR and restriction enzyme cleavage (MAPREC) for oral poliovirus (Sabin) vaccine*) is available from WHO, Quality and Safety of Biologicals (QSB), Geneva. A laboratory must demonstrate to the competent authority that it is competent to perform the assay. The manufacturer and the competent authority shall agree on the procedure and the criteria for deciding whether a monovalent pooled harvest contains significantly more 472-C than the International Standard.

Acceptance/rejection criteria for assessment of consistency of production are determined for each manufacturer and for each working seed lot by agreement with the competent authority. These criteria are updated as each new bulk is prepared and analysed. An investigation of consistency occurs if a monovalent pooled harvest gives results that are inconsistent with previous production history.

As the MAPREC assay for type 3 poliovirus (Sabin) is highly predictive of *in vivo* neurovirulence, if a filtered monovalent pooled harvest of type 3 poliovirus (Sabin) fails the MAPREC assay then this triggers an investigation of the consistency of the manufacturing process. This investigation also includes a consideration of the suitability of the working seed lot.

Monovalent pooled harvests passing the MAPREC assay are subsequently tested for *in vivo* neurovirulence.

For poliovirus type 3, results from the MAPREC assay and the monkey neurovirulence test (*2.6.19*) are used concomitantly to assess the impact of changes in the production process or when a new manufacturer starts production.

Pending validation of MAPREC assays for poliovirus types 1 and 2, for these viruses filtered bulk suspension is tested for the property of reproducing at temperatures of 36 °C and 40 °C. A ratio of the replication capacities of the virus in the monovalent pooled harvest is obtained over a temperature range between 36 °C and 40 °C in comparison with the seed lot or a reference preparation for the marker tests and with appropriate rct/40– and rct/40+ strains of poliovirus of the same type. The incubation temperatures used in this test are controlled to within ± 0.1 °C. The monovalent pooled harvest passes the test if, for both the virus in the harvest and the appropriate reference material, the titre determined at 36 °C is at least 5.0 log greater than that determined at 40 °C. If growth at 40 °C is so low that a valid comparison cannot be established, a temperature in the region of 39.0-39.5 °C is used, at which temperature the reduction in titre of the reference material must be in the range 3.0-5.0 log of its value at 36 °C; the acceptable minimum reduction is determined for each virus strain at a given temperature. If the titres obtained for 1 or more of the reference viruses are not concordant with the expected values, the test must be repeated.

Neurovirulence (*2.6.19*). Each monovalent pooled harvest complies with the test for neurovirulence of poliomyelitis vaccine (oral). If the monkey neurovirulence test is carried out only by the manufacturer, the test slides are provided to the competent authority for assessment. The TgPVR21 transgenic mouse model provides a suitable alternative to the monkey neurovirulence test for neurovirulence testing of types 1, 2 or 3 vaccines once a laboratory qualifies as being competent to perform the test and the experience gained is to the satisfaction of the competent authority. The test is carried out using a standard operating procedure approved by the competent authority. A suitable procedure (*Neurovirulence test of type 1, 2 or 3 live poliomyelitis vaccines (oral) in transgenic mice susceptible to poliovirus*) is available from WHO, Quality and Safety of Biologicals, Geneva.

Primary monkey kidney cell cultures. *The following special requirements apply to monovalent pooled harvests derived from primary monkey kidney cell cultures.*

Retroviruses. The monovalent pooled harvest is examined using a reverse transcriptase assay. No indication of the presence of retroviruses is found.

Test in rabbits. A sample of the monovalent pooled harvest is tested for cercopithecid herpesvirus 1 (B virus) and other viruses by injection of not less than 100 ml into not fewer than 10 healthy rabbits each weighing 1.5-2.5 kg. Each rabbit receives not less than 10 ml and not more than 20 ml, of which 1 ml is given intradermally at multiple sites since the maximum volume to be given intradermally at each site is 0.1 ml, and the remainder subcutaneously. The rabbits are observed for at least 3 weeks for death or signs of illness.

All rabbits that die after the first 24 h of the test and those showing signs of illness are examined by autopsy, and the brain and organs removed for detailed examination to establish the cause of death.

The test is not valid if more than 20 per cent of the inoculated rabbits show signs of intercurrent infection during the observation period. The monovalent pooled harvest passes the test if none of the rabbits shows evidence of infection with B virus or with other extraneous agents or lesions of any kind attributable to the bulk suspension.

If the presence of B virus is demonstrated, the measures concerning vaccine production described above under Cell cultures are taken.

Test in guinea-pigs. If the primary monkey kidney cell cultures are not derived from monkeys kept in a closed colony, the monovalent pooled harvest shall be shown to comply with the following test. Administer to each of not fewer than 5 guinea-pigs, each weighing 350-450 g, 0.1 ml of the monovalent pooled harvest by intracerebral injection (0.05 ml in each cerebral hemisphere) and 0.5 ml by intraperitoneal injection. Measure the rectal temperature of each animal on each working day for 6 weeks. At the end of the observation period carry out autopsy on each animal.

In addition, administer to not fewer than 5 guinea-pigs 0.5 ml by intraperitoneal injection and observe as described above for 2-3 weeks. At the end of the observation period, carry out a passage from these animals to not fewer than 5 guinea-pigs using blood and a suspension of liver or spleen tissue. Measure the rectal temperature of the latter guinea-pigs for 2-3 weeks. Examine by autopsy all animals that, after the first day of the test, die or are euthanised because they show disease, or show on 3 consecutive days a body temperature higher than 40.1 °C; carry out histological examination to detect infection with filoviruses; in addition, inject a suspension of liver or spleen tissue or of blood intraperitoneally into not fewer than 3 guinea-pigs. If any signs of infection with filoviruses are noted, confirmatory serological tests are carried out on the blood of the affected animals. The monovalent pooled harvest complies with the test if not fewer than 80 per cent of the guinea-pigs survive to the end of the observation period and remain in good health, and no animal shows signs of infection with filoviruses.

FINAL BULK VACCINE

The final bulk vaccine is prepared from one or more satisfactory monovalent pooled harvests and may contain more than one virus type. Suitable flavouring substances and stabilisers may be added.

Only a final bulk vaccine that complies with the following requirement may be used in the preparation of the final lot.

Bacterial and fungal contamination. Carry out the test for sterility (*2.6.1*), using 10 ml for each medium.

FINAL LOT

Only a final lot that complies with the following requirement for thermal stability and is satisfactory with respect to each of the requirements given below under Identification, Tests and Assay may be released for use.

IDENTIFICATION

The vaccine is shown to contain poliovirus of each type stated on the label, using specific antibodies.

TESTS

Bacterial and fungal contamination. The vaccine complies with the test for sterility (*2.6.1*).

Thermal stability. Maintain not fewer than 3 vials of the final lot at 37 ± 1 °C for 48 h. Determine the total virus concentration as described under Assay in parallel for the heated vaccine and for vaccine maintained at the temperature recommended for storage. The estimated difference between the total virus concentration of the unheated and heated vaccines is not greater than 0.5 log infectious virus units ($CCID_{50}$) per single human dose.

ASSAY

Titrate the vaccine for infectious virus, using not fewer than 3 separate vials of vaccine, following the method described below. Titrate 1 vial of an appropriate virus reference preparation in triplicate to validate each assay. The virus concentration of the reference preparation is monitored using a control chart and a titre is established on a historical basis by each laboratory. If the vaccine contains more than one poliovirus type, titrate each type separately, using an appropriate type-specific antiserum (or preferably a monoclonal antibody) to neutralise each of the other types present.

Calculate the individual virus concentration for each vial of vaccine and for each replicate of the reference preparation as well as the corresponding combined virus concentrations, using the usual statistical methods (for example, *5.3*).

For a trivalent vaccine, the combined estimated virus titres per single human dose must be:

- not less than 6.0 log infectious virus units ($CCID_{50}$) for type 1;
- not less than 5.0 log infectious virus units ($CCID_{50}$) for type 2; and
- not less than 5.5 log infectious virus units ($CCID_{50}$) for type 3.

For a monovalent or divalent vaccine, the minimum virus titres are decided by the competent authority.

Method. Inoculate a suitable number of wells in a microtitre plate with a suitable volume of each of the selected dilutions of virus followed by a suitable volume of a cell suspension of the Hep-2 (Cincinnati) line. Examine the cultures between days 7 and 9.

The assay is not valid if:

- the confidence interval (P = 0.95) of the estimated virus concentration of the reference preparation for the 3 replicates combined is greater than ± 0.3 log $CCID_{50}$;
- the virus concentration of the reference preparation differs by more than 0.5 log $CCID_{50}$ from the established value. The relation with the appropriate European Pharmacopoeia Biological Reference Preparation is established and monitored at regular intervals when a manufacturer's reference preparation is used.

The assay is repeated if the confidence interval (P = 0.95) of the combined virus concentration of the vaccine is greater than ± 0.3 log $CCID_{50}$; data obtained from valid assays only are combined by the usual statistical methods (for example, *5.3*) to calculate the virus concentration of the sample. The confidence interval (P = 0.95) of the combined virus concentration is not greater than ± 0.3 log $CCID_{50}$.

Poliomyelitis vaccine (oral) BRP is suitable for use as a reference preparation.

Where justified and authorised, different assay designs may be used; this may imply the application of different validity and acceptance criteria. However, the vaccine must comply if tested as described above.

LABELLING

The label states:

- the types of poliovirus contained in the vaccine;
- the minimum amount of virus of each type contained in a single human dose;
- the cell substrate used for the preparation of the vaccine;
- that the vaccine is not to be injected.

04/2008:0216

RABIES VACCINE FOR HUMAN USE PREPARED IN CELL CULTURES

Vaccinum rabiei ex cellulis ad usum humanum

DEFINITION

Rabies vaccine for human use prepared in cell cultures is a freeze-dried preparation of a suitable strain of fixed rabies virus grown in cell cultures and inactivated by a validated method.

The vaccine is reconstituted immediately before use as stated on the label to give a clear liquid that may be coloured owing to the presence of a pH indicator.

PRODUCTION

GENERAL PROVISIONS

The production of the vaccine is based on a virus seed-lot system and, if a cell line is used for virus propagation, a cell-bank system. The production method shall have been shown to yield consistently vaccines that comply with the requirements for immunogenicity, safety and stability. Unless otherwise justified and authorised, the virus in the final vaccine must not have undergone more passages from the master seed lot than were used to prepare the vaccine shown in clinical studies to be satisfactory with respect to safety and efficacy; even with authorised exceptions, the number of passages beyond the level used for clinical studies must not exceed 5.

The production method is validated to demonstrate that the product, if tested, would comply with the test for abnormal toxicity for immunosera and vaccines for human use (*2.6.9*).

SUBSTRATE FOR VIRUS PROPAGATION

The virus is propagated in a human diploid cell line (*5.2.3*), in a continuous cell line approved by the competent authority, or in cultures of chick-embryo cells derived from a flock free from specified pathogens (*5.2.2*).

SEED LOTS

The strain of rabies virus used shall be identified by historical records that include information on the origin of the strain and its subsequent manipulation.

Working seed lots are prepared by not more than 5 passages from the master seed lot.

Only a working seed lot that complies with the following tests may be used for virus propagation.

Identification. Each working seed lot is identified as rabies virus using specific antibodies.

Virus concentration. The virus concentration of each working seed lot is determined by a cell culture method using immunofluorescence, to ensure consistency of production.

Extraneous agents (*2.6.16*). The working seed lot complies with the requirements for virus seed lots. If the virus has been passaged in mouse brain, specific tests for murine viruses are carried out.

VIRUS PROPAGATION AND HARVEST

All processing of the cell bank and subsequent cell cultures is done under aseptic conditions in an area where no other cells are handled. Approved animal (but not human) serum may be used in the media, but the final medium for maintaining cell growth during virus multiplication does not contain animal serum; the media may contain human albumin. Serum and trypsin used in the preparation of cell suspensions and media are shown to be free from extraneous agents. The cell culture media may contain a pH indicator such as phenol red and approved antibiotics at the lowest effective concentration. Not less than 500 ml of the cell cultures employed for vaccine production are set aside as uninfected cell cultures (control cells). The virus suspension is harvested on one or more occasions during incubation. Multiple harvests from the same production cell culture may be pooled and considered as a single harvest.

Only a single harvest that complies with the following requirements may be used in the preparation of the inactivated viral harvest.

Identification. The single harvest contains virus that is identified as rabies virus using specific antibodies.

Virus concentration. Titrate for infective virus in cell cultures; the titre is used to monitor consistency of production.

Control cells. The control cells of the production cell culture from which the single harvest is derived comply with a test for identification and with the requirements for extraneous agents (*2.6.16*).

PURIFICATION AND INACTIVATION

The virus harvest may be concentrated and/or purified by suitable methods; the virus harvest is inactivated by a validated method at a fixed, well-defined stage of the process, which may be before, during or after any concentration or purification. The method shall have been shown to be capable of inactivating rabies virus without destruction of the immunogenic activity. If betapropiolactone is used, the concentration shall at no time exceed 1:3500.

Only an inactivated viral suspension that complies with the following requirements may be used in the preparation of the final bulk vaccine.

Residual infectious virus. Carry out an amplification test for residual infectious rabies virus immediately after inactivation or using a sample frozen immediately after inactivation and stored at – 70 °C. Inoculate a quantity of inactivated viral suspension equivalent to not less than 25 human doses of vaccine into cell cultures of the same type as those used for production of the vaccine. A passage may be made after 7 days. Maintain the cultures for a total of 21 days and then examine the cell cultures for rabies virus using an immunofluorescence test. The inactivated virus harvest complies with the test if no rabies virus is detected.

Residual host-cell DNA. If a continuous cell line is used for virus propagation, the content of residual host-cell DNA, determined using a suitable method as described in *Products of recombinant DNA technology (0784)*, is not greater than 10 ng per single human dose.

FINAL BULK VACCINE

The final bulk vaccine is prepared from one or more inactivated viral suspensions. An approved stabiliser may be added to maintain the activity of the product during and after freeze-drying.

Only a final bulk vaccine that complies with the following requirements may be used in the preparation of the final lot.

Glycoprotein content. Determine the glycoprotein content by a suitable immunochemical method (*2.7.1*), for example, single-radial immunodiffusion, enzyme-linked immunosorbent assay or an antibody-binding test. The content is within the limits approved for the particular product.

Sterility (*2.6.1*). The final bulk vaccine complies with the test for sterility, carried out using 10 ml for each medium.

FINAL LOT

The final bulk vaccine is distributed aseptically into sterile containers and freeze-dried to a moisture content shown to be favourable to the stability of the vaccine. The containers are then closed so as to avoid contamination and the introduction of moisture.

Only a final lot that complies with each of the requirements given below under Identification, Tests and Assay may be released for use. Provided that the test for residual infectious virus has been carried out with satisfactory results on the inactivated viral suspension and the test for bovine serum albumin has been carried out with satisfactory results on the final bulk vaccine, these tests may be omitted on the final lot.

IDENTIFICATION

The vaccine is shown to contain rabies virus antigen by a suitable immunochemical method (*2.7.1*) using specific antibodies, preferably monoclonal; alternatively, the assay serves also to identify the vaccine.

TESTS

Residual infectious virus. Inoculate a quantity equivalent to not less than 25 human doses of vaccine into cell cultures of the same type as those used for production of the vaccine. A passage may be made after 7 days. Maintain the cultures for a total of 21 days and then examine the cell cultures for rabies virus using an immunofluorescence test. The vaccine complies with the test if no rabies virus is detected.

Bovine serum albumin: maximum 50 ng per single human dose, determined by a suitable immunochemical method (*2.7.1*).

Sterility (*2.6.1*). It complies with the test.

Bacterial endotoxins (*2.6.14*): less than 25 IU per single human dose.

Pyrogens (*2.6.8*). It complies with the test. Unless otherwise justified and authorised, inject into each rabbit a single human dose of the vaccine diluted to 10 times its volume.

Water (*2.5.12*): maximum 3.0 per cent.

ASSAY

The potency of rabies vaccine is determined by comparing the dose necessary to protect mice against the effects of a lethal dose of rabies virus, administered intracerebrally, with the quantity of a reference preparation of rabies vaccine necessary to provide the same protection. For this comparison a reference preparation of rabies vaccine, calibrated in International Units, and a suitable preparation of rabies virus for use as the challenge preparation are necessary.

The International Unit is the activity contained in a stated quantity of the International Standard. The equivalence in International Units of the International Standard is stated by the World Health Organisation.

The test described below uses a parallel-line model with at least 3 points for the vaccine to be examined and the reference preparation. Once the analyst has experience with the method for a given vaccine, it is possible to carry out a simplified test using a single dilution of the vaccine to be examined. Such a test enables the analyst to determine that the vaccine has a potency significantly higher than the required minimum, but does not give full information on the validity of each individual potency determination. The use of a single dilution allows a considerable reduction in the number of animals required for the test and must be considered by each laboratory in accordance with the provisions of the European Convention for the Protection of Vertebrate Animals used for Experimental and other Scientific Purposes.

Selection and distribution of the test animals. Use healthy female mice, about 4 weeks old, each weighing 11-15 g, and from the same stock. Distribute the mice into 6 groups of a size suitable to meet the requirements for validity of the test and, for titration of the challenge suspension, 4 groups of 5.

Preparation of the challenge suspension. Inoculate mice intracerebrally with the Challenge Virus Standard (CVS) strain of rabies virus and when the mice show signs of rabies, but before they die, euthanise them, then remove the brains and prepare a homogenate of the brain tissue in a suitable diluent. Separate gross particulate matter by centrifugation and use the supernatant liquid as the challenge suspension. Distribute the suspension in small volumes in ampoules, seal and store at a temperature below − 60 °C. Thaw one ampoule of the suspension and make serial dilutions in a suitable diluent. Allocate each dilution to a group of 5 mice and inject intracerebrally into each mouse 0.03 ml of the dilution allocated to its group. Observe the mice for 14 days. Calculate the LD_{50} of the undiluted suspension using the number in each group that, between the 5th and 14th days, die or develop signs of rabies.

Determination of potency of the vaccine. Prepare 3 fivefold serial dilutions of the vaccine to be examined and 3 fivefold serial dilutions of the reference preparation. Prepare the dilutions such that the most concentrated suspensions may be expected to protect more than 50 per cent of the animals to which they are administered and the least concentrated suspensions may be expected to protect less than 50 per cent of the animals to which they are administered. Allocate the 6 dilutions, 1 to each of the 6 groups of mice, and inject by the intraperitoneal route into each mouse 0.5 ml of the dilution allocated to its group. After 7 days, prepare 3 identical dilutions of the vaccine to be examined and of the reference preparation and repeat the injections. 7 days after the second injection, prepare a suspension of the challenge virus such that, on the basis of the preliminary titration, 0.03 ml contains about 50 LD_{50}. Inject intracerebrally into each vaccinated mouse 0.03 ml of this suspension. Prepare 3 suitable serial dilutions of the challenge suspension. Allocate the challenge suspension and the 3 dilutions, 1 to each of the 4 groups of 5 control mice, and inject intracerebrally into each mouse 0.03 ml of the suspension or dilution allocated to its group. Observe the animals in each group for 14 days and record the number in each group that die or show signs of rabies in the period 5-14 days after challenge.

The test is not valid unless:

- for both the vaccine to be examined and the reference preparation the 50 per cent protective dose lies between the largest and smallest doses given to the mice;
- the titration of the challenge suspension shows that 0.03 ml of the suspension contained not less than 10 LD_{50};
- the statistical analysis shows a significant slope and no significant deviations from linearity or parallelism of the dose-response curves;
- the confidence limits (P = 0.95) are not less than 25 per cent and not more than 400 per cent of the estimated potency.

The vaccine complies with the test if the estimated potency is not less than 2.5 IU per human dose.

Application of alternative end-points. Once a laboratory has established the above assay for routine use, the lethal end-point is replaced by an observation of clinical signs and application of an end-point earlier than death to reduce animal suffering. The following is given as an example.

The progress of rabies infection in mice following intracerebral injection can be represented by 5 stages defined by typical clinical signs:

Stage 1: ruffled fur, hunched back;

Stage 2: slow movements, loss of alertness (circular movements may also occur);

Stage 3: shaky movements, trembling, convulsions;

Stage 4: signs of paresis or paralysis;

Stage 5: moribund state.

Mice are observed at least twice daily from day 4 after challenge. Clinical signs are recorded using a chart such as that shown in Table 0216.-1. Experience has shown that using stage 3 as an end-point yields assay results equivalent

Vaccines

to those found when a lethal end-point is used. This must be verified by each laboratory by scoring a suitable number of assays using both the clinical signs and the lethal end-point.

Table 0216.-1. – *Example of a chart used to record clinical signs in the rabies vaccine potency test*

	Days after challenge							
Clinical signs	**4**	**5**	**6**	**7**	**8**	**9**	**10**	**11**
Ruffled fur Hunched back								
Slow movements Loss of alertness Circular movements								
Shaky movements Trembling Convulsions								
Paresis Paralysis								
Moribund state								

LABELLING

The label states the biological origin of the cells used for the preparation of the vaccine.

04/2008:0162

RUBELLA VACCINE (LIVE)

Vaccinum rubellae vivum

DEFINITION

Rubella vaccine (live) is a freeze-dried preparation of a suitable attenuated strain of rubella virus. The vaccine is reconstituted immediately before use, as stated on the label, to give a clear liquid that may be coloured owing to the presence of a pH indicator.

PRODUCTION

The production of vaccine is based on a virus seed-lot system and a cell-bank system. The production method shall have been shown to yield consistently live rubella vaccines of adequate immunogenicity and safety in man. Unless otherwise justified and authorised, the virus in the final vaccine shall have undergone no more passages from the master seed lot than were used to prepare the vaccine shown in clinical studies to be satisfactory with respect to safety and efficacy.

The potential neurovirulence of the vaccine strain is considered during preclinical development, based on available epidemiological data on neurovirulence and neurotropism, primarily for the wild-type virus. In light of this, a risk analysis is carried out. Where necessary and if available, a test is carried out on the vaccine strain using an animal model that differentiates wild-type and attenuated virus; tests on strains of intermediate attenuation may also be needed.

The production method is validated to demonstrate that the product, if tested, would comply with the test for abnormal toxicity for immunosera and vaccines for human use (*2.6.9*).

SUBSTRATE FOR VIRUS PROPAGATION

The virus is propagated in human diploid cells (*5.2.3*).

SEED LOT

The strain of rubella virus used shall be identified by historical records that include information on the origin of the strain and its subsequent manipulation. Virus seed lots are prepared in large quantities and stored at temperatures below – 20 °C if freeze-dried, or below – 60 °C if not freeze-dried.

Only a seed lot that complies with the following requirements may be used for virus propagation.

Identification. The master and working seed lots are identified as rubella virus by serum neutralisation in cell culture, using specific antibodies.

Virus concentration. The virus concentration of the master and working seed lots is determined to ensure consistency of production.

Extraneous agents (*2.6.16*). The working seed lot complies with the requirements for seed lots.

PROPAGATION AND HARVEST

All processing of the cell bank and subsequent cell cultures is done under aseptic conditions in an area where no other cells are handled during the production. Suitable animal (but not human) serum may be used in the growth medium, but the final medium for maintaining cell growth during virus multiplication does not contain animal serum. Serum and trypsin used in the preparation of cell suspensions and culture media are shown to be free from extraneous agents. The cell culture medium may contain a pH indicator such as phenol red and suitable antibiotics at the lowest effective concentration. It is preferable to have a substrate free from antibiotics during production. Not less than 500 ml of the production cell cultures is set aside as uninfected cell cultures (control cells). The temperature of incubation is controlled during the growth of the virus. The virus suspension is harvested, on one or more occasions, within 28 days of inoculation. Multiple harvests from the same production cell culture may be pooled and considered as a single harvest.

Only a single harvest that complies with the following requirements may be used in the preparation of the final bulk vaccine.

Identification. The single harvest contains virus that is identified as rubella virus by serum neutralisation in cell culture, using specific antibodies.

Virus concentration. The virus concentration in the single harvest is determined as prescribed under Assay to monitor consistency of production and to determine the dilution to be used for the final bulk vaccine.

Extraneous agents (*2.6.16*). The single harvest complies with the tests for extraneous agents.

Control cells. The control cells comply with a test for identification and with the tests for extraneous agents (*2.6.16*).

FINAL BULK VACCINE

Single harvests that comply with the above tests are pooled and clarified to remove cells. A suitable stabiliser may be added and the pooled harvests diluted as appropriate.

Only a final bulk vaccine that complies with the following requirement may be used in the preparation of the final lot.

Bacterial and fungal contamination. The final bulk vaccine complies with the test for sterility (*2.6.1*), carried out using 10 ml for each medium.

FINAL LOT

A minimum virus concentration for release of the product is established such as to ensure, in light of stability data, that the minimum concentration stated on the label will be present at the end of the period of validity.

Only a final lot that complies with the requirements for minimum virus concentration for release, with the following requirement for thermal stability and with each of the requirements given below under Identification and Tests may be released for use. Provided that the test for bovine serum albumin has been carried out with satisfactory results on the final bulk vaccine, it may be omitted on the final lot.

Thermal stability. Maintain at least 3 vials of the final lot of freeze-dried vaccine in the dry state at 37 ± 1 °C for 7 days. Determine the virus concentration as described under Assay in parallel for the heated vaccine and for vaccine stored at the temperature recommended for storage. The virus concentration of the heated vaccine is not more than 1.0 log lower than that of the unheated vaccine.

IDENTIFICATION

When the vaccine reconstituted as stated on the label is mixed with specific rubella antibodies, it is no longer able to infect susceptible cell cultures.

TESTS

Bacterial and fungal contamination. The reconstituted vaccine complies with the test for sterility (*2.6.1*).

Bovine serum albumin. Not more than 50 ng per single human dose, determined by a suitable immunochemical method (*2.7.1*).

Water (*2.5.12*). Not more than 3.0 per cent, determined by the semi-micro determination of water.

ASSAY

Titrate the vaccine for infective virus, using at least 3 separate vials of vaccine and inoculating a suitable number of wells for each dilution step. Titrate 1 vial of an appropriate virus reference preparation in triplicate to validate each assay. The virus concentration of the reference preparation is monitored using a control chart and a titre is established on a historical basis by each laboratory. The relation with the appropriate European Pharmacopoeia Biological Reference Preparation is established and monitored at regular intervals if a manufacturer's reference preparation is used. Calculate the individual virus concentration for each vial of vaccine and for each replicate of the reference preparation as well as the corresponding combined virus concentrations, using the usual statistical methods (for example, *5.3*). The combined estimate of the virus concentration for the 3 vials of vaccine is not less than that stated on the label; the minimum virus concentration stated on the label is not less than 3.0 log $CCID_{50}$ per single human dose.

The assay is not valid if:

- the confidence interval (P = 0.95) of the estimated virus concentration of the reference preparation for the 3 replicates combined is greater than ± 0.3 log $CCID_{50}$;
- the virus concentration of the reference preparation differs by more than 0.5 log $CCID_{50}$ from the established value.

The assay is repeated if the confidence interval (P = 0.95) of the combined virus concentration of the vaccine is greater than ± 0.3 log $CCID_{50}$; data obtained from valid assays only are combined by the usual statistical methods (for example, *5.3*) to calculate the virus concentration of the sample. The confidence interval (P = 0.95) of the combined virus concentration is not greater than ± 0.3 log $CCID_{50}$.

Rubella vaccine (live) BRP is suitable for use as a reference preparation.

Where justified and authorised, different assay designs may be used; this may imply the application of different validity and acceptance criteria. However, the vaccine must comply if tested as described above.

LABELLING

The label states:

- the strain of virus used for the preparation of the vaccine;
- the type and origin of the cells used for the preparation of the vaccine;
- the minimum virus concentration;
- that contact between the vaccine and disinfectants is to be avoided;
- that the vaccine must not be given to a pregnant woman and that a woman must not become pregnant within 2 months after having the vaccine.

04/2008:0164

SMALLPOX VACCINE (LIVE)

Vaccinum variolae vivum

DEFINITION

Smallpox vaccine (live) is a liquid or freeze-dried preparation of live vaccinia virus grown *in ovo* in the membranes of the chick embryo, in cell cultures or in the skin of living animals.

This monograph applies to vaccines produced using strains of confirmed efficacy in man, in particular those used during eradication of smallpox, for example the Lister strain (sometimes referred to as the Lister/Elstree strain) and the New York City Board of Health (NYCBOH) strain. It does not apply to non-replicative strains such as Modified Virus Ankara (MVA).

PRODUCTION

GENERAL PROVISIONS

The production method shall have been shown to yield consistently smallpox vaccines of adequate safety and immunogenicity in man. The strain used shall have been shown to produce typical vaccinia skin lesions in man. Production is based on a seed-lot system.

The production method is validated to demonstrate that the product, if tested, would comply with the test for abnormal toxicity of immunosera and vaccines for human use (*2.6.9*).

The International Reference Preparation for smallpox vaccine is suitable for use as a reference preparation in virus titration.

SUBSTRATE FOR VIRUS PROPAGATION

Animals used for production of skin-derived vaccines. If the vaccine is prepared in animals skins, the animals used are of a species approved by the competent authority, are in good health, are kept in closed or intensively monitored colonies, and have not previously been employed for experimental purposes. Only animals susceptible to infection by dermal inoculations with vaccinia virus may be used for vaccine production.

The animals are kept in well-constructed and adequately ventilated animals rooms with cages spaced as far apart as possible. Adequate precautions are taken to prevent cross-infection between cages. Not more than 1 large animal is housed per stall. Not more than 2 small animals are housed per cage and cage-mates must not be interchanged. The animals must be kept in the country of production of

Vaccines

the vaccine in quarantine groups for a period of not less than 6 weeks before use.

If at any time during the quarantine period the overall death rate of the group reaches 5 per cent, no animals from that entire group may be used for vaccine production.

The groups are kept continuously in isolation, as in quarantine, even after completion of the quarantine period, until the animals are used. After the last animal of a group has been taken, the room that housed the group is thoroughly cleaned and decontaminated before receiving a new group.

Animals that are to be inoculated are anaesthetised and thoroughly examined. If an animal shows any pathological lesion, it is not used in the preparation of a seed lot or a vaccine, nor are any of the remaining animals of the quarantine group concerned unless it is evident that their use will not impair the safety of the product.

The prophylactic and diagnostic measures adopted to exclude the presence of infectious disease are approved by the competent authority. According to the species of animals used and the diseases to which that animal is liable in the country where the vaccine is being produced, these measures may vary. Consideration must also be given to the danger of spreading diseases to other countries to which the vaccine may be shipped. Special attention must always be given to foot-and-mouth disease, brucellosis, Q fever, tuberculosis and dermatomycosis, and it may also be necessary to consider diseases such as contagious pustular dermatitis (orf), anthrax, rinderpest, haemorrhagic septicaemia, Rift valley fever and others.

Vaccines

Embryonated eggs. Embryonated eggs used for production are obtained from a flock free from specified pathogens (SPF) (*5.2.2*).

Human diploid cells, continuous cell lines. Human diploid cells and continuous cell lines comply with the requirements for cell substrates (*5.2.3*).

Primary chick embryo cells. Primary chick embryo cells are derived from an SPF flock (*5.2.2*).

Primary rabbit kidney cells. Only healthy rabbits derived from a closed colony approved by the competent authority are used as a source. The animals, preferably 2-4 weeks old, are tested to ensure freedom from specified pathogens or their antibodies.

Where new animals are introduced into the colony, they are maintained in quarantine for a minimum of 2 months and shown to be free from specified pathogens. Animals to be used to provide kidneys shall not have been previously employed for experimental purposes, especially those involving infectious agents. The colony is monitored for zoonotic viruses and markers of contamination at regular intervals.

At the time the colony is established, all animals are tested to determine freedom from antibodies to possible viral contaminants for which there is evidence of capacity for infecting humans or evidence of capacity to replicate *in vitro* in cells of human origin. A test for retroviruses using a sensitive polymerase chain reaction (PCR)-based reverse transcriptase assay is also included. Nucleic acid amplification tests (*2.6.21*) for retroviruses may also be used.

After the colony is established, it is monitored by testing a representative group of at least 5 per cent of the animals, which are then bled at suitable (for example monthly) intervals. In addition, the colony is screened for pathogenic micro-organisms, including mycobacteria, fungi and mycoplasmas. The screening programme is designed to ensure that all animals are tested within a given period of time.

Any animal that dies is examined to determine the cause of death. If the presence of a causative infectious agent is demonstrated in the colony, the production of smallpox vaccine is discontinued.

At the time of kidney harvest, the animals are examined for the presence of abnormalities and, if any are noted, the animals are not used for vaccine production.

Each set of control cultures derived from a single group of animals used to produce a single virus harvest must remain identifiable as such until all testing, especially for extraneous agents, is completed.

VIRUS SEED LOT

The vaccinia virus isolate used for the master seed lot is identified by historical records that include information on its origin and the tests used in its characterisation.

Virus from the working seed lot must have the same characteristics as the strain that was used to prepare the master seed lot. The number of passages required to produce single harvests from the original isolate is limited and approved by the competent authority. Vaccine is produced from the working seed with a minimum number of intervening passages.

Since cell culture production and clonal selection (for example, plaque purification) may lead to altered characteristics of the virus, the master seed virus must be characterised as fully as possible, for example by comparing the safety profile and biological characteristics of the strain with that of the parental isolate. The characterisation shall include the following:

- antigenic analyses using specific antisera and/or monoclonal antibodies;
- biological studies such as infectivity titre, chorioallantoic membrane (CAM) assay, *in vitro* yield and *in vivo* growth characteristics in a suitable animal model;
- genetic analyses such as restriction mapping/southern blotting, PCR analyses and limited sequencing studies;
- phenotypic and genetic stability upon passage in the substrate;
- neurovirulence testing and immunogenicity studies.

The characterisation tests are also carried out on each working seed lot and on 3 batches of vaccine from the first working seed lot to verify genetic stability of the vaccine strain.

Only a virus seed that complies with the following requirements may be used for virus propagation.

Identification. Each working seed lot is identified as vaccinia virus using specific antibodies and molecular tests. Suitable tests are conducted to exclude the presence of variola virus and other orthopoxviruses.

Virus concentration. Determine by the CAM assay or by a suitable validated *in vitro* assay (plaque assay or $CCID_{50}$ assay). The virus concentration is the basis for the quantity of virus used in the neurovirulence test.

Extraneous agents (*2.6.16*). If the working seed lot is produced in embryonated eggs, human diploid cells, or in a continuous cell line, it complies with the requirements for seed lots for virus vaccines. Seed lots produced in embryonated eggs and seed lots produced in primary cell cultures comply with the additional requirements described below.

Where the tests prescribed cannot be carried out because complete neutralisation of the seed virus is not possible, the seed lot may be diluted to a concentration equivalent to that of the dilution used as inoculum for production of vaccine prior to testing for extraneous viruses. Supplementary specific testing for extraneous viruses using validated nucleic acid amplification techniques (*2.6.21*) or immunochemical methods (*2.7.1*) may be envisaged. Where the indicator cell culture method for mycoplasma detection (*2.6.7*) cannot be carried out, nucleic acid amplification testing is performed instead.

Seed lots to be used for embryonated egg or cell culture production are in addition to be tested for carry-over of potential extraneous agents from the original seed. Given that the complete passage history of the original seed is unlikely to be known and that more than one species may have been used, this additional testing must at least cover important extraneous agents of concern.

The bioburden of master and working seed lots prepared in animal skins is limited by meticulous controls of facilities, personnel, and animals used for production, and by specific tests on the seeds. However, it may be difficult to ensure that seed lots produced in animal skins are totally free from extraneous agents, and consideration must be given to production procedures which remove or reduce them. Such lots must comply with the requirements indicated below. The absence of specific human pathogens is confirmed by additional testing procedures, for example, bacterial and fungal cultures, virus culture, nucleic acid amplification testings (*2.6.21*) for viral agents.

Neurovirulence. The neurovirulence of master and working seed lots is assessed using a suitable animal model, for example in monkeys or mice. The parental isolate is used as comparator. Where the original isolate is not available for this purpose, equivalent materials may be used.

VIRUS PROPAGATION AND HARVEST

VACCINE PRODUCED IN LIVING ANIMALS

Before inoculation the animals are cleaned and thereafter kept in scrupulously clean stalls until the vaccinia material is harvested. For 5 days before inoculation and during incubation the animals remain under veterinary supervision and must remain free from any sign of disease; daily rectal temperatures are recorded. If any abnormal rise in temperature occurs or any clinical sign of disease is observed, the production of vaccine from the group of animals concerned must be suspended until the cause has been resolved.

The inoculation of seed virus is carried out on such parts of the animal that are not liable to be soiled by urine and faeces. The surface used for inoculation is shaved and cleaned so as to achieve conditions that are as close as possible to surgical asepsis. If any antiseptic substance deleterious to the virus is used in the cleaning process it is removed by thorough rinsing with sterile water prior to inoculation. During inoculation the exposed surface of the animal not used for inoculation is covered with a sterile covering. By historical experience the ventral surface of female animals is appropriate for inoculation and inoculation of male animals is more appropriate on the flank.

Before the collection of the vaccinia material, any antibiotic is removed and the inoculated area is cleaned. The uninoculated surfaces are covered with a sterile covering. Before harvesting the animals are euthanised and exsanguinated to avoid heavy mixtures of the vaccinia material with blood. The vaccinia material from each animal is collected separately with aseptic precautions. All animals used in the production of vaccine are examined by autopsy. If evidence of any generalised or systemic disease other than vaccinia is found, the vaccinia material from that animal is discarded. If the disease is considered to be a communicable one, the harvest from the entire group of animals exposed must be discarded unless otherwise justified and authorised.

VACCINE PRODUCED IN EGGS

All processing of embryonated eggs is done under aseptic conditions in an area where no other infectious agents or cells are handled at the same time. After inoculation and incubation at a controlled temperature only living and suitable chick embryos are harvested. The age of the embryos at the time of virus harvest is reckoned from the initial introduction of the egg into the incubator and shall be not more than 12 days. After homogenisation and clarification by centrifugation, the extract of embryonic pulp is tested as described below and kept at – 70 °C or below until further processing. Virus harvests that comply with the prescribed tests may be pooled. No human protein is added to the virus suspension at any stage during production. If stabilisers are added, they shall have been shown to have no antigenic or sensitising properties for man.

Only a single harvest that complies with the following requirements may be used in the preparation of the final bulk vaccine.

Control eggs. Control eggs comply with the tests for extraneous agents (*2.6.16*). A sample of 2 per cent of uninoculated embryonated eggs (not less than 20 and not more than 50) from the batch used for vaccine production shall be incubated under the same conditions as the inoculated eggs. At the time of virus harvest the uninoculated eggs are processed in the same manner as the inoculated eggs.

Sterility (*2.6.1*). It complies with the test for sterility, carried out using 10 ml for each medium.

VACCINE PRODUCED IN CELL CULTURES (PRIMARY CHICK EMBRYO CELLS, PRIMARY RABBIT KIDNEY CELLS, HUMAN DIPLOID CELLS OR CONTINUOUS CELL LINES)

All processing of the cell bank and subsequent cell cultures is done under aseptic conditions in an area where no other cells are handled at the same time during production. Suitable animal (but not human) serum may be used in the culture media, but the final medium for maintaining cell growth during virus multiplication does not contain animal serum. Serum and trypsin used in the preparation of cell suspensions and media are shown to be free from extraneous agents. The cell culture medium may contain a pH indicator such as phenol red and suitable antibiotics at the lowest effective concentration. It is preferable to have a substrate free from antibiotics during production. On the day of inoculation with the virus working seed lot, not less than 5 per cent or 1000 ml, whichever is the least, of the cell cultures employed for vaccine production are set aside as uninfected cell cultures (control cells); special requirements, given below, apply to control cells when the vaccine is produced in primary rabbit kidney cell cultures.

After inoculation of the production cell culture with the working seed lot, inoculated cells are maintained at a suitable fixed temperature, and the virus suspension is harvested after a suitable incubation period.

Only a single harvest that complies with the following requirements may be used in the preparation of the monovalent pooled harvest.

Control cells. The control cells of the production cell culture from which the virus harvest is derived comply with a test for identity and with the requirements for extraneous agents (*2.6.16*) or, where primary rabbit kidney cells cultures are used, with specific tests as mentioned hereafter. The test is invalid if more than 20 per cent of the control cell cultures have been discarded at the end of the observation period.

Extraneous agents (*2.6.16*). The single harvest complies with the tests for extraneous agents. Complete neutralisation of vaccinia virus may be difficult to achieve at high virus concentration. In this case specific tests such as nucleic acid amplification (*2.6.21*) and immunochemical tests (*2.7.1*) can replace non-specific testing in cell culture or eggs. To save biological reagents such as vaccinia neutralising antisera, testing for extraneous agents may be performed on the final bulk instead of on the single harvests.

Vaccine prepared in primary chick embryo cells. A sample of fluids pooled from the control cultures is tested for adenoviruses and for avian retroviruses such as avian leukosis virus. In addition, a volume of each neutralised virus pool equivalent to 100 human doses of vaccine or 10 ml, whichever is the greater, is tested in a group of fertilised eggs by the allantoic route of inoculation, and a similar sample is tested in a separate group of eggs by the yolk-sac route of inoculation. In both cases 0.5 ml of inoculum is used per egg. The virus pool passes the test if, after 3-7 days, there is no evidence of the presence of any extraneous agent.

Vaccine prepared in primary rabbit kidney cell cultures. The following special requirements apply to virus propagation, harvest and testing. On the day of inoculation with virus working seed, a sample of at least 30 ml of the pooled fluid is removed from the cell cultures of the kidneys of each group of animals used to prepare the primary cell suspension. The pooled fluid is inoculated in primary kidney cell cultures in such a way that the dilution of the pooled fluid does not exceed 1 in 4. The cultures are incubated at a temperature of 34-36 °C and observed for a period of at least 4 weeks. During this observation period and after not less than 2 weeks of incubation, at least 1 subculture of fluid is made from each of these cultures and observed also for a period of 2 weeks. The test is invalid if more than 20 per cent of the cultures are discarded. If evidence is found of the presence of an extraneous agent, no cell cultures from the entire group may be used for vaccine production.

Vaccines

- *Control cell cultures.* Cultures prepared on the day of inoculation with the working virus seed lot from 25 per cent of the cell suspensions obtained from the kidneys of each group of animals are maintained as controls. These control cell cultures are incubated under the same conditions as the inoculated cultures for at least 2 weeks. The test is invalid if more than 20 per cent of the control cell cultures are discarded for non-specific reasons.
- *Test for haemadsorbing viruses.* At the time of harvest or not more than 4 days after the day of inoculation of the production cultures with the virus working seed, a sample of 4 per cent of the control cell cultures is tested for haemadsorbing viruses by addition of guinea-pig red blood cells.
- *Test for other extraneous agents.* At the time of harvest or not more than 7 days after the day of inoculation of the production cultures with the virus working seed, a sample of at least 20 ml of the pooled fluid from each group of control cultures is tested for other extraneous agents.
- *Tests of neutralised single harvest in primary rabbit kidney cell cultures.* Each neutralised single harvest is additionally tested in primary kidney cell cultures prepared from a different group of animals to that used for production.

POOLED HARVEST

Only a pooled harvest that complies with the following requirements and is within the limits approved for the product may be used in the preparation of the final lot.

Identity. The vaccinia virus in the pooled harvest is identified by serological methods, which may be supplemented by molecular methods. Molecular tests such as restriction fragment length polymorphism or partial sequencing, especially of terminal DNA sequences which show the greatest variation between vaccinia strains, may be useful.

Virus concentration. The vaccinia virus concentration of the pooled harvest is determined by chick egg CAM assay or in cell cultures. A reference preparation is assayed in the same system in parallel for validation of the pooled harvest titration. The virus concentration serves as the basis for the quantity of virus used in the neurovirulence test in mice.

Consistency of virus characteristics. Vaccinia virus in the pooled harvest or the final bulk is examined by tests that are able to determine that the phenotypic and genetic characteristics of the vaccinia virus have not undergone changes during the multiplication in the production system. The master seed or an equivalent preparation is used as a comparator in these tests and the comparator and the tests to be used are approved by the competent authority.

Neurovirulence. The neurovirulence of the pooled harvest is assessed versus a comparator original seed (or equivalent) by intracerebral inoculation into suckling mice. Other tests may be useful to discriminate between acceptable and unacceptable batches.

Residual DNA. For viruses grown in continuous cells the pooled harvest is tested for residual DNA. The production process demonstrates a level of cellular DNA of less than 10 ng per human dose.

Bacterial and fungal contamination. For vaccines other than those prepared on animal skins, the final bulk complies with the test for sterility (*2.6.1*) using 10 ml for each medium.

Mycoplasma (*2.6.7*). For vaccines other than those prepared on animal skins, the final bulk complies with the test for mycoplasma, carried out using 10 ml.

FINAL BULK VACCINE

A minimum virus concentration for release of the product is established such as to ensure, in the light of stability data, that the minimum concentration stated on the label will be present at the end of the period of validity.

VACCINE PRODUCED IN LIVING ANIMALS

The pooled harvest is centrifuged. If the vaccine is intended for issue in the liquid form, treatment to reduce the presence of extraneous agents may consist of the addition of glycerol or another suitable diluent, with or without an antimicrobial substance, and temporary storage at a suitable temperature. If the vaccine is intended for issue in the dried form, the treatment may consist of the addition of a suitable antimicrobial substance. The following special requirements apply to the bulk vaccine for vaccines produced in living animals.

Only a final bulk vaccine that complies with the following requirements may be used in the preparation of the final lot.

Total bacterial count: for vaccines produced on animal skins only, maximum 50 per millilitre, determined by plate count using a suitable volume of the final bulk vaccine.

Escherichia coli. At least 1 ml samples of a 1:100 dilution of the final bulk vaccine is cultured on plates of a medium suitable for differentiating *E. coli* from other bacteria. The plates are incubated at 35-37 °C for 48 h. If *E. coli* is detected the final bulk is discarded or, subject to approval by the competent authority, processed further.

Haemolytic streptococci, coagulase-positive staphylococci or any other pathogenic micro-organisms which are known to be harmful to man by vaccination. At least 1 ml samples of a 1:100 dilution of the final bulk vaccine are cultured on blood agar. The plates are incubated at 35-37 °C for 48 h. If micro-organisms are detected, the final bulk vaccine is discarded.

Bacillus anthracis. Any colony seen on any of the plates that morphologically resembles *B. anthracis* is examined. If the organisms contained in the colony are non-motile, further tests for the cultural character of *B. anthracis* are carried out, including pathogenicity tests in suitable animals. If *B. anthracis* is found to be present, the final bulk vaccine and any other associated bulks are discarded. Additional validated molecular testing may be performed.

***Clostridium tetani* and other pathogenic spore-forming anaerobes**. A total volume of not less than 10 ml of the final bulk vaccine is distributed in equal amounts into 10 tubes, each containing not less than 10 ml of suitable medium for the growth of anaerobic micro-organisms. The tubes are kept at 65 °C for 1 h in order to reduce the content of non-spore-forming organisms, after which they are anaerobically incubated at 35-37 °C for at least 1 week. From every tube or plate showing growth, subcultures are made on plates of a suitable medium. Tubes and plates are incubated anaerobically at the same temperature. All anaerobic colonies are examined and identified and if *C. tetani* or other pathogenic spore-forming anaerobes are present, the final bulk is discarded.

VACCINE PRODUCED IN EGGS

The pooled harvest is clarified and may be further purified.

VACCINE PRODUCED IN CELL CULTURES (PRIMARY CHICK EMBRYOS FIBROBLASTS, HUMAN DIPLOID CELLS OR CONTINUOUS CELL LINES)

The pooled harvest is clarified to remove cells and may be further purified.

FINAL LOT

Only a final lot that complies with the requirements for minimum virus concentration for release, with the following requirement for thermal stability and with each of the requirements given below under Identification, Tests and Assay may be released for use. Provided that the tests for antimicrobial preservative, protein content, bovine serum albumin and ovalbumin have been carried out with satisfactory results on the final bulk vaccine, they may be omitted on the final lot.

Thermal stability. Representative final containers of the vaccine are incubated at an elevated temperature for a defined period.

For liquid products, the conditions of the test and the requirements are approved by the competent authority.

For freeze-dried vaccines, maintain at least 3 vials of the final lot in the dry state at 37 ± 1 °C for 28 days. The total virus content in the 3 treated vials is determined as described under Assay in parallel alongside 3 vials of vaccine maintained at the recommended storage temperature. An appropriate reference preparation is also included to validate each assay. The vaccine complies with the test if the loss in titre after exposure at elevated temperature is not greater than 1.0 log infectious units per human dose and if the virus concentration after exposure at elevated temperature is not less than the minimum stated on the label.

IDENTIFICATION

The vaccinia virus is identified by an appropriate method.

TESTS

Antimicrobial preservative. Where applicable determine the amount of antimicrobial preservative by a suitable chemical method. The content is not less than the minimum amount shown to be effective and is not greater than 115 per cent of the quantity stated on the label.

Phenol (*2.5.15*): maximum 0.5 per cent, if phenol is used.

Protein content. The protein content of each filling lot, if not done on the final bulk, is determined and is within the limits approved by the competent authority.

Bovine serum albumin: maximum 50 ng per single human dose, determined by a suitable immunochemical method (*2.7.1*), where bovine serum albumin is used during cell culture.

Ovalbumin. For vaccines produced in embryonated eggs, the ovalbumin content is within the limits approved by the competent authority.

Residual moisture. The residual moisture content of each final lot of freeze-dried vaccines is within the limits approved by the competent authority.

Bacterial count. For skin-derived vaccines, examine the vaccine by suitable microscopic and culture methods for micro-organisms pathogenic for man and, in particular, haemolytic streptococci, staphylococci, pathogenic spore-bearing organisms, especially *B. anthracis*, and *E. coli*. The vaccine is free from such contaminants. The total number of non-pathogenic bacteria does not exceed 50 per millilitre.

Sterility (*2.6.1*). Except for skin-derived vaccines, the vaccine complies with the test for sterility.

Bacterial endotoxins (*2.6.14*). The vaccine complies with the specification approved by the competent authority.

ASSAY

Reconstitue the vaccine if necessary and titrate for infectious virus using at least 3 separate vials of vaccine. Titrate 1 vial of an appropriate virus reference preparation in triplicate to validate each assay. The virus concentration of the reference preparation is monitored using a control chart and a titre is established on a historical basis by each laboratory. Calculate the individual virus concentration for each vial of vaccine and for each replicate of the reference preparation as well as the corresponding combined virus concentrations, using the usual statistical methods (for example, *5.3*). The combined virus concentration for the 3 vials of vaccine is not less than 8.0 log pock-forming units per millilitre or the validated equivalent in plaque-forming units or 50 per cent cell culture infective doses, unless a lower titre is justified by clinical studies.

The assay is not valid if:

- the confidence interval (P = 0.95) of the estimated virus concentration of the reference preparation for the 3 replicates combined is greater than ± 0.5 log infectious units;
- the virus concentration of the reference preparation differs by more than 0.5 log infectious units from the established value.

The assay is repeated if the confidence interval (P = 0.95) of the combined virus concentration of the vaccine is greater than ± 0.5 log infectious units; data obtained from valid assays only are combined by the usual statistical methods (for example, *5.3*) to calculate the virus concentration of the sample. The confidence interval (P = 0.95) of the combined virus concentration is not greater than ± 0.5 log infectious units.

Where justified and authorised, different assay designs may be used; this may imply the application of different validity and acceptance criteria. However, the vaccine must comply if tested as described above.

LABELLING

The label states:

- the designation of the vaccinia virus strain;
- the minimum amount of virus per millilitre;
- the substrate used for the preparation of the vaccine;
- the nature and amount of stabiliser, preservative or additive present in the vaccine and/or in the diluent.

04/2008:0648

VARICELLA VACCINE (LIVE)

Vaccinum varicellae vivum

DEFINITION

Varicella vaccine (live) is a freeze-dried preparation of a suitable attenuated strain of *Herpesvirus varicellae*. The vaccine is reconstituted immediately before use, as stated on the label, to give a clear liquid that may be coloured owing to the presence of a pH indicator.

PRODUCTION

The production of vaccine is based on a virus seed-lot system and a cell-bank system. The production method shall have been shown to yield consistently live varicella vaccines of adequate immunogenicity and safety in man. The virus in the final vaccine shall not have been passaged in cell cultures beyond the 38th passage from the original isolated virus.

The potential neurovirulence of the vaccine strain is considered during preclinical development, based on available epidemiological data on neurovirulence and neurotropism, primarily for the wild-type virus. In light of this, a risk analysis is carried out. Where necessary and if available, a test is carried out on the vaccine strain using an animal model that differentiates wild-type and attenuated virus; tests on strains of intermediate attenuation may also be needed.

The production method is validated to demonstrate that the product, if tested, would comply with the test for abnormal toxicity for immunosera and vaccines for human use (*2.6.9*).

SUBSTRATE FOR VIRUS PROPAGATION

The virus is propagated in human diploid cells (*5.2.3*).

VIRUS SEED LOT

The strain of varicella virus used shall be identified as being suitable by historical records that include information on the origin of the strain and its subsequent manipulation. The virus shall at no time have been passaged in continuous cell lines. Seed lots are prepared in the same kind of cells as those used for the production of the final vaccine. Virus seed lots are prepared in large quantities and stored at temperatures below − 20 °C if freeze-dried, or below − 60 °C if not freeze-dried.

Only a virus seed lot that complies with the following requirements may be used for virus propagation.

Identification. The master and working seed lots are identified as varicella virus by serum neutralisation in cell culture, using specific antibodies.

Virus concentration. The virus concentration of the master and working seed lots is determined as prescribed under Assay to monitor consistency of production.

Extraneous agents (*2.6.16*). The working seed lot complies with the requirements for seed lots for live virus vaccines; a sample of 50 ml is taken for the test in cell cultures.

VIRUS PROPAGATION AND HARVEST

All processing of the cell bank and subsequent cell cultures is done under aseptic conditions in an area where no other cells are handled during the production. Suitable animal (but not human) serum may be used in the culture media. Serum and trypsin used in the preparation of cell suspensions and media are shown to be free from extraneous agents. The cell culture medium may contain a pH indicator such as phenol red and suitable antibiotics at the lowest effective concentration. It is preferable to have a substrate free from antibiotics during production. 5 per cent, but not less than 50 ml, of the cell cultures employed for vaccine production is set aside as uninfected cell cultures (control cells). The infected cells constituting a single harvest are washed, released from the support surface and pooled. The cell suspension is disrupted by sonication.

Only a virus harvest that complies with the following requirements may be used in the preparation of the final bulk vaccine.

Identification. The virus harvest contains virus that is identified as varicella virus by serum neutralisation in cell culture, using specific antibodies.

Virus concentration. The concentration of infective virus in virus harvests is determined as prescribed under Assay to monitor consistency of production and to determine the dilution to be used for the final bulk vaccine.

Extraneous agents (*2.6.16*). Use 50 ml for the test in cell cultures.

Control cells. The control cells of the production cell culture from which the single harvest is derived comply with a test for identity and with the requirements for extraneous agents (*2.6.16*).

FINAL BULK VACCINE

Virus harvests that comply with the above tests are pooled and clarified to remove cells. A suitable stabiliser may be added and the pooled harvests diluted as appropriate.

Only a final bulk vaccine that complies with the following requirements may be used in the preparation of the final lot.

Bacterial and fungal contamination. Carry out the test for sterility (*2.6.1*) using 10 ml for each medium.

FINAL LOT

The final bulk vaccine is distributed aseptically into sterile, tamper-proof containers and freeze-dried to a moisture content shown to be favourable to the stability of the vaccine. The containers are then closed so as to prevent contamination and the introduction of moisture.

Only a final lot that is satisfactory with respect to each of the requirements given below under Identification, Tests and Assay may be released for use. Provided that the test for bovine serum albumin has been carried out with satisfactory results on the final bulk vaccine, it may be omitted on the final lot.

IDENTIFICATION

When the vaccine reconstituted as stated on the label is mixed with specific *Herpesvirus varicellae* antibodies, it is no longer able to infect susceptible cell cultures.

TESTS

Bacterial and fungal contamination. The reconstituted vaccine complies with the test for sterility (*2.6.1*).

Bovine serum albumin. Not more than 0.5 µg per human dose, determined by a suitable immunochemical method (*2.7.1*).

Water (*2.5.12*). Not more than 3.0 per cent, determined by the semi-micro determination of water.

ASSAY

Titrate the vaccine for infective virus, using at least 3 separate vials of vaccine. Titrate 1 vial of an appropriate virus reference preparation in triplicate to validate each assay. The virus concentration of the reference preparation is monitored using a control chart and a titre is established on a historical basis by each laboratory. Calculate the individual virus concentration for each vial of vaccine and for each replicate of the reference preparation as well as the corresponding combined virus concentrations, using the usual statistical methods (for example, *5.3*). The combined estimate of the virus concentration for the 3 vials of vaccine is not less than that stated on the label.

The assay is not valid if:

- the confidence interval (P = 0.95) of the estimated virus concentration of the reference preparation for the 3 replicates combined is greater than ± 0.3 log PFU;
- the virus concentration of the reference preparation differs by more than 0.5 log PFU from the established value.

The assay is repeated if the confidence interval (P = 0.95) of the combined virus concentration of the vaccine is greater than ± 0.3 log PFU; data obtained from valid assays only are combined by the usual statistical methods (for example, *5.3*) to calculate the virus concentration of the sample. The confidence interval (P = 0.95) of the combined virus concentration is not greater than ± 0.3 log PFU.

Where justified and authorised, different assay designs may be used; this may imply the application of different validity and acceptance criteria. However, the vaccine must comply if tested as described above.

LABELLING

The label states:

- the strain of virus used for the preparation of the vaccine;
- the type and origin of the cells used for the preparation of the vaccine;
- the minimum virus concentration;
- that contact between the vaccine and disinfectants is to be avoided;
- that the vaccine is not to be administered to pregnant women.

04/2008:0537

YELLOW FEVER VACCINE (LIVE)

Vaccinum febris flavae vivum

DEFINITION

Yellow fever vaccine (live) is a freeze-dried preparation of the 17D strain of yellow fever virus grown in fertilised hen eggs. The vaccine is reconstituted immediately before use, as stated on the label, to give a clear liquid.

PRODUCTION

The production of vaccine is based on a virus seed-lot system. The production method shall have been shown to yield consistently yellow fever vaccine (live) of acceptable immunogenicity and safety for man.

The production method is validated to demonstrate that the product, if tested, would comply with the test for abnormal toxicity for immunosera and vaccines for human use (*2.6.9*) modified as follows for the test in guinea-pigs: inject 10 human doses into each guinea-pig at 2 different injection sites and observe for 21 days.

Reference preparation. In the test for neurotropism, a suitable batch of vaccine known to have satisfactory properties in man is used as the reference preparation.

SUBSTRATE FOR VIRUS PROPAGATION

Virus for the preparation of master and working seed lots and of all vaccine batches is grown in the tissues of chick embryos from a flock free from specified pathogens (SPF) (*5.2.2*).

SEED LOTS

The 17D strain shall be identified by historical records that include information on the origin of the strain and its subsequent manipulation. Virus seed lots are prepared in large quantities and stored at a temperature below – 60 °C. Master and working seed lots shall not contain any human protein or added serum.

Unless otherwise justified and authorised, the virus in the final vaccine shall be between passage levels 204 and 239 from the original isolate of strain 17D. A working seed lot shall be only 1 passage from a master seed lot. A working seed lot shall be used without intervening passage as the inoculum for infecting the tissues used in the production of a vaccine lot, so that no vaccine virus is more than 1 passage from a seed lot that has passed all the safety tests.

Only a virus seed lot that complies with the following requirements may be used for virus propagation.

Identification. The master and working seed lots are identified as containing yellow fever virus by serum neutralisation in cell culture, using specific antibodies.

Extraneous agents (*2.6.16*). Each master seed lot complies with the following tests:

- test in guinea-pigs (as described in chapter *2.6.16* under Virus seed lot);
- bacterial and fungal sterility (as described in chapter *2.6.16* under Virus seed lot and virus harvests);
- mycoplasmas (as described in chapter *2.6.16* under Virus seed lot and virus harvests).

Avian leucosis viruses (*2.6.24*). Each master seed lot complies with the test for avian leucosis viruses.

Extraneous agents (*2.6.16*). Each working seed lot complies with the following tests:

- test in adult mice (intraperitoneal inoculation only) (as described in chapter *2.6.16* under Virus seed lot);
- test in guinea-pigs (as described in chapter *2.6.16* under Virus seed lot);
- bacterial and fungal sterility (as described in chapter *2.6.16* under Virus seed lot and virus harvests);
- mycoplasmas (as described in chapter *2.6.16* under Virus seed lot and virus harvests);
- mycobacteria (as described in chapter *2.6.16* under Virus seed lot and virus harvests);
- test in cell culture for other extraneous agents (as described in chapter *2.6.16* under Virus seed lot and virus harvests);
- avian viruses (as described in chapter *2.6.16* under Virus seed lot and virus harvests).

Avian leucosis viruses (*2.6.24*). Each working seed lot complies with the test for avian leucosis viruses.

Tests in monkeys. Each master and working seed lot complies with the following tests in monkeys for viraemia (viscerotropism), immunogenicity and neurotropism.

The monkeys shall be *Macaca* sp. susceptible to yellow fever virus and shall have been shown to be non-immune to yellow fever at the time of injecting the seed virus. They shall be healthy and shall not have received previously intracerebral or intraspinal inoculation. Furthermore, they shall not have been inoculated by other routes with neurotropic viruses or with antigens related to yellow fever virus. Not fewer than 10 monkeys are used for each test.

Use a test dose of 0.25 ml containing the equivalent of not less than 5000 mouse LD_{50} and not more than 50 000 mouse LD_{50}, determined by a titration for infectious virus and using the established equivalence between virus concentration and mouse LD_{50} (see under Assay). Inject the test dose into 1 frontal lobe of each monkey under anaesthesia and observe the monkeys for not less than 30 days.

Viraemia (Viscerotropism). Viscerotropism is indicated by the amount of virus present in serum. Take blood from each of the test monkeys on the 2nd, 4th and 6th days after inoculation and prepare serum from each sample. Prepare 1:10, 1:100 and 1:1000 dilutions from each serum and inoculate each dilution into a group of at least 6 cell culture vessels used for the determination of the virus concentration. The seed lot complies with the test if none of the sera contains more than the equivalent of 500 mouse LD_{50} in 0.03 ml and at most 1 serum contains more than the equivalent of 100 mouse LD_{50} in 0.03 ml.

Immunogenicity. Take blood from each monkey 30 days after the injection of the test dose and prepare serum from each sample. The seed lot complies with the test if at least 90 per cent of the test monkeys are shown to be immune, as determined by examining their sera in the test for neutralisation of yellow fever virus described below.

It has been shown that a low dilution of serum (for example, 1:10) may contain non-specific inhibitors that influence this test; such serum shall be treated to remove inhibitors. Mix dilutions of at least 1:10, 1:40 and 1:160 of serum from each monkey with an equal volume of 17D vaccine virus at a dilution that will yield an optimum number of plaques with the titration method used. Incubate the serum-virus mixtures in a water-bath at 37 °C for 1 h and then cool in iced water; add 0.2 ml of each serum-virus mixture to each of 4 cell-culture plates and proceed as for the determination of virus concentration. Inoculate similarly 10 plates with the same amount of virus, plus an equal volume of a 1:10 dilution of monkey serum known to contain no neutralising antibodies to yellow fever virus. At the end of the observation period, compare the mean number of plaques in the plates receiving virus plus non-immune serum with the mean number of plaques in the plates receiving virus plus dilutions of each monkey serum. Not more than 10 per cent of the test monkeys have serum that fails to reduce the number of plaques by 50 per cent at the 1:10 dilution.

Neurotropism. Neurotropism is assessed from clinical evidence of encephalitis, from incidence of clinical manifestations and by evaluation of histological lesions, in comparison with 10 monkeys injected with the reference preparation. The seed lot is not acceptable if either the onset and duration of the febrile reaction or the clinical signs of encephalitis and pathological findings are such as to indicate a change in the properties of the virus.

Clinical evaluation

The monkeys are examined daily for 30 days by personnel familiar with clinical signs of encephalitis in primates (if necessary, the monkeys are removed from their cage and examined for signs of motor weakness or spasticity). The seed lot is not acceptable if in the monkeys injected with it the incidence of severe signs of encephalitis, such as paralysis or inability to stand when stimulated, or mortality is greater than for the reference vaccine. These and other signs of encephalitis, such as paresis, incoordination, lethargy, tremors or spasticity are assigned numerical values for the severity of symptoms by a grading method. Each day each monkey in the test is given a score based on the following scale:

- grade 1: rough coat, not eating;
- grade 2: high-pitched voice, inactive, slow moving;
- grade 3: shaky, tremors, unco-ordinated, limb weakness;
- grade 4: inability to stand, limb paralysis or death (a dead monkey receives a daily score of 4 from the day of death until day 30).

A clinical score for a particular monkey is the average of its daily scores; the clinical score for the seed lot is the mean of the individual monkey scores. The seed lot is not acceptable if the mean of the clinical severity scores for the group of monkeys inoculated with it is significantly greater ($P = 0.95$) than the mean for the group of monkeys injected with the reference preparation. In addition, special consideration is given to any animal showing unusually severe signs when deciding on the acceptability of the seed lot.

Histological evaluation

5 levels of the brain are examined including:

- block I: the corpus striatum at the level of the optic chiasma;
- block II: the thalamus at the level of the mamillary bodies;
- block III: the mesencephalon at the level of the superior colliculi;
- block IV: the pons and cerebellum at the level of the superior olives;
- block V: the medulla oblongata and cerebellum at the level of the mid-inferior olivary nuclei.

Cervical and lumbar enlargements of the spinal cord are each divided equally into 6 blocks; 15 µm sections are cut from the tissue blocks embedded in paraffin wax and stained with gallocyanin. Numerical scores are given to each hemisection of the cord and to structures in each hemisection of the brain as listed below. Lesions are scored as follows:

- grade 1 - minimal: 1 to 3 small focal inflammatory infiltrates; degeneration or loss of a few neurons;
- grade 2 - moderate: 4 or more focal inflammatory infiltrates; degeneration or loss of neurons affecting not more than one third of cells;
- grade 3 - severe: moderate focal or diffuse inflammatory infiltration; degeneration or loss of up to two thirds of the neurons;
- grade 4 - overwhelming: variable but often severe inflammatory reaction; degeneration or loss of more than 90 per cent of neurons.

It has been found that inoculation of yellow fever vaccine into the monkey brain causes histological lesions in different anatomical formations of the central nervous system with varying frequency and severity (I. S. Levenbook *et al.*, *Journal of Biological Standardization*, 1987, 15, 305-313). Based on these 2 indicators, the anatomical structures can be divided into target, spared and discriminator areas. Target areas are those which show more severe specific lesions in a majority of monkeys irrespective of the degree of neurovirulence of the seed lot. Spared areas are those which show only minimal specific lesions and in a minority of monkeys. Discriminator areas are those where there is a significant increase in the frequency of more severe specific lesions with seed lots having a higher degree of neurovirulence. Discriminator and target areas for *Macaca cynomolgus* and *Macaca rhesus* monkeys are shown in the table below.

Type of monkey	Discriminator areas	Target areas
Macaca cynomolgus	Globus pallidus	Substantia nigra
	Putamen	
	Anterior/median thalamic nucleus	
	Lateral thalamic nucleus	
Macaca rhesus	Caudate nucleus	Substantia nigra
	Globus pallidus	Cervical enlargement
	Putamen	Lumbar enlargement
	Anterior/median thalamic nucleus	
	Lateral thalamic nucleus	
	Cervical enlargement	
	Lumbar enlargement	

Scores for discriminator and target areas are used for the final evaluation of the seed lot. The individual monkey score is calculated from the sum of individual target area scores in each hemisection divided by the number of areas examined. A separate score is calculated similarly for the discriminator areas.

Mean scores for the test group are calculated in 2 ways: (1) by dividing the sum of the individual monkey discriminator scores by the number of monkeys and (2) by dividing the sum of the individual monkey target and discriminator scores by the number of monkeys. These 2 mean scores are taken into account when deciding on the acceptability of the seed lot. The seed lot is not acceptable if either of the mean lesion scores is significantly greater ($P = 0.95$) than for the reference preparation.

PROPAGATION AND HARVEST

All processing of the fertilised eggs is done under aseptic conditions in an area where no other infectious agents or cells are handled at the same time. At least 2 per cent but not less than 20 and not more than 80 eggs are maintained as uninfected control eggs. After inoculation and incubation at a controlled temperature, only living and typical chick embryos are harvested. At the time of harvest, the control eggs are treated in the same way as the inoculated eggs to obtain a control embryonic pulp. The age of the embryo at the time of virus harvest is reckoned from the initial introduction of the egg into the incubator and shall be not more than 12 days. After homogenisation and clarification by centrifugation, the extract of embryonic pulp is tested as described below and kept at – 70 °C or colder until further processing. Virus harvests that comply with the prescribed tests may be pooled. No human protein is added to the virus suspension at any stage during production. If stabilisers are added, they shall have been shown to have no antigenic or sensitising properties for man.

Only a single harvest that complies with the following requirements may be used in the preparation of the final bulk vaccine.

Identification. The single harvest contains virus that is identified as yellow fever virus by serum neutralisation in cell culture, using specific antibodies.

Bacterial and fungal contamination (*2.6.1*). The harvest complies with the test for sterility, carried out using 10 ml for each medium.

Mycoplasmas (*2.6.7*).The single harvest complies with the test for mycoplasma, carried out using 10 ml.

Mycobacteria (*2.6.2*). A 5 ml single harvest sample is tested for the presence of *Mycobacterium spp.* by culture methods known to be sensitive for the detection of these organisms.

Embryonic pulp of control eggs. The extract of the control eggs shows no evidence of the presence of any extraneous agents in the tests described below.

Test in cell culture for other extraneous agents. Inoculate a 5 ml sample of embryonic pulp of the control eggs into continuous simian kidney and human cell cultures as well as into primary chick-embryo-fibroblast cells. The cells are incubated at 36 ± 1 °C and observed for a period of 14 days. The embryonic pulp of the control eggs passes the test if there is no evidence of the presence of any extraneous agents. The test is not valid unless at least 80 per cent of the cell cultures remain viable.

Avian viruses. Using 0.1 ml per egg, inoculate the embryonic pulp of control eggs: by the allantoic route into a group of 10 fertilised SPF eggs (*5.2.2*) (9 to 11 days old); into the yolk sac of a group of 10 fertilised SPF eggs (*5.2.2*), 5 to 7 days old. Incubate for 7 days. The embryonic pulp lot of the control eggs complies if the allantoic and yolk sac fluids show no signs of haemagglutinating agents and if the embryos and chorio-allantoic membranes examined to detect any macroscopic pathology are typical. The test is not valid unless at least 80 per cent of the inoculated eggs survive during the 7 day observation period.

Virus concentration. In order to calculate the dilution for formulation of the final bulk, each single harvest is titrated as described under Assay.

FINAL BULK VACCINE

Single harvests that comply with the tests prescribed above are pooled and clarified again. A test for protein nitrogen content is carried out. A suitable stabiliser may be added and the pooled harvests diluted as appropriate.

Only a final bulk vaccine that complies with the following requirements may be used in the preparation of the final lot.

Bacterial and fungal contamination (*2.6.1*). The final bulk vaccine complies with the test for sterility, carried out using 10 ml for each medium.

Protein nitrogen content: maximum 0.25 mg per human dose before the addition of any stabiliser.

FINAL LOT

The final bulk vaccine is distributed aseptically into sterile, tamper-proof containers and freeze-dried to a moisture content shown to be favourable to the stability of the vaccine. The containers are then closed so as to prevent contamination and the introduction of moisture.

Only a final lot that is satisfactory with respect to thermal stability and each of the requirements given below under Identification, Tests and Assay may be released for use. Provided that the test for ovalbumin has been performed with satisfactory results on the final bulk vaccine, it may be omitted on the final lot.

Thermal stability. Maintain samples of the final lot of freeze-dried vaccine in the dry state at 37 °C for 14 days. Determine the virus concentration as described under Assay in parallel for the heated vaccine and for unheated vaccine. The difference in the virus concentration between unheated and heated vaccine does not exceed 1.0 log and the virus concentration of the heated vaccine is not less than the number of plaque-forming units (PFU) equivalent to 3.0 log mouse LD_{50} per human dose.

IDENTIFICATION

When the vaccine reconstituted as stated on the label is mixed with specific yellow fever virus antibodies, there is a significant reduction in its ability to infect susceptible cell cultures.

TESTS

Ovalbumin: maximum 5 μg of ovalbumin per human dose, determined by a suitable immunochemical method (*2.7.1*).

Water (*2.5.12*): maximum 3.0 per cent.

Bacterial and fungal contamination (*2.6.1*). The reconstituted vaccine complies with the test for sterility.

Bacterial endotoxins (*2.6.14*): less than 5 IU per single human dose.

ASSAY

Titrate for infective virus in cell cultures using at least 3 separate vials of vaccine. Titrate 1 vial of an appropriate virus reference preparation in triplicate to validate each assay. The virus concentration of the reference preparation is monitored using a control chart and a titre is established on a historical basis by each laboratory. Calculate the individual virus concentration for each vial of vaccine and for each replicate of the reference preparation as well as the corresponding combined virus concentrations using the usual statistical methods (for example, *5.3*). The combined virus concentration for the 3 vials of vaccine is not less than the equivalent in PFU of 3.0 log mouse LD_{50} per human dose. The relationship between mouse LD_{50} and PFU is established by each laboratory and approved by the competent authority.

The assay is not valid if:

- the confidence interval (P = 0.95) of the estimated virus concentration of the reference preparation for the 3 replicates combined is greater than ± 0.3 log PFU;
- the virus concentration of the reference preparation differs by more than 0.5 log PFU from the established value.

The assay is repeated if the confidence interval (P = 0.95) of the combined virus concentration of the vaccine is greater than ± 0.3 log PFU; data obtained from valid assays only are combined by the usual statistical methods (for example, *5.3*) to calculate the virus concentration of the sample. The confidence interval (P = 0.95) of the combined virus concentration is not greater than ± 0.3 log PFU.

Where justified and authorised, different assay designs may be used; this may imply the application of different validity and acceptance criteria. However, the vaccine must comply if tested as described above.

The method shown below, or another suitable technique, may be used to determine the mouse LD_{50}.

Suggested method for determination of the mouse LD_{50}

Mouse LD_{50}. The statistically calculated quantity of virus suspension that is expected to produce fatal specific encephalitis in 50 per cent of mice of a highly susceptible strain, 4 to 6 weeks of age, after intracerebral inoculation.

Appropriate serial dilutions of the reconstituted vaccine are made in diluent for yellow fever virus (a 7.5 g/l solution of *bovine albumin R* in *phosphate buffered saline pH 7.4 R*, or any other diluent that has been shown to be equivalent for maintaining the infectivity of the virus).

Mice of a highly susceptible strain, 4 to 6 weeks of age, are injected intracerebrally under anaesthesia with 0.03 ml of the vaccine dilution. Groups of not fewer than 6 mice are used for each dilution; the series of dilutions is chosen so as to cover the range 0-100 per cent mortality of the mice. Injection of the mice is performed immediately after the dilutions have been made. The mice are observed for 21 days and all deaths are recorded.

Only survivors and deaths caused by typical yellow fever infections are counted in the computations. Mice paralysed on the 21st day of observation are counted as survivors.

LABELLING

The label states:

- the strain of virus used in preparation of the vaccine;
- that the vaccine has been prepared in chick embryos;
- the minimum virus concentration;
- that contact between the vaccine and disinfectants is to be avoided.

VACCINES FOR VETERINARY USE

04/2008:0442

AVIAN INFECTIOUS BRONCHITIS VACCINE (LIVE)

Vaccinum bronchitidis infectivae aviariae vivum

1. DEFINITION

Avian infectious bronchitis vaccine (live) is a preparation of one or more suitable strains of different types of avian infectious bronchitis virus. This monograph applies to vaccines intended for administration to chickens for active immunisation against respiratory disease caused by avian infectious bronchitis virus.

2. PRODUCTION

2-1. *PREPARATION OF THE VACCINE*

The vaccine virus is grown in embryonated hens' eggs or in cell cultures.

2-2. *SUBSTRATE FOR VIRUS PROPAGATION*

2-2-1. **Embryonated hens' eggs**. If the vaccine virus is grown in embryonated hens' eggs, they are obtained from flocks free from specified pathogens (SPF) (*5.2.2*).

2-2-2. **Cell cultures**. If the vaccine virus is grown in cell cultures, they comply with the requirements for cell cultures for production of veterinary vaccines (*5.2.4*).

2-3. *SEED LOTS*

2-3-1. **Extraneous agents**. The master seed lot complies with the tests for extraneous agents in seed lots (*2.6.24*). In these tests on the master seed lot, the organisms used are not more that 5 passages from the master seed lot at the start of the test.

2-4. *CHOICE OF VACCINE VIRUS*

The vaccine virus shall be shown to be satisfactory with respect to safety (*5.2.6*) and efficacy (*5.2.7*) for the chickens for which it is intended.
The following tests for safety (section 2-4-1), increase in virulence (section 2-4-2) and immunogenicity (section 2-4-3) may be used during the demonstration of safety and efficacy.

2-4-1. **Safety**

2-4-1-1. *Safety for the respiratory tract and kidneys.* Carry out the test in chickens not older than the minimum age to be recommended for vaccination. Use vaccine virus at the least attenuated passage level that will be present between the master seed lot and a batch of the vaccine.

Use not fewer than 15 chickens of the same origin and from an SPF flock (*5.2.2*). Administer to each chicken by the oculonasal route a quantity of the vaccine virus equivalent to not less than 10 times the maximum virus titre likely to be contained in 1 dose of the vaccine. On each of days 5, 7 and 10 after administration of the virus, euthanise not fewer than 5 of the chickens and take samples of trachea and kidney. Fix kidney samples for histological examination. Remove the tracheas and prepare 3 transverse sections from the upper part, 4 from the middle part and 3 from the lower part of the trachea of each chicken; examine all tracheal explants as soon as possible and at the latest 2 h after sampling by low-magnification microscopy for ciliary activity. Score for ciliostasis on a scale from 0 (100 per cent ciliary activity) to 4 (no activity, complete ciliostasis); calculate the mean ciliostasis score (the maximum for each trachea being 40) for the 5 chickens euthanised on each of days 5, 7 and 10. The test is not valid if more than 10 per cent of the chickens die from causes not attributable to the vaccine virus. The vaccine virus complies with the test if:

- no chicken shows notable clinical signs of avian infectious bronchitis or dies from causes attributable to the vaccine virus;
- any inflammatory lesions seen during the kidney histological examination are, at most, moderate.

A risk/benefit analysis is carried out, taking into account the average ciliostasis scores obtained and the benefits expected from the use of the vaccine.

2-4-1-2. *Safety for the reproductive tract.* If the recommendations for use state or imply that the vaccine may be used in females less than 3 weeks old that are subsequently kept to sexual maturity, it shall be demonstrated that there is no damage to the development of the reproductive tract when the vaccine is given to chickens of the minimum age to be recommended for vaccination.

The following test may be carried out: use not fewer than 40 female chickens from an SPF flock (*5.2.2*) that are not older than the minimum age recommended for vaccination; use the vaccine virus at the least attenuated passage level that will be present in a batch of vaccine; administer to each chicken by a recommended route a quantity of virus equivalent to not less than the maximum titre likely to be present in 1 dose of vaccine; at least 10 weeks after administration of the vaccine virus, euthanise the chickens and carry out a macroscopic examination of the oviducts. The vaccine virus complies with the test if abnormalities are present in not more than 5 per cent of the oviducts.

2-4-2. **Increase in virulence**. The test for increase in virulence consists of the administration of the vaccine virus, at the least attenuated virus passage level that will be present between the master seed lot and a batch of the vaccine, to a group of 5 two-week-old chickens from an SPF flock (*5.2.2*); sequential passages, 5 times where possible, to further similar groups and testing of the final recovered virus for increase in virulence. If the properties of the vaccine virus allow sequential passage to 5 groups via natural spreading, this method may be used, otherwise, passage as described below is carried out and the maximally passaged virus that has been recovered is tested for increase in virulence. Care must be taken to avoid contamination by virus from previous passages.

Administer to each chicken by eye-drop a quantity of the vaccine virus that will allow recovery of virus for the passages described below. 2-4 days after administration of the vaccine virus, prepare a suspension from the mucosa of the trachea of each chicken and pool these samples. Administer 0.05 ml of the pooled samples by eye-drop to each of 5 other two-week-old chickens from an SPF flock (*5.2.2*). Carry out this passage operation not fewer than 5 times; verify the presence of the virus at each passage. If the virus is not found at a passage level, carry out a second series of passages. Carry out the test for safety for the respiratory tract and kidney (section 2-4-1-1) and, where applicable, the test for safety for the reproductive tract (section 2-4-1-2) using the unpassaged vaccine virus and the maximally passaged virus that has been recovered. Administer the virus by the route to be recommended for vaccination that is likely to be the least safe.

The vaccine virus complies with the test if no indication of an increase in virulence of the maximally passaged virus compared with the unpassaged virus is observed. If virus is not recovered at any passage level in the 1st and 2nd series of passages, the vaccine virus also complies with the test.

2-4-3. **Immunogenicity**. Immunogenicity is demonstrated for each strain of virus to be included in the vaccine. A test is carried out for each route and method of administration to be recommended using in each case chickens from an SPF flock (*5.2.2*) that are not older than the minimum age to be recommended for vaccination. The quantity of the vaccine virus administered to each chicken is not greater than the minimum virus titre to be stated on the label and the virus is at the most attenuated passage level that will be present in a batch of the vaccine.

Either or both of the tests below may be used during the demonstration of immunogenicity.

2-4-3-1. *Ciliary activity of tracheal explants*. Use not fewer than 25 chickens of the same origin and from an SPF flock (*5.2.2*). Vaccinate by a recommended route not fewer than 20 chickens. Maintain not fewer than 5 chickens as controls. Challenge each chicken after 21 days by eye-drop with a sufficient quantity of virulent avian infectious bronchitis virus of the same type as the vaccine virus to be tested. Euthanise the chickens 4-7 days after challenge and prepare 3 transverse sections from the upper part, 4 from the middle part, and 3 from the lower part of the trachea of each chicken. Examine all tracheal explants as soon as possible and at the latest 2 h after sampling by low-magnification microscopy for ciliary activity. For a given tracheal section, ciliary activity is considered as normal when at least 50 per cent of the internal ring shows vigorous ciliary movement. A chicken is considered not affected if not fewer than 9 out of 10 rings show normal ciliary activity.

Vaccines

The test is not valid if:

- fewer than 80 per cent of the control chickens show cessation or extreme loss of vigour of ciliary activity;
- and/or during the period between the vaccination and challenge, more than 10 per cent of vaccinated or control chickens show abnormal clinical signs or die from causes not attributable to the vaccine.

The vaccine virus complies with the test if not fewer than 80 per cent of the vaccinated chickens show normal ciliary activity.

2-4-3-2. *Virus recovery from tracheal swabs*. Use not fewer than 30 chickens of the same origin and from an SPF flock (*5.2.2*). Vaccinate by a recommended route not fewer than 20 chickens. Maintain not fewer than 10 chickens as controls. Challenge each chicken after 21 days by eye-drop with a sufficient quantity of virulent avian infectious bronchitis virus of the same type as the vaccine virus to be tested. Euthanise the chickens 4-7 days after challenge and prepare a suspension from swabs of the tracheal mucosa of each chicken. Inoculate 0.2 ml of the suspension into the allantoic cavity of each of 5 embryonated hens' eggs, 9-11 days old, from an SPF flock (*5.2.2*). Incubate the eggs for 6-8 days after inoculation. Eggs that after 1 day of incubation do not contain a live embryo are eliminated and considered as non-specific deaths. Record the other eggs containing a dead embryo and after 6-8 days' incubation examine each egg containing a live embryo for lesions characteristic of avian infectious bronchitis. Make successively 3 such passages. If 1 embryo of a series of eggs dies or shows characteristic lesions, the inoculum is considered to be a carrier of avian infectious bronchitis virus. The examination of a series of eggs is considered to be definitely negative if no inoculum concerned is a carrier. The test is not valid if:

- the challenge virus is re-isolated from fewer than 80 per cent of the control chickens;
- and/or during the period between vaccination and challenge, more than 10 per cent of the vaccinated or control chickens show abnormal clinical signs or die from causes not attributable to the vaccine;
- and/or more than 1 egg in any group is eliminated because of non-specific embryo death.

The vaccine virus complies with the test if the challenge virus is re-isolated from not more than 20 per cent of the vaccinated chickens.

3. BATCH TESTS

3-1. **Identification**

3-1-1. *Vaccines containing one type of virus*. The vaccine, diluted if necessary and mixed with avian infectious bronchitis virus antiserum specific for the virus type, no longer infects embryonated hens' eggs from an SPF flock (*5.2.2*) or susceptible cell cultures (*5.2.4*) into which it is inoculated.

3-1-2. *Vaccines containing more than one type of virus*. The vaccine, diluted if necessary and mixed with type-specific antisera against each strain present in the vaccine except that to be identified, infects embryonated hens' eggs from an SPF flock (*5.2.2*) or susceptible cell cultures (*5.2.4*) into which it is inoculated, whereas after further admixture with type-specific antiserum against the strain to be identified it no longer produces such infection.

3-2. **Bacteria and fungi**

Vaccines intended for administration by injection comply with the test for sterility prescribed in the monograph *Vaccines for veterinary use (0062)*.

Vaccines not intended for administration by injection comply either with the test for sterility prescribed in the monograph *Vaccines for veterinary use (0062)* or with the following test: carry out a quantitative test for bacterial and fungal contamination; carry out identification tests for micro-organisms detected in the vaccine; the vaccine does not contain pathogenic micro-organisms and contains not more than 1 non-pathogenic micro-organism per dose.

Any liquid supplied with the vaccine complies with the test for sterility prescribed in the monograph *Vaccines for veterinary use (0062)*.

3-3. **Mycoplasmas**. The vaccine complies with the test for mycoplasmas (*2.6.7*).

3-4. **Extraneous agents**. The vaccine complies with the tests for extraneous agents in batches of finished product (*2.6.25*).

3-5. **Safety**. Use not fewer than 10 chickens from an SPF flock (*5.2.2*) and of the minimum age recommended for vaccination. Administer by a recommended route to each chicken 10 doses of the vaccine. Observe the chickens at least daily for 21 days. The test is invalid if more than 20 per cent of the chickens show abnormal clinical signs or die from causes not attributable to the vaccine.

The vaccine complies with the test if no chicken shows notable clinical signs of disease or dies from causes attributable to the vaccine.

3-6. **Virus titre**. Titrate the vaccine virus by inoculation into embryonated hens' eggs from an SPF flock (*5.2.2*) or into suitable cell cultures (*5.2.4*). If the vaccine contains more than 1 strain of virus, titrate each strain after having neutralised the others with type-specific avian infectious bronchitis antisera. The vaccine complies with the test if 1 dose contains for each vaccine virus not less than the minimum titre stated on the label.

3-7. **Potency**. The vaccine complies with the requirements of 1 of the tests prescribed under Immunogenicity (section 2-4-3) when administered according to the recommended schedule by a recommended route and method. It is not necessary to carry out the potency test for each batch of the vaccine if it has been carried out on a representative batch using a vaccinating dose containing not more than the minimum virus titre stated on the label.

01/2008:1361
corrected 6.1

PORCINE PROGRESSIVE ATROPHIC RHINITIS VACCINE (INACTIVATED)

Vaccinum rhinitidis atrophicantis ingravescentis suillae inactivatum

1. DEFINITION

Porcine progressive atrophic rhinitis vaccine (inactivated) is a preparation containing either the dermonecrotic exotoxin of *Pasteurella multocida*, treated to render it harmless while maintaining adequate immunogenic properties, or a genetically modified form of the exotoxin which has adequate immunogenic properties and which is free from toxic properties; the vaccine may also contain cells and/or antigenic components of one or more suitable strains of *P. multocida* and/or *Bordetella bronchiseptica*. This monograph applies to vaccines intended for the active immunisation of sows and gilts for passive protection of their progeny against porcine progressive atrophic rhinitis.

2. PRODUCTION

2-1. *PREPARATION OF THE VACCINE*

The bacterial strains used for production are cultured separately in suitable media. The toxins and/or cells are treated to render them safe. The vaccine may be adjuvanted.

2-2. *DETOXIFICATION*

A test for detoxification of the dermonecrotic exotoxin of *P. multocida* is carried out immediately after detoxification. The concentration of detoxified exotoxin used in the test is not less than that in the vaccine. The suspension complies with the test if no toxic dermonecrotic exotoxin is detected. The test for detoxification is not required where the vaccine is prepared using a toxin-like protein free from toxic properties, produced by expression of a modified form of the corresponding gene.

2-3. *ANTIGEN CONTENT*

The content of the dermonecrotic exotoxin of *P. multocida* in the detoxified suspension or the toxin-like protein in the harvest is determined by a suitable immunochemical method (*2.7.1*), such as an enzyme-linked immunosorbent assay and the value found is used in the formulation of the vaccine. The content of other antigens stated on the label is also determined (*2.7.1*).

2-4. *CHOICE OF VACCINE COMPOSITION*

The strains used for the preparation of the vaccine are shown to be satisfactory with respect to the production of the dermonecrotic exotoxin and the other antigens claimed to be protective. The vaccine is shown to be satisfactory with respect to safety (*5.2.6*) and efficacy (*5.2.7*) for the sows and gilts for which it is intended.

The following tests for production of antigens (section 2-4-1), safety (section 2-4-2) and immunogenicity (section 2-4-3) may be used during the demonstration of safety and efficacy.

2-4-1. **Production of antigens**. The production of antigens claimed to be protective is verified by a suitable bioassay or immunochemical method (*2.7.1*), carried out on the antigens obtained from each of the vaccine strains under the conditions to be used for the production of the vaccine.

2-4-2. **Safety**

2-4-2-1. *Laboratory test.* Carry out the test for each route and method of administration to be recommended for vaccination. Use a batch containing not less than the maximum potency that may be expected in a batch of vaccine.

For each test, use not fewer than 10 pregnant sows or gilts that do not have antibodies against the components of the vaccine, from a herd or herds where there are no signs of atrophic rhinitis and that have not been vaccinated against atrophic rhinitis. Administer to each pig a double dose of the vaccine at the stage of pregnancy to be recommended, then one dose after the interval to be recommended. Observe the pigs at least daily until farrowing. Record body temperature the day before vaccination, at vaccination, 2 h, 4 h and 6 h later and then daily for 4 days; note the maximum temperature increase for each pig.

The vaccine complies with the test if no pig shows abnormal local or systemic reactions or dies from causes attributable to the vaccine, if the average temperature increase for all pigs does not exceed 1.5 °C and no pig shows a rise greater than 2 °C and if no adverse effects on the pregnancy and offspring are noted.

2-4-2-2. *Field studies.* The pigs used for field trials are also used to evaluate safety. Use not fewer than 3 groups each of not fewer than 20 pigs with corresponding groups of not fewer than 10 controls. Examine the injection site for local reactions after vaccination. Record body temperature the day before vaccination, at vaccination, at the time interval after which a rise in temperature, if any, was seen in test 2-4-2-1, and daily during the 2 days following vaccination; note the maximum temperature increase for each pig.

The vaccine complies with the test if no pig shows abnormal local or systemic reactions or dies from causes attributable to the vaccine and if the average temperature increase for all pigs does not exceed 1.5 °C and no pig shows a rise greater than 2 °C.

2-4-3. **Immunogenicity**. Each test is carried out for each route and method of administration to be recommended, using in each case pigs that do not have antibodies against the components of the vaccine, that are from a herd or herds where there are no signs of atrophic rhinitis and that have not been vaccinated against atrophic rhinitis. The vaccine administered to each pig is of minimum potency.

2-4-3-1. *Vaccines containing dermonecrotic exotoxin of* P. multocida *(with or without cells of* P. multocida*).* Use not fewer than 12 breeder pigs. Vaccinate not fewer than 6 randomly chosen pigs at the stage of pregnancy or non-pregnancy and according to the schedule to be recommended. Maintain not fewer than 6 pigs as controls. From birth allow all the piglets from the vaccinated and unvaccinated breeder pigs to feed from their own dam. Constitute from the progeny 2 challenge groups each of not fewer than 30 piglets chosen randomly, taking not fewer than 3 piglets from each litter. On the 2 consecutive days preceding challenge, the mucosa of the nasal cavity of the piglets may be treated by instillation of 0.5 ml of a solution of acetic acid (10 g/l $C_2H_4O_2$) in isotonic buffered saline pH 7.2.

Challenge each piglet at 10 days of age by the intranasal route with a sufficient quantity of a toxigenic strain of *P. multocida*. At the age of 42 days, euthanise the piglets of the 2 groups and dissect the nose of each of them transversally at premolar-1. Examine the ventral and dorsal turbinates and the nasal septum for evidence of atrophy or distortion and grade the observations on the following scales:

Turbinates

0 no atrophy

1 slight atrophy

2 moderate atrophy

3 severe atrophy

4 very severe atrophy with almost complete disappearance of the turbinate

The maximum score is 4 for each turbinate and 16 for the sum of the 2 dorsal and 2 ventral turbinates.

Nasal septum

0 no deviation

1 very slight deviation

2 deviation of the septum

The maximum total score for the turbinates and the nasal septum is 18.

The test is invalid if fewer than 80 per cent of the progeny of each litter of the unvaccinated breeder pigs have a total score of at least 10. The vaccine complies with the test if a significant reduction in the total score has been demonstrated in the group from the vaccinated breeder pigs compared to that from the unvaccinated breeder pigs.

2-4-3-2. *Vaccines containing* P. multocida *dermonecrotic exotoxin (with or without cells of* P. multocida*) and cells and/or antigenic components of* B. bronchiseptica. Use not fewer than 24 breeder pigs. Vaccinate not fewer than 12 randomly chosen pigs at the stage of pregnancy or non-pregnancy and according to the schedule to be recommended. Maintain not fewer than 12 pigs as controls. From birth allow all the piglets from the vaccinated and unvaccinated breeder pigs to feed from their own dam. Using groups of not fewer than 6 pigs, constitute from their progeny 2 challenge groups from vaccinated pigs and 2 groups from control pigs each group consisting of not fewer than 30 piglets chosen randomly, taking not fewer than 3 piglets from each litter. On the 2 consecutive days preceding challenge, the mucosa of the nasal cavity of the piglets may be treated by instillation of 0.5 ml of a solution of acetic acid (10 g/l $C_2H_4O_2$) in isotonic buffered saline pH 7.2. For a group of piglets from not fewer than 6 vaccinated pigs and a group from not fewer than 6 controls, challenge each piglet by the intranasal route at 10 days of age with a sufficient quantity of a toxigenic strain of *P. multocida*. For the other group of piglets from not fewer than 6 vaccinated pigs and the other group from not fewer than 6 controls, challenge each piglet at 7 days of age by the intranasal route with a sufficient quantity of *B. bronchiseptica*. In addition, challenge each piglet at 10 days of age by the intranasal route with a sufficient quantity of a toxigenic strain of *P. multocida*. At the age of 42 days, euthanise the piglets of the 4 groups and dissect the nose of each of them transversally at premolar-1. Examine the ventral and dorsal turbinates and the nasal septum for evidence of atrophy or distortion and grade the observations on the scale described above.

The test is invalid if fewer than 80 per cent of the progeny of each litter of the unvaccinated breeder pigs have a total score of at least 10. The vaccine complies with the test if a significant reduction in the total score has been demonstrated in the groups from the vaccinated breeder pigs compared to the corresponding group from the unvaccinated breeder pigs.

2-5. *MANUFACTURER'S TESTS*

2-5-1. **Batch potency test**. It is not necessary to carry out the Potency test (section 3-4) for each batch of vaccine if it has been carried out using a batch of vaccine with a minimum potency. Where the test is not carried out, an alternative validated method is used, the criteria for acceptance being set with reference to a batch of vaccine that has given satisfactory results in the test described under Potency. The following test may be used.

Use not fewer than 7 pigs not less than 3 weeks old and that do not have antibodies against the components of the vaccine. Vaccinate not fewer than 5 pigs by a recommended route and according to the recommended schedule. Maintain not fewer than 2 pigs of the same origin as controls under the same conditions. Alternatively, if the nature of the antigens allows reproducible results to be obtained, a test in laboratory animals that do not have antibodies against the components of the vaccine may be carried out. To obtain a valid assay, it may be necessary to carry out a test using several groups of animals, each receiving a different quantity of vaccine. For each quantity of vaccine, carry out the test as follows: vaccinate not fewer than 5 animals with a suitable quantity of vaccine. Maintain not fewer than 2 animals of the same species and origin as controls. Where the recommended schedule requires a booster injection to be given, a booster vaccination may also be given in this test provided it has been demonstrated that this will still provide a suitably sensitive test system. At a given interval within the range of 14-21 days after the last administration, collect blood from each animal and prepare serum samples. Use a validated test such as an enzyme-linked immunosorbent assay to measure the antibody response to each of the antigens stated on the label.

The test is invalid if there is a significant antibody titre in the controls. The vaccine complies with the test if the antibody responses of the vaccinated animals are not significantly less than those obtained with a batch of vaccine that has given satisfactory results in the test or tests (as applicable) described under Potency.

Where animals that do not have antibodies against the antigens stated on the label are not available, seropositive animals may be used in the above test. During the development of a test with seropositive animals, particular care will be required during the validation of the test system to establish that the test is suitably sensitive and to specify acceptable pass, fail and retest criteria. It will be necessary to take into account the range of prevaccination antibody titres and to establish the acceptable minimum antibody titre rise after vaccination in relation to these.

2-5-2. **Bacterial endotoxins**. A test for bacterial endotoxins (*2.6.14*) is carried out on the batch or, where the nature of the adjuvant prevents performance of a satisfactory test, on the bulk antigen or the mixture of bulk antigens immediately before addition of the adjuvant. The maximum acceptable amount of bacterial endotoxins is that found for a batch of vaccine shown satisfactory in safety test 2-4-2-1 given under Choice of vaccine composition or in the safety test described under Tests, carried out using 10 pigs. Where the latter test is used, note the maximum temperature increase for each pig; the vaccine complies with the test if the average temperature increase for all pigs does not exceed 1.5 °C. The method chosen for determining the amount of bacterial endotoxin present in the vaccine batch used in the safety test for determining the maximum acceptable level of endotoxin is used subsequently for testing of each batch.

3. BATCH TESTS

3-1. **Identification**. In animals that do not have specific antibodies against the antigens stated on the label, the vaccine stimulates the production of such antibodies.

3-2. **Bacteria and fungi**. The vaccine and, where applicable, the liquid supplied with it comply with the test for sterility prescribed in the monograph *Vaccines for veterinary use (0062)*.

3-3. **Safety**. Use not fewer than 2 pigs that do not have antibodies against *P. multocida* and that preferably do not have antibodies against *B. bronchiseptica*. Administer to each pig by a recommended route a double dose of the vaccine. Observe the pigs at least daily for 14 days. Record body temperature the day before vaccination, at vaccination, 2 h, 4 h and 6 h later and then daily for 2 days.

The vaccine complies with the test if no pig shows notable signs of disease or dies from causes attributable to the vaccine; a transient temperature increase not exceeding 2 °C may occur.

3-4. **Potency**. The vaccine complies with the requirements of the tests mentioned under Immunogenicity (section 2-4-3) when administered by a recommended route and method.

04/2008:0451

RABIES VACCINE (INACTIVATED) FOR VETERINARY USE

Vaccinum rabiei inactivatum ad usum veterinarium

1. DEFINITION

Rabies vaccine (inactivated) for veterinary use is a preparation of a suitable strain of fixed rabies virus, inactivated while maintaining adequate immunogenic properties. This monograph applies to vaccines intended for the active immunisation of animals against rabies.

2. PRODUCTION

2-1. *PREPARATION OF THE VACCINE*

The vaccine is prepared from virus grown either in suitable cell lines or in primary cell cultures from healthy animals (*5.2.4*). The virus suspension is harvested on one or more occasions within 28 days of inoculation. Multiple harvests from a single production cell culture may be pooled and considered as a single harvest.

The virus harvest is inactivated. The vaccine may be adjuvanted.

2-2. *SUBSTRATE FOR VIRUS PROPAGATION*

2-2-1. **Cell cultures**. The cell cultures comply with the requirements for cell cultures for production of veterinary vaccines (*5.2.4*).

2-3. *CHOICE OF VACCINE COMPOSITION*

The vaccine virus is shown to be satisfactory with respect to safety (*5.2.6*) and efficacy (*5.2.7*) for the species for which it is intended.

The following test for Immunogenicity (section 2-3-1) may be used during the demonstration of efficacy in cats and dogs.

The suitability of the vaccine with respect to Immunogenicity (section 2-3-1) for carnivores (cats and dogs) is demonstrated by direct challenge. For other species, if a challenge test has been carried out for the vaccine in cats or dogs, an indirect test is carried out by determining the antibody level following vaccination of not fewer than 20 animals according to the schedule to be recommended; the vaccine is satisfactory if, after the period to be claimed for protection, the mean rabies virus antibody level in the serum of the animals is not less than 0.5 IU/ml and if not more than 10 per cent of the animals have an antibody level less than 0.1 IU/ml.

2-3-1. **Immunogenicity**. Each test is carried out for each route and method of administration to be recommended, using in each case animals of the minimum age to be recommended for vaccination. The vaccine administered to each animal is of minimum potency.

Use for the test not fewer than 35 animals. Take a blood sample from each animal and test individually for antibodies against rabies virus to determine susceptibility. Vaccinate not fewer than 25 animals, according to the schedule to be recommended. Maintain not fewer than 10 animals as controls. Observe all the animals for a period equal to the claimed duration of immunity. No animal shows signs of rabies. On the last day of the claimed period for duration of immunity or later, challenge each animal by intramuscular injection with a sufficient quantity of virulent rabies virus of a strain approved by the competent authority. Observe the animals at least daily for 90 days after challenge. Animals that die from causes not attributable to rabies are eliminated. The test is invalid if the number of such deaths reduces the number of vaccinated animals in the test to fewer than 25 and the test is invalid unless at least 8 control animals (or a statistically equivalent number if more than 10 control animals are challenged) show signs of rabies and the presence of rabies virus in their brain is demonstrated by the fluorescent-antibody test or some other suitable method. The vaccine complies with the test if not more than 2 of the 25 vaccinated animals (or a statistically equivalent number if more than 25 vaccinated animals are challenged) show signs of rabies.

2-4. MANUFACTURER'S TESTS

2-4-1. **Residual live virus**. The test for residual live virus is carried out by inoculation of the inactivated virus into the same type of cell culture as that used in the production of the vaccine or a cell culture shown to be at least as sensitive. The quantity of inactivated virus harvest used is equivalent to not less than 25 doses of the vaccine. After incubation for 4 days, a subculture is made using trypsinised cells; after incubation for a further 4 days, the cultures are examined for residual live rabies virus by an immunofluorescence test. The inactivated virus harvest complies with the test if no live virus is detected.

2-4-2. **Antigen content of the harvest**. The content of rabies virus glycoprotein is determined by a suitable immunochemical method (*2.7.1*). The content is within the limits approved for the particular preparation.

2-4-3. **Batch potency test**. It is not necessary to carry out the potency test (section 3-5) for each batch of vaccine if it has been carried out using a batch of vaccine with a minimum potency. Where the test is not carried out, an alternative validated method is used, the criteria for acceptance being set with reference to a batch of vaccine that has given satisfactory results in the test described under Potency. The following test may be used.

Use 5 mice each weighing 18-20 g. Vaccinate each mouse by a subcutaneous or intramuscular route using 1/5 of the recommended dose volume. Take blood samples 14 days after the injection and test the sera individually for rabies antibody using the rapid fluorescent focus inhibition test described for *Human rabies immunoglobulin (0723)*.

Vaccines

The vaccine complies with the test if the antibody titre is not less than that obtained with a batch of vaccine that gave satisfactory results in the test described under Potency.

2-4-4. **Antigen content of the batch**. The quantity of rabies virus glycoprotein per dose, determined by a suitable immunochemical method (*2.7.1*), is not significantly lower than that of a batch of vaccine that gave satisfactory results in the test described under Potency.

3. BATCH TESTS

3-1. **Identification**. Administered to animals that do not have antibodies against rabies virus, the vaccine stimulates the production of such antibodies.

3-2. **Bacteria and fungi**. The vaccine and, where applicable, the liquid supplied with it, comply with the test for sterility prescribed in the monograph *Vaccines for veterinary use (0062)*.

3-3. **Residual live virus**. Carry out the test using a pool of the contents of 5 containers.

For vaccines which do not contain an adjuvant, carry out a suitable amplification test for residual live virus using the same type of cell culture as that used in the production of the vaccine or a cell culture shown to be at least as sensitive. The vaccine complies with the test if no live virus is detected.

For vaccines that contain an adjuvant, inject intracerebrally into each of not fewer than 10 mice each weighing 11-15 g, 0.03 ml of a pool of at least 5 times the smallest stated dose. To avoid interference from any antimicrobial preservative or the adjuvant, the vaccine may be diluted not more than 10 times before injection. In this case or if the vaccine strain is pathogenic only for unweaned mice, carry out the test on mice 1 to 4 days old. Observe the animals for 21 days. If more than 2 animals die during the first 48 h, repeat the test. The vaccine complies with the test if, from the 3rd to the 21st days following the injection, the animals show no signs of rabies and immunofluorescence tests carried out on the brains of the animals show no indication of the presence of rabies virus.

Vaccines

3-4. **Safety**. If the vaccine is intended for more than one species including one belonging to the order of Carnivora, carry out the test in dogs. Otherwise use one of the species for which the vaccine is intended. Use 2 animals, that preferably do not have antibodies against rabies virus. Administer to each animal by a recommended route a double dose of the vaccine. Observe the animals at least daily for 14 days.

The vaccine complies with the test if no animal shows notable signs of disease or dies from causes attributable to the vaccine.

3-5. **Potency**.

The potency of rabies vaccine is determined by comparing the dose necessary to protect mice against the clinical effects of the dose of rabies virus defined below, administered intracerebrally, with the quantity of a reference preparation, calibrated in International Units, necessary to provide the same protection.

The International Unit is the activity of a stated quantity of the International Standard. The equivalence in International Units of the International Standard is stated by the World Health Organisation.

Rabies vaccine (inactivated) for veterinary use BRP is calibrated in International Units against the International Standard.

The test described below uses a parallel-line model with at least 3 points for the vaccine to be examined and the reference preparation. Once the analyst has experience with the method for a given vaccine, it is possible to carry out a simplified test using one dilution of the vaccine to be examined. Such a test enables the analyst to determine that the vaccine has a potency significantly higher than the required minimum but will not give full information on the validity of each individual potency determination. It allows a considerable reduction in the number of animals required for the test and should be considered by each laboratory in accordance with the provisions of the European Convention for the Protection of Vertebrate Animals used for Experimental and other Scientific Purposes.

Selection and distribution of the test animals. Use in the test healthy female mice about 4 weeks old and from the same stock. Distribute the mice into at least 10 groups of not fewer than 10 mice.

Preparation of the challenge suspension. Inoculate a group of mice intracerebrally with the CVS strain of rabies virus and when the mice show signs of rabies, but before they die, euthanise the mice and remove the brains and prepare a homogenate of the brain tissue in a suitable diluent. Separate gross particulate matter by centrifugation and use the supernatant liquid as challenge suspension. Distribute the suspension in small volumes in ampoules, seal and store at a temperature below − 60 °C. Thaw one ampoule of the suspension and make serial dilutions in a suitable diluent. Allocate each dilution to a group of mice and inject intracerebrally into each mouse 0.03 ml of the dilution allocated to its group. Observe the animals at least daily for 14 days and record the number in each group that, between the 5th and the 14th days, develop signs of rabies. Calculate the ID_{50} of the undiluted suspension.

Determination of potency of the vaccine to be examined. Prepare at least 3 serial dilutions of the vaccine to be examined and 3 similar dilutions of the reference preparation. Prepare the dilutions such that those containing the largest quantity of vaccine may be expected to protect more than 50 per cent of the animals into which they are injected and those containing the smallest quantities of vaccine may be expected to protect less than 50 per cent of the animals into which they are injected. Allocate each dilution to a different group of mice and inject by the intraperitoneal route into each mouse 0.5 ml of the dilution allocated to its group. 14 days after the injection prepare a suspension of the challenge virus such that, on the basis of the preliminary titration, it contains about 50 ID_{50} in each 0.03 ml. Inject intracerebrally into each vaccinated mouse 0.03 ml of this suspension. Prepare 3 suitable serial dilutions of the challenge suspension. Allocate the challenge suspension and the 3 dilutions one to each of 4 groups of 10 unvaccinated mice and inject intracerebrally into each mouse 0.03 ml of the suspension or one of the dilutions allocated to its group. Observe the animals in each group at least daily for 14 days. The test is invalid if more than 2 mice of any group die within the first 4 days after challenge. Record the numbers in each group that show signs of rabies in the period 5 days to 14 days after challenge.

The test is invalid unless:

- for both the vaccine to be examined and the reference preparation the 50 per cent protective dose lies between the smallest and the largest dose given to the mice;
- the titration of the challenge suspension shows that 0.03 ml of the suspension contained at least 10 ID_{50};
- the confidence limits ($P = 0.95$) are not less than 25 per cent and not more than 400 per cent of the estimated potency;

- the statistical analysis shows a significant slope and no significant deviations from linearity or parallelism of the dose-response lines.

The vaccine complies with the test if the estimated potency is not less than 1 IU in the smallest prescribed dose.

Application of alternative end-points. Once a laboratory has established the above assay for routine use, the lethal end-point is replaced by an observation of clinical signs and application of an end-point earlier than death to reduce animal suffering. The following is given as an example.

The progress of rabies infection in mice following intracerebral injection can be represented by 5 stages defined by typical clinical signs:

Stage 1: ruffled fur, hunched back;

Stage 2: slow movements, loss of alertness (circular movements may also occur);

Stage 3: shaky movements, trembling, convulsions;

Stage 4: signs of paresis or paralysis;

Stage 5: moribund state.

Mice are observed at least twice daily from day 4 after challenge. Clinical signs are recorded using a chart such as that shown in Table 0451.-1. Experience has shown that using stage 3 as an end-point yields assay results equivalent to those found when a lethal end-point is used. This must be verified by each laboratory by scoring a suitable number of assays using both clinical signs and the lethal end-point.

Table 0451.-1. – *Example of a chart used to record clinical signs in the rabies vaccine potency test*

	Days after challenge							
Clinical signs	**4**	**5**	**6**	**7**	**8**	**9**	**10**	**11**
Ruffled fur Hunched back								
Slow movements Loss of alertness Circular movements								
Shaky movements Trembling Convulsions								
Paresis Paralysis								
Moribund state								

4. LABELLING

The label states:

- the type of cell culture used to prepare the vaccine and the species of origin;
- the minimum number of International Units per dose;
- the minimum period for which the vaccine provides protection.

RADIOPHARMACEUTICAL PREPARATIONS

01/2008:2351
corrected 6.1

IOBENGUANE SULPHATE FOR RADIOPHARMACEUTICAL PREPARATIONS

Iobenguani sulfas ad radiopharmaceutica

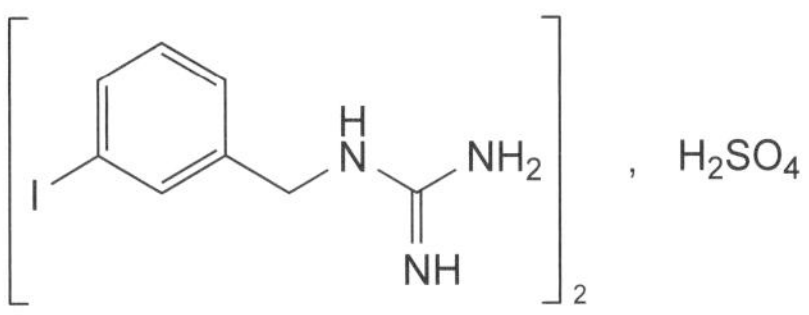

$C_{16}H_{22}I_2N_6O_4S$ M_r 648

DEFINITION

Bis[(3-iodobenzyl)guanidine] sulphate.

Content: 98.0 per cent to 102.0 per cent.

CHARACTERS

Appearance: white or almost white crystals.

IDENTIFICATION

A. Infrared absorption spectrophotometry (*2.2.24*).

Comparison: *Ph. Eur. reference spectrum of iobenguane sulphate.*

B. Dissolve about 10 mg in 1 ml of *water R* with gentle heating. The solution gives reaction (a) of sulphates (*2.3.1*).

TESTS

Related substances. Liquid chromatography (*2.2.29*). *Prepare the solutions immediately before use.*

Test solution. Dissolve 10.0 mg of the substance to be examined in 1 ml of *ethanol (96 per cent) R* with gentle heating and dilute to 5.0 ml with the same solvent.

Reference solution (a). Dissolve 10.0 mg of *iobenguane sulphate CRS* in 1 ml of *ethanol (96 per cent) R* with gentle heating and dilute to 5.0 ml with the same solvent.

Reference solution (b). Dissolve 23.1 mg of *3-iodobenzylammonium chloride R* (salt of impurity A) in 1 ml of *ethanol (96 per cent) R* with gentle heating and dilute to 10.0 ml with the same solvent.

Reference solution (c). Mix 1 ml of reference solution (a) and 1 ml of reference solution (b).

Reference solution (d). Dilute 0.1 ml of reference solution (b) to 10.0 ml with *ethanol (96 per cent) R*.

Column:

– *size*: *l* = 0.25 m, Ø = 4.0 mm;
– *stationary phase*: *silica gel for chromatography R* (5 µm);
– *temperature*: maintain at a constant temperature between 20 °C and 30 °C.

Mobile phase: mix 40 ml of an 80 g/l solution of *ammonium nitrate R*, 80 ml of *dilute ammonia R2* and 1080 ml of *methanol R*.

Flow rate: 1 ml/min.

Detection: spectrophotometer at 254 nm.

Injection: 20 µl of the test solution and reference solutions (c) and (d).

Run time: 15 min.

Relative retention with reference to iobenguane (retention time = about 7 min): impurity A = about 0.2.

System suitability: reference solution (c):

– *resolution*: minimum 4.0 between the peaks due to iobenguane and impurity A.

Limit:

– *impurity A*: not more than the area of the corresponding peak in the chromatogram obtained with reference solution (d) (1.0 per cent).

ASSAY

Liquid chromatography (*2.2.29*) as described in the test for related substances with the following modification.

Injection: test solution and reference solution (a).

Calculate the percentage content of $C_{16}H_{22}I_2N_6O_4S$ from the declared content of *iobenguane sulphate CRS*.

STORAGE

Protected from light, at a temperature below 25 °C.

LABELLING

The label recommends testing the substance in a production test before its use for the manufacture of radiopharmaceutical preparations. This ensures that, under specified production conditions, the substance yields the radiopharmaceutical preparation in the desired quantity and quality specified.

IMPURITIES

Specified impurities: A.

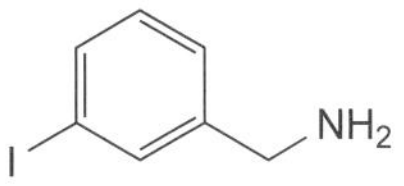

A. 1-(3-iodophenyl)methanamine.

Radiopharmaceutical preparations

HOMOEOPATHIC PREPARATIONS

01/2008:2371
corrected 6.1

METHODS OF PREPARATION OF HOMOEOPATHIC STOCKS AND POTENTISATION

Via praeparandi stirpes homoeopathicas et potentificandi

Homoeopathic stocks are prepared, using suitable methods, from raw materials that comply with the requirements of the monograph *Homoeopathic preparations (1038).* The methods described below, combined with established methods for potentisation, are examples of methods, but other methods described in an official national pharmacopoeia of a Member State may equally be used.

Where material of animal origin is to be used, particular reference is made to the requirements concerning the use of raw material of zoological or human origin in the monograph *Homoeopathic preparations (1038).*

In the preparation of liquid dilutions, the ethanol of the concentration prescribed in the method may, if necessary, be replaced by ethanol (30 per cent *m/m*) [ethanol (36 per cent *V/V*)] or ethanol (15 per cent *m/m*) [ethanol (18 per cent *V/V*)].

When the individual monograph allows that the mother tincture be prepared from more than one plant species, the mother tincture can be prepared from the specified parts of an individual plant species or from any mixture thereof.

Unless otherwise stated, mother tinctures are prepared by maceration. Maceration lasts not less than 10 days and not more than 30 days.

Maceration may be replaced by long maceration (maximum 60 days) or very long maceration (maximum 180 days), provided it is demonstrated that the quality of the resulting mother tincture is the same as that of the mother tincture prepared by maceration.

Unless otherwise stated in the individual monograph, the term 'part(s)' denotes 'mass part(s)'. Unless otherwise stated in the method, the maximum temperature for the preparation is 25 °C.

METHOD 1a

Method 1a is used for fresh herbal drugs containing generally more than 70 per cent of expressed juice and no essential oil or resin or mucilage. Mother tinctures prepared according to Method 1a are mixtures of equal parts of expressed juices and ethanol (86 per cent *m/m*) [ethanol (90 per cent *V/V*)].

Express the comminuted herbal drug. Immediately mix the expressed juice with an equal mass of ethanol (86 per cent *m/m*) [ethanol (90 per cent *V/V*)]. Allow to stand in a closed container at a temperature not exceeding 20 °C for not less than 5 days, then filter.

Adjustment to any value specified in the individual monograph

Determine the percentage dry residue (*2.8.16*) or, where prescribed, the percentage assay content of the above-mentioned filtrate. Calculate the amount (A_1), in kilograms, of ethanol (43 per cent *m/m*) [ethanol (50 per cent *V/V*)] required, using the following expression:

$$\frac{m \times (N_x - N_0)}{N_0}$$

m = mass of filtrate, in kilograms;

N_0 = percentage dry residue or percentage assay content as required in the individual monograph;

N_x = percentage dry residue or percentage assay content of the filtrate.

Mix the filtrate with the calculated amount of ethanol (43 per cent *m/m*) [ethanol (50 per cent *V/V*)]. Allow to stand at a temperature not exceeding 20 °C for not less than 5 days, then filter if necessary.

Potentisation

The 1st 'decimal' dilution (D1) is made from:

2 parts of the mother tincture;

8 parts of ethanol (43 per cent *m/m*) [ethanol (50 per cent *V/V*)].

The 2nd decimal dilution (D2) is made from:

1 part of the 1st 'decimal' dilution;

9 parts of ethanol (43 per cent *m/m*) [ethanol (50 per cent *V/V*)].

Subsequent decimal dilutions are produced as stated for D2.

The 1st 'centesimal' dilution (C1) is made from:

2 parts of the mother tincture;

98 parts of ethanol (43 per cent *m/m*) [ethanol (50 per cent *V/V*)].

The 2nd centesimal dilution (C2) is made from:

1 part of the 1st 'centesimal' dilution;

99 parts of ethanol (43 per cent *m/m*) [ethanol (50 per cent *V/V*)].

Subsequent centesimal dilutions are produced as stated for C2.

METHOD 1b

Method 1b is used where the latex of a herbal drug is to be processed.

Mother tinctures prepared according to Method 1b are mixtures of fresh plant latex with ethanol (30 per cent *m/m*) [ethanol (36 per cent *V/V*)]. Mix the fresh latex with 2 parts by mass of ethanol (30 per cent *m/m*) [ethanol (36 per cent *V/V*)] and filter.

Adjustment to any value specified in the individual monograph

Determine the percentage dry residue (*2.8.16*) or, where prescribed, the percentage assay content of the above-mentioned filtrate. Calculate the amount (A_1), in kilograms, of ethanol (30 per cent *m/m*) [ethanol (36 per cent *V/V*)] required, using the following expression:

$$\frac{m \times (N_x - N_0)}{N_0}$$

m = mass of filtrate, in kilograms;

N_0 = percentage dry residue or percentage assay content as required in the individual monograph;

N_x = percentage dry residue or percentage assay content of the filtrate.

Mix the filtrate with the calculated amount of ethanol (30 per cent *m/m*) [ethanol (36 per cent *V/V*)]. Allow to stand at a temperature not exceeding 20 °C for not less than 5 days, then filter if necessary.

Potentisation

The 1st 'decimal' dilution (D1) is made from:

3 parts of the mother tincture;

7 parts of ethanol (30 per cent *m/m*) [ethanol (36 per cent *V/V*)].

The 2nd decimal dilution (D2) is made from:

1 part of the 1st 'decimal' dilution;

9 parts of ethanol (15 per cent *m/m*) [ethanol (18 per cent *V/V*)].

Subsequent decimal dilutions are produced as stated for D2.

METHOD 2a

Method 2a is used for fresh herbal drugs containing generally less than 70 per cent of expressed juice and more than 60 per cent moisture (loss on drying) and no essential oil or resin.

Mother tinctures prepared according to Method 2a (ethanol content approximately 43 per cent *m/m* or 50 per cent *V/V*) are prepared by maceration as described below.

Comminute the herbal drug. Take a sample and determine the loss on drying (*2.2.32*). Unless otherwise prescribed, determine the loss on drying on 2.00-5.00 g of comminuted raw material in a flat-bottomed tared vessel, 45-55 mm in diameter, that has been previously dried as indicated for the raw material. Dry the raw material at 100-105 °C for 2 h then allow to cool in a desiccator.

To the comminuted herbal drug immediately add not less than half the mass of ethanol (86 per cent *m/m*) [ethanol (90 per cent *V/V*)] and store in well-closed containers at a temperature not exceeding 20 °C.

Use the following expression to calculate the amount (A_2), in kilograms, of ethanol (86 per cent *m/m*) [ethanol (90 per cent *V/V*)] required for the mass (m) of raw material, then subtract the amount of ethanol (86 per cent *m/m*) [ethanol (90 per cent *V/V*)] already added and add the difference to the mixture.

$$\frac{m \times T}{100}$$

m = mass of raw material, in kilograms;

T = percentage loss on drying of the sample.

Allow to stand at a temperature not exceeding 20 °C for not less than 10 days, swirling from time to time, then express the mixture and filter the resulting liquid.

Adjustment to any value specified in the individual monograph

Determine the percentage dry residue (*2.8.16*) or, where prescribed, the percentage assay content of the above-mentioned filtrate. Calculate the amount (A_1), in kilograms, of ethanol (43 per cent *m/m*) [ethanol (50 per cent *V/V*)] required, using the following expression:

$$\frac{m \times (N_x - N_0)}{N_0}$$

m = mass of filtrate, in kilograms;

N_0 = percentage dry residue or percentage assay content as required in the individual monograph;

N_x = percentage dry residue or percentage assay content of the filtrate.

Mix the filtrate with the calculated amount of ethanol (43 per cent *m/m*) [ethanol (50 per cent *V/V*)]. Allow to stand at a temperature not exceeding 20 °C for not less than 5 days, then filter if necessary.

Potentisation

The 1st 'decimal' dilution (D1) is made from:

2 parts of the mother tincture;

8 parts of ethanol (43 per cent *m/m*) [ethanol (50 per cent *V/V*)].

The 2nd decimal dilution (D2) is made from:

1 part of the 1st 'decimal' dilution;

9 parts of ethanol (43 per cent *m/m*) [ethanol (50 per cent *V/V*)].

Subsequent decimal dilutions are produced as stated for D2.

The 1st 'centesimal' dilution (C1) is made from:

2 parts of the mother tincture;

98 parts of ethanol (43 per cent *m/m*) [ethanol (50 per cent *V/V*)].

The 2nd centesimal dilution (C2) is made from:

1 part of the 1st 'centesimal' dilution;

99 parts of ethanol (43 per cent *m/m*) [ethanol (50 per cent *V/V*)].

Subsequent centesimal dilutions are produced as stated for C2.

METHOD 2b

Method 2b is used for fresh herbal drugs containing generally less than 70 per cent of expressed juice and more than 60 per cent moisture (loss on drying) and no essential oil or resin.

Mother tinctures prepared according to Method 2b (ethanol content approximately 30 per cent *m/m* or 36 per cent *V/V*) are prepared by maceration as described below.

Comminute the herbal drug. Take a sample and determine the loss on drying (*2.2.32*). Unless otherwise prescribed, determine the loss on drying on 2.00-5.00 g of comminuted raw material in a flat-bottomed tared vessel, 45-55 mm in diameter, that has been previously dried as indicated for the raw material. Dry the raw material at 100-105 °C for 2 h then allow to cool in a desiccator.

To the comminuted herbal drug immediately add not less than half the mass of ethanol (62 per cent *m/m*) [ethanol (70 per cent *V/V*)] and store in well-closed containers at a temperature not exceeding 20 °C.

Use the following expression to calculate the amount (A_2), in kilograms, of ethanol (62 per cent *m/m*) [ethanol (70 per cent *V/V*)] required for the mass (m) of raw material, then subtract the amount of ethanol (62 per cent *m/m*) [ethanol (70 per cent *V/V*)] already added and add the difference to the mixture.

$$\frac{m \times T}{100}$$

m = mass of raw material, in kilograms;

T = percentage loss on drying of the sample.

Allow to stand at a temperature not exceeding 20 °C for not less than 10 days, swirling from time to time, then express the mixture and filter the resulting liquid.

Adjustment to any value specified in the individual monograph

Determine the percentage dry residue (*2.8.16*) or, where prescribed, the percentage assay content of the above-mentioned filtrate. Calculate the amount (A_1), in kilograms, of ethanol (30 per cent *m/m*) [ethanol (36 per cent *V/V*)] required, using the following expression:

$$\frac{m \times (N_x - N_0)}{N_0}$$

m = mass of filtrate, in kilograms;

N_0 = percentage dry residue or percentage assay content as required in the individual monograph;

N_x = percentage dry residue or percentage assay content of the filtrate.

Mix the filtrate with the calculated amount of ethanol (30 per cent *m/m*) [ethanol (36 per cent *V/V*)]. Allow to stand at a temperature not exceeding 20 °C for not less than 5 days, then filter if necessary.

Potentisation

The 1st 'decimal' dilution (D1) is made from:

2 parts of the mother tincture;

8 parts of ethanol (30 per cent *m/m*) [ethanol (36 per cent *V/V*)].

The 2nd decimal dilution (D2) is made from:

1 part of the 1st 'decimal' dilution;

9 parts of ethanol 15 per cent (*m/m*) [ethanol (18 per cent *V/V*)].

Subsequent decimal dilutions are produced as stated for D2.

METHOD 3a

Method 3a is used for fresh herbal drugs containing essential oil or resin, or generally less than 60 per cent moisture (loss on drying).

Mother tinctures prepared according to Method 3a (ethanol content approximately 60 per cent *m/m* or 68 per cent *V/V*) are prepared by maceration as described below.

Comminute the herbal drug. Take a sample and determine the loss on drying (*2.2.32*). Unless otherwise prescribed, determine the loss on drying on 2.00-5.00 g of comminuted raw material in a flat-bottomed tared vessel, 45-55 mm in diameter, that has been previously dried as indicated for the raw material. Dry the raw material at 100-105 °C for 2 h then allow to cool in a desiccator.

To the comminuted herbal drug immediately add not less than half the mass of ethanol (86 per cent *m/m*) [ethanol (90 per cent *V/V*)] and store in well-closed containers at a temperature not exceeding 20 °C.

Use the following expression to calculate the amount (A_3), in kilograms, of ethanol (86 per cent *m/m*) [ethanol (90 per cent *V/V*)] required for the mass (m) of raw material, then subtract the amount of ethanol (86 per cent *m/m*) [ethanol (90 per cent *V/V*)] already added and add the difference to the mixture.

$$\frac{2 \times m \times T}{100}$$

m = mass of raw material, in kilograms;

T = percentage loss on drying of the sample.

Allow to stand at a temperature not exceeding 20 °C for not less than 10 days, swirling from time to time, then express the mixture and filter the resulting liquid.

Adjustment to any value specified in the individual monograph

Determine the percentage dry residue (*2.8.16*) or, where prescribed, the percentage assay content of the above-mentioned filtrate. Calculate the amount (A_1), in kilograms, of ethanol (62 per cent *m/m*) [ethanol (70 per cent *V/V*)] required, using the following expression:

$$\frac{m \times (N_x - N_0)}{N_0}$$

m = mass of filtrate, in kilograms;

N_0 = percentage dry residue or percentage assay content as required in the individual monograph;

N_x = percentage dry residue or percentage assay content of the filtrate.

Mix the filtrate with the calculated amount of ethanol (62 per cent *m/m*) [ethanol (70 per cent *V/V*)]. Allow to stand at a temperature not exceeding 20 °C for not less than 5 days, then filter if necessary.

Potentisation

The 1st 'decimal' dilution (D1) is made from:

3 parts of the mother tincture;

7 parts of ethanol (62 per cent *m/m*) [ethanol (70 per cent *V/V*)].

The 2nd decimal dilution (D2) is made from:

1 part of the 1st 'decimal' dilution;

9 parts of ethanol (62 per cent *m/m*) [ethanol (70 per cent *V/V*)].

Subsequent dilutions are produced as stated for D2. Use ethanol (43 per cent *m/m*) [ethanol (50 per cent *V/V*)] for dilutions from D4 onwards.

The 1st 'centesimal' dilution (C1) is made from:

3 parts of the mother tincture;

97 parts of ethanol (62 per cent *m/m*) [ethanol (70 per cent *V/V*)].

The 2nd 'centesimal' dilution (C2) is made from:

1 part of the 1st 'centesimal' dilution;

99 parts of ethanol (43 per cent *m/m*) [ethanol (50 per cent *V/V*)].

Subsequent dilutions are produced as stated for C2.

METHOD 3b

Method 3b is used for fresh herbal drugs containing essential oils or resins or generally less than 60 per cent moisture (loss on drying).

Mother tinctures prepared according to Method 3b (ethanol content approximately 43 per cent *m/m* or 50 per cent *V/V*) are prepared by maceration as described below.

Comminute the herbal drug. Take a sample and determine the loss on drying (*2.2.32*). Unless otherwise prescribed, determine the loss on drying on 2.00-5.00 g of comminuted raw material in a flat-bottomed tared vessel, 45-55 mm in diameter, that has been previously dried as indicated for the raw material. Dry the raw material at 100-105 °C for 2 h then allow to cool in a desiccator.

To the comminuted herbal drug immediately add not less than half the mass of ethanol (73 per cent *m/m*) [ethanol (80 per cent *V/V*)] and store in well-closed containers at a temperature not exceeding 20 °C.

Use the following expression to calculate the amount (A_3), in kilograms, of ethanol (73 per cent *m/m*) [ethanol (80 per cent *V/V*)] required for the mass (m) of raw material, then subtract the amount of ethanol (73 per cent *m/m*) [ethanol (80 per cent *V/V*)] already added and add the difference to the mixture.

$$\frac{2 \times m \times T}{100}$$

m = mass of raw material, in kilograms;

T = percentage loss on drying of the sample.

Allow to stand at a temperature not exceeding 20 °C for not less than 10 days, swirling from time to time, then express the mixture and filter the resulting liquid.

Adjustment to any value specified in the individual monograph

Determine the percentage dry residue (*2.8.16*) or, where prescribed, the percentage assay content of the above-mentioned filtrate. Calculate the amount (A_1), in kilograms, of ethanol (43 per cent *m/m*) [ethanol 50 per cent *V/V*)] required, using the following expression:

$$\frac{m \times (N_x - N_0)}{N_0}$$

m = mass of filtrate, in kilograms;

N_0 = percentage dry residue or percentage assay content as required in the individual monograph;

N_x = percentage dry residue or percentage assay content of the filtrate.

Mix the filtrate with the calculated amount of ethanol (43 per cent *m/m*) [ethanol (50 per cent *V/V*)]. Allow to stand at a temperature not exceeding 20 °C for not less than 5 days, then filter if necessary.

Potentisation

The 1st 'decimal' dilution (D1) is made from:

3 parts of the mother tincture;

7 parts of ethanol (43 per cent *m/m*) [ethanol (50 per cent *V/V*)].

The 2nd decimal dilution (D2) is made from:

1 part of the 1st 'decimal' dilution;

9 parts of ethanol (30 per cent *m/m*) [ethanol (36 per cent *V/V*)].

The 3rd decimal dilution (D3) is made from:

1 part of the 2nd decimal dilution;

9 parts of ethanol (15 per cent *m/m*) [ethanol (19 per cent *V/V*)].

Subsequent decimal dilutions are produced as stated for D3.

METHOD 3c

Method 3c is used for fresh herbal drugs containing generally less than 60 per cent moisture (loss on drying).

Mother tinctures prepared according to Method 3c (ethanol content approximately 30 per cent *m/m* or 36 per cent *V/V*) are prepared by maceration as described below.

Comminute the herbal drug. Take a sample and determine the loss on drying (*2.2.32*). Unless otherwise prescribed, determine the loss on drying on 2.00-5.00 g of comminuted raw material in a flat-bottomed tared vessel, 45-55 mm in diameter, that has been previously dried as indicated for the raw material. Dry the raw material at 100-105 °C for 2 h then allow to cool in a desiccator.

To the comminuted herbal drug immediately add not less than half the mass of ethanol (43 per cent *m/m*) [ethanol (50 per cent *V/V*)] and store in well-closed containers at a temperature not exceeding 20 °C.

Use the following expression to calculate the amount (A_3), in kilograms, of ethanol (43 per cent *m/m*) [ethanol (50 per cent *V/V*)] required for the mass (*m*) of raw material, then subtract the amount of ethanol (43 per cent *m/m*) [ethanol (50 per cent *V/V*)] already added and add the difference to the mixture.

$$\frac{2 \times m \times T}{100}$$

m = mass of raw material, in kilograms;

T = percentage loss on drying of the sample.

Allow to stand at a temperature not exceeding 20 °C for not less than 10 days, swirling from time to time, then express the mixture and filter the resulting liquid.

Adjustment to any value specified in the individual monograph

Determine the percentage dry residue (*2.8.16*) or, where prescribed, the percentage assay content of the above-mentioned filtrate. Calculate the amount (A_1), in kilograms, of ethanol (30 per cent *m/m*) [ethanol (36 per cent *V/V*)] required, using the following expression:

$$\frac{m \times (N_x - N_0)}{N_0}$$

m = mass of filtrate, in kilograms;

N_0 = percentage dry residue or percentage assay content as required in the individual monograph;

N_x = percentage dry residue or percentage assay content of the filtrate.

Mix the filtrate with the calculated amount of ethanol (30 per cent *m/m*) [ethanol (36 per cent *V/V*)]. Allow to stand at a temperature not exceeding 20 °C for not less than 5 days, then filter if necessary.

Potentisation

The 1st 'decimal' dilution (D1) is made from:

3 parts of the mother tincture;

7 parts of ethanol (30 per cent *m/m*) [ethanol (36 per cent *V/V*)].

The 2nd decimal dilution (D2) is made from:

1 part of the 1st 'decimal' dilution;

9 parts of ethanol (15 per cent *m/m*) [ethanol (18 per cent *V/V*)].

Subsequent decimal dilutions are produced as stated for D2.

METHOD 4a

Method 4a is generally used for dried herbal drugs.

Mother tinctures prepared according to Method 4a are prepared by maceration or percolation as described below, using 1 part of dried herbal drug and 10 parts of ethanol of the appropriate concentration (anhydrous, 94 per cent *m/m* - 96 per cent *V/V*, 86 per cent *m/m* - 90 per cent *V/V*, 73 per cent *m/m* - 80 per cent *V/V*, 62 per cent *m/m* - 70 per cent *V/V*, 43 per cent *m/m* - 50 per cent *V/V*, 30 per cent *m/m* - 36 per cent *V/V*, 15 per cent *m/m* - 18 per cent *V/V*), unless otherwise prescribed in the individual monograph.

Production by maceration. Unless otherwise prescribed, comminute the herbal drug, mix thoroughly with ethanol of the appropriate concentration and allow to stand in a closed container for an appropriate time. Separate the residue from the ethanol and, if necessary, press out. In the latter case, combine the 2 liquids obtained.

Production by percolation. If necessary, comminute the herbal drug. Mix thoroughly with a portion of ethanol of the appropriate concentration and allow to stand for an appropriate time. Transfer to a percolator and allow the percolate to flow slowly, at room temperature, making sure that the herbal drug to be extracted is always covered with the remaining ethanol. The residue may be pressed out and the expressed liquid combined with the percolate.

If adjustment to a given concentration is necessary, calculate the amount (A_1), in kilograms, of ethanol of the appropriate concentration required to obtain the concentration specified or used for production, using the following expression:

$$\frac{m \times (N_x - N_0)}{N_0}$$

m = mass of percolate or macerate, in kilograms;

N_0 = percentage dry residue or percentage assay content as required in the individual monograph;

N_x = percentage dry residue or percentage assay content of the percolate or macerate.

Mix the macerate or percolate with the calculated amount of ethanol of the appropriate concentration. Allow to stand at a temperature not exceeding 20 °C for not less than 5 days, then filter if necessary.

Potentisation

The mother tincture corresponds to the 1st decimal solution (Ø = D1).

The 2nd decimal dilution (D2) is made from:

1 part of the mother tincture (D1);

9 parts of ethanol of the same concentration.

The 3rd decimal dilution (D3) is made from:

1 part of the 2nd decimal dilution;

9 parts of ethanol of the same concentration.

Unless a different ethanol concentration is specified, use ethanol (43 per cent *m/m*) [ethanol (50 per cent *V/V*)] for subsequent decimal dilutions from D4 onwards and proceed as stated for D3.

The 1st 'centesimal' dilution (C1) is made from:

10 parts of the mother tincture (D1);

90 parts of ethanol of the same concentration.

The 2nd centesimal dilution (C2) is made from:

1 part of the 1st 'centesimal' dilution;

99 parts of ethanol (43 per cent *m/m*) [ethanol (50 per cent *V/V*)], unless a different ethanol concentration is specified.

Subsequent centesimal dilutions are produced as stated for C2.

METHOD 4b

Method 4b is generally used for animal matter.

Mother tinctures prepared according to Method 4b are prepared by maceration or percolation as described below, using 1 part of animal matter and 10 parts of ethanol of the appropriate concentration (anhydrous, 94 per cent *m/m* - 96 per cent *V/V*, 86 per cent *m/m* - 90 per cent *V/V*, 73 per cent *m/m* - 80 per cent *V/V*, 62 per cent *m/m* - 70 per cent *V/V*, 43 per cent *m/m* - 50 per cent *V/V*, 30 per cent *m/m* - 36 per cent *V/V*, 15 per cent *m/m* - 18 per cent *V/V*), unless otherwise prescribed in the individual monograph.

Production by maceration. Unless otherwise prescribed, comminute the animal matter, mix thoroughly with ethanol of the appropriate concentration and allow to stand in a closed container for an appropriate time. Separate the residue from the ethanol and, if necessary, press out. In the latter case, combine the 2 liquids obtained.

Production by percolation. If necessary, comminute the animal matter. Mix thoroughly with a portion of ethanol of the appropriate concentration and allow to stand for an appropriate time. Transfer to a percolator and allow the percolate to flow slowly at room temperature, making sure that the animal matter to be extracted is always covered with the remaining ethanol. The residue may be pressed out and the expressed liquid combined with the percolate.

If adjustment to a given concentration is necessary, calculate the amount (A_1), in kilograms, of ethanol of the appropriate concentration required to obtain the concentration specified or used for production, using the following expression:

$$\frac{m \times (N_x - N_0)}{N_0}$$

m = mass of percolate or macerate, in kilograms;

N_0 = percentage dry residue or percentage assay content as required in the individual monograph;

N_x = percentage dry residue or percentage assay content of the percolate or macerate.

Mix the macerate or percolate with the calculated amount of ethanol of the appropriate concentration. Allow to stand at a temperature not exceeding 20 °C for not less than 5 days, then filter if necessary.

Potentisation

The mother tincture corresponds to the 1st decimal solution (Ø = D1).

The 2nd decimal dilution (D2) is made from:

1 part of the mother tincture (D1);

9 parts of ethanol of the same concentration.

The 3rd decimal dilution (D3) is made from:

1 part of the 2nd decimal dilution;

9 parts of ethanol of the same concentration.

Unless a different ethanol concentration is specified, use ethanol (43 per cent *m/m*) [ethanol (50 per cent *V/V*)] for subsequent decimal dilutions from D4 onwards and proceed as stated for D3.

The 1st 'centesimal' dilution (C1) is made from:

10 parts of the mother tincture (D1);

90 parts of ethanol of the same concentration.

The 2nd centesimal dilution (C2) is made from:

1 part of the 1st 'centesimal' dilution;

99 parts of ethanol (43 per cent *m/m*) [ethanol (50 per cent *V/V*)], unless a different ethanol concentration is specified.

Subsequent centesimal dilutions are produced as stated for C2.

METHOD 4c

Method 4c is generally used for herbal drugs. The state of the herbal drug, fresh or dried, is specified in the individual monograph.

Mother tinctures prepared according to Method 4c are prepared by maceration.

Comminute appropriately the herbal drug. Take a sample and determine the loss on drying at 100-105 °C for 2 h (*2.2.32*) or the water content (*2.2.13*). Taking this value into account, calculate and add to the herbal drug the quantities of ethanol of the appropriate concentration required to produce, unless otherwise prescribed, a 1 in 10 mother tincture (1:10 mother tincture) with a suitable ethanol content. Allow to macerate for at least 10 days, with sufficient shaking.

Separate the residue from the ethanol and strain at a pressure of about 10^7 Pa. Allow the combined liquids to stand for 48 h and filter. For mother tinctures with a required assay content, adjustment may be carried out, if necessary, by adding ethanol of the same concentration as used for the preparation of the tincture.

Potentisation

The 1st decimal dilution (D1) is made from:

1 part of the mother tincture;

9 parts of ethanol of the appropriate concentration.

The 2nd decimal dilution (D2) is made from:

1 part of the 1st decimal dilution;

9 parts of ethanol of the appropriate concentration.

Subsequent decimal dilutions are produced as stated for D2, using ethanol of the appropriate concentration.

The 1st centesimal dilution (C1) is made from:

1 part of the mother tincture;

99 parts of ethanol of the appropriate concentration.

The 2nd centesimal dilution (C2) is made from:

1 part of the 1st centesimal dilution;

99 parts of ethanol of the appropriate concentration.

Subsequent centesimal dilutions are produced as stated for C2, using ethanol of the appropriate concentration.

METHOD 4d

Method 4d is generally used for animal matter.

Mother tinctures prepared according to Method 4d are prepared by maceration.

The mass ratio of raw material to mother tincture is usually 1 to 20. To the raw material, appropriately comminuted, add the quantity of ethanol of the appropriate concentration required to produce a 1 in 20 mother tincture. Allow to macerate for at least 10 days, with sufficient shaking. Decant and filter. Allow to stand for 48 h and filter again.

Potentisation

The 1st decimal dilution (D1) is made from:

1 part of the mother tincture;

9 parts of ethanol of the appropriate concentration.

The 2nd decimal dilution (D2) is made from:

1 part of the 1st decimal dilution;

9 parts of ethanol of the appropriate concentration.

Subsequent decimal dilutions are produced as stated for D2, using ethanol of the appropriate concentration.

The 1st centesimal dilution (C1) is made from:

1 part of the mother tincture;

99 parts of ethanol of the appropriate concentration.

The 2nd centesimal dilution (C2) is made from:

1 part of the 1st centesimal dilution;

99 parts of ethanol of the appropriate concentration.

Subsequent centesimal dilutions are produced as stated for C2, using ethanol of the appropriate concentration.

A

04/2008:1686

ACEMETACIN

Acemetacinum

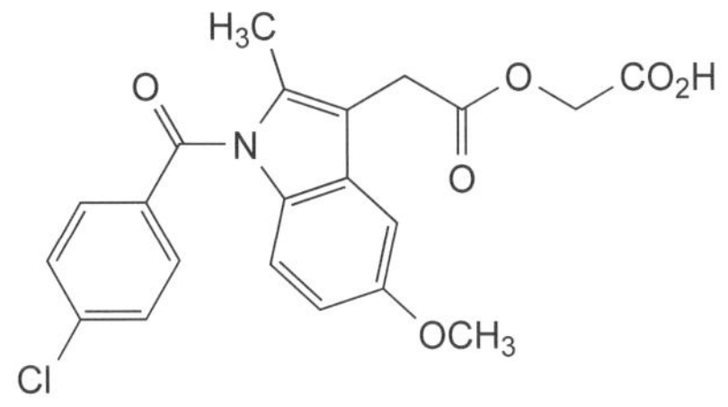

$C_{21}H_{18}ClNO_6$ M_r 415.8

[53164-05-9]

DEFINITION

[[[1-(4-Chlorobenzoyl)-5-methoxy-2-methyl-1*H*-indol-3-yl]acetyl]oxy]acetic acid.

Content: 99.0 per cent to 101.0 per cent (dried substance).

CHARACTERS

Appearance: yellow or greenish-yellow, crystalline powder.

Solubility: practically insoluble in water, soluble in acetone, slightly soluble in anhydrous ethanol.

It shows polymorphism (*5.9*).

IDENTIFICATION

Infrared absorption spectrophotometry (*2.2.24*).

Comparison: *acemetacin CRS.*

If the spectra obtained in the solid state show differences, dissolve the substance to be examined and the reference substance separately in *acetone R*, evaporate to dryness and record new spectra using the residues.

TESTS

Related substances. Liquid chromatography (*2.2.29*).

Test solution. Dissolve 0.100 g of the substance to be examined in *acetonitrile for chromatography R* and dilute to 20.0 ml with the same solvent.

Reference solution (a). Dilute 5.0 ml of the test solution to 50.0 ml with *acetonitrile for chromatography R.* Dilute 1.0 ml of this solution to 100.0 ml with *acetonitrile for chromatography R.*

Reference solution (b). Dissolve 5.0 mg of *acemetacin impurity A CRS* and 10.0 mg of *indometacin CRS* (impurity B) in *acetonitrile for chromatography R,* and dilute to 50.0 ml with the same solvent.

Reference solution (c). Dilute 1.0 ml of reference solution (b) to 20.0 ml with *acetonitrile for chromatography R.*

Reference solution (d). To 1 ml of reference solution (b), add 10 ml of the test solution and dilute to 20 ml with *acetonitrile for chromatography R.*

Reference solution (e). Dissolve the contents of a vial of *acemetacin impurity mixture CRS* (containing impurities C, D, E and F) in 2 ml of the test solution.

Column:

- *size*: *l* = 0.25 m, Ø = 4 mm;
- *stationary phase*: spherical *end-capped octadecylsilyl silica gel for chromatography R* (5 µm);
- *temperature*: 40 °C.

Mobile phase:

- *mobile phase A*: dissolve 1.0 g of *potassium dihydrogen phosphate R* in 900 ml of *water R,* adjust to pH 6.5 with *1 M sodium hydroxide* and dilute to 1000 ml with *water R*;
- *mobile phase B*: *acetonitrile for chromatography R*;

Time (min)	Mobile phase A (per cent *V/V*)	Mobile phase B (per cent *V/V*)
0 - 5	95	5
5 - 9	95 → 65	5 → 35
9 - 16	65	35
16 - 28	65 → 20	35 → 80
28 - 34	20	80

Flow rate: 1.0 ml/min.

Detection: spectrophotometer at 235 nm.

Injection: 20 µl.

Identification of impurities:

- use the chromatogram supplied with *acemetacin impurity mixture CRS* and the chromatogram obtained with reference solution (e) to identify the peaks due to impurities C, D, E and F;
- use the chromatogram obtained with reference solution (b) to identify the peak due to impurity B.

Relative retention with reference to acemetacin (retention time = about 15 min): impurity A = about 0.7; impurity B = about 0.9; impurity F = about 1.2; impurity C = about 1.3; impurity D = about 1.5; impurity E = about 2.2.

System suitability: reference solution (d):

- *peak-to-valley ratio*: minimum 15, where H_p = height above the baseline of the peak due to impurity B and H_v = height above the baseline of the lowest point of the curve separating this peak from the peak due to acemetacin.

Limits:

- *correction factors*: for the calculation of content, multiply the peak areas of the following impurities by the corresponding correction factor: impurity C = 1.3; impurity D = 1.4; impurity F = 1.3;
- *impurity E*: not more than 3 times the area of the principal peak in the chromatogram obtained with reference solution (a) (0.3 per cent);
- *impurity B*: not more than the area of the corresponding peak in the chromatogram obtained with reference solution (c) (0.2 per cent);
- *impurity A*: not more than the area of the corresponding peak in the chromatogram obtained with reference solution (c) (0.1 per cent);
- *impurities C, D, F*: for each impurity, not more than the area of the principal peak in the chromatogram obtained with reference solution (a) (0.1 per cent);
- *unspecified impurities*: for each impurity, not more than the area of the principal peak in the chromatogram obtained with reference solution (a) (0.10 per cent);
- *total*: not more than 4 times the area of the principal peak in the chromatogram obtained with reference solution (a) (0.4 per cent);
- *disregard limit*: 0.5 times the area of the principal peak in the chromatogram obtained with reference solution (a) (0.05 per cent).

Heavy metals : maximum 20 ppm.

Solvent mixture: *methanol R, acetone R* (10:90 *V/V*).

Test solution. Dissolve 0.250 g of the substance to be examined in 20 ml of the solvent mixture.

Reference solution. Dilute 0.5 ml of *lead standard solution (10 ppm Pb) R* to 20 ml with the solvent mixture.

Blank solution: 20 ml of the solvent mixture.

Monitor solution. Dissolve 0.250 g of the substance to be examined in 0.5 ml of *lead standard solution (10 ppm Pb) R* and dilute to 20 ml with the solvent mixture.

To each solution, add 2 ml of *buffer solution pH 3.5 R*. Mix and add to 1.2 ml of *thioacetamide reagent R*. Mix immediately. Filter the solutions through a membrane filter (pore size 0.45 µm) (*2.4.8*). Compare the spots on the filters obtained with the different solutions. The test is invalid if the reference solution does not show a slight brown colour compared to the blank solution. The substance to be examined complies with the test if the brown colour of the spot resulting from the test solution is not more intense than that of the spot resulting from the reference solution.

Loss on drying (*2.2.32*): maximum 0.5 per cent, determined on 1.000 g by drying in an oven at 105 °C.

Sulphated ash (*2.4.14*): maximum 0.1 per cent, determined on 1.0 g.

ASSAY

Dissolve 0.350 g in 20 ml of *acetone R* and add 10 ml of *water R*. Titrate with *0.1 M sodium hydroxide*, determining the end-point potentiometrically (*2.2.20*).

1 ml of *0.1 M sodium hydroxide* is equivalent to 41.58 mg of $C_{21}H_{18}ClNO_6$.

STORAGE

Protected from light.

IMPURITIES

Specified impurities: A, B, C, D, E, F.

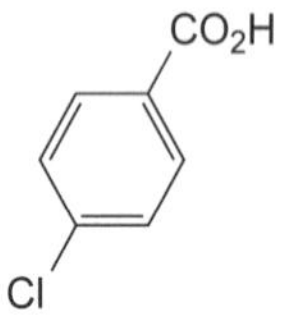

A. 4-chlorobenzoic acid,

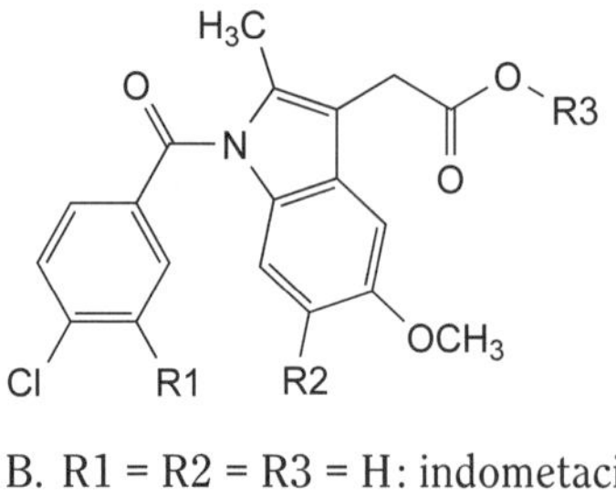

B. R1 = R2 = R3 = H: indometacin,

C. R1 = Cl, R2 = H, R3 = CH_2-CO_2H: [[[1-(3,4-dichlorobenzoyl)-5-methoxy-2-methyl-1*H*-indol-3-yl]acetyl]oxy]acetic acid,

D. R1 = H, R2 = $C(CH_3)_3$, R3 = CH_2-CO_2H: [[[1-(4-chlorobenzoyl)-6-(1,1-dimethylethyl)-5-methoxy-2-methyl-1*H*-indol-3-yl]acetyl]oxy]acetic acid,

E. R1 = R2 = H, R3 = CH_2-CO-O-$C(CH_3)_3$: 1,1-dimethylethyl [[[1-(4-chlorobenzoyl)-5-methoxy-2-methyl-1*H*-indol-3-yl]acetyl]oxy]acetate,

F. R1 = R2 = H, R3 = CH_2-CO-O-CH_2-CO_2H: [[[[[1-(4-chlorobenzoyl)-5-methoxy-2-methyl-1*H*-indol-3-yl]acetyl]oxy]acetyl]oxy]acetic acid.

04/2008:1287

ALFUZOSIN HYDROCHLORIDE

Alfuzosini hydrochloridum

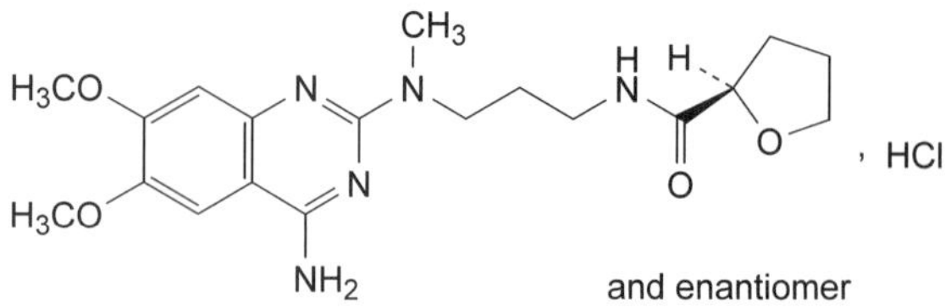

and enantiomer

$C_{19}H_{28}ClN_5O_4$ M_r 425.9
[81403-68-1]

DEFINITION

(2*RS*)-*N*-[3-[(4-Amino-6,7-dimethoxyquinazolin-2-yl)methylamino]propyl]tetrahydrofuran-2-carboxamide hydrochloride.

Content: 99.0 per cent to 101.0 per cent (anhydrous substance).

CHARACTERS

Appearance: white or almost white, crystalline powder, slightly hygroscopic.

Solubility: freely soluble in water, sparingly soluble in ethanol (96 per cent), practically insoluble in methylene chloride.

IDENTIFICATION

A. Infrared absorption spectrophotometry (*2.2.24*).

Comparison: *alfuzosin hydrochloride CRS.*

B. It gives reaction (a) of chlorides (*2.3.1*).

TESTS

pH (*2.2.3*): 4.0 to 5.5.

Dissolve 0.500 g in *carbon dioxide-free water R* and dilute to 25.0 ml with the same solvent. Use a freshly prepared solution.

Related substances. Liquid chromatography (*2.2.29*).

Test solution. Dissolve 40 mg of the substance to be examined in the mobile phase and dilute to 100.0 ml with the mobile phase.

Reference solution (a). Dilute 1.0 ml of the test solution to 100.0 ml with the mobile phase. Dilute 1.0 ml of this solution to 10.0 ml with the mobile phase.

Reference solution (b). Dissolve 4 mg of *alfuzosin for system suitability CRS* (containing impurities A and D) in the mobile phase and dilute to 10 ml with the mobile phase.

Column:

– *size*: *l* = 0.15 m, Ø = 4.6 mm;
– *stationary phase*: *end-capped octadecylsilyl silica gel for chromatography R* (5 µm).

Mobile phase: mix 1 volume of *tetrahydrofuran R*, 20 volumes of *acetonitrile R* and 80 volumes of a solution prepared as follows: dilute 5.0 ml of *perchloric acid R* in 900 ml of *water R*, adjust to pH 3.5 with *dilute sodium hydroxide solution R* and dilute to 1000 ml with *water R*.

Flow rate: 1.5 ml/min.

Detection: spectrophotometer at 254 nm.

Injection: 10 µl.

Run time: twice the retention time of alfuzosin.

Identification of impurities: use the chromatogram supplied with *alfuzosin for system suitability CRS* and the chromatogram obtained with reference solution (b) to identify the peaks due to impurities A and D.

Relative retention with reference to alfuzosin (retention time = about 8 min): impurity D = about 0.4; impurity A = about 1.2.

System suitability: reference solution (b):

- *peak-to-valley ratio*: minimum 5.0, where H_p = height above the baseline of the peak due to impurity A and H_v = height above the baseline of the lowest point of the curve separating this peak from the peak due to alfuzosin.

Limits:

- *impurity D*: not more than twice the area of the principal peak in the chromatogram obtained with reference solution (a) (0.2 per cent);
- *unspecified impurities*: for each impurity, not more than the area of the principal peak in the chromatogram obtained with reference solution (a) (0.10 per cent);
- *total*: not more than 3 times the area of the principal peak in the chromatogram obtained with reference solution (a) (0.3 per cent);
- *disregard limit*: 0.5 times the area of the principal peak in the chromatogram obtained with reference solution (a) (0.05 per cent).

Water (*2.5.12*) : maximum 0.5 per cent, determined on 1.000 g.

Sulphated ash (*2.4.14*): maximum 0.1 per cent, determined on 1.0 g.

ASSAY

Dissolve 0.300 g in a mixture of 40 ml of *anhydrous acetic acid R* and 40 ml of *acetic anhydride R*. Titrate with *0.1 M perchloric acid,* determining the end-point potentiometrically (*2.2.20*).

1 ml of *0.1 M perchloric acid* is equivalent to 42.59 mg of $C_{19}H_{28}ClN_5O_4$.

STORAGE

In an airtight container, protected from light.

IMPURITIES

Specified impurities: D.

Other detectable impurities (the following substances would, if present at a sufficient level, be detected by one or other of the tests in the monograph. They are limited by the general acceptance criterion for other/unspecified impurities and/or by the general monograph *Substances for pharmaceutical use (2034)*. It is therefore not necessary to identify these impurities for demonstration of compliance. See also *5.10. Control of impurities in substances for pharmaceutical use*): *A, B, C, E.*

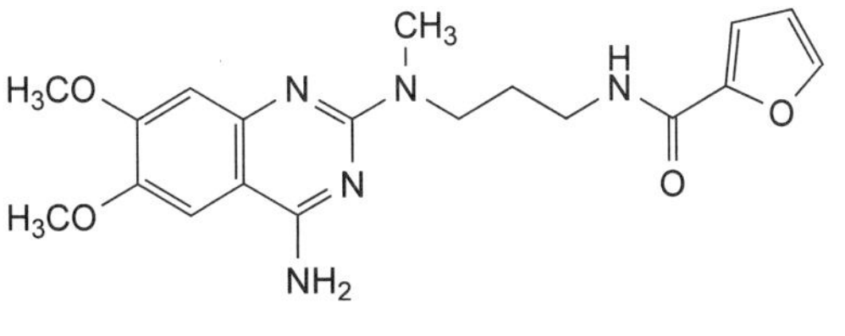

A. *N*-[3-[(4-amino-6,7-dimethoxyquinazolin-2-yl)methylamino]propyl]furan-2-carboxamide,

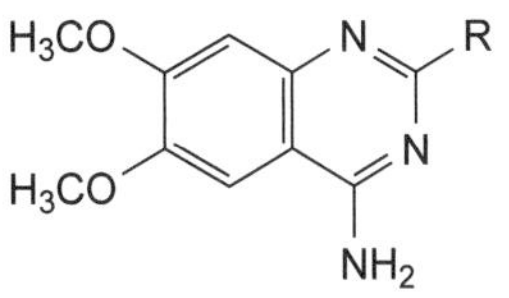

B. R = Cl: 2-chloro-6,7-dimethoxyquinazolin-4-amine,

D. R = $N(CH_3)$-$[CH_2]_3$-NH_2: *N*-(4-amino-6,7-dimethoxyquinazolin-2-yl)-*N*-methylpropane-1,3-diamine,

E. R = $N(CH_3)$-$[CH_2]_3$-NH-CO-H: *N*-[3-[(4-amino-6,7-dimethoxyquinazolin-2-yl)methylamino]propyl]formamide,

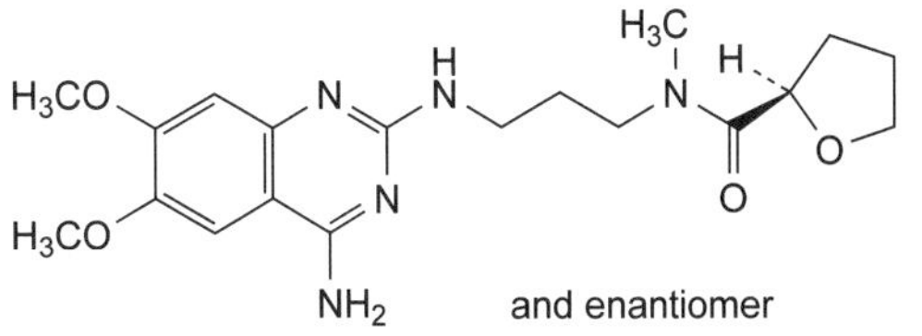

C. (2*RS*)-*N*-[3-[(4-amino-6,7-dimethoxyquinazolin-2-yl)amino]propyl]-*N*-methyltetrahydrofuran-2-carboxamide.

04/2008:1664

ALUMINIUM HYDROXIDE, HYDRATED, FOR ADSORPTION

Aluminii hydroxidum hydricum ad adsorptionem

$[AlO(OH)],nH_2O$

DEFINITION

Content: 90.0 per cent to 110.0 per cent of the content of aluminium stated on the label.

NOTE: shake the gel vigorously for at least 30 s immediately before examining.

CHARACTERS

Appearance: white or almost white, translucent, viscous, colloidal gel. A supernatant may be formed upon standing.

Solubility: a clear or almost clear solution is obtained with alkali hydroxide solutions and mineral acids.

IDENTIFICATION

Solution S (see Tests) gives the reaction of aluminium.

To 10 ml of solution S add about 0.5 ml of *dilute hydrochloric acid R* and about 0.5 ml of *thioacetamide reagent R*. No precipitate is formed. Add dropwise 5 ml of *dilute sodium hydroxide solution R*. Allow to stand for 1 h. A gelatinous white precipitate is formed which dissolves upon addition of 5 ml of *dilute sodium hydroxide solution R*. Gradually add 5 ml of *ammonium chloride solution R* and allow to stand for 30 min. The gelatinous white precipitate is re-formed.

TESTS

Solution S. Add 1 g to 4 ml of *hydrochloric acid R*. Heat at 60 °C for 1 h, cool, dilute to 50 ml with *distilled water R* and filter if necessary.

pH (*2.2.3*): 5.5 to 8.5.

Adsorption power. Dilute the substance to be examined with *distilled water R* to obtain an aluminium concentration of 5 mg/ml. Prepare *bovine albumin R* solutions with the following concentrations of bovine albumin: 0.5 mg/ml, 1 mg/ml, 2 mg/ml, 3 mg/ml, 5 mg/ml and 10 mg/ml. If necessary, adjust the gel and the *bovine albumin R* solutions to pH 6.0 with *dilute hydrochloric acid R* or *dilute sodium hydroxide solution R*.

For adsorption, mix 1 part of the diluted gel with 4 parts of each of the solutions of *bovine albumin R* and allow to stand at room temperature for 1 h. During this time shake the mixture vigorously at least 5 times. Centrifuge or filter through a non-protein-retaining filter. Immediately determine the protein content (*2.5.33, Method 2*) of either the supernatant or the filtrate.

It complies with the test if no bovine albumin is detectable in the supernatant or filtrate of the 2 mg/ml *bovine albumin R* solution (maximum level of adsorption) and in the supernatant or filtrate of *bovine albumin R* solutions of lower concentrations. Solutions containing 3 mg/ml, 5 mg/ml and 10 mg/ml *bovine albumin R* may show bovine albumin in the supernatant or filtrate, proportional to the amount of bovine albumin in the solutions.

Sedimentation. If necessary, adjust the substance to be examined to pH 6.0 using *dilute hydrochloric acid R* or dilute *sodium hydroxide solution R*. Dilute with *distilled water R* to obtain an aluminium concentration of approximately 5 mg/ml. If the aluminium content of the substance to be examined is lower than 5 mg/ml, adjust to pH 6.0 and dilute with a 9 g/l solution of *sodium chloride R* to obtain an aluminium concentration of about 1 mg/ml. After shaking for at least 30 s, place 25 ml of the preparation in a 25 ml graduated cylinder and allow to stand for 24 h.

It complies with the test if the volume of the clear supernatant is less than 5 ml for the gel with an aluminium content of about 5 mg/ml.

It complies with the test if the volume of the clear supernatant is less than 20 ml for the gel with an aluminium content of about 1 mg/ml.

Chlorides (*2.4.4*): maximum 0.33 per cent.

Dissolve 0.5 g in 10 ml of *dilute nitric acid R* and dilute to 500 ml with *water R*.

Nitrates: maximum 100 ppm.

Place 5 g in a test-tube immersed in ice-water, add 0.4 ml of a 100 g/l solution of *potassium chloride R*, 0.1 ml of *diphenylamine solution R* and, dropwise with shaking, 5 ml of *sulphuric acid R*. Transfer the tube to a water-bath at 50 °C. After 15 min, any blue colour in the solution is not more intense than that in a standard prepared at the same time and in the same manner using 5 ml of *nitrate standard solution (100 ppm NO_3) R*.

Sulphates (*2.4.13*): maximum 0.5 per cent.

Dilute 2 ml of solution S to 20 ml with *water R*.

Ammonium (*2.4.1, Method B*): maximum 50 ppm, determined on 1.0 g.

Prepare the standard using 0.5 ml of *ammonium standard solution (100 ppm NH_4) R*.

Arsenic (*2.4.2, Method A*): maximum 1 ppm, determined on 1 g.

Iron (*2.4.9*): maximum 15 ppm, determined on 0.67 g.

Heavy metals (*2.4.8*): maximum 20 ppm.

Dissolve 2.0 g in 10 ml of *dilute nitric acid R* and dilute to 20 ml with *water R*. The solution complies with test A. Prepare the reference solution using *lead standard solution (2 ppm Pb) R*.

Bacterial endotoxins (*2.6.14*): less than 5 IU of endotoxin per milligram of aluminium, if intended for use in the manufacture of an adsorbed product without a further appropriate procedure for the removal of bacterial endotoxins.

ASSAY

Dissolve 2.50 g in 10 ml of *hydrochloric acid R*, heating for 30 min at 100 °C on a water-bath. Cool and dilute to 20 ml with *water R*. To 10 ml of the solution, add *concentrated ammonia R* until a precipitate is obtained. Add the smallest quantity of *hydrochloric acid R* needed to dissolve the precipitate and dilute to 20 ml with *water R*. Carry out the complexometric titration of aluminium (*2.5.11*). Carry out a blank titration.

STORAGE

At a temperature not exceeding 30 °C. Do not allow to freeze. If the substance is sterile, store in a sterile, airtight, tamper-proof container.

LABELLING

The label states the declared content of aluminium.

01/2008:1289
corrected 6.1

AMIKACIN

Amikacinum

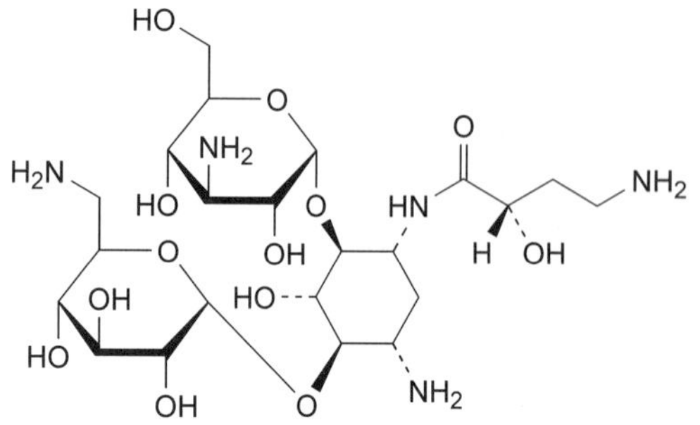

$C_{22}H_{43}N_5O_{13}$ M_r 585.6
[37517-28-5]

DEFINITION

6-*O*-(3-Amino-3-deoxy-α-D-glucopyranosyl)-4-*O*-(6-amino-6-deoxy-α-D-glucopyranosyl)-1-*N*-[(2*S*)-4-amino-2-hydroxybutanoyl]-2-deoxy-D-streptamine.

Antimicrobial substance obtained from kanamycin A.

Semi-synthetic product derived from a fermentation product.

Content: 96.5 per cent to 102.0 per cent (anhydrous substance).

CHARACTERS

Appearance: white or almost white powder.

Solubility: sparingly soluble in water, slightly soluble in methanol, practically insoluble in acetone and in ethanol (96 per cent).

IDENTIFICATION

A. Infrared absorption spectrophotometry (*2.2.24*).
   Comparison: *amikacin CRS*.

B. Thin-layer chromatography (*2.2.27*).

Test solution. Dissolve 25 mg of the substance to be examined in *water R* and dilute to 10 ml with the same solvent.

Reference solution (a). Dissolve 25 mg of *amikacin CRS* in *water R* and dilute to 10 ml with the same solvent.

Reference solution (b). Dissolve 5 mg of *kanamycin monosulphate CRS* in 1 ml of the test solution and dilute to 10 ml with *water R*.

Plate: *TLC silica gel plate R*.

Mobile phase: the lower layer of a mixture of equal volumes of *concentrated ammonia R*, *methanol R* and *methylene chloride R*.

Application: 5 μl.

Development: over a path of 15 cm.

Drying: in air.

Detection: spray with *ninhydrin solution R1* and heat at 110 °C for 5 min.

System suitability: reference solution (b):

– the chromatogram shows 2 clearly separated spots.

Results: the principal spot in the chromatogram obtained with the test solution is similar in position, colour and size to the principal spot in the chromatogram obtained with reference solution (a).

TESTS

pH (*2.2.3*): 9.5 to 11.5.

Dissolve 0.1 g in *carbon dioxide-free water R* and dilute to 10 ml with the same solvent.

Specific optical rotation (*2.2.7*): + 97 to + 105 (anhydrous substance).

Dissolve 0.50 g in *water R* and dilute to 25.0 ml with the same solvent.

Related substances. Liquid chromatography (*2.2.29*). *Maintain the solutions at 10 °C.*

Test solution (a). Dissolve 0.100 g of the substance to be examined in *water R* and dilute to 10.0 ml with the same solvent. In a ground-glass-stoppered vial, add 0.2 ml of this solution to 2.0 ml of a 10 g/l solution of *2,4,6-trinitrobenzene sulphonic acid R*. Then add 3.0 ml of *pyridine R* and close the vial tightly. Shake vigorously for 30 s and heat in a water-bath at 75 °C for 45 min. Cool in cold water for 2 min and add 2 ml of *glacial acetic acid R*. Shake vigorously for 30 s.

Test solution (b). Dissolve 50.0 mg of the substance to be examined in *water R* and dilute to 50.0 ml with the same solvent. Then prepare as prescribed for test solution (a).

Reference solution (a). Dissolve 5.0 mg of *amikacin impurity A CRS* in *water R* and dilute to 50.0 ml with the same solvent. Then prepare as prescribed for test solution (a).

Reference solution (b). Dissolve 50.0 mg of *amikacin CRS* in *water R* and dilute to 50.0 ml with the same solvent. Then prepare as prescribed for test solution (a).

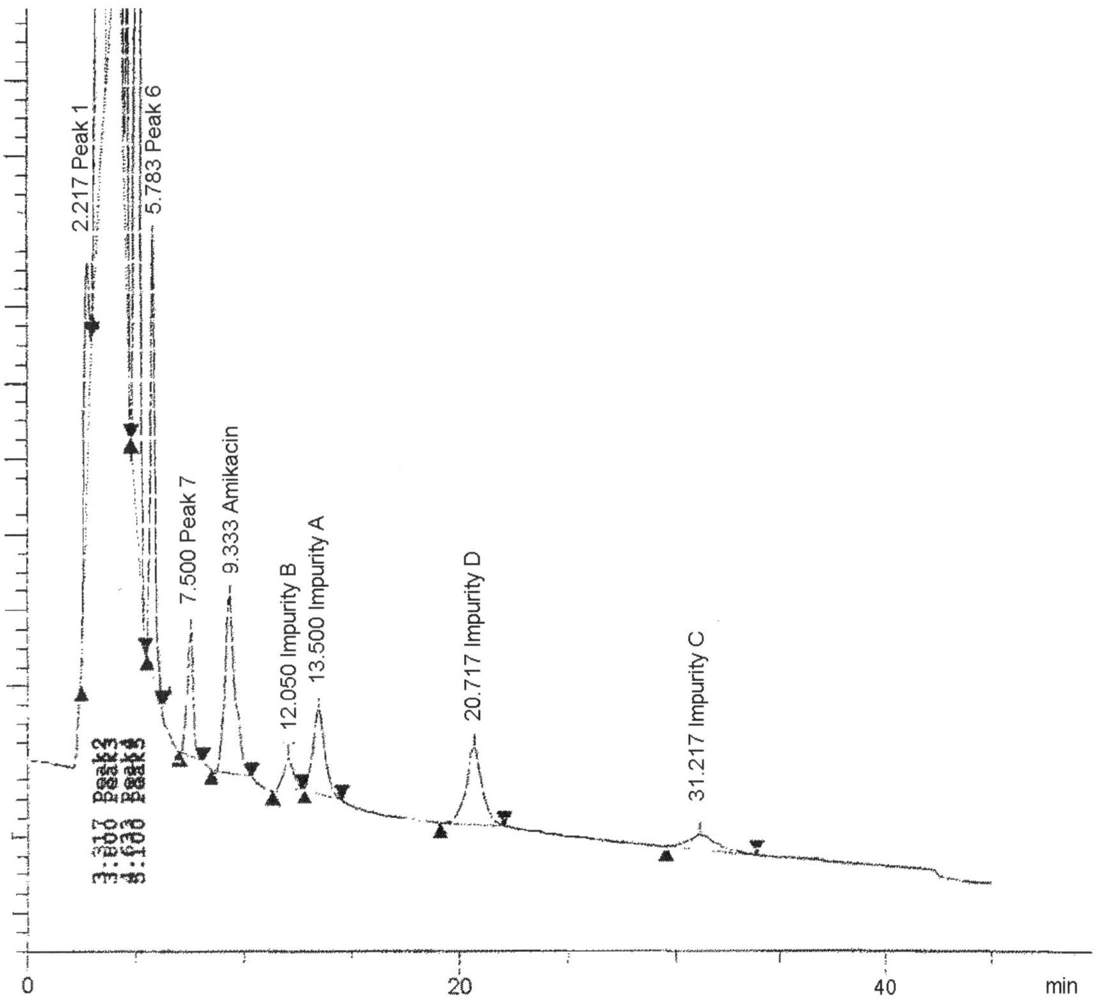

Figure 1289.-1. – *Chromatogram for the test for related substances of amikacin*

Reference solution (c). Dissolve 2 mg of *amikacin CRS* and 2 mg of *amikacin impurity A CRS* in *water R* and dilute to 20 ml with the same solvent. Then prepare as prescribed for test solution (a).

Blank solution. Prepare as described for test solution (a) using 0.2 ml of *water R*.

Column:

- *size*: l = 0.25 m, Ø = 4.6 mm;
- *stationary phase*: *octadecylsilyl silica gel for chromatography R* (5 μm);
- *temperature*: 30 °C.

Mobile phase: mix 30 volumes of a 2.7 g/l solution of *potassium dihydrogen phosphate R*, adjusted to pH 6.5 with a 22 g/l solution of *potassium hydroxide R*, and 70 volumes of *methanol R*.

Flow rate: 1 ml/min.

Detection: spectrophotometer at 340 nm.

Injection: 20 μl of test solution (a) and reference solutions (a) and (c).

Run time: 4 times the retention time of amikacin.

System suitability: reference solution (c):

- *resolution*: minimum 3.5 between the peaks due to amikacin and impurity A (see Figure 1289.-1).

Limits:

- *impurity A*: not more than the area of the principal peak in the chromatogram obtained with reference solution (a) (1 per cent);
- *any other impurity*: for each impurity, not more than 0.5 times the area of the principal peak in the chromatogram obtained with reference solution (a) (0.5 per cent);
- *sum of impurities other than A*: not more than 1.5 times the area of the principal peak in the chromatogram obtained with reference solution (a) (1.5 per cent);
- *disregard limit*: 0.1 times the area of the principal peak in the chromatogram obtained with reference solution (a) (0.1 per cent); disregard any peak due to the blank.

Water (*2.5.12*): maximum 8.5 per cent, determined on 0.200 g.

Sulphated ash (*2.4.14*): maximum 0.5 per cent, determined on 1.0 g.

ASSAY

Liquid chromatography (*2.2.29*) as described in the test for related substances with the following modifications.

Injection: test solution (b) and reference solution (b).

System suitability:

- *repeatability*: maximum relative standard deviation of 2.0 per cent after 6 injections of reference solution (b).

Calculate the percentage content of $C_{22}H_{43}N_5O_{13}$ from the declared content of *amikacin CRS*.

IMPURITIES

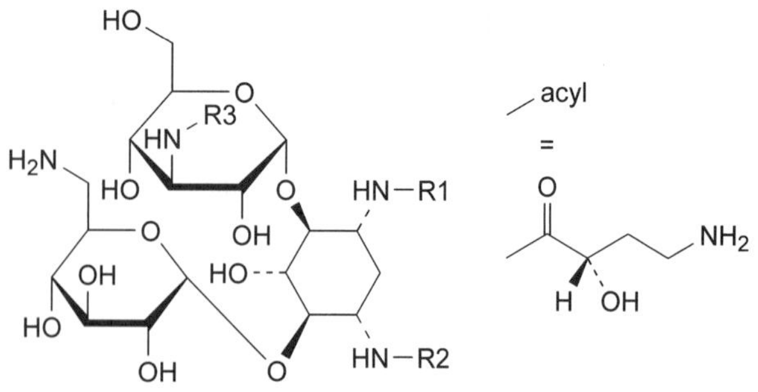

A. R1 = R3 = H, R2 = acyl: 4-*O*-(3-amino-3-deoxy-α-D-glucopyranosyl)-6-*O*-(6-amino-6-deoxy-α-D-glucopyranosyl)-1-*N*-[(2*S*)-4-amino-2-hydroxybutanoyl]-2-deoxy-L-streptamine,

B. R1 = R2 = acyl, R3 = H: 4-*O*-(3-amino-3-deoxy-α-D-glucopyranosyl)-6-*O*-(6-amino-6-deoxy-α-D-glucopyranosyl)-1,3-*N*-bis[(2*S*)-4-amino-2-hydroxybutanoyl]-2-deoxy-L-streptamine,

C. R1 = R2 = H, R3 = acyl: 4-*O*-(6-amino-6-deoxy-α-D-glucopyranosyl)-6-*O*-[3-[[(2*S*)-4-amino-2-hydroxybutanoyl]amino]-3-deoxy-α-D-glucopyranosyl]-2-deoxy-D-streptamine,

D. R1 = R2 = R3 = H: kanamycin.

01/2008:1290
corrected 6.1

AMIKACIN SULPHATE

Amikacini sulfas

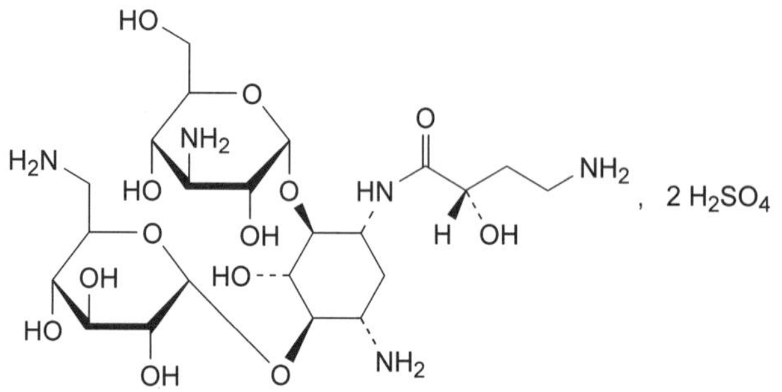

$C_{22}H_{47}N_5O_{21}S_2$ M_r 782
[39831-55-5]

DEFINITION

6-*O*-(3-Amino-3-deoxy-α-D-glucopyranosyl)-4-*O*-(6-amino-6-deoxy-α-D-glucopyranosyl)-1-*N*-[(2*S*)-4-amino-2-hydroxybutanoyl]-2-deoxy-D-streptamine sulphate.

Antimicrobial substance obtained from kanamycin A.

Semi-synthetic product derived from a fermentation product.

Content: 96.5 per cent to 102.0 per cent (dried substance).

CHARACTERS

Appearance: white or almost white powder.

Solubility: freely soluble in water, practically insoluble in acetone and in ethanol (96 per cent).

IDENTIFICATION

A. Infrared absorption spectrophotometry (*2.2.24*).
Comparison: *amikacin sulphate CRS*.

B. Thin-layer chromatography (*2.2.27*).

Test solution. Dissolve 25 mg of the substance to be examined in *water R* and dilute to 10 ml with the same solvent.

Reference solution (a). Dissolve 25 mg of *amikacin sulphate CRS* in *water R* and dilute to 10 ml with the same solvent.

Reference solution (b). Dissolve 5 mg of *kanamycin monosulphate CRS* in 1 ml of the test solution and dilute to 10 ml with *water R.*

Plate: *TLC silica gel plate R.*

Mobile phase: the lower layer of a mixture of equal volumes of *concentrated ammonia R, methanol R* and *methylene chloride R.*

Application: 5 μl.

Development: over a path of 15 cm.

Drying: in air.

Detection: spray with *ninhydrin solution R1* and heat at 110 °C for 5 min.

System suitability: reference solution (b):

– the chromatogram shows 2 clearly separated spots.

Results: the principal spot in the chromatogram obtained with the test solution is similar in position, colour and size to the principal spot in the chromatogram obtained with reference solution (a).

C. It gives reaction (a) of sulphates (*2.3.1*).

TESTS

pH (*2.2.3*): 2.0 to 4.0.

Dissolve 0.1 g in *carbon dioxide-free water R* and dilute to 10 ml with the same solvent.

Specific optical rotation (*2.2.7*): + 76 to + 84 (dried substance).

Dissolve 0.50 g in *water R* and dilute to 25.0 ml with the same solvent.

Related substances. Liquid chromatography (*2.2.29*). *Maintain the solutions at 10 °C.*

Test solution (a). Dissolve 0.100 g of the substance to be examined in *water R* and dilute to 10.0 ml with the same solvent. In a ground-glass-stoppered vial, add 0.2 ml of this solution to 2.0 ml of a 10 g/l solution of *2,4,6-trinitrobenzene sulphonic acid R*. Then add 3.0 ml of *pyridine R* and close the vial tightly. Shake vigorously for 30 s and heat on a water-bath at 75 °C for 2 h. Cool in cold water for 2 min and add 2 ml of *glacial acetic acid R*. Shake vigorously for 30 s.

Test solution (b). Dissolve 50.0 mg of the substance to be examined in *water R* and dilute to 50.0 ml with the same solvent. Then prepare as prescribed for test solution (a).

Reference solution (a). Dissolve 5.0 mg of *amikacin impurity A CRS* in *water R* and dilute to 50.0 ml with the same solvent. Then prepare as prescribed for test solution (a).

Reference solution (b). Dissolve 50.0 mg of *amikacin sulphate CRS* in *water R* and dilute to 50.0 ml with the same solvent. Then prepare as prescribed for test solution (a).

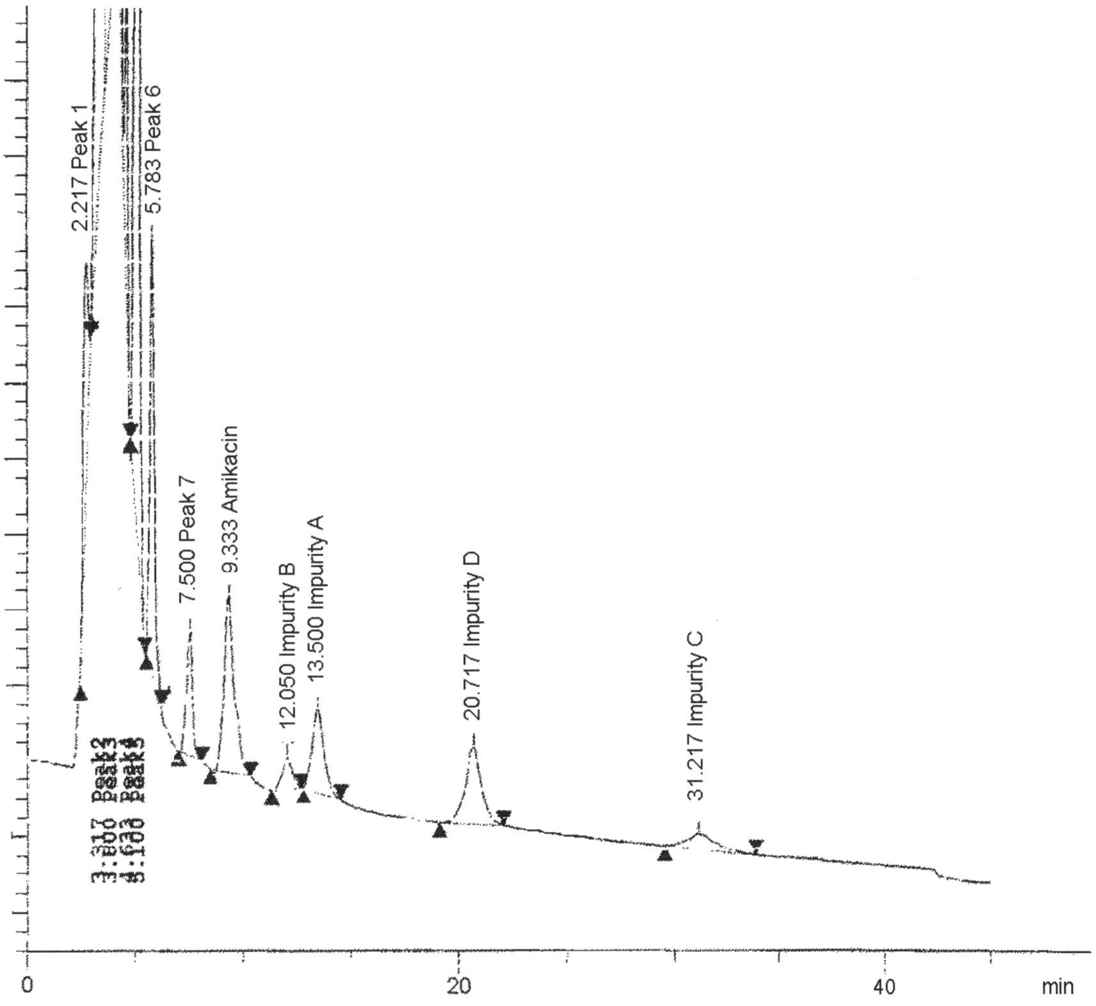

Figure 1290.-1. – *Chromatogram for the test for related substances of amikacin sulphate*

Reference solution (c). Dissolve 2 mg of *amikacin sulphate CRS* and 2 mg of *amikacin impurity A CRS* in *water R* and dilute to 20 ml with the same solvent. Then prepare as prescribed for test solution (a).

Blank solution. Prepare as described for test solution (a) using 0.2 ml of *water R*.

Column:

- *size*: *l* = 0.25 m, Ø = 4.6 mm;
- *stationary phase*: *octadecylsilyl silica gel for chromatography R* (5 μm);
- *temperature*: 30 °C.

Mobile phase: mix 30 volumes of a 2.7 g/l solution of *potassium dihydrogen phosphate R*, adjusted to pH 6.5 with a 22 g/l solution of *potassium hydroxide R*, and 70 volumes of *methanol R*.

Flow rate: 1 ml/min.

Detection: spectrophotometer at 340 nm.

Injection: 20 μl of test solution (a) and reference solutions (a) and (c).

Run time: 4 times the retention time of amikacin.

System suitability: reference solution (c):

- *resolution*: minimum 3.5 between the peaks due to amikacin and impurity A (see Figure 1290.-1).

Limits:

- *impurity A*: not more than the area of the principal peak in the chromatogram obtained with reference solution (a) (1.0 per cent);
- *any other impurity*: for each impurity, not more than 0.5 times the area of the principal peak in the chromatogram obtained with reference solution (a) (0.5 per cent);
- *sum of impurities other than A*: not more than 1.5 times the area of the principal peak in the chromatogram obtained with reference solution (a) (1.5 per cent);
- *disregard limit*: 0.1 times the area of the principal peak in the chromatogram obtained with reference solution (a) (0.1 per cent); disregard any peak due to the blank and any peak eluting before the principal peak.

Sulphate: 23.3 per cent to 25.8 per cent (dried substance).

Dissolve 0.250 g in 100 ml of *water R* and adjust the solution to pH 11 using *concentrated ammonia R*. Add 10.0 ml of *0.1 M barium chloride* and about 0.5 mg of *phthalein purple R*. Titrate with *0.1 M sodium edetate* adding 50 ml of *ethanol (96 per cent) R* when the colour of the solution begins to change and continue the titration until the violet-blue colour disappears.

1 ml of *0.1 M barium chloride* is equivalent to 9.606 mg of sulphate (SO_4).

Loss on drying (*2.2.32*): maximum 13.0 per cent, determined on 0.500 g by drying in an oven at 105 °C at a pressure not exceeding 0.7 kPa for 3 h.

Pyrogens (*2.6.8*). If intended for use in the manufacture of parenteral dosage forms without a further appropriate procedure for the removal of pyrogens, it complies with the test for pyrogens. Inject per kilogram of the rabbit's mass 5 ml of a solution containing 25 mg of the substance to be examined in *water for injections R*.

ASSAY

Liquid chromatography (*2.2.29*) as described in the test for related substances with the following modifications.

Injection: test solution (b) and reference solution (b).

System suitability:

- *repeatability*: maximum relative standard deviation of 2.0 per cent after 6 injections of reference solution (b).

Calculate the percentage content of $C_{22}H_{47}N_5O_{21}S_2$ from the declared content of *amikacin sulphate CRS*.

STORAGE

If the substance is sterile, store in a sterile, airtight, tamper-proof container.

IMPURITIES

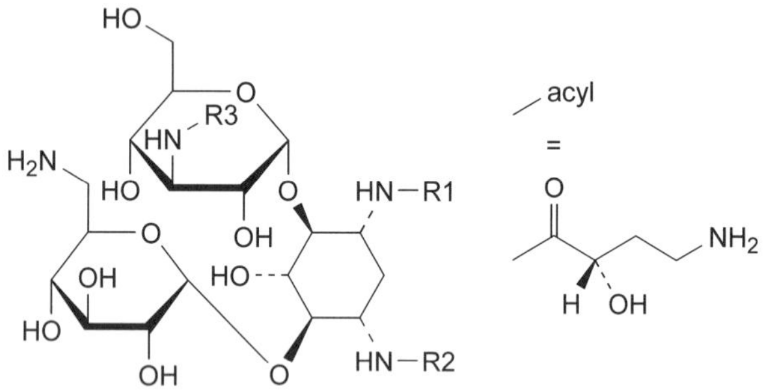

A. R1 = R3 = H, R2 = acyl: 4-*O*-(3-amino-3-deoxy-α-D-glucopyranosyl)-6-*O*-(6-amino-6-deoxy-α-D-glucopyranosyl)-1-*N*-[(2*S*)-4-amino-2-hydroxybutanoyl]-2-deoxy-L-streptamine,

B. R1 = R2 = acyl, R3 = H: 4-*O*-(3-amino-3-deoxy-α-D-glucopyranosyl)-6-*O*-(6-amino-6-deoxy-α-D-glucopyranosyl)-1,3-*N*-bis[(2*S*)-4-amino-2-hydroxybutanoyl]-2-deoxy-L-streptamine,

C. R1 = R2 = H, R3 = acyl: 4-*O*-(6-amino-6-deoxy-α-D-glucopyranosyl)-6-*O*-[3-[[(2*S*)-4-amino-2-hydroxybutanoyl]amino]-3-deoxy-α-D-glucopyranosyl]-2-deoxy-D-streptamine,

D. R1 = R2 = R3 = H: kanamycin.

04/2008:1391

ARNICA FLOWER

Arnicae flos

DEFINITION

Whole or partially broken, dried flower-heads of *Arnica montana* L.

Content: minimum 0.40 per cent *m/m* of total sesquiterpene lactones, expressed as dihydrohelenalin tiglate (dried drug).

CHARACTERS

Aromatic odour.

The capitulum, when spread out, is about 20 mm in diameter and about 15 mm deep, and has a peduncle 2-3 cm long. The involucre consists of 18-24 elongated lanceolate bracts, with acute apices, arranged in 1-2 rows: the bracts, about 8-10 mm long, are green with yellowish-green external hairs visible under a lens. The receptacle, about 6 mm in diameter, is convex, alveolate and covered with hairs. Its periphery bears about 20 ligulate florets 20-30 mm long; the disc bears a greater number of tubular florets about 15 mm long. The ovary, 4-8 mm long, is crowned by a pappus of whitish bristles 4-8 mm long. Some brown achenes, crowned or not by a pappus, may be present.

IDENTIFICATION

A. The involucre consists of elongated oval bracts with acute apices; the margin is ciliated. The ligulate floret has a reduced calyx crowned by fine, shiny, whitish bristles, bearing small coarse trichomes. The orange-yellow corolla bears 7-10 parallel veins and ends in 3 small lobes. The stamens, with free anthers, are incompletely developed. The narrow, brown ovary bears a stigma divided into 2 branches curving outwards. The tubular floret is actinomorphic. The ovary and the calyx are similar to those of the ligulate floret. The short corolla has 5 reflexed triangular lobes; the 5 fertile stamens are fused at the anthers.

B. Separate the capitulum into its different parts. Examine under a microscope using *chloral hydrate solution R*. The powder shows the following diagnostic characters: the epidermises of the bracts of the involucre have stomata and trichomes, more abundant on the outer (abaxial) surface. There are several different types of trichomes: uniseriate multicellular covering trichomes, varying in length from 50-500 µm, particularly abundant on the margins of the bract; secretory trichomes with uni- or biseriate multicellular stalks and with multicellular, globular heads, about 300 µm long, abundant on the outer surface of the bract; secretory trichomes with uniseriate multicellular stalks and with multicellular, globular heads, about 80 µm long, abundant on the inner surface of the bract. The epidermis of the ligulate corolla consists of lobed or elongated cells, a few stomata and trichomes of different types: covering trichomes, with very sharp ends, whose length may exceed 500 µm, consisting of 1-3 proximal cells with thickened walls and 2-4 distal cells with thin walls; secretory trichomes with biseriate multicellular heads; secretory trichomes with multicellular stalks and multicellular globular heads. The ligule ends in rounded papillose cells. The epidermis of the ovary is covered with trichomes: secretory trichomes with short stalks and multicellular globular heads; twinned covering trichomes usually consisting of 2 longitudinally united cells, with common punctuated walls; their ends are sharp and sometimes bifid. The epidermises of the calyx consist of elongated cells bearing short, unicellular, covering trichomes pointing towards the upper end of the bristle. The pollen grains have a diameter of about 30 µm, are rounded, with a spiny exine, and have 3 germinal pores.

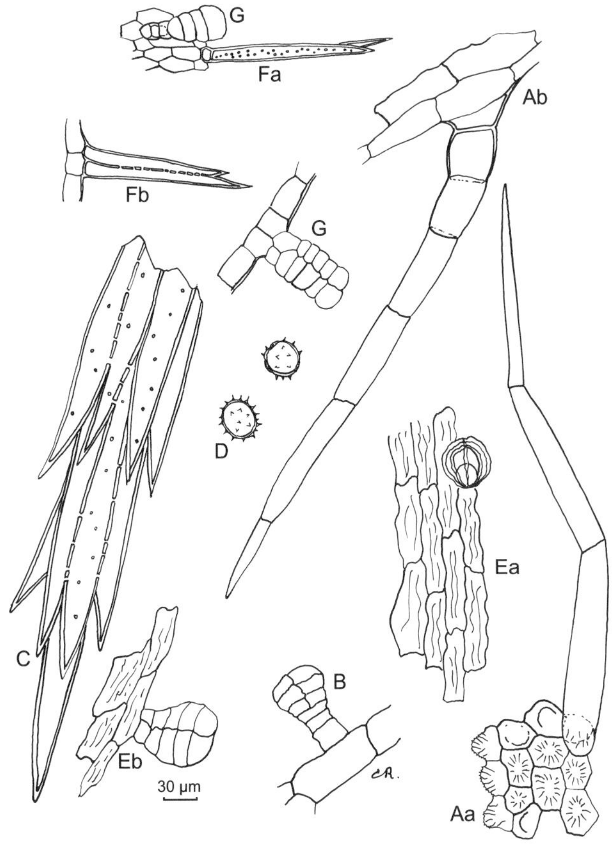

A. Epidermis of the ligulate corolla with covering trichome in surface view (Aa) and in side view (Ab)

B. Secretory trichome with multicellular head

C. Bristles of the calyx

D. Pollen grain

E. Epidermis of the corolla with striated cuticle and biseriate secretory trichome in surface view (Ea) and in side view (Eb)

F. Covering trichome of the ovary in surface view (Fa) and in side view (Fb)

G. Secretory trichome of the ovary

Figure 1391.-1. – *Illustration of powdered herbal drug of arnica flower (see Identification B)*

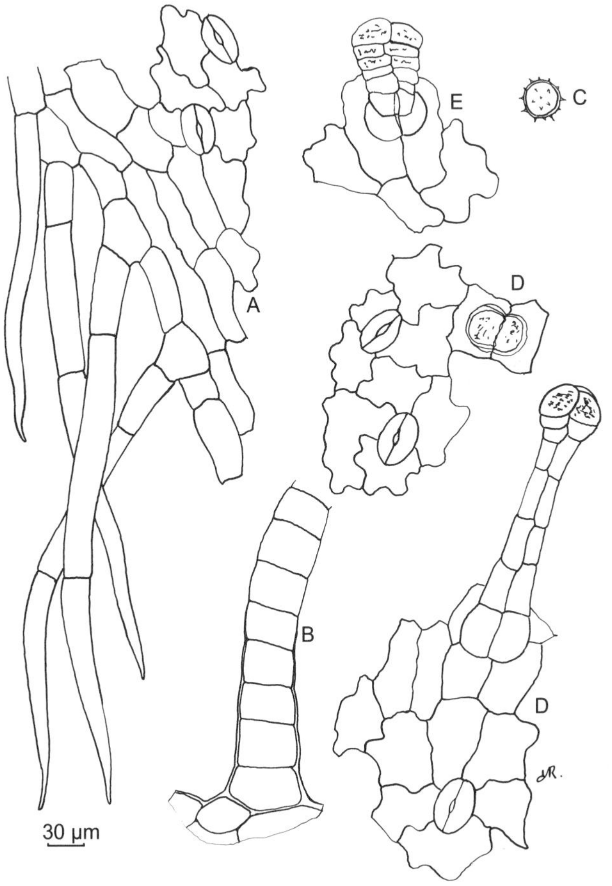

A. Epidermis of the bracts of the involucre with covering trichomes and stomata

B. Multicellular stalk of covering trichome

C. Pollen grain

D. Epidermis of bracts of the involucre with stomata and biseriate secretory trichome

E. Secretory trichome

Figure 1391.-2. – *Illustration of powdered herbal drug of arnica flower (see Identification B)*

Monographs A-C

C. Examine the chromatograms obtained in the test for *Calendula officinalis* L. - *Heterotheca inuloides* Cass.

Results: the chromatogram obtained with the test solution shows, in the middle, a fluorescent blue zone corresponding to the zone due to chlorogenic acid in the chromatogram obtained with the reference solution; it shows, above this zone, 3 fluorescent yellowish-brown or orange-yellow zones, and above these 3 zones a fluorescent greenish-yellow zone due to astragalin. The zone located below the astragalin zone is due to isoquercitroside; the zone located just below this zone is due to luteolin-7-glucoside. It also shows a fluorescent greenish-blue zone below the zone due to caffeic acid in the chromatogram obtained with the reference solution.

TESTS

Foreign matter (*2.8.2*): maximum 5.0 per cent.

***Calendula officinalis* L. - *Heterotheca inuloides* Cass.** Thin-layer chromatography (*2.2.27*).

Test solution. To 2.00 g of the powdered drug (710) (*2.9.12*) add 10 ml of *methanol R*. Heat in a water-bath at 60 °C for 5 min with shaking. Cool and filter.

Reference solution. Dissolve 2.0 mg of *caffeic acid R*, 2.0 mg of *chlorogenic acid R* and 5.0 mg of *rutin R* in *methanol R* and dilute to 30 ml with the same solvent.

Plate: *TLC silica gel plate R.*

Mobile phase: *anhydrous formic acid R, water R, methyl ethyl ketone R, ethyl acetate R* (10:10:30:50 *V/V/V/V*).

Application: 15 µl, as bands.

Development: over a path of 15 cm.

Drying: in air for a few minutes.

Detection: spray with a 10 g/l solution of *diphenylboric acid aminoethyl ester R* in *methanol R*, and then with a 50 g/l solution of *macrogol 400 R* in *methanol R*. Heat at 100-105 °C for 5 min. Allow to dry in air and examine in ultraviolet light at 365 nm.

Results: the chromatogram obtained with the reference solution shows in the lower part an orange-yellow fluorescent zone due to rutin, in the middle part a fluorescent zone due to chlorogenic acid and in the upper part a light bluish fluorescent zone due to caffeic acid. The chromatogram obtained with the test solution does not show a fluorescent orange-yellow zone corresponding to the zone due to rutin in the chromatogram obtained with the reference solution, nor does it show a zone below this.

Loss on drying (*2.2.32*): maximum 10.0 per cent, determined on 1.000 g of the powdered drug (355) (*2.9.12*) by drying in an oven at 105 °C for 2 h.

Total ash (*2.4.16*): maximum 10.0 per cent.

ASSAY

Liquid chromatography (*2.2.29*).

Internal standard solution. Dissolve immediately before use 0.010 g of *santonin R*, accurately weighed in 10.0 ml of *methanol R*.

Test solution. Introduce 1.00 g of the powdered drug (355) (*2.9.12*) into a 250 ml round-bottomed flask, add 50 ml of a mixture of equal volumes of *methanol R* and *water R* and heat under a reflux condenser in a water-bath at 50-60 °C for 30 min, shaking frequently. Allow to cool and filter through a paper filter. Add the paper filter, cut into pieces, to the residue in the round-bottomed flask, add 50 ml of a mixture of equal volumes of *methanol R* and *water R* and heat under a reflux condenser in a water-bath at 50-60 °C for 30 min, shaking frequently. Repeat this procedure twice. To the combined filtrate add 3.00 ml of the internal standard solution and evaporate to 18 ml under reduced pressure. Rinse the round-bottomed flask with *water R* and dilute, with the washings, to 20.0 ml. Transfer the solution to a chromatography column about 0.15 m long and about 30 mm in internal diameter containing 15 g of *kieselguhr for chromatography R*. Allow to stand for 20 min. Elute with 200 ml of a mixture of equal volumes of *ethyl acetate R* and *methylene chloride R*. Evaporate the eluate to dryness in a 250 ml round-bottomed flask. Dissolve the residue in 10.0 ml of *methanol R* and add 10.0 ml of *water R*. Add 7.0 g of *neutral aluminium oxide R*, shake for 120 s, centrifuge at 5000 *g* for 10 min and filter through a paper filter. Evaporate 10.0 ml of the filtrate to dryness. Dissolve the residue in 3.0 ml of a mixture of equal volumes of *methanol R* and *water R* and filter.

Column:

- *size*: l = 0.12 m, Ø = 4 mm;
- *stationary phase*: *octadecylsilyl silica gel for chromatography R* (4 µm).

Mobile phase:

- *mobile phase A*: *water R*;
- *mobile phase B*: *methanol R*;

Time (min)	Mobile phase A (per cent *V/V*)	Mobile phase B (per cent *V/V*)
0 - 3	62	38
3 - 20	62 → 55	38 → 45
20 - 30	55	45
30 - 55	55 → 45	45 → 55
55 - 57	45 → 0	55 → 100
57 - 70	0	100
70 - 90	62	38

Flow rate: 1.2 ml/min.

Detection: spectrophotometer at 225 nm.

Injection: a 20 µl loop injector.

Calculate the percentage content of total sesquiterpene lactones, expressed as dihydrohelenalin tiglate, using the following expression:

$$\frac{S_{LS} \times C \times V \times 1.187 \times 100}{S_S \times m \times 1000}$$

S_{LS} = area of all peaks due to sesquiterpene lactones appearing after the santonin peak in the chromatogram obtained with the test solution;

S_S = area of the peak due to santonin in the chromatogram obtained with the test solution;

m = mass of the drug to be examined, in grams;

C = concentration of santonin in the internal standard solution used for the test solution, in milligrams per millilitre;

V = volume of the internal standard solution used for the test solution, in millilitres;

1.187 = peak correlation factor between dihydrohelenalin tiglate and santonin.

Monographs A-C

04/2008:2056

ATROPINE

Atropinum

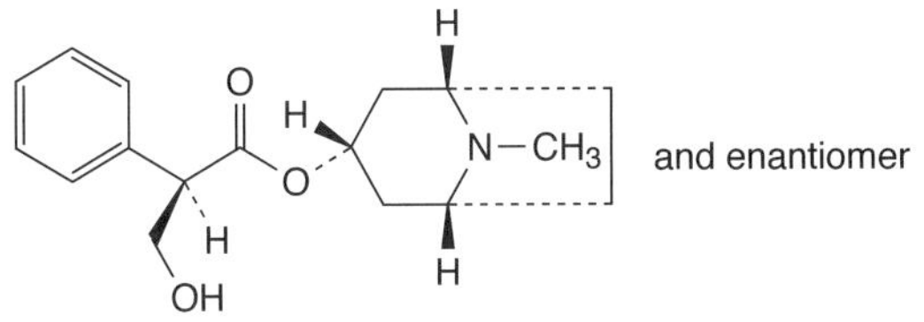

$C_{17}H_{23}NO_3$ M_r 289.4
[51-55-8]

DEFINITION

(1*R*,3*r*,5*S*)-8-Methyl-8-azabicyclo[3.2.1]oct-3-yl (2*RS*)-3-hydroxy-2-phenylpropanoate.

Content: 99.0 per cent to 101.0 per cent (dried substance).

CHARACTERS

Appearance: white or almost white, crystalline powder or colourless crystals.

Solubility: very slightly soluble in water, freely soluble in ethanol (96 per cent) and in methylene chloride.

IDENTIFICATION

First identification: A, B, E.

Second identification: A, C, D, E.

A. Melting point (*2.2.14*): 115 °C to 119 °C.

B. Infrared absorption spectrophotometry (*2.2.24*).

Comparison: *atropine CRS.*

C. Thin-layer chromatography (*2.2.27*).

Test solution. Dissolve 10 mg of the substance to be examined in *methanol R* and dilute to 10 ml with the same solvent.

Reference solution. Dissolve 10 mg of *atropine CRS* in *methanol R* and dilute to 10 ml with the same solvent.

Plate: *TLC silica gel plate R.*

Mobile phase: *concentrated ammonia R, water R, acetone R* (3:7:90 *V/V/V*).

Application: 10 µl.

Development: over half of the plate.

Drying: at 100-105 °C for 15 min.

Detection: after cooling, spray with *dilute potassium iodobismuthate solution R.*

Results: the principal spot in the chromatogram obtained with the test solution is similar in position, colour and size to the principal spot in the chromatogram obtained with the reference solution.

D. Place about 3 mg in a porcelain crucible and add 0.2 ml of *fuming nitric acid R*. Evaporate to dryness on a water-bath. Dissolve the residue in 0.5 ml of a 30 g/l solution of *potassium hydroxide R* in *methanol R*; a violet colour develops.

E. Optical rotation (see Tests).

TESTS

Optical rotation (*2.2.7*): – 0.70° to + 0.05° (measured in a 2 dm tube).

Dissolve 1.25 g in *ethanol (96 per cent) R* and dilute to 25.0 ml with the same solvent.

Related substances. Liquid chromatography (*2.2.29*).

Test solution. Dissolve 24 mg of the substance to be examined in mobile phase A and dilute to 100.0 ml with mobile phase A.

Reference solution (a). Dilute 1.0 ml of the test solution to 100.0 ml with mobile phase A. Dilute 1.0 ml of this solution to 10.0 ml with mobile phase A.

Reference solution (b). Dissolve 5 mg of *atropine impurity B CRS* in the test solution and dilute to 20 ml with the test solution. Dilute 5 ml of this solution to 25 ml with mobile phase A.

Reference solution (c). Dissolve 5 mg of *atropine for peak identification CRS* (containing impurities A, B, D, E, F, G and H) in mobile phase A and dilute to 20 ml with mobile phase A.

Reference solution (d). Dissolve 5 mg of *tropic acid R* (impurity C) in mobile phase A and dilute to 10 ml with mobile phase A. Dilute 1 ml of the solution to 100 ml with mobile phase A. Dilute 1 ml of this solution to 10 ml with mobile phase A.

Column:
- *size*: *l* = 0.10 m, Ø = 4.6 mm;
- *stationary phase*: *octadecylsilyl silica gel for chromatography R* (3 µm).

Mobile phase:
- *mobile phase A*: dissolve 3.5 g of *sodium dodecyl sulphate R* in 606 ml of a 7.0 g/l solution of *potassium dihydrogen phosphate R* previously adjusted to pH 3.3 with *0.05 M phosphoric acid,* and mix with 320 ml of *acetonitrile R1*;
- *mobile phase B*: *acetonitrile R1*;

Time (min)	Mobile phase A (per cent *V/V*)	Mobile phase B (per cent *V/V*)
0 - 2	95	5
2 - 20	95 → 70	5 → 30

Flow rate: 1 ml/min.

Detection: spectrophotometer at 210 nm.

Injection: 10 µl.

Identification of impurities: use the chromatogram supplied with *atropine for peak identification CRS* and the chromatogram obtained with reference solution (c) to identify the peaks due to impurities A, B, D, E, F, G and H. Use the chromatogram obtained with reference solution (d) to identify the peak due to impurity C.

Relative retention with reference to atropine (retention time = about 11 min): impurity C = about 0.2; impurity E = about 0.67; impurity D = about 0.73; impurity F = about 0.8; impurity B = about 0.89; impurity H = about 0.93; impurity G = about 1.1; impurity A = about 1.7.

System suitability: reference solution (b):
- *resolution*: minimum 2.5 between the peaks due to impurity B and atropine.

Limits:
- *correction factors*: for the calculation of content, multiply the peak areas of the following impurities by the corresponding correction factor: impurity A = 0.6; impurity C = 0.6;
- *impurities E, H*: for each impurity, not more than 3 times the area of the principal peak in the chromatogram obtained with reference solution (a) (0.3 per cent);
- *impurities A, B, C, D, F, G*: for each impurity, not more than twice the area of the principal peak in the chromatogram obtained with reference solution (a) (0.2 per cent);

Monographs A-C

- *unspecified impurities*: for each impurity, not more than the area of the principal peak in the chromatogram obtained with reference solution (a) (0.10 per cent);
- *total*: not more than 5 times the area of the principal peak in the chromatogram obtained with reference solution (a) (0.5 per cent);
- *disregard limit*: 0.5 times the area of the principal peak in the chromatogram obtained with reference solution (a) (0.05 per cent).

Loss on drying (*2.2.32*): maximum 0.2 per cent, determined on 1.000 g by drying in an oven at 105 °C for 2 h.

ASSAY

Dissolve 0.250 g in 40 ml of *anhydrous acetic acid R*, warming if necessary. Allow the solution to cool. Titrate with *0.1 M perchloric acid*, determining the end-point potentiometrically (*2.2.20*).

1 ml of *0.1 M perchloric acid* is equivalent to 28.94 mg of $C_{17}H_{23}NO_3$.

STORAGE

Protected from light.

IMPURITIES

Specified impurities: *A, B, C, D, E, F, G, H.*

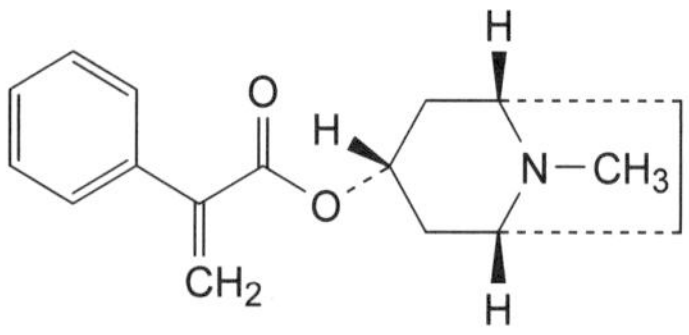

A. (1*R*,3*r*,5*S*)-8-methyl-8-azabicyclo[3.2.1]oct-3-yl 2-phenylpropenoate (apoatropine),

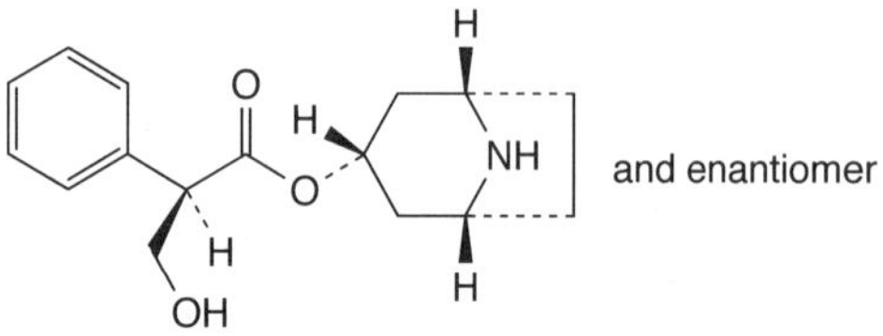

B. (1*R*,3*r*,5*S*)-8-azabicyclo[3.2.1]oct-3-yl (2*RS*)-3-hydroxy-2-phenylpropanoate (noratropine),

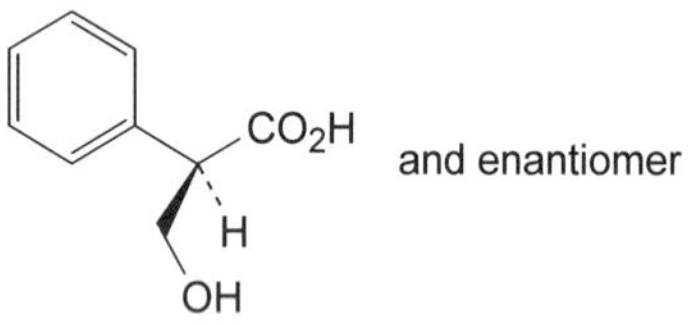

C. (2*RS*)-3-hydroxy-2-phenylpropanoic acid (tropic acid),

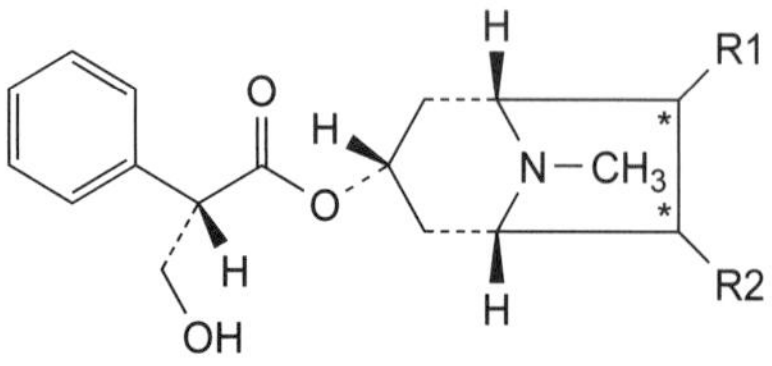

D. R1 = OH, R2 = H: (1*R*,3*S*,5*R*,6*RS*)-6-hydroxy-8-methyl-8-azabicyclo[3.2.1]oct-3-yl (2*S*)-3-hydroxy-2-phenylpropanoate (6-hydroxyhyoscyamine),

E. R1 = H, R2 = OH: (1*S*,3*R*,5*S*,6*RS*)-6-hydroxy-8-methyl-8-azabicyclo[3.2.1]oct-3-yl (2*S*)-3-hydroxy-2-phenylpropanoate (7-hydroxyhyoscyamine),

F. hyoscine,

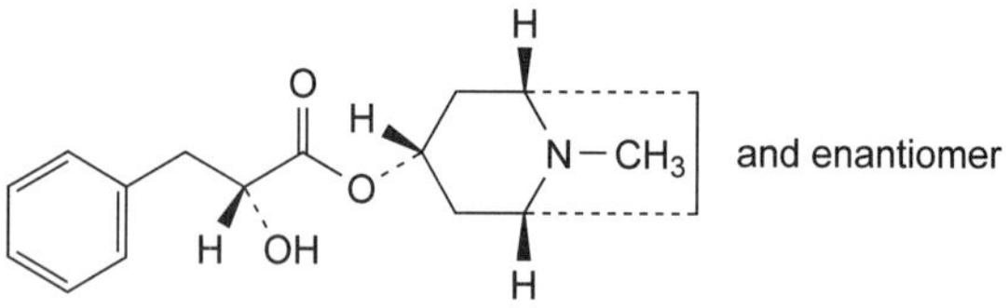

G. (1*R*,3*r*,5*S*)-8-methyl-8-azabicyclo[3.2.1]oct-3-yl (2*RS*)-2-hydroxy-3-phenylpropanoate (littorine),

H. unknown structure.

04/2008:0068

ATROPINE SULPHATE

Atropini sulfas

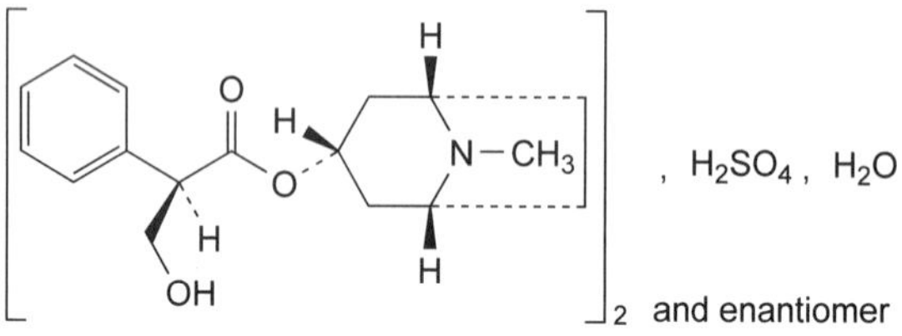

$C_{34}H_{48}N_2O_{10}S,H_2O$ M_r 695
[5908-99-6]

DEFINITION

Bis[(1*R*,3*r*,5*S*)-8-methyl-8-azabicyclo[3.2.1]oct-3-yl (2*RS*)-3-hydroxy-2-phenylpropanoate] sulphate monohydrate.

Content: 99.0 per cent to 101.0 per cent (anhydrous substance).

CHARACTERS

Appearance: white or almost white, crystalline powder or colourless crystals.

Solubility: very soluble in water, freely soluble in ethanol (96 per cent).

IDENTIFICATION

First identification: A, B, E.

Second identification: C, D, E, F.

A. Optical rotation (see Tests).

B. Infrared absorption spectrophotometry (*2.2.24*).

Comparison: *atropine sulphate CRS*.

C. Dissolve about 50 mg in 5 ml of *water R* and add 5 ml of *picric acid solution R*. The precipitate, washed with *water R* and dried at 100-105 °C for 2 h, melts (*2.2.14*) at 174 °C to 179 °C.

D. To about 1 mg add 0.2 ml of *fuming nitric acid R* and evaporate to dryness in a water-bath. Dissolve the residue in 2 ml of *acetone R* and add 0.1 ml of a 30 g/l solution of *potassium hydroxide R* in *methanol R*. A violet colour develops.

E. It gives the reactions of sulphates (*2.3.1*).

F. It gives the reaction of alkaloids (*2.3.1*).

TESTS

pH (*2.2.3*): 4.5 to 6.2.

Dissolve 0.6 g in *carbon dioxide-free water R* and dilute to 30 ml with the same solvent.

Optical rotation (*2.2.7*): – 0.50° to + 0.05° (measured in a 2 dm tube).

Dissolve 2.50 g in *water R* and dilute to 25.0 ml with the same solvent.

Related substances. Liquid chromatography (*2.2.29*).

Test solution. Dissolve 24 mg of the substance to be examined in mobile phase A and dilute to 100.0 ml with mobile phase A.

Reference solution (a). Dilute 1.0 ml of the test solution to 100.0 ml with mobile phase A. Dilute 1.0 ml of this solution to 10.0 ml with mobile phase A.

Reference solution (b). Dissolve 5 mg of *atropine impurity B CRS* in the test solution and dilute to 20 ml with the test solution. Dilute 5 ml of this solution to 25 ml with mobile phase A.

Reference solution (c). Dissolve 5 mg of *atropine for peak identification CRS* (containing impurities A, B, D, E, F, G and H) in mobile phase A and dilute to 20 ml with mobile phase A.

Reference solution (d). Dissolve 5 mg of *tropic acid R* (impurity C) in mobile phase A and dilute to 10 ml with mobile phase A. Dilute 1 ml of the solution to 100 ml with mobile phase A. Dilute 1 ml of this solution to 10 ml with mobile phase A.

Column:

- *size*: *l* = 0.10 m, Ø = 4.6 mm;
- *stationary phase*: *octadecylsilyl silica gel for chromatography R* (3 µm).

Mobile phase:

- *mobile phase A*: dissolve 3.5 g of *sodium dodecyl sulphate R* in 606 ml of a 7.0 g/l solution of *potassium dihydrogen phosphate R* previously adjusted to pH 3.3 with *0.05 M phosphoric acid,* and mix with 320 ml of *acetonitrile R1*;
- *mobile phase B*: *acetonitrile R1*;

Time (min)	Mobile phase A (per cent *V/V*)	Mobile phase B (per cent *V/V*)
0 - 2	95	5
2 - 20	95 → 70	5 → 30

Flow rate: 1 ml/min.

Detection: spectrophotometer at 210 nm.

Injection: 10 µl.

Identification of impurities: use the chromatogram supplied with *atropine for peak identification CRS* and the chromatogram obtained with reference solution (c) to identify the peaks due to impurities A, B, D, E, F, G and H. Use the chromatogram obtained with reference solution (d) to identify the peak due to impurity C.

Relative retention with reference to atropine (retention time = about 11 min): impurity C = about 0.2; impurity E = about 0.67; impurity D = about 0.73; impurity F = about 0.8; impurity B = about 0.89; impurity H = about 0.93; impurity G = about 1.1; impurity A = about 1.7.

System suitability: reference solution (b):

- *resolution*: minimum 2.5 between the peaks due to impurity B and atropine.

Limits:

- *correction factors*: for the calculation of content, multiply the peak areas of the following impurities by the corresponding correction factor: impurity A = 0.6; impurity C = 0.6;
- *impurities E, H*: for each impurity, not more than 3 times the area of the principal peak in the chromatogram obtained with reference solution (a) (0.3 per cent);
- *impurities A, B, C, D, F, G*: for each impurity, not more than twice the area of the principal peak in the chromatogram obtained with reference solution (a) (0.2 per cent);
- *unspecified impurities*: for each impurity, not more than the area of the principal peak in the chromatogram obtained with reference solution (a) (0.10 per cent);
- *total*: not more than 5 times the area of the principal peak in the chromatogram obtained with reference solution (a) (0.5 per cent);
- *disregard limit*: 0.5 times the area of the principal peak in the chromatogram obtained with reference solution (a) (0.05 per cent).

Water (*2.5.12*): 2.0 per cent to 4.0 per cent, determined on 0.500 g.

Sulphated ash (*2.4.14*): maximum 0.1 per cent, determined on 1.0 g.

ASSAY

Dissolve 0.500 g in 30 ml of *anhydrous acetic acid R,* warming if necessary. Cool the solution. Titrate with *0.1 M perchloric acid,* determining the end-point potentiometrically (*2.2.20*).

1 ml of *0.1 M perchloric acid* is equivalent to 67.68 mg of $C_{34}H_{48}N_2O_{10}S$.

STORAGE

Protected from light.

IMPURITIES

Specified impurities: A, B, C, D, E, F, G, H.

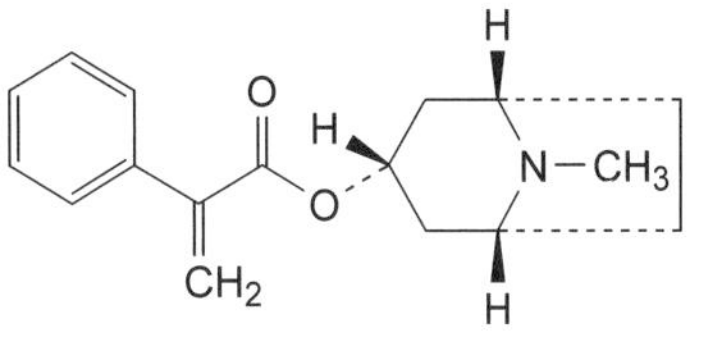

A. (1*R*,3*r*,5*S*)-8-methyl-8-azabicyclo[3.2.1]oct-3-yl 2-phenylpropenoate (apoatropine),

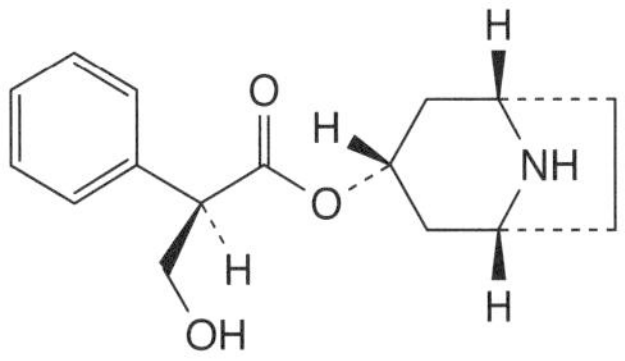

and enantiomer

B. (1*R*,3*r*,5*S*)-8-azabicyclo[3.2.1]oct-3-yl (2*RS*)-3-hydroxy-2-phenylpropanoate (noratropine),

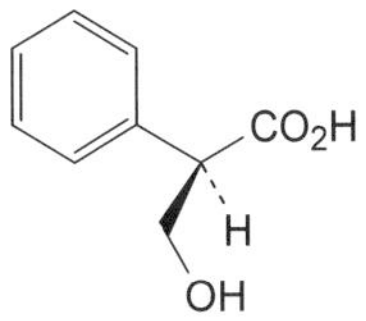

and enantiomer

C. (2*RS*)-3-hydroxy-2-phenylpropanoic acid (tropic acid),

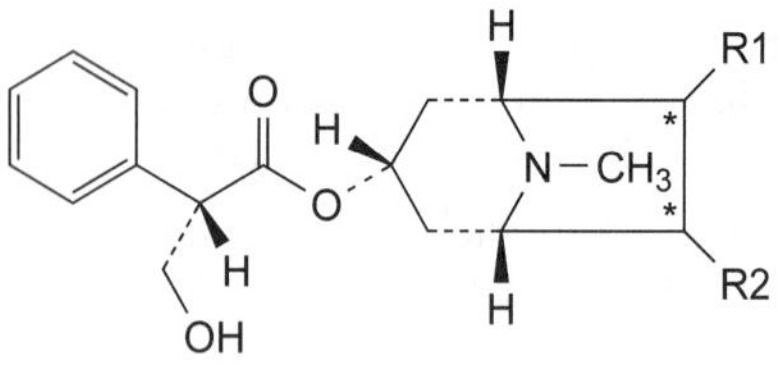

D. R1 = OH, R2 = H: (1*R*,3*S*,5*R*,6*RS*)-6-hydroxy-8-methyl-8-azabicyclo[3.2.1]oct-3-yl (2*S*)-3-hydroxy-2-phenylpropanoate (6-hydroxyhyoscyamine),

E. R1 = H, R2 = OH: (1*S*,3*R*,5*S*,6*RS*)-6-hydroxy-8-methyl-8-azabicyclo[3.2.1]oct-3-yl (2*S*)-3-hydroxy-2-phenylpropanoate (7-hydroxyhyoscyamine),

F. hyoscine,

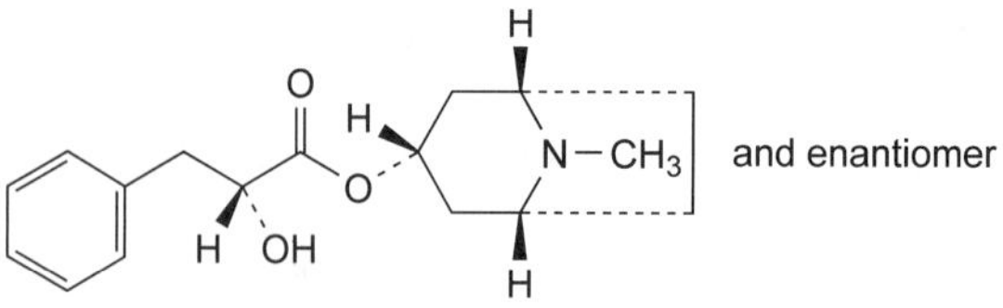

G. (1*R*,3*r*,5*S*)-8-methyl-8-azabicyclo[3.2.1]oct-3-yl (2*RS*)-2-hydroxy-3-phenylpropanoate (littorine).

H. unknown structure.

B

01/2008:0808
corrected 6.1

BACAMPICILLIN HYDROCHLORIDE

Bacampicillini hydrochloridum

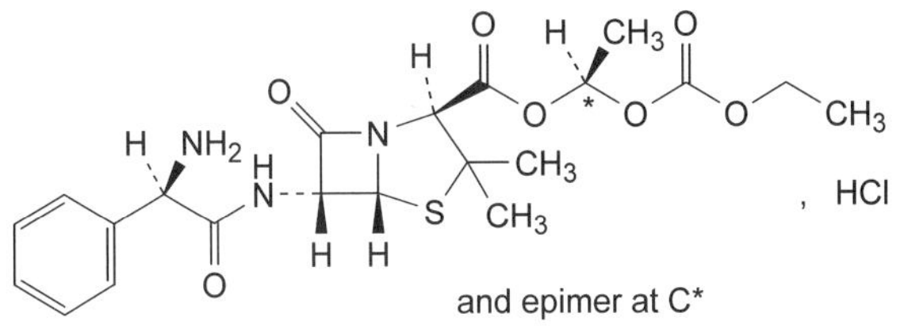

$C_{21}H_{28}ClN_3O_7S$ M_r 502.0

[37661-08-8]

DEFINITION

(1*RS*)-1-[(Ethoxycarbonyl)oxy]ethyl (2*S*,5*R*,6*R*)-6-[[(2*R*)-2-amino-2-phenylacetyl]amino]-3,3-dimethyl-7-oxo-4-thia-1-azabicyclo[3.2.0]heptane-2-carboxylate hydrochloride.

Semi-synthetic product derived from a fermentation product.

Content: 95.0 per cent to 102.0 per cent (anhydrous substance).

CHARACTERS

Appearance: white or almost white powder or granules, hygroscopic.

Solubility: soluble in water, freely soluble in ethanol (96 per cent), soluble in methylene chloride.

IDENTIFICATION

First identification: A, D.

Second identification: B, C, D.

A. Infrared absorption spectrophotometry (*2.2.24*).

Comparison: *bacampicillin hydrochloride CRS.*

B. Thin-layer chromatography (*2.2.27*).

Test solution. Dissolve 10 mg of the substance to be examined in 2 ml of *methanol R*.

Reference solution (a). Dissolve 10 mg of *bacampicillin hydrochloride CRS* in 2 ml of *methanol R*.

Reference solution (b). Dissolve 10 mg of *bacampicillin hydrochloride CRS*, 10 mg of *talampicillin hydrochloride CRS* and 10 mg of *pivampicillin CRS* in 2 ml of *methanol R*.

Plate: *TLC silanised silica gel plate R.*

Mobile phase: mix 10 volumes of a 272 g/l solution of *sodium acetate R* adjusted to pH 5.0 with *glacial acetic acid R*, 40 volumes of *water R* and 50 volumes of *ethanol (96 per cent) R*.

Application: 1 µl.

Development: over a path of 15 cm.

Drying: in a current of warm air.

Detection: spray with *ninhydrin solution R1* and heat at 60 °C for 10 min.

System suitability: reference solution (b):

– the chromatogram shows 3 clearly separated spots.

Results: the principal spot in the chromatogram obtained with the test solution is similar in position, colour and size to the principal spot in the chromatogram obtained with reference solution (a).

C. Place about 2 mg in a test-tube about 150 mm long and 15 mm in diameter. Moisten with 0.05 ml of *water R* and add 2 ml of *sulphuric acid-formaldehyde reagent R*. Mix the contents of the tube by swirling; the solution is practically colourless. Place the test-tube on a water-bath for 1 min; a dark yellow colour develops.

D. Dissolve about 25 mg in 2 ml of *water R*. Add 2 ml of *dilute sodium hydroxide solution R* and shake. Wait a few minutes and add 3 ml of *dilute nitric acid R* and 0.5 ml of *silver nitrate solution R1*. A white precipitate is formed. Add 0.5 ml of *concentrated ammonia R*. The precipitate dissolves.

TESTS

Appearance of solution. Dissolve 0.200 g in 20 ml of *water R*; the solution is not more opalescent than reference suspension II (*2.2.1*). Dissolve 0.500 g in 10 ml of *water R*; the absorbance (*2.2.25*) of the solution at 430 nm is not greater than 0.10.

pH (*2.2.3*): 3.0 to 4.5.

Dissolve 1.0 g in *carbon dioxide-free water R* and dilute to 50 ml with the same solvent.

Specific optical rotation (*2.2.7*): + 175 to + 195 (anhydrous substance).

Dissolve 0.250 g in *water R* and dilute to 25.0 ml with the same solvent.

Related substances. Liquid chromatography (*2.2.29*). *Prepare the test solution and reference solutions (a), (b) and (d) immediately before use.*

Phosphate buffer A. Dissolve 1.4 g of *sodium dihydrogen phosphate monohydrate R* in *water R* and dilute to about 800 ml with the same solvent. Adjust to pH 3.0 with *dilute phosphoric acid R* and dilute to 1000.0 ml with *water R*.

Phosphate buffer B. Dissolve 2.75 g of *sodium dihydrogen phosphate monohydrate R* and 2.3 g of *disodium hydrogen phosphate dihydrate R* in *water R* and dilute to about 1800 ml with the same solvent. Adjust to pH 6.8, if necessary, using *dilute phosphoric acid R* or *dilute sodium hydroxide solution R* and dilute to 2000.0 ml with *water R*.

Test solution. Dissolve 30.0 mg of the substance to be examined in phosphate buffer A and dilute to 100.0 ml with phosphate buffer A.

Reference solution (a). Dissolve 30.0 mg of *bacampicillin hydrochloride CRS* in phosphate buffer A and dilute to 100.0 ml with phosphate buffer A.

Reference solution (b). Dilute 1.0 ml of reference solution (a) to 100.0 ml with phosphate buffer A.

Reference solution (c). Dissolve 30 mg of the substance to be examined in phosphate buffer B and dilute to 100 ml with phosphate buffer B. Heat at 80 °C for about 30 min.

Reference solution (d). Dissolve 20 mg of *ampicillin trihydrate CRS* (impurity I) in phosphate buffer A and dilute to 250 ml with phosphate buffer A. Dilute 5 ml of this solution to 100 ml with phosphate buffer A.

Column:

– *size*: *l* = 0.05 m, Ø = 3.9 mm;

– *stationary phase*: *octadecylsilyl silica gel for chromatography R* (5 µm).

Mobile phase: mix 30 volumes of *acetonitrile R1* and 70 volumes of a 0.06 per cent *m/m* solution of *tetrahexylammonium hydrogen sulphate R* in phosphate buffer B.

Flow rate: 1.0 ml/min.

Detection: spectrophotometer at 220 nm.

Injection: 20 µl of the test solution and reference solutions (b), (c) and (d).

Run time: 3.5 times the retention time of bacampicillin.

Monographs A-C

System suitability:

- the peak due to impurity I is separated from the peaks due to the solvent in the chromatogram obtained with reference solution (d);
- *relative retention* with reference to bacampicillin: degradation product eluting just after bacampicillin = 1.12 to 1.38 in the chromatogram obtained with reference solution (c); if necessary, adjust the concentration of tetrahexylammonium hydrogen sulphate in the mobile phase.

Limits:

- *any impurity*: for each impurity, not more than 1.5 times the area of the principal peak in the chromatogram obtained with reference solution (b) (1.5 per cent);
- *total*: not more than 3 times the area of the principal peak in the chromatogram obtained with reference solution (b) (3 per cent);
- *disregard limit*: 0.1 times the area of the principal peak in the chromatogram obtained with reference solution (b) (0.1 per cent).

Butyl acetate and ethyl acetate (*2.4.24, System A*): maximum 2.0 per cent of butyl acetate, maximum 4.0 per cent of ethyl acetate and maximum 5.0 per cent for the sum of the contents.

Sample solution. Dissolve 50.0 mg of the substance to be examined in *water R* and dilute to 10.0 ml with the same solvent.

Use the method of standard additions.

Static head-space conditions that may be used:

- *equilibration temperature*: 60 °C;
- *equilibration time*: 20 min.

***N,N*-Dimethylaniline** (*2.4.26, Method A*): maximum 20 ppm.

Water (*2.5.12*): maximum 0.8 per cent, determined on 0.300 g.

Sulphated ash (*2.4.14*): maximum 1.5 per cent, determined on 1.0 g.

ASSAY

Liquid chromatography (*2.2.29*) as described in the test for related substances with the following modifications.

Injection: test solution and reference solution (a).

System suitability: reference solution (a):

- *repeatability*: maximum relative standard deviation of 1.0 per cent after 6 injections.

Calculate the percentage content of $C_{21}H_{28}ClN_3O_7S$ from the declared content of *bacampicillin hydrochloride CRS*.

STORAGE

In an airtight container.

IMPURITIES

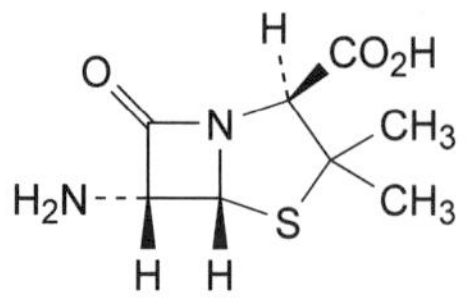

A. (2*S*,5*R*,6*R*)-6-amino-3,3-dimethyl-7-oxo-4-thia-1-azabicyclo-[3.2.0]heptane-2-carboxylic acid (6-aminopenicillanic acid),

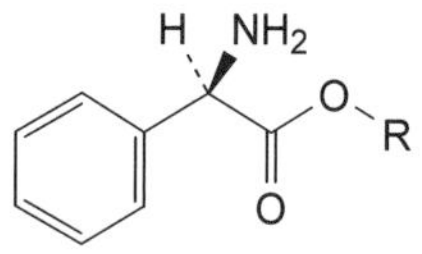

B. R = H: (2*R*)-2-amino-2-phenylacetic acid (D-phenylglycine),

G. R = CH_3: methyl (2*R*)-2-amino-2-phenylacetate (methyl D-phenylglycinate),

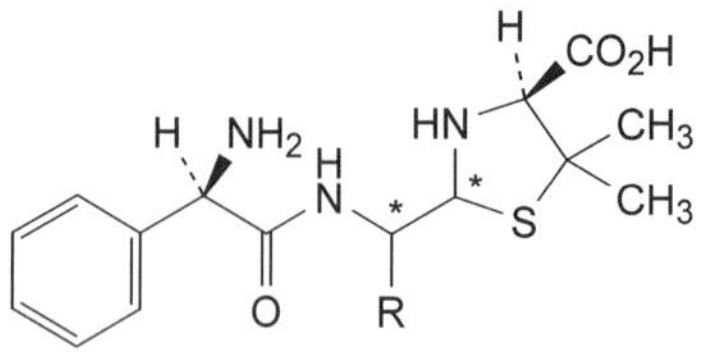

C. R = H: (2*RS*,4*S*)-2-[[[(2*R*)-2-amino-2-phenylacetyl]amino]-methyl]-5,5-dimethylthiazolidine-4-carboxylic acid (penilloic acids of ampicillin),

D. R = CO_2H: (4*S*)-2-[[[(2*R*)-2-amino-2-phenylacetyl]amino]-carboxymethyl]-5,5-dimethylthiazolidine-4-carboxylic acid (penicilloic acids of ampicillin),

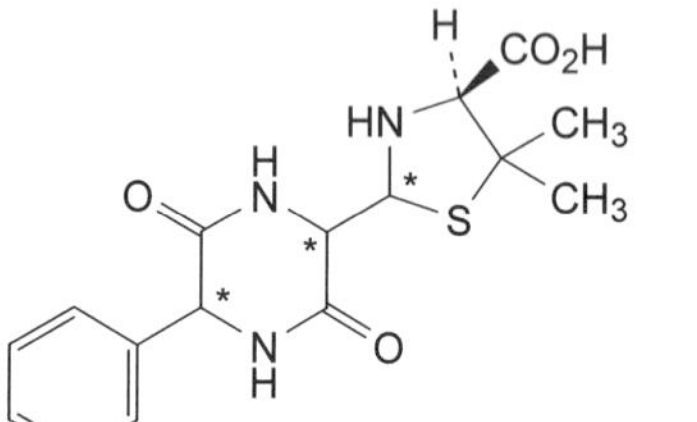

E. (4*S*)-2-(3,6-dioxo-5-phenylpiperazin-2-yl)-5,5-dimethylthia-zolidine-4-carboxylic acid (diketopiperazines of ampicillin),

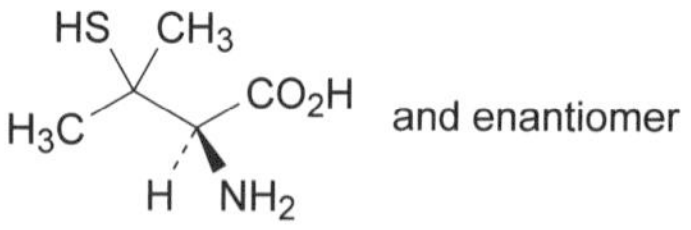

F. (2*RS*)-2-amino-3-methyl-3-sulphanylbutanoic acid (DL-penicillamine),

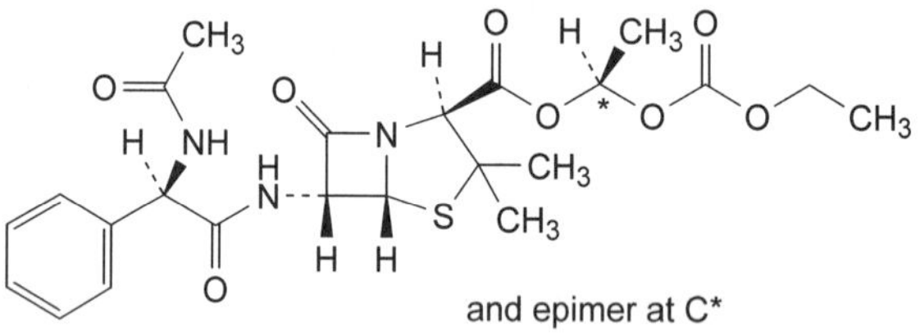

H. (1*RS*)-1-[(ethoxycarbonyl)oxy]ethyl (2*S*,5*R*,6*R*)-6-[[(2*R*)-2-(acetylamino)-2-phenylacetyl]amino]-3,3-dimethyl-7-oxo-4-thia-1-azabicyclo[3.2.0]heptane-2-carboxylate (*N*-acetylbacampicillin),

I. ampicillin.

04/2008:1054

BEARBERRY LEAF

Uvae ursi folium

DEFINITION

Whole or cut, dried leaf of *Arctostaphylos uva-ursi* (L.) Spreng.

Content: minimum 7.0 per cent of anhydrous arbutin ($C_{12}H_{16}O_7$; M_r 272.3) (dried drug).

IDENTIFICATION

A. The leaf, shiny and dark green on the adaxial surface, lighter on the abaxial surface, is normally 7-30 mm long and 5-12 mm wide. The entire leaf is obovate with smooth margins, somewhat reflexed downwards, narrowing at the base into a short petiole. The leaf is obtuse or retuse at its apex. The lamina is thick and coriaceous. The venation, pinnate and finely reticulate, is clearly visible on both surfaces. The adaxial surface is marked with sunken veinlets, giving it a characteristic grainy appearance. Only the young leaf has ciliated margins. Old leaves are glabrous.

B. Reduce to a powder (355) (*2.9.12*). The powder is green to greenish-grey or yellowish-green. Examine under a microscope using *chloral hydrate solution R*. The powder shows the following diagnostic characters: fragments of epidermises, which, seen in surface view, show polygonal cells covered by a thick smooth cuticle, and with straight, thick and irregularly pitted walls; anomocytic stomata (*2.8.3*), surrounded by 5-11 subsidiary cells and scars of hair bases only on the abaxial epidermis; fragments of palisade parenchyma, with 3 or 4 layers of cells of unequal lengths, and spongy parenchyma; groups of lignified fibres from the pericycle, with rows of cells containing prisms of calcium oxalate; occasional conical, unicellular covering trichomes.

C. Thin-layer chromatography (*2.2.27*).

Test solution. To 0.5 g of the powdered drug (355) (*2.9.12*) add 5 ml of a mixture of equal volumes of *methanol R* and *water R*, and heat under a reflux condenser for 10 min. Filter whilst hot. Wash the flask and the filter with a mixture of equal volumes of *methanol R* and *water R* and dilute to 5 ml with the same mixture of solvents.

Reference solution. Dissolve 25 mg of *arbutin R*, 25 mg of *gallic acid R* and 25 mg of *hydroquinone R* in *methanol R* and dilute to 10.0 ml with the same solvent.

Plate: *TLC silica gel G plate R.*

Mobile phase: *anhydrous formic acid R, water R, ethyl acetate R* (6:6:88 *V/V/V*).

Application: 10 µl of the reference solution and 20 µl of the test solution, as bands.

Development: over a path of 15 cm.

Drying: at 105-110 °C until the mobile phase has evaporated.

Detection: spray with a 10 g/l solution of *dichloroquinonechlorimide R* in *methanol R*, then spray with a 20 g/l solution of *anhydrous sodium carbonate R*.

Results: see below the sequence of zones present in the chromatograms obtained with the reference solution and the test solution. Furthermore, 2 or 3 blue bands and several brown or brownish-grey bands may be present in the chromatogram obtained with the test solution.

Top of the plate	
Hydroquinone: a blue zone	A blue zone
Gallic acid: a brownish zone	A brownish zone
_______	_______
_______	_______
Arbutin: a light blue zone	A light blue zone (arbutin)
Reference solution	**Test solution**

TESTS

Foreign matter (*2.8.2*): maximum 5 per cent of stems and maximum 3 per cent of other foreign matter.

Leaves of different colour: maximum 10 per cent, determined in the same manner as foreign matter (*2.8.2*).

Loss on drying (*2.2.32*): maximum 10.0 per cent, determined on 1.000 g of the powdered drug (355) (*2.9.12*) by drying in an oven at 105 °C for 2 h.

Total ash (*2.4.16*): maximum 5.0 per cent.

ASSAY

Liquid chromatography (*2.2.29*).

Test solution. In a 100 ml flask with a ground-glass neck, place 0.800 g of the powdered drug (250) (*2.9.12*). Add 20 ml of *water R* and heat under a reflux condenser on a water-bath for 30 min. Allow to cool and filter the liquid through a plug of absorbent cotton. Add the absorbent cotton to the residue in the 100 ml flask and extract with 20 ml of *water R* under a reflux condenser on a water-bath for 30 min. Allow to cool and filter through a paper filter. Combine the filtrates and dilute to 50.0 ml with *water R*. Filter the liquid through a paper filter. Discard the first 10 ml of the filtrate.

Reference solution (a). Dissolve 50.0 mg of *arbutin CRS* in the mobile phase and dilute to 50.0 ml with the mobile phase.

Reference solution (b). Dissolve 2.5 mg of *hydroquinone R* in the mobile phase and dilute to 10.0 ml with the mobile phase. To 5.0 ml of this solution add 2.5 ml of reference solution (a) and dilute to 10.0 ml with the mobile phase.

Column:

- *size*: l = 0.25 m, Ø = 4 mm;
- *stationary phase*: *base-deactivated octadecylsilyl silica gel for chromatography R* (5 µm).

Mobile phase: *methanol R, water R* (10:90 *V/V*).

Flow rate: 1.2 ml/min.

Detection: spectrophotometer at 280 nm.

Injection: 20 µl.

System suitability:

- *resolution*: minimum 4.0 between the peaks due to arbutin and hydroquinone in the chromatogram obtained with reference solution (b).

Calculate the percentage content of arbutin using the following expression:

$$\frac{F_1 \times m_2 \times p}{F_2 \times m_1}$$

F_1 = area of the peak due to arbutin in the chromatogram obtained with the test solution;

F_2 = area of the peak due to arbutin in the chromatogram obtained with the reference solution;

m_1 = mass of the drug to be examined used to prepare the test solution, in grams;

m_2 = mass of *arbutin CRS* used to prepare the reference solution, in grams;

p = percentage content of arbutin in *arbutin CRS*.

01/2008:1602
corrected 6.1

BILBERRY FRUIT, FRESH

Myrtilli fructus recens

DEFINITION

Fresh or frozen, ripe fruit of *Vaccinium myrtillus* L.

Content: minimum 0.30 per cent of anthocyanins, expressed as cyanidin 3-*O*-glucoside chloride (chrysanthemin, $C_{21}H_{21}ClO_{11}$; M_r 484.8) (dried drug).

CHARACTERS

Sweet and slightly astringent taste.

IDENTIFICATION

A. The fresh fruit is a blackish-blue globular berry about 5 mm in diameter. Its lower end shows a scar or, rarely, a fragment of the pedicel. The upper end is flattened and surmounted by the remains of the persistent style and of the calyx, which appears as a circular fold. The violet, fleshy mesocarp includes 4 to 5 locules containing numerous small, brown, ovoid seeds.

B. The crushed fresh fruit is violet-red. Examine under a microscope using *chloral hydrate solution R*. It shows violet-pink sclereids from the endocarp and the mesocarp, usually aggregated, with thick, channelled walls; reddish-brown fragments of the epicarp consisting of polygonal cells with moderately thickened walls; brownish-yellow fragments of the outer layer of the testa composed of elongated cells with U-shaped thickened walls; cluster crystals of calcium oxalate.

C. Thin-layer chromatography (*2.2.27*).

Test solution. To 5 g of the freshly crushed drug, add 20 ml of *methanol R*. Stir for 15 min and filter.

Reference solution. Dissolve 5 mg of *chrysanthemin R* in 10 ml of *methanol R*.

Plate: *TLC silica gel plate R*.

Mobile phase: *anhydrous formic acid R, water R, butanol R* (16:19:65 *V/V/V*).

Application: 10 µl, as bands.

Development: over a path of 10 cm.

Drying: in air.

Detection: examine in daylight.

Results: see below the sequence of the zones present in the chromatograms obtained with the reference solution and the test solution.

Top of the plate	
	A violet-red zone
Chrysanthemin: a violet-red zone	A principal violet-red zone
	A compact set of other principal zones: – a violet-red zone – several violet-blue zones
Reference solution	**Test solution**

TESTS

Total ash (*2.4.16*): maximum 0.6 per cent.

Loss on drying (*2.2.32*): 80.0 per cent to 90.0 per cent, determined on 5.000 g of the freshly crushed drug by drying in an oven at 105 °C.

ASSAY

Crush 50 g extemporaneously. To about 5.00 g of the crushed, accurately weighed drug, add 95 ml of *methanol R*. Stir mechanically for 30 min. Filter into a 100.0 ml volumetric flask. Rinse the filter and dilute to 100.0 ml with *methanol R*. Prepare a 50-fold dilution of this solution in a 0.1 per cent *V/V* solution of *hydrochloric acid R* in *methanol R*.

Measure the absorbance (*2.2.25*) of the solution at 528 nm, using a 0.1 per cent *V/V* solution of *hydrochloric acid R* in *methanol R* as the compensation liquid.

Calculate the percentage content of anthocyanins, expressed as cyanidin 3-*O*-glucoside chloride, using the following expression:

$$\frac{A \times 5000}{718 \times m}$$

718 = specific absorbance of cyanidin 3-*O*-glucoside chloride at 528 nm;

A = absorbance at 528 nm;

m = mass of the substance to be examined in grams.

STORAGE

When frozen, store at or below – 18 °C.

04/2008:1710

BISOPROLOL FUMARATE

Bisoprololi fumaras

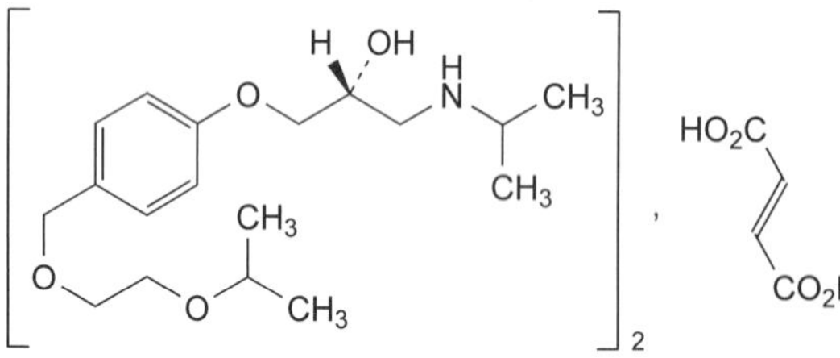

and enantiomer

$C_{40}H_{66}N_2O_{12}$ M_r 767
[66722-44-9]

DEFINITION

(*RS*)-1-[4-[[2-(1-Methylethoxy)ethoxy]methyl]phenoxy]-3-[(1-methylethyl)amino]propan-2-ol fumarate.

Content: 99.0 per cent to 101.0 per cent (anhydrous substance).

CHARACTERS

Appearance: white or almost white, slightly hygroscopic powder.

Solubility: very soluble in water, freely soluble in methanol.

It shows polymorphism (*5.9*).

IDENTIFICATION

Infrared absorption spectrophotometry (*2.2.24*).

Comparison: *bisoprolol fumarate CRS*.

If the spectra obtained in the solid state show differences, dissolve the substance to be examined and the reference substance separately in *methanol R*, evaporate and dry the residue at 60 °C at a pressure not exceeding 700 Pa and record new spectra using the residues.

TESTS

Related substances.

A. Impurities A and E. Liquid chromatography (*2.2.29*).

Test solution. Dissolve 25 mg of the substance to be examined in mobile phase A and dilute to 25.0 ml with mobile phase A.

Reference solution (a). Dilute 1.0 ml of the test solution to 100.0 ml with mobile phase A. Dilute 1.0 ml of this solution to 10.0 ml with mobile phase A.

Reference solution (b). Dissolve the contents of a vial of *bisoprolol for system suitability method A CRS* (containing impurities A, B and E) in 1.0 ml of mobile phase A.

Column:

- *size*: *l* = 0.25 m, Ø = 4.6 mm;
- *stationary phase*: *octadecylsilyl silica gel for chromatography R* (5 µm);
- *temperature*: 30 °C.

Mobile phase:

- *mobile phase A*: mix 10 volumes of *acetonitrile R1* and 90 volumes of a solution containing 0.4 ml/l of *triethylamine R1* and 3.12 g/l of *sodium dihydrogen phosphate R*, previously adjusted to pH 4.2 with *dilute phosphoric acid R*;
- *mobile phase B*: mix 25 volumes of a solution containing 0.4 ml/l of *triethylamine R1* and 3.12 g/l of *sodium dihydrogen phosphate R*, previously adjusted to pH 4.2 with *dilute phosphoric acid R* and 75 volumes of *acetonitrile R1*;

Time (min)	Mobile phase A (per cent *V/V*)	Mobile phase B (per cent *V/V*)
0 - 40	95 → 10	5 → 90
40 - 45	10	90
45 - 50	10 → 95	90 → 5
50 - 60	95	5

Flow rate: 1.0 ml/min.

Detection: spectrophotometer at 225 nm.

Injection: 10 µl.

Identification of impurities: use the chromatogram supplied with *bisoprolol for system suitability method A CRS* and the chromatogram obtained with reference solution (b) to identify the peaks due to fumaric acid and impurities A, B and E.

Relative retention with reference to bisoprolol (retention time = about 14.5 min): impurity A = about 0.25; impurity G = about 1.05; impurity B = about 1.1; impurity E = about 1.3.

System suitability: reference solution (b):

- *resolution*: minimum 5.0 between the peaks due to bisoprolol and impurity B.

Limits:

- *impurity A*: not more than 3 times the area of the principal peak in the chromatogram obtained with reference solution (a) (0.3 per cent);
- *impurity E*: not more than twice the area of the principal peak in the chromatogram obtained with reference solution (a) (0.2 per cent);
- *unspecified impurities*: for each impurity, not more than the area of the principal peak in the chromatogram obtained with reference solution (a) (0.10 per cent);
- *total*: not more than 3 times the area of the principal peak in the chromatogram obtained with reference solution (a) (0.3 per cent);
- *disregard limit*: 0.5 times the area of the principal peak in the chromatogram obtained with reference solution (a) (0.05 per cent); disregard the peak due to fumaric acid and any peak due to impurity G.

B. Impurities A and G. Liquid chromatography (*2.2.29*).

Solvent mixture: *acetonitrile R1, water for chromatography R* (20:80 *V/V*).

Test solution. Dissolve 25 mg of the substance to be examined in the solvent mixture and dilute to 25.0 ml with the solvent mixture.

Reference solution (a). Dilute 1.0 ml of the test solution to 100.0 ml with the solvent mixture. Dilute 2.0 ml of this solution to 10.0 ml with the solvent mixture.

Reference solution (b). Dissolve the contents of a vial of *bisoprolol for system suitability method B CRS* (containing impurities A and G) in 1.0 ml of the solvent mixture.

Column:

- *size*: *l* = 0.25 m, Ø = 4.6 mm;
- *stationary phase*: *octadecylsilyl silica gel for chromatography R* (5 µm);
- *temperature*: 30 °C.

Mobile phase:

- *mobile phase A*: 10 g/l solution of *phosphoric acid R*;
- *mobile phase B*: 10 g/l solution of *phosphoric acid R* in *acetonitrile R1*;

Time (min)	Mobile phase A (per cent *V/V*)	Mobile phase B (per cent *V/V*)
0 - 35	90 → 20	10 → 80
35 - 40	20 → 90	80 → 10
40 - 50	90	10

Flow rate: 1.0 ml/min.

Detection: spectrophotometer at 225 nm.

Injection: 10 µl.

Identification of impurities: use the chromatogram supplied with *bisoprolol for system suitability method B CRS* and the chromatogram obtained with reference solution (b) to identify the peaks due to fumaric acid and impurities A and G.

Relative retention with reference to bisoprolol (retention time = about 13.4 min): impurity A = about 0.4; impurity G = about 1.02; impurity E = about 1.2.

System suitability: reference solution (b):

- *peak-to-valley ratio*: minimum 2.5, where H_p = height above the baseline of the peak due to impurity G, and H_v = height above the baseline of the lowest point of the curve separating this peak from the peak due to bisoprolol.

Limits:

- *impurity G*: not more than 2.5 times the area of the principal peak in the chromatogram obtained with reference solution (a) (0.5 per cent);
- *impurity A*: not more than 1.5 times the area of the principal peak in the chromatogram obtained with reference solution (a) (0.3 per cent);
- *unspecified impurities*: for each impurity, not more than 0.5 times the area of the principal peak in the chromatogram obtained with reference solution (a) (0.10 per cent);
- *total*: not more than 2.5 times the area of the principal peak in the chromatogram obtained with reference solution (a) (0.5 per cent);
- *disregard limit*: 0.25 times the area of the principal peak in the chromatogram obtained with reference solution (a) (0.05 per cent); disregard the peak due to fumaric acid and any peak due to impurity E.

Water (*2.5.12*): maximum 0.5 per cent, determined on 1.000 g.

Sulphated ash (*2.4.14*): maximum 0.1 per cent, determined on 1.0 g.

ASSAY

Dissolve 0.300 g in 50 ml of *anhydrous acetic acid R*. Titrate with *0.1 M perchloric acid,* determining the end-point potentiometrically (*2.2.20*).

1 ml of *0.1 M perchloric acid* is equivalent to 38.35 mg of $C_{40}H_{66}N_2O_{12}$.

STORAGE

In an airtight container, protected from light.

IMPURITIES

Specified impurities: A, E, G.

Other detectable impurities (the following substances would, if present at a sufficient level, be detected by one or other of the tests in the monograph. They are limited by the general acceptance criterion for other/unspecified impurities and/or by the general monograph *Substances for pharmaceutical use (2034).* It is therefore not necessary to identify these impurities for demonstration of compliance. See also *5.10. Control of impurities in substances for pharmaceutical use*):

- *by method A: B, C, D, F;*
- *by method B: B, K, L, N, Q, R, S, T, U.*

Monographs A-C

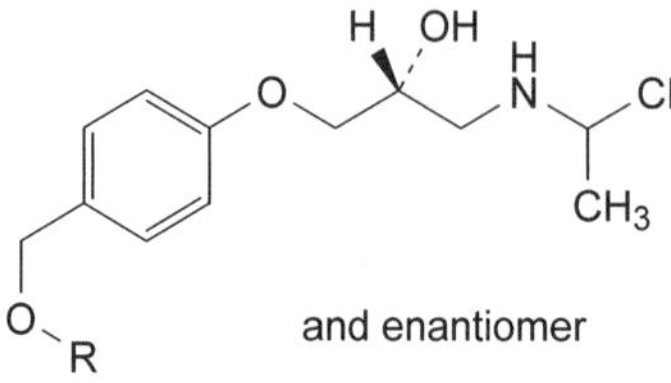

A. R = H: (*RS*)-1-(4-hydroxymethyl-phenoxy)-3-isopropylaminopropan-2-ol,

B. R = CH_2-CH_2-O-[CH_2]$_2$-CH_3: (*RS*)-1-isopropylamino-3-[4-(2-propoxy-ethoxymethyl)phenoxy]propan-2-ol,

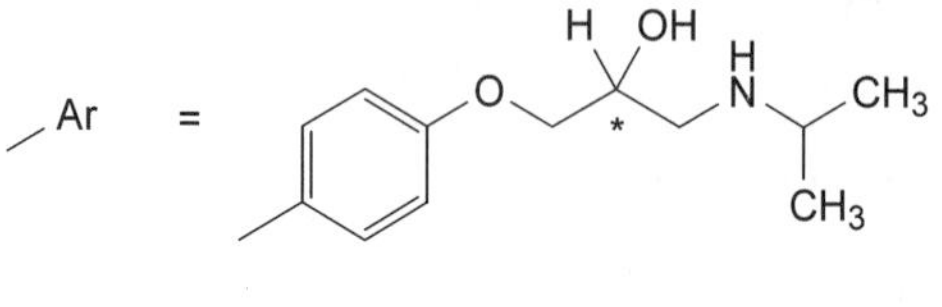

C. Ar-CH_2-Ar: (*RS*)-1-[4-[4-(2-hydroxy-3-isopropylamino-propoxy)benzyl]phenoxy]-3-isopropylaminopropan-2-ol,

D. Ar-CH_2-O-CH_2-Ar: (*RS*)-1-[4-[4-(2-hydroxy-3-isopropylaminopropoxy)benzyloxylmethyl]phenoxy]-3-isopropylaminopropan-2-ol,

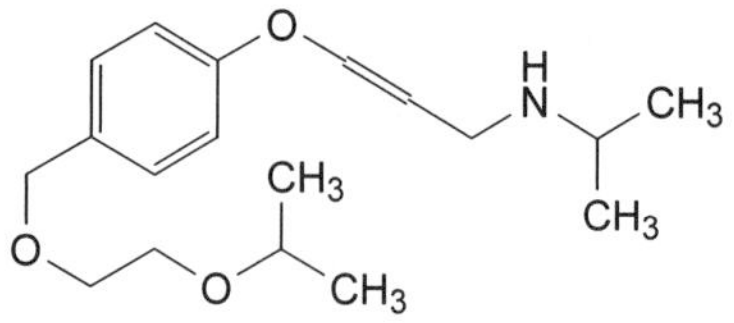

E. (*EZ*)-[3-[4-(2-isopropoxy-ethoxymethyl)phenoxy]allyl] isopropylamine,

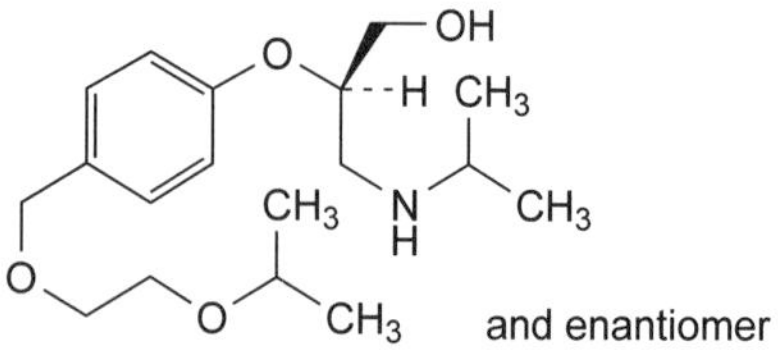

F. (*RS*)-2-[4-(2-isopropoxy-ethoxymethyl)phenoxy]-3-isopropylaminopropan-2-ol,

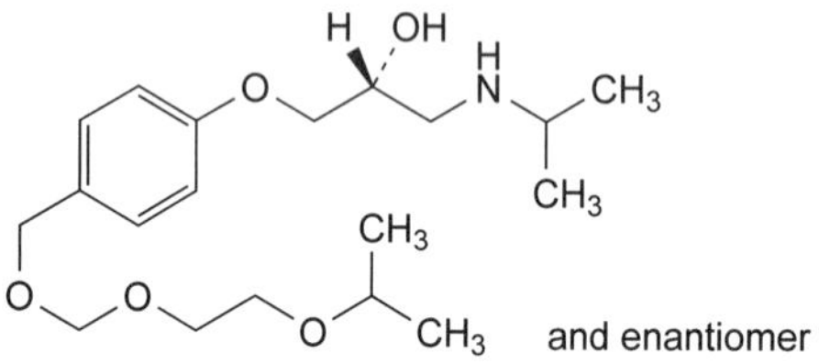

G. (2*RS*)-1-[4-[[(2-isopropoxyethoxy)methoxy]methyl] phenoxy]-3-isopropylaminopropan-2-ol,

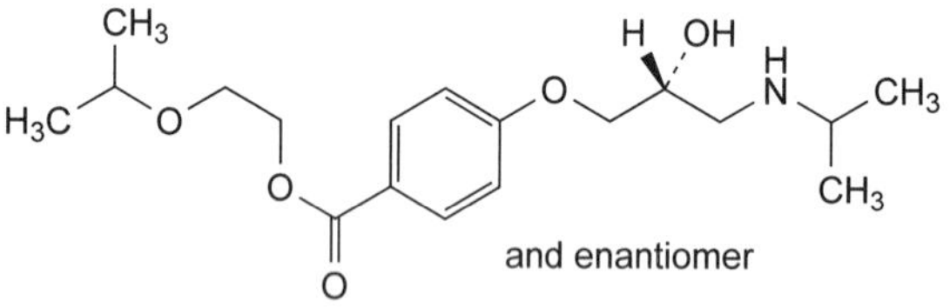

K. 2-isopropoxyethyl 4-[[(2*RS*)-2-hydroxy-3-(isopropylamino)propyl]oxy]benzoate,

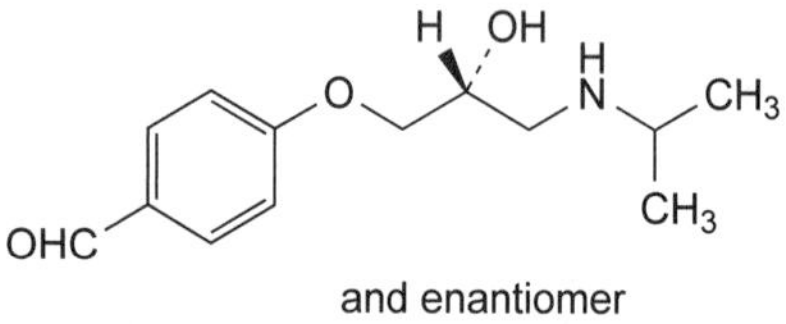

L. 4-[[(2*RS*)-2-hydroxy-3-(isopropylamino)propyl]oxy]-benzaldehyde,

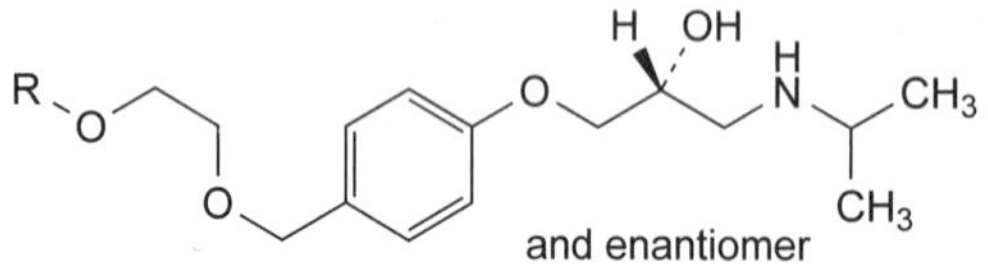

N. R = C_2H_5: [(2*RS*)-1-[4-[(2-ethoxyethoxy)methyl]phenoxy]-3-isopropylaminopropan-2-ol,

Q. R = CH_3: (2*RS*)-1-(isopropylamino)-3-[4-(2-methoxyethoxy)methyl]phenoxypropan-2-ol,

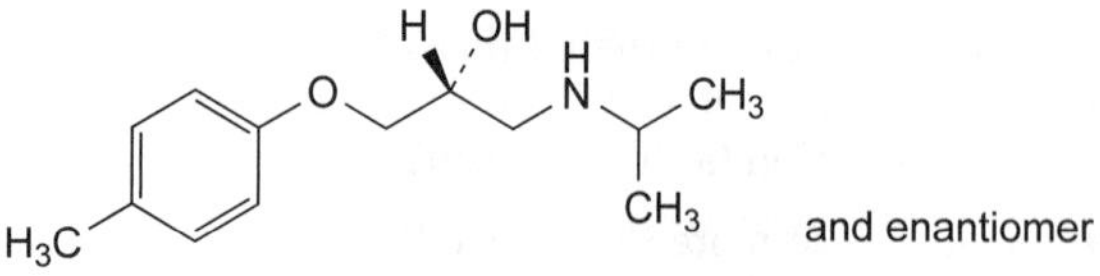

R. (2*RS*)-1-(isopropylamino)-3-(4-methylphenoxy)propan-2-ol,

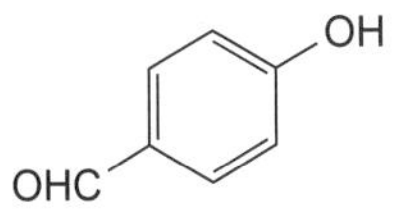

S. 4-hydroxybenzaldehyde,

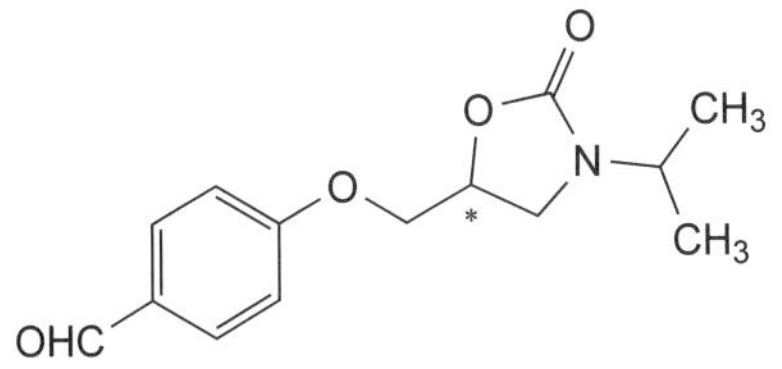

T. 4-[(3-isopropyl-2-oxo-1,3-oxazolidin-5-yl)methoxy]-benzaldehyde,

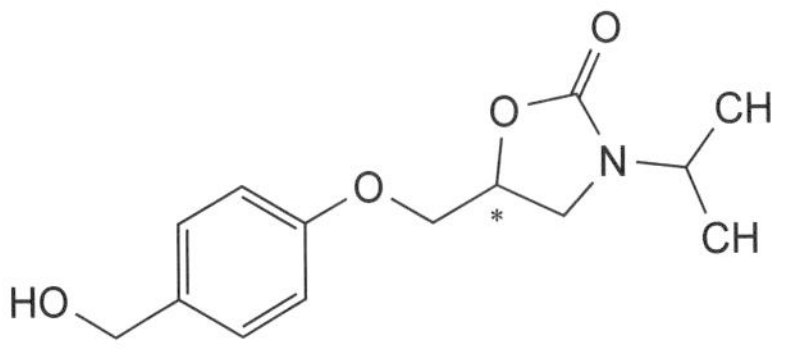

U. 5-[[4-(hydroxymethyl)phenoxy]methyl]-3-isopropyl-1,3-oxazolidin-2-one.

04/2008:1816

BOLDO LEAF DRY EXTRACT

Boldi folii extractum siccum

DEFINITION

Extract produced from *Boldo leaf (1396).*

Content:

- *for aqueous extracts*: minimum 0.5 per cent of total alkaloids, expressed as boldine ($C_{19}H_{21}NO_4$; M_r 327.4) (dried extract);
- *for hydroalcoholic extracts*: minimum 1.0 per cent of total alkaloids, expressed as boldine ($C_{19}H_{21}NO_4$; M_r 327.4) (dried extract).

PRODUCTION

The extract is produced from the herbal drug by a suitable procedure using either hot water at not less than 65 °C or a hydroalcoholic solvent equivalent in strength to ethanol (45-75 per cent *V/V*).

CHARACTERS

Appearance: brown or greenish-brown, hygroscopic powder.

IDENTIFICATION

Thin-layer chromatography (*2.2.27*).

Test solution. To 0.5 g of the extract to be examined add 1 ml of *hydrochloric acid R* and 20 ml of *water R*. Sonicate for 10 min. Transfer the liquid to a separating funnel and make alkaline with 2 ml of *dilute ammonia R1*. Shake with 2 quantities, each of 20 ml, of *methylene chloride R*. Evaporate the combined organic layers to dryness. Dissolve the residue in 1 ml of *methanol R*.

Reference solution. Dissolve 2 mg of *boldine R* and 10 mg of *hyoscine hydrobromide R* in 5 ml of *methanol R*.

Plate: *TLC silica gel plate R* (5-40 µm) [or *TLC silica gel plate R* (2-10 µm)].

Mobile phase: *diethylamine R, methanol R, toluene R* (10:10:80 *V/V/V*).

Application: 20 µl [or 3 µl], as bands of 15 mm [or 8 mm].

Development: over a path of 15 cm [or 6 cm].

Drying: in air.

Detection: spray with *potassium iodobismuthate solution R2*, allow to dry in air for 5 min and spray with *sodium nitrite solution R*; examine in daylight after 30 min.

Results: see below the sequence of zones present in the chromatograms obtained with the reference solution and the test solution. Furthermore, other faint zones may be present in the chromatogram obtained with the test solution.

Top of the plate	
———	———
	A yellowish-brown zone
	An orange-yellow zone
Hyoscine: a pale brown zone	
	An orange zone
	An orange zone
———	———
Boldine: a brown zone	A brown zone (boldine)
	Several orange zones
Reference solution	**Test solution**

ASSAY

Liquid chromatography (*2.2.29*).

Test solution. To 1.000 g of the extract to be examined add 50 ml of *dilute hydrochloric acid R* and sonicate for 10 min. Transfer to a separating funnel and wash with 10 ml of a mixture of equal volumes of *ethyl acetate R* and *hexane R*. Adjust the aqueous phase to pH 9.5 with *dilute ammonia R1*. After cooling, shake successively with 100 ml, 50 ml, and a further 50 ml of *methylene chloride R*, taking care not to form an emulsion. Evaporate the combined lower layers to dryness under reduced pressure. Dissolve the residue in the mobile phase and transfer the solution to a volumetric flask. Rinse and dilute to 10.0 ml with the mobile phase.

Reference solution. Dissolve 12.0 mg of *boldine CRS* in the mobile phase and dilute to 100.0 ml with the mobile phase.

Column:

- *size*: *l* = 0.25 m, Ø = 4.6 mm;
- *stationary phase*: *octadecylsilyl silica gel for chromatography R* (5 µm).

Solution A. Mix 0.2 ml of *diethylamine R* with 99.8 ml of *acetonitrile R*.

Solution B. Mix 0.2 ml of *diethylamine R* with 99.8 ml of *water R* and adjust to pH 3 with *anhydrous formic acid R*.

Mobile phase: solution A, solution B (16:84 *V/V*).

Flow rate: 1.5 ml/min.

Detection: spectrophotometer at 304 nm.

Injection: 20 µl.

Relative retention with reference to boldine (retention time = about 6 min): isoboldine = about 0.9; isocorydine *N*-oxide = about 1.8; laurotetanine = about 2.2; isocorydine = about 2.8; *N*-methyllaurotetanine = about 3.2. Additional peaks may be present.

System suitability: test solution:

- *resolution*: minimum 1.0 between the peaks due to isoboldine and boldine.

Calculate the percentage content of total alkaloids, expressed as boldine, using the following expression:

$$\frac{(\sum A_1) \times m_2 \times p}{A_2 \times m_1 \times 10}$$

ΣA_1 = sum of the areas of the peaks due to the 6 alkaloids identified in the chromatogram obtained with the test solution;

A_2 = area of the peak due to boldine in the chromatogram obtained with the reference solution;

m_1 = mass of the extract to be examined used to prepare the test solution, in grams;

m_2 = mass of *boldine CRS* used to prepare the reference solution, in grams;

p = percentage content of boldine in *boldine CRS*.

04/2008:1847

BUTCHER'S BROOM

Rusci rhizoma

DEFINITION

Dried, whole or fragmented underground parts of *Ruscus aculeatus* L.

Content: minimum 1.0 per cent of total sapogenins, expressed as ruscogenins [mixture of neoruscogenin ($C_{27}H_{40}O_4$; M_r 428.6) and ruscogenin ($C_{27}H_{42}O_4$; M_r 430.6)] (dried drug).

IDENTIFICATION

A. The rhizome consists of yellowish, branched, articulated, somewhat knotty pieces, cylindrical or subconical, about 5-10 cm long and about 5 mm thick. The surface is marked with thin annulations about 1-3 mm wide, separated from one another; rounded scars of the aerial stems are present on the upper surface. On the lower surface numerous roots, or their scars, occur; the roots are about 2 mm in diameter and similar in colour to the rhizome. The outer layer is easily detached, revealing a yellowish-white, very hard central cylinder.

B. Reduce to a powder (355) (*2.9.12*). The powder is yellowish. Examine under a microscope using *chloral hydrate solution R*. The powder shows groups of sclereids of the rhizome, variously-shaped cells, ranging from rounded to elongated or rectangular; the walls are moderately thickened and distinctly beaded, with large, rounded to oval pits. Fragments of the endodermis composed of a single layer of irregularly-thickened cells. Groups of rounded parenchymatous cells, thickened at the corners, with small, triangular intercellular spaces; thin-walled parenchyma containing raphides of calcium oxalate. Groups of thick-walled fibres and small vessels, up to about 50 µm in diameter, the walls showing numerous small, slit-shaped pits.

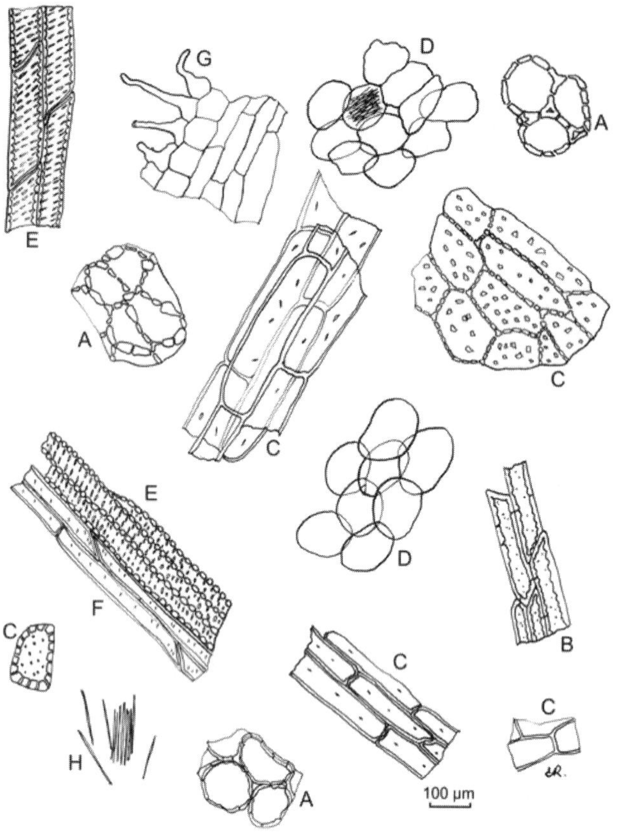

A. Thick-walled parenchymatous cells
B. Endodermis fragment
C. Variously-shaped sclereid cells
D. Parenchyma, some cells of which contain raphides of calcium oxalate
E. Small vessels sometimes accompanied by fibres (F)
F. Thick-walled fibres
G. Dermal tissue of the root
H. Raphides of calcium oxalate
I. Thin-walled parenchyma

Figure 1847.-1. – *Illustration of powdered herbal drug of butcher's broom (see Identification B)*

C. Thin-layer chromatography (*2.2.27*)

Test solution. Introduce 1.0 g of the powdered drug (355) (*2.9.12*) and 50 ml of *dilute hydrochloric acid R* into a 100 ml flask with a ground-glass neck. Heat on a water-bath under a reflux condenser for 40 min. Allow to cool and extract the unfiltered mixture with 3 quantities, each of 25 ml, of *methylene chloride R*. Combine the organic solutions and dry over *anhydrous sodium sulphate R*. Filter and evaporate to dryness. Dissolve the residue in 5 ml of *methanol R*.

Reference solution. Dissolve 1 mg of *ruscogenins CRS* and 1 mg of *stigmasterol R* in *methanol R* and dilute to 5 ml with the same solvent.

Plate: *TLC silica gel plate R*.

Mobile phase: *methanol R, methylene chloride R* (7:93 *V/V*).

Application: 10 µl as bands.

Development: over a path of 15 cm.

Drying: in air.

Detection: spray with *vanillin reagent R*, dry the plate in an oven at 100-105 °C for 1 min and examine in daylight.

Results: see below the sequence of the zones present in the chromatograms obtained with the reference solution and the test solution. Furthermore, other weak zones may be present in the chromatogram obtained with the test solution.

Top of the plate	
	Several zones of various colours
Stigmasterol: a violet zone	A violet zone
_______	_______
	A violet zone
Ruscogenins: a yellow zone	A yellow zone (ruscogenins)
	Several zones of various colours
_______	_______
Reference solution	**Test solution**

TESTS

Foreign matter (*2.8.2*): maximum 5 per cent.

Loss on drying (*2.2.32*): maximum 12.0 per cent, determined on 1.000 g of the powdered drug (355) (*2.9.12*) by drying in an oven at 105 °C for 2 h.

Total ash (*2.4.16*): maximum 12.0 per cent.

Ash insoluble in hydrochloric acid (*2.8.1*): maximum 5.0 per cent.

ASSAY

Liquid chromatography (*2.2.29*).

Test solution. To 2.000 g of the powdered drug (355) (*2.9.12*), add 60 ml of *anhydrous ethanol R*, 15 ml of *water R* and 0.2 g of *potassium hydroxide R*. Extract under reflux on a water-bath for 4 h. Allow to cool and filter into a 100 ml volumetric flask. Rinse the extraction flask and the residue in the filter with 3 quantities, each of 10 ml, of *anhydrous ethanol R* and add the rinsings to the volumetric flask. Dilute to 100.0 ml with *anhydrous ethanol R*. Introduce 25.0 ml of the solution into a round-bottomed flask fitted to a rotary evaporator and evaporate to dryness. Dissolve the residue in 10 ml of *butanol R*, add 3 ml of *hydrochloric acid R1* and 8 ml of *water R*. Heat under reflux on a water-bath for 1 h. Allow to cool and transfer the liquid into a separating funnel, rinse the round-bottomed flask with 2 quantities, each of 10 ml, of *butanol R*. Add the rinsings to the separating funnel. Extract with 3 quantities, each of 20 ml, of *butanol R* saturated with *water R*. Combine the butanolic extracts and evaporate to dryness using a rotary evaporator. Dissolve the residue in 20 ml of *methanol R* and transfer to a 100 ml volumetric flask. Rinse the extraction flask with 2 quantities, each of 20 ml then 10 ml of *methanol R* and add the rinsings to the volumetric flask. Dilute to 100 ml with *methanol R*.

Reference solution. Dissolve 5.0 mg of *ruscogenins CRS* in 100 ml of *methanol R*.

Column:

- *size*: l = 0.25 m, Ø = 4.6 mm;
- *stationary phase*: *octadecylsilyl silica gel for chromatography R* (5 µm).

Mobile phase:

- *mobile phase A*: *water R*;
- *mobile phase B*: *acetonitrile for chromatography R*;

Time (min)	**Mobile phase A (per cent *V/V*)**	**Mobile phase B (per cent *V/V*)**
0 - 25	40	60
25 - 27	40 → 0	60 → 100
27 - 37	0	100
37 - 39	0 → 40	100 → 60
39 - 42	40	60

Flow rate: 1.2 ml/min.

Detection: spectrophotometer at 203 nm.

Injection: 20 µl.

Retention time with reference to neoruscogenin (retention time = about 16 min): ruscogenin = about 1.2.

System suitability: reference solution:

- *resolution*: minimum 1.5 between the peaks due to neoruscogenin and ruscogenin.

Calculate the percentage content of sapogenins expressed as ruscogenins (neoruscogenin and ruscogenin) in the test solution by comparing the areas of the peaks in the chromatograms obtained with the test solution and the reference solution.

C

04/2008:0267

CAFFEINE

Coffeinum

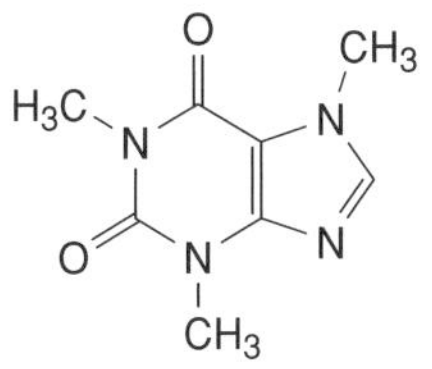

$C_8H_{10}N_4O_2$ M_r 194.2
[58-08-2]

DEFINITION

1,3,7-Trimethyl-3,7-dihydro-1*H*-purine-2,6-dione.

Content: 98.5 per cent to 101.5 per cent (dried substance).

CHARACTERS

Appearance: white or almost white, crystalline powder or silky, white or almost white, crystals.

Solubility: sparingly soluble in water, freely soluble in boiling water, slightly soluble in ethanol (96 per cent). It dissolves in concentrated solutions of alkali benzoates or salicylates.

It sublimes readily.

IDENTIFICATION

First identification: A, B, E.

Second identification: A, C, D, E, F.

A. Melting point (*2.2.14*): 234 °C to 239 °C.

B. Infrared absorption spectrophotometry (*2.2.24*).
Comparison: *caffeine CRS.*

C. To 2 ml of a saturated solution add 0.05 ml of *iodinated potassium iodide solution R*. The solution remains clear. Add 0.1 ml of *dilute hydrochloric acid R*; a brown precipitate is formed. Neutralise with *dilute sodium hydroxide solution R*; the precipitate dissolves.

D. In a ground-glass-stoppered tube, dissolve about 10 mg in 0.25 ml of a mixture of 0.5 ml of *acetylacetone R* and 5 ml of *dilute sodium hydroxide solution R*. Heat in a water-bath at 80 °C for 7 min. Cool and add 0.5 ml of *dimethylaminobenzaldehyde solution R2*. Heat again in a water-bath at 80 °C for 7 min. Allow to cool and add 10 ml of *water R*; an intense blue colour develops.

E. Loss on drying (see Tests).

F. It gives the reaction of xanthines (*2.3.1*).

TESTS

Solution S. Dissolve 0.5 g with heating in 50 ml of *carbon dioxide-free water R* prepared from *distilled water R*, cool and dilute to 50 ml with the same solvent.

Appearance of solution. Solution S is clear (*2.2.1*) and colourless (*2.2.2, Method II*).

Acidity. To 10 ml of solution S add 0.05 ml of *bromothymol blue solution R1*; the solution is green or yellow. Not more than 0.2 ml of *0.01 M sodium hydroxide* is required to change the colour of the indicator to blue.

Related substances. Liquid chromatography (*2.2.29*).

Test solution. Dissolve 0.100 g of the substance to be examined in the mobile phase and dilute to 50.0 ml with the mobile phase. Dilute 1.0 ml of this solution to 10.0 ml with the mobile phase.

Reference solution (a). Dilute 2.0 ml of the test solution to 100.0 ml with the mobile phase. Dilute 1.0 ml of this solution to 10.0 ml with the mobile phase.

Reference solution (b). Dissolve 5 mg of *caffeine for system suitability CRS* (containing impurities A, C, D and F) in the mobile phase and dilute to 5 ml with the mobile phase. Dilute 2 ml of this solution to 10 ml with the mobile phase.

Column:

– *size*: *l* = 0.15 m, Ø = 4.6 mm;
– *stationary phase*: *base-deactivated end-capped octadecylsilyl silica gel for chromatography R* (5 μm).

Mobile phase: dissolve 1.64 g of *anhydrous sodium acetate R* in *water R* and dilute to 2000 ml with the same solvent. Adjust 1910 ml of this solution to pH 4.5 with *glacial acetic acid R* and add 50 ml of *acetonitrile R* and 40 ml of *tetrahydrofuran R*.

Flow rate: 1.0 ml/min.

Detection: spectrophotometer at 275 nm.

Injection: 10 μl.

Run time: 1.5 times the retention time of caffeine.

Identification of impurities: use the chromatogram supplied with *caffeine for system suitability CRS* and the chromatogram obtained with reference solution (b) to identify the peaks due to impurities A, C, D and F.

Retention time: caffeine = about 8 min.

System suitability: reference solution (b):

– *resolution*: minimum 2.5 between the peaks due to impurities C and D and minimum 2.5 between the peaks due to impurities F and A.

Limits:

– *unspecified impurities*: for each impurity, not more than 0.5 times the area of the principal peak in the chromatogram obtained with reference solution (a) (0.10 per cent);
– *total*: not more than 0.5 times the area of the principal peak in the chromatogram obtained with reference solution (a) (0.1 per cent);
– *disregard limit*: 0.25 times the area of the principal peak in the chromatogram obtained with reference solution (a) (0.05 per cent).

Sulphates (*2.4.13*): maximum 500 ppm, determined on 15 ml of solution S.

Prepare the standard using a mixture of 7.5 ml of *sulphate standard solution (10 ppm SO_4) R* and 7.5 ml of *distilled water R*.

Heavy metals (*2.4.8*): maximum 20 ppm.

1.0 g complies with test C. Prepare the reference solution using 2 ml of *lead standard solution (10 ppm Pb) R*.

Loss on drying (*2.2.32*): maximum 0.5 per cent, determined on 1.000 g by drying in an oven at 105 °C for 1 h.

Sulphated ash (*2.4.14*): maximum 0.1 per cent, determined on 1.0 g.

ASSAY

Dissolve 0.170 g with heating in 5 ml of *anhydrous acetic acid R*. Allow to cool, add 10 ml of *acetic anhydride R* and 20 ml of *toluene R*. Titrate with *0.1 M perchloric acid*, determining the end-point potentiometrically (*2.2.20*).

1 ml of *0.1 M perchloric acid* is equivalent to 19.42 mg of $C_8H_{10}N_4O_2$.

IMPURITIES

Other detectable impurities (the following substances would, if present at a sufficient level, be detected by one or other of the tests in the monograph. They are limited by the general acceptance criterion for other/unspecified impurities and/or by the general monograph *Substances for pharmaceutical use (2034)*. It is therefore not necessary to identify these impurities for demonstration of compliance. See also *5.10. Control of impurities in substances for pharmaceutical use*): *A, B, C, D, E, F*.

A. theophylline,

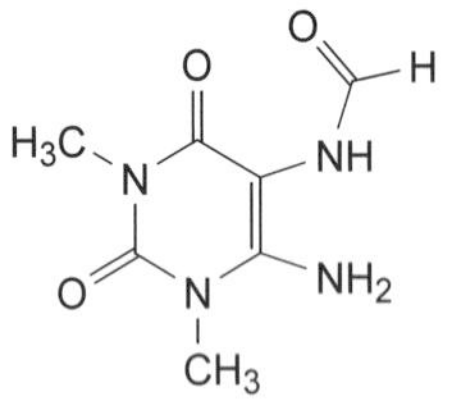

B. *N*-(6-amino-1,3-dimethyl-2,4-dioxo-1,2,3,4-tetrahydropyrimidin-5-yl)formamide,

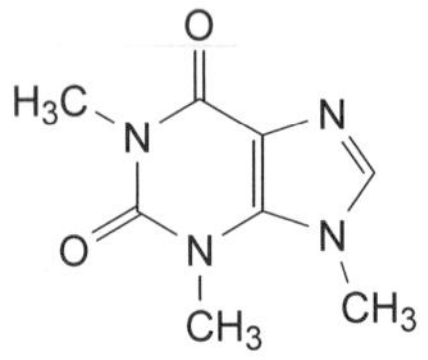

C. 1,3,9-trimethyl-3,9-dihydro-1*H*-purine-2,6-dione (isocaffeine),

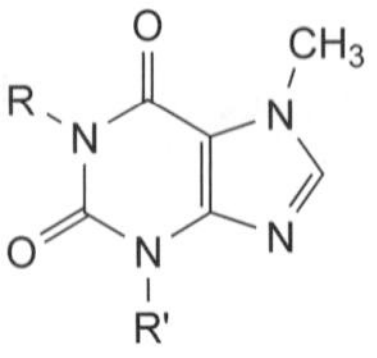

D. R = H, R′ = CH_3: theobromine,

F. R = CH_3, R′ = H: 1,7-dimethyl-3,7-dihydro-1*H*-purine-2,6-dione,

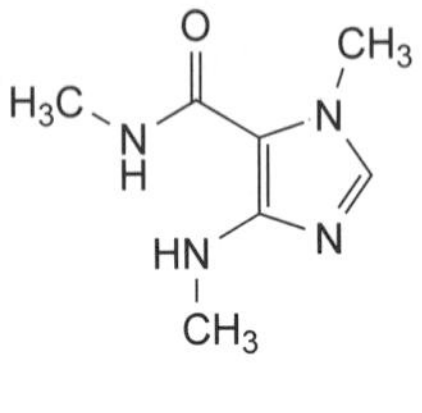

E. *N*,1-dimethyl-4-(methylamino)-1*H*-imidazole-5-carboxamide (caffeidine).

04/2008:1299

CARBOMERS

Carbomera

DEFINITION

High-molecular-mass polymers of acrylic acid cross-linked with polyalkenyl ethers of sugars or polyalcohols.

Content: 56.0 per cent to 68.0 per cent of carboxylic acid (-CO_2H) groups (dried substance).

CHARACTERS

Appearance: white or almost white, fluffy, hygroscopic, powder.

Solubility: swells in water and in other polar solvents after dispersion and neutralisation with sodium hydroxide solution.

IDENTIFICATION

First identification: A, E.

Second identification: B, C, D, E.

A. Infrared absorption spectrophotometry (*2.2.24*).

Main bands: at 1710 ± 5 cm^{-1}, 1454 ± 5 cm^{-1}, 1414 ± 5 cm^{-1}, 1245 ± 5 cm^{-1}, 1172 ± 5 cm^{-1}, 1115 ± 5 cm^{-1} and 801 ± 5 cm^{-1}, with the strongest band at 1710 ± 5 cm^{-1}.

B. Adjust a 10 g/l dispersion to about pH 7.5 with *1 M sodium hydroxide*. A highly viscous gel is formed.

C. Add 2 ml of a 100 g/l solution of *calcium chloride R* with continuous stirring to 10 ml of the gel from identification test B. A white precipitate is immediately produced.

D. Add 0.5 ml of *thymol blue solution R* to 10 ml of a 10 g/l dispersion; an orange colour is produced. Add 0.5 ml of *cresol red solution R* to 10 ml of a 10 g/l dispersion. A yellow colour is produced.

E. It complies with the nominal apparent viscosity indicated on the label.

TESTS

Apparent viscosity: the nominal apparent viscosity is between 300 mPa·s and 115 000 mPa·s. For a product with a nominal apparent viscosity of 20 000 mPa·s or greater, the apparent viscosity is 70.0 per cent to 130.0 per cent of the value stated on the label; for a product with a nominal apparent viscosity of less than 20 000 mPa·s, the apparent viscosity is 50.0 per cent to 150.0 per cent of the value stated on the label.

Dry the substance to be examined *in vacuo* at 80 °C for 1 h. Carefully add 2.50 g of the previously dried substance to be examined to 500 ml of *water R* in a 1000 ml beaker while stirring continuously at 1000 ± 50 r/min, with the stirrer shaft set at an angle of 60° to one side of the beaker. Add the previously dried substance over a period of 45-90 s, at a uniform rate, ensuring that loose aggregates of powder are broken up, and continue stirring at 1000 ± 50 r/min for 15 min. Remove the stirrer and place the beaker containing the dispersion in a water-bath at 25 ± 0.2 °C for 30 min. Insert the stirrer to a depth necessary to ensure that air is not drawn into the dispersion and, while stirring at 300 ± 25 r/min, titrate with a glass-calomel electrode system to pH 7.3-7.8 by adding a 180 g/l solution of *sodium hydroxide R* below the surface, determining the end-point potentiometrically (*2.2.20*). The total volume of the 180 g/l solution of *sodium hydroxide R* used is about 6.2 ml. Allow 2-3 min before the final pH determination. If the final pH exceeds 7.8, discard the preparation and prepare another using a smaller amount of sodium hydroxide for titration. Return the neutralised preparation to the water-bath at 25 °C for 1 h, then perform the viscosity determination without delay to avoid slight viscosity changes that occur 75 min after neutralisation. Determine the viscosity (*2.2.10*) using a rotating viscometer with a spindle rotating at 20 r/min, using a spindle suitable for the expected apparent viscosity.

Free acrylic acid. Liquid chromatography (*2.2.29*).

Test solution. Mix 0.125 g of the substance to be examined with a 25 g/l solution of *aluminium potassium sulphate R* and dilute to 25.0 ml with the same solution. Heat the suspension at 50 °C for 20 min with shaking. Then shake the suspension at room temperature for 60 min. Centrifuge and use the clear supernatant solution as the test solution.

Reference solution. Dissolve 62.5 mg of *acrylic acid R* in a 25 g/l solution of *aluminium potassium sulphate R* and dilute to 100.0 ml with the same solution. Dilute 1.0 ml of this solution to 50.0 ml with a 25 g/l solution of *aluminium potassium sulphate R*.

Column:

- *size*: *l* = 0.12 m, Ø = 4.6 mm;
- *stationary phase*: *octadecylsilyl silica gel for chromatography R* (5 µm).

Mobile phase:

- *mobile phase A*: 1.361 g/l solution of *potassium dihydrogen phosphate R*, adjusted to pH 2.5 using *dilute phosphoric acid R*;
- *mobile phase B*: 1.361 g/l solution of *potassium dihydrogen phosphate R, acetonitrile for chromatography R* (50:50 *V/V*);

Time (min)	Mobile phase A (per cent *V/V*)	Mobile phase B (per cent *V/V*)
0 - 8	100	0
8 - 9	100 → 0	0 → 100
9 - 20	0	100
20 - 21	0 → 100	100 → 0
21 - 30	100	0

Flow rate: 1 ml/min.

Detection: spectrophotometer at 205 nm.

Injection: 20 µl.

Retention time: acrylic acid = about 6.0 min.

Limit:

- *acrylic acid*: not more than the area of the corresponding peak in the chromatogram obtained with the reference solution (0.25 per cent).

Benzene. Gas chromatography (*2.4.24, System A*).

Solution A. Dissolve 0.100 g of *benzene R* in *dimethyl sulphoxide R* and dilute to 100.0 ml with the same solvent. Dilute 1.0 ml of the solution to 100.0 ml with *water R*. Dilute 1.0 ml of this solution to 100.0 ml with *water R*.

Test solution. Weigh 50.0 mg of the substance to be examined into an injection vial and add 5.0 ml of *water R* and 1.0 ml of *dimethyl sulphoxide R*.

Reference solution. Weigh 50.0 mg of the substance to be examined into an injection vial and add 4.0 ml of *water R*, 1.0 ml of *dimethyl sulphoxide R* and 1.0 ml of solution A.

Close the vials with a tight rubber membrane stopper coated with polytetrafluoroethylene and secure with an aluminium crimped cap. Shake to obtain a homogeneous dispersion.

Static head-space conditions that may be used:

- *equilibration temperature*: 80 °C;
- *equilibration time*: 60 min;
- *transfer line temperature*: 90 °C.

Injection: 1 ml of the gaseous phase of the test solution and 1 ml of the gaseous phase of the reference solution; repeat these injections twice more.

System suitability:

- *repeatability*: maximum relative standard deviation of the differences in area between the analyte peaks obtained from the 3 replicate pair injections of the reference solution and the test solution is 15 per cent.

Limit:

- *benzene*: the mean area of the peak due to benzene in the chromatograms obtained with the test solution is not greater than 0.5 times the mean area of the peak due to benzene in the chromatograms obtained with the reference solution (2 ppm).

Heavy metals (*2.4.8*): maximum 20 ppm.

1.0 g complies with test C. Prepare the reference solution using 2 ml of *lead standard solution (10 ppm Pb) R*.

Loss on drying (*2.2.32*): maximum 3.0 per cent, determined on 1.000 g by drying *in vacuo* at 80 °C for 60 min.

Sulphated ash (*2.4.14*): maximum 4.0 per cent, determined on 1.0 g.

ASSAY

Slowly add 50 ml of *water R* to 0.120 g whilst stirring and heating at 60 °C for 15 min. Stop heating, add 150 ml of *water R* and continue stirring for 30 min. Add 2 g of *potassium chloride R* and titrate with *0.2 M sodium hydroxide,* determining the end-point potentiometrically (*2.2.20*).

1 ml of *0.2 M sodium hydroxide* is equivalent to 9.0 mg of carboxylic acid (-CO_2H) groups.

STORAGE

In an airtight container.

LABELLING

The label states the nominal apparent viscosity.

04/2008:0813

CEFADROXIL MONOHYDRATE

Cefadroxilum monohydricum

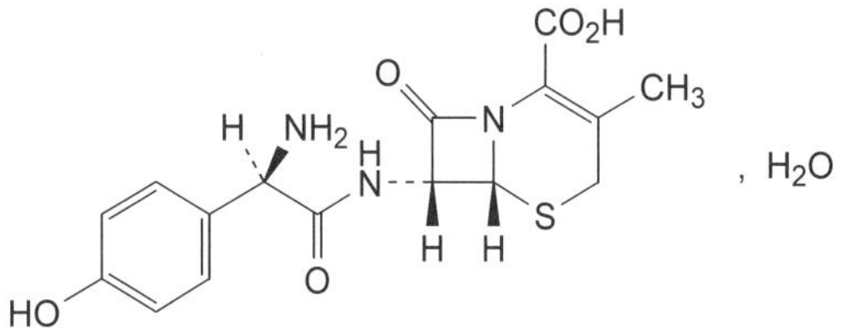

$C_{16}H_{17}N_3O_5S,H_2O$ M_r 381.4

[50370-12-2]

DEFINITION

(6*R*,7*R*)-7-[[(2*R*)-2-Amino-2-(4-hydroxyphenyl)acetyl]amino]-3-methyl-8-oxo-5-thia-1-azabicyclo[4.2.0]oct-2-ene-2-carboxylic acid monohydrate.

Semi-synthetic product derived from a fermentation product.

Content: 95.0 per cent to 102.0 per cent (anhydrous substance).

CHARACTERS

Appearance: white or almost white powder.

Solubility: slightly soluble in water, very slightly soluble in ethanol (96 per cent).

IDENTIFICATION

Infrared absorption spectrophotometry (*2.2.24*).

Monographs A-C

Comparison: *cefadroxil CRS.*

TESTS

pH (*2.2.3*): 4.0 to 6.0.

Suspend 1.0 g in *carbon dioxide-free water R* and dilute to 20 ml with the same solvent.

Specific optical rotation (*2.2.7*): + 165 to + 178 (anhydrous substance).

Dissolve 0.500 g in *water R* and dilute to 50.0 ml with the same solvent.

Related substances. Liquid chromatography (*2.2.29*).

Test solution. Dissolve 50.0 mg of the substance to be examined in mobile phase A and dilute to 50.0 ml with mobile phase A.

Reference solution (a). Dissolve 10.0 mg of *D-α-(4-hydroxyphenyl)glycine CRS* (impurity A) in mobile phase A and dilute to 10.0 ml with mobile phase A.

Reference solution (b). Dissolve 10.0 mg of *7-aminodesacetoxycephalosporanic acid CRS* (impurity B) in *phosphate buffer solution pH 7.0 R5* and dilute to 10.0 ml with the same buffer solution.

Reference solution (c). Dilute 1.0 ml of reference solution (a) and 1.0 ml of reference solution (b) to 100.0 ml with mobile phase A.

Reference solution (d). Dissolve 10 mg of *dimethylformamide R* and 10 mg of *dimethylacetamide R* in mobile phase A and dilute to 10.0 ml with mobile phase A. Dilute 1.0 ml of this solution to 100.0 ml with mobile phase A.

Reference solution (e). Dilute 1.0 ml of reference solution (c) to 25.0 ml with mobile phase A.

Column:

- *size*: *l* = 0.10 m, Ø = 4.6 mm,
- *stationary phase*: spherical *octadecylsilyl silica gel for chromatography R* (5 μm).

Mobile phase:

- *mobile phase A*: *phosphate buffer solution pH 5.0 R,*
- *mobile phase B*: *methanol R2,*

Time (min)	Mobile phase A (per cent *V/V*)	Mobile phase B (per cent *V/V*)
0 - 1	98	2
1 - 20	98 → 70	2 → 30
20 - 23	70 → 98	30 → 2
23 - 30	98	2

Flow rate: 1.5 ml/min.

Detection: spectrophotometer at 220 nm.

Injection: 20 μl of the test solution and reference solutions (c), (d) and (e).

Relative retention with reference to cefadroxil (retention time = about 6 min): dimethylformamide = about 0.4; dimethylacetamide = about 0.75.

System suitability:

- *resolution*: minimum 5.0 between the peaks due to impurities A and B in the chromatogram obtained with reference solution (c),
- *signal-to-noise ratio*: minimum 10 for the 2nd peak in the chromatogram obtained with reference solution (e).

Limits:

- *impurity A*: not more than the area of the 1st peak in the chromatogram obtained with reference solution (c) (1.0 per cent),
- *any other impurity*: for each impurity, not more than the area of the 2nd peak in the chromatogram obtained with reference solution (c) (1.0 per cent),
- *total*: not more than 3 times the area of the 2nd peak in the chromatogram obtained with reference solution (c) (3.0 per cent),
- *disregard limit*: 0.05 times the area of the 2nd peak in the chromatogram obtained with reference solution (c) (0.05 per cent); disregard the peaks due to dimethylformamide and dimethylacetamide.

***N,N*-Dimethylaniline** (*2.4.26, Method B*): maximum 20 ppm.

Water (*2.5.12*): 4.0 per cent to 6.0 per cent, determined on 0.200 g.

Sulphated ash (*2.4.14*): maximum 0.5 per cent, determined on 1.0 g.

ASSAY

Liquid chromatography (*2.2.29*).

Test solution. Dissolve 50.0 mg of the substance to be examined in the mobile phase and dilute to 100.0 ml with the mobile phase.

Reference solution (a). Dissolve 50.0 mg of *cefadroxil CRS* in the mobile phase and dilute to 100.0 ml with the mobile phase.

Reference solution (b). Dissolve 5 mg of *cefadroxil CRS* and 50 mg of *amoxicillin trihydrate CRS* in the mobile phase and dilute to 100 ml with the mobile phase.

Column:

- *size*: *l* = 0.25 m, Ø = 4.6 mm,
- *stationary phase*: *octadecylsilyl silica gel for chromatography R* (5 μm).

Mobile phase: *acetonitrile R*, a 2.72 g/l solution of *potassium dihydrogen phosphate R* (4:96 *V/V*).

Flow rate: 1 ml/min.

Detection: spectrophotometer at 254 nm.

Injection: 20 μl.

System suitability: reference solution (b):

- *resolution*: minimum 5.0 between the peaks due to cefadroxil and to amoxicillin.

Calculate the percentage content of cefadroxil.

STORAGE

Protected from light.

IMPURITIES

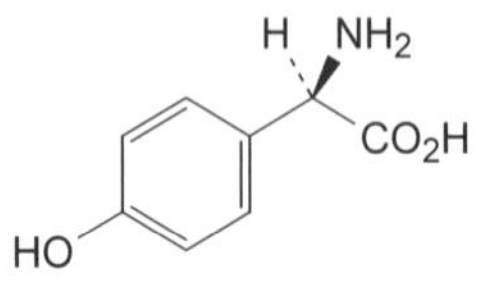

A. (2*R*)-2-amino-2-(4-hydroxyphenyl)acetic acid,

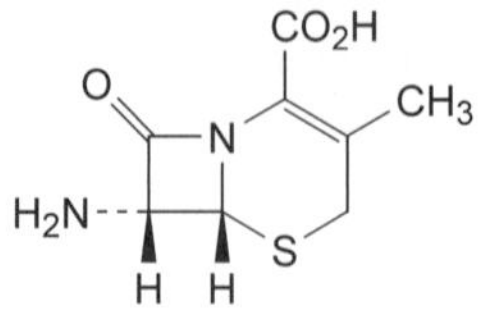

B. (6*R*,7*R*)-7-amino-3-methyl-8-oxo-5-thia-1-aza-bicyclo[4.2.0]oct-2-ene-2-carboxylic acid (7-ADCA),

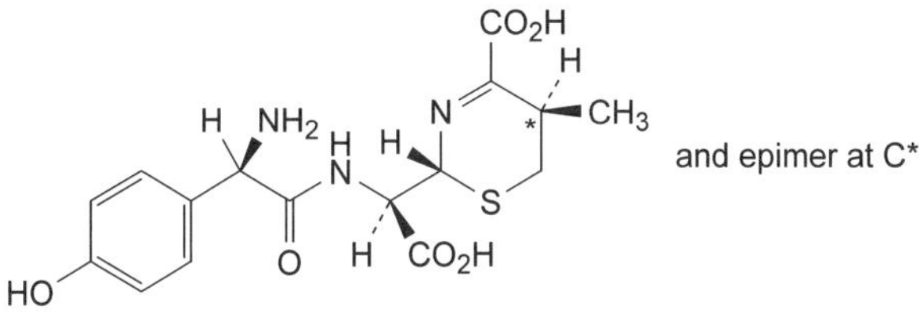

C. (2*R*,5*RS*)-2-[(*R*)-[[(2*R*)-2-amino-2-(4-hydroxyphenyl)-acetyl]amino]carboxymethyl]-5-methyl-5,6-dihydro-2*H*-1,3-thiazine-4-carboxylic acid,

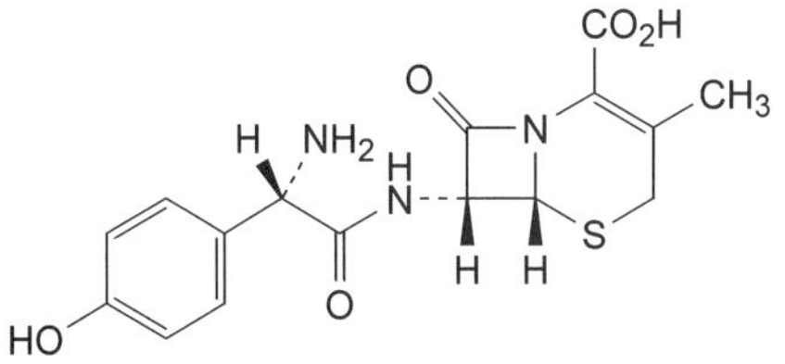

D. (6*R*,7*R*)-7-[[(2*S*)-2-amino-2-(4-hydroxyphenyl)-acetyl]amino]-3-methyl-8-oxo-5-thia-1-azabicyclo-[4.2.0]oct-2-ene-2-carboxylic acid (L-cefadroxil),

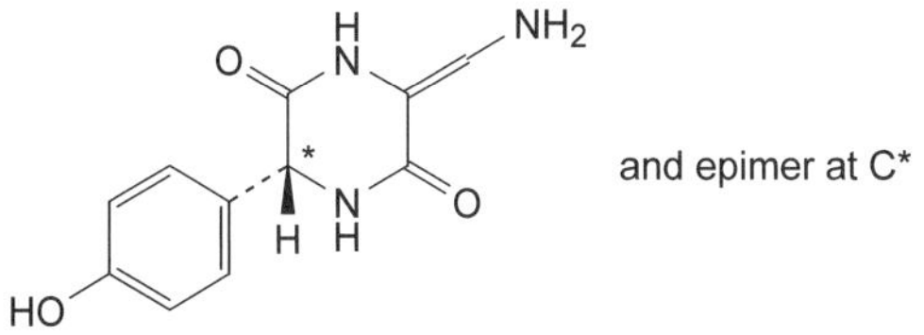

E. (6*RS*)-3-(aminomethylene)-6-(4-hydroxyphenyl)piperazine-2,5-dione,

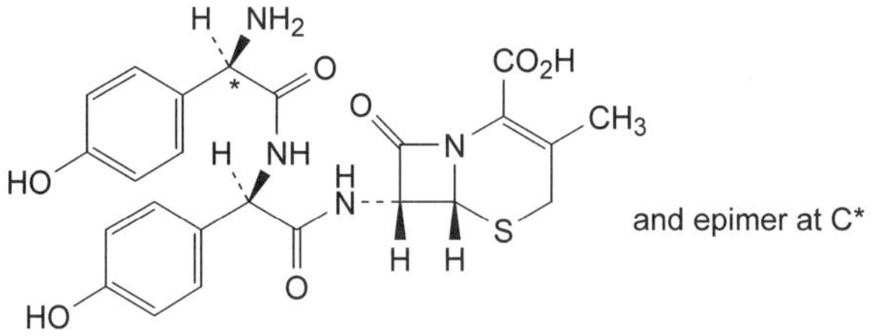

F. (6*R*,7*R*)-7-[[(2*R*)-2-[[(2*RS*)-2-amino-2-(4-hydroxyphenyl)-acetyl]amino]-2-(4-hydroxyphenyl)acetyl]amino]-3-methyl-8-oxo-5-thia-1-azabicyclo[4.2.0]oct-2-ene-2-carboxylic acid,

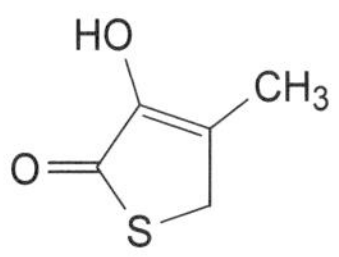

G. 3-hydroxy-4-methylthiophen-2(5*H*)-one,

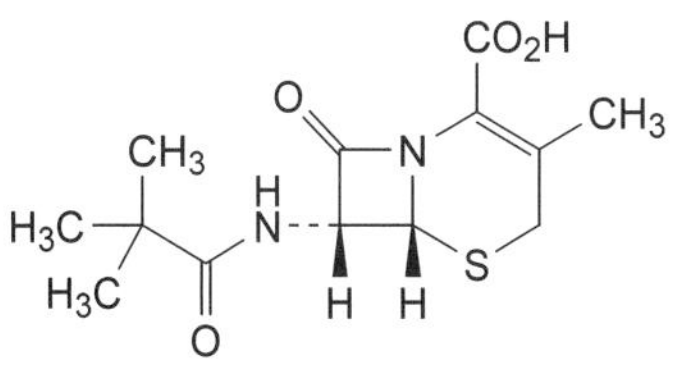

H. (6*R*,7*R*)-7-[(2,2-dimethylpropanoyl)amino]-3-methyl-8-oxo-5-thia-1-azabicyclo[4.2.0]oct-2-ene-2-carboxylic acid (7-ADCA pivalamide).

04/2008:0708

CEFALEXIN MONOHYDRATE

Cefalexinum monohydricum

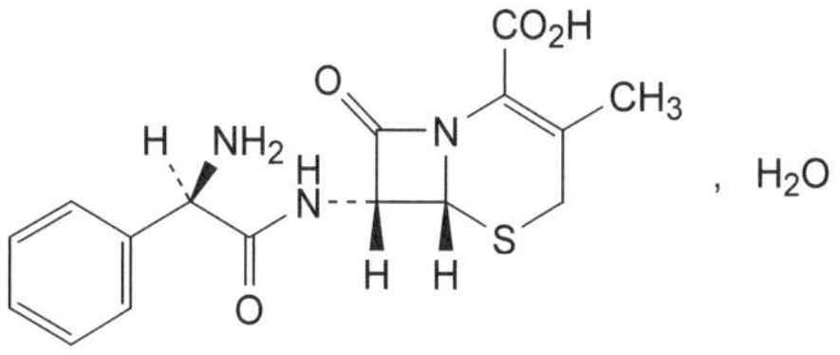

$C_{16}H_{17}N_3O_4S,H_2O$ M_r 365.4

[23325-78-2]

DEFINITION

(6*R*,7*R*)-7-[[(2*R*)-2-Amino-2-phenylacetyl]amino]-3-methyl-8-oxo-5-thia-1-azabicyclo[4.2.0]oct-2-ene-2-carboxylic acid monohydrate.

Semi-synthetic product derived from a fermentation product.

Content: 95.0 per cent to 102.0 per cent (anhydrous substance).

CHARACTERS

Appearance: white or almost white, crystalline powder.

Solubility: sparingly soluble in water, practically insoluble in ethanol (96 per cent).

IDENTIFICATION

Infrared absorption spectrophotometry (*2.2.24*).

Comparison: *cefalexin monohydrate CRS*.

TESTS

pH (*2.2.3*): 4.0 to 5.5.

Dissolve 50 mg in *carbon dioxide-free water R* and dilute to 10 ml with the same solvent.

Specific optical rotation (*2.2.7*): + 149 to + 158 (anhydrous substance).

Dissolve 0.125 g in *phthalate buffer solution pH 4.4 R* and dilute to 25.0 ml with the same solvent.

Related substances. Liquid chromatography (*2.2.29*).

Test solution. Dissolve 50.0 mg of the substance to be examined in mobile phase A and dilute to 50.0 ml with mobile phase A.

Reference solution (a). Dissolve 10.0 mg of *D-phenylglycine R* in mobile phase A and dilute to 10.0 ml with mobile phase A.

Reference solution (b). Dissolve 10.0 mg of *7-aminodesacetoxycephalosporanic acid CRS* in *phosphate buffer solution pH 7.0 R5* and dilute to 10.0 ml with mobile phase A.

Reference solution (c). Dilute 1.0 ml of reference solution (a) and 1.0 ml of reference solution (b) to 100.0 ml with mobile phase A.

Reference solution (d). Dissolve 10 mg of *dimethylformamide R* and 10 mg of *dimethylacetamide R* in mobile phase A and dilute to 10.0 ml with mobile phase A. Dilute 1.0 ml of this solution to 100.0 ml with mobile phase A.

Reference solution (e). Dilute 1.0 ml of reference solution (c) to 20.0 ml with mobile phase A.

Monographs A-C

Reference solution (f). Dissolve 10 mg of *cefotaxime sodium CRS* in mobile phase A and dilute to 10.0 ml with mobile phase A. To 1.0 ml of this solution add 1.0 ml of the test solution and dilute to 100 ml with mobile phase A.

Column:

- *size*: *l* = 0.10 m, Ø = 4.6 mm;
- *stationary phase*: spherical *octadecylsilyl silica gel for chromatography R* (5 μm).

Mobile phase:

- *mobile phase A*: *phosphate buffer solution pH 5.0 R*;
- *mobile phase B*: *methanol R2*;

Time (min)	Mobile phase A (per cent *V/V*)	Mobile phase B (per cent *V/V*)
0 - 1	98	2
1 - 20	98 → 70	2 → 30
20 - 23	70 → 98	30 → 2
23 - 30	98	2

Flow rate: 1.5 ml/min.

Detection: spectrophotometer at 220 nm.

Injection: 20 μl of the test solution and reference solutions (c), (d), (e) and (f).

System suitability:

- *resolution*: minimum 2.0 between the peaks due to impurities A and B in the chromatogram obtained with reference solution (c) and minimum 1.5 between the peaks due to cefalexin and cefotaxime in the chromatogram obtained with reference solution (f).

Limits:

- *impurity B*: not more than the area of the 2nd peak in the chromatogram obtained with reference solution (c) (1.0 per cent);
- *any other impurity*: not more than the area of the 1st peak in the chromatogram obtained with reference solution (c) (1.0 per cent);
- *total*: not more than 3 times the area of the 1st peak in the chromatogram obtained with reference solution (c) (3.0 per cent);
- *disregard limit*: the area of the 2nd peak in the chromatogram obtained with reference solution (e) (0.05 per cent); disregard any peaks due to dimethylformamide or dimethylacetamide.

***N,N*-Dimethylaniline** (*2.4.26, Method B*): maximum 20 ppm.

Water (*2.5.12*): 4.0 per cent to 8.0 per cent, determined on 0.300 g.

Sulphated ash (*2.4.14*): maximum 0.2 per cent, determined on 1.0 g.

ASSAY

Liquid chromatography (*2.2.29*).

Test solution. Dissolve 50.0 mg of the substance to be examined in *water R* and dilute to 100.0 ml with the same solvent.

Reference solution (a). Dissolve 50.0 mg of *cefalexin monohydrate CRS* in *water R* and dilute to 100.0 ml with the same solvent.

Reference solution (b). Dissolve 10 mg of *cefradine CRS* in 20 ml of reference solution (a) and dilute to 100 ml with *water R*.

Column:

- *size*: *l* = 0.25 m, Ø = 4.6 mm;
- *stationary phase*: *octadecylsilyl silica gel for chromatography R* (5 μm).

Mobile phase: *methanol R, acetonitrile R*, 13.6 g/l solution of *potassium dihydrogen phosphate R, water R* (2:5:10:83 *V/V/V/V*).

Flow rate: 1.5 ml/min.

Detection: spectrophotometer at 254 nm.

Injection: 20 μl.

System suitability: reference solution (b):

- *resolution*: minimum 4.0 between the peaks due to cefalexin and cefradine.

Calculate the percentage content of cefalexin monohydrate.

STORAGE

Protected from light.

IMPURITIES

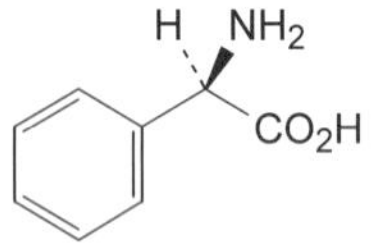

A. (2*R*)-2-amino-2-phenylacetic acid (D-phenylglycine),

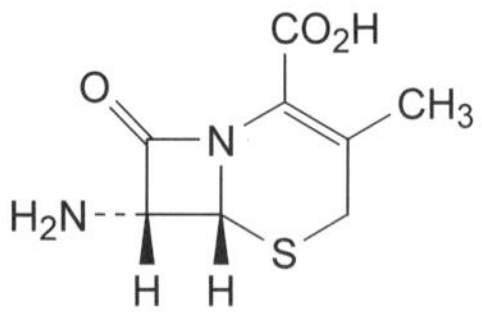

B. (6*R*,7*R*)-7-amino-3-methyl-8-oxo-5-thia-1-azabicyclo[4.2.0]oct-2-ene-2-carboxylic acid (7-aminodesacetoxycephalosporanic acid, 7-ADCA),

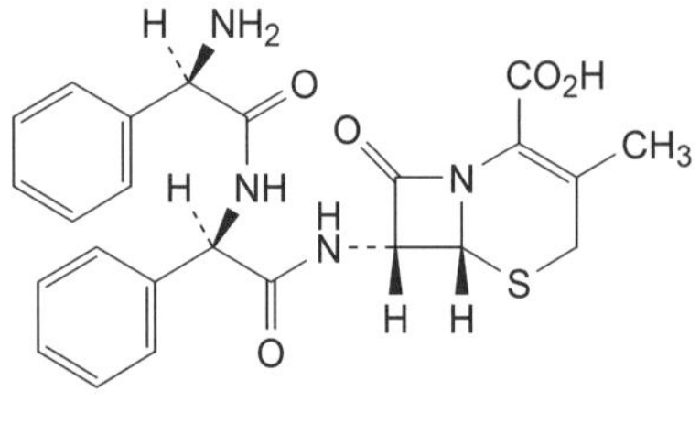

C. (6*R*,7*R*)-7-[[(2*R*)-2-[[(2*R*)-2-amino-2-phenylacetyl]amino]-2-phenylacetyl]amino]-3-methyl-8-oxo-5-thia-1-azabicyclo[4.2.0]oct-2-ene-2-carboxylic acid,

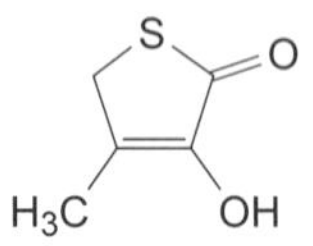

D. 3-hydroxy-4-methylthiophen-2(5*H*)-one,

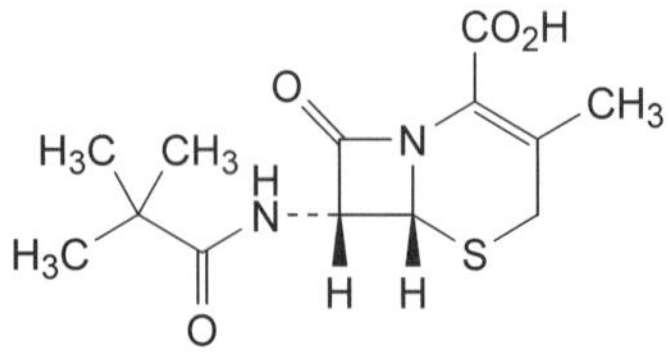

E. (6*R*,7*R*)-7-[(2,2-dimethylpropanoyl)amino]-3-methyl-8-oxo-5-thia-1-azabicyclo[4.2.0]oct-2-ene-2-carboxylic acid (7-ADCA pivalamide),

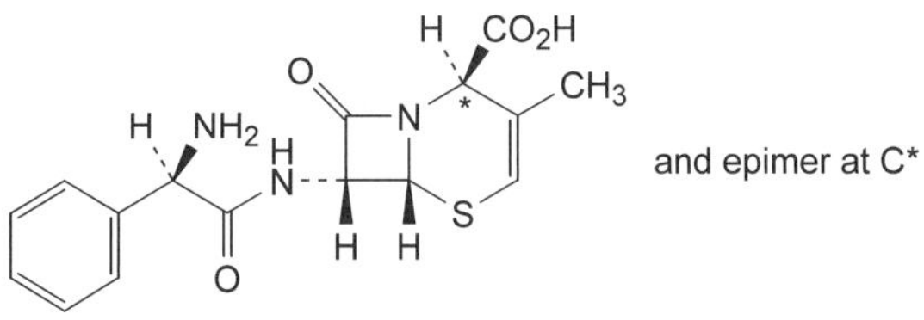

F. (2*RS*,6*R*,7*R*)-7-[[(2*R*)-2-amino-2-phenylacetyl]amino]-3-methyl-8-oxo-5-thia-1-azabicyclo[4.2.0]oct-3-ene-2-carboxylic acid (delta-2-cefalexin).

04/2008:0386

CHLORPHENAMINE MALEATE

Chlorphenamini maleas

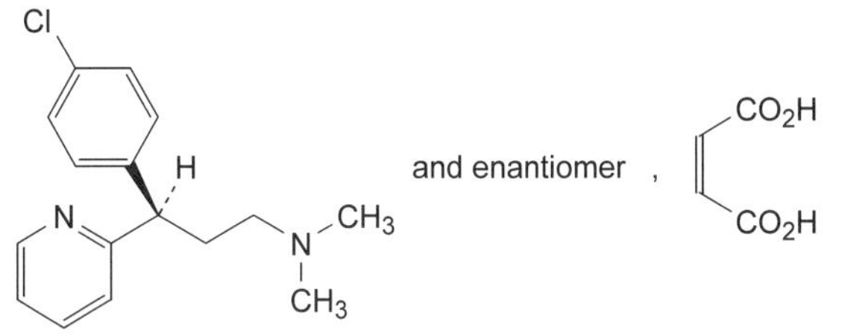

$C_{20}H_{23}ClN_2O_4$ M_r 390.9

[113-92-8]

DEFINITION

(3*RS*)-3-(4-Chlorophenyl)-*N*,*N*-dimethyl-3-(pyridin-2-yl)propan-1-amine hydrogen (*Z*)-butenedioate.

Content: 98.0 per cent to 101.0 per cent (dried substance).

CHARACTERS

Appearance: white or almost white, crystalline powder.

Solubility: freely soluble in water, soluble in ethanol (96 per cent).

IDENTIFICATION

A. Melting point (*2.2.14*): 130 °C to 135 °C.

B. Infrared absorption spectrophotometry (*2.2.24*).

Comparison: *chlorphenamine maleate CRS.*

C. Optical rotation (see Tests).

TESTS

Solution S. Dissolve 2.0 g in *water R* and dilute to 20.0 ml with the same solvent.

Appearance of solution. Solution S is clear (*2.2.1*) and not more intensely coloured than reference solution BY_6 (*2.2.2, Method II*).

Optical rotation (*2.2.7*): – 0.10° to + 0.10°, determined on solution S.

Related substances. Liquid chromatography (*2.2.29*).

Test solution. Dissolve 0.100 g of the substance to be examined in the mobile phase and dilute to 100.0 ml with the mobile phase.

Reference solution (a). Dilute 0.5 ml of the test solution to 100.0 ml with the mobile phase.

Reference solution (b). Dilute 1.0 ml of reference solution (a) to 10.0 ml with the mobile phase.

Reference solution (c). Dissolve 5 mg of *chlorphenamine impurity C CRS* in 5 ml of the test solution and dilute to 50.0 ml with the mobile phase. Dilute 2 ml of this solution to 20 ml with the mobile phase.

Reference solution (d). Dissolve 5 mg of *2,2′-dipyridylamine R* (impurity B) in the mobile phase and dilute to 100 ml with the mobile phase.

Reference solution (e). Dissolve the contents of a vial of *chlorphenamine impurity A CRS* in 2 ml of the test solution. Sonicate for 5 min.

Column:

– *size*: *l* = 0.30 m, Ø = 3.9 mm;

– *stationary phase*: *octadecylsilyl silica gel for chromatography R* (10 µm).

Mobile phase: mix 20 volumes of *acetonitrile R* and 80 volumes of a 8.57 g/l solution of *ammonium dihydrogen phosphate R* previously adjusted to pH 3.0 with *phosphoric acid R.*

Flow rate: 1.2 ml/min.

Detection: spectrophotometer at 225 nm.

Injection: 20 µl.

Run time: 3.5 times the retention time of chlorphenamine.

Relative retention with reference to chlorphenamine (retention time = about 11 min): maleic acid = about 0.2; impurity A = about 0.3; impurity B = about 0.4; impurity C = about 0.9; impurity D = about 3.0.

System suitability: reference solution (c):

– *resolution*: minimum 1.5 between the peaks due to impurity C and chlorphenamine.

Limits:

– *correction factors*: for the calculation of contents, multiply the peak areas of the following impurities by the corresponding correction factor: impurity A = 1.5; impurity B = 1.4;

– *impurity A*: not more than 0.4 times the area of the principal peak in the chromatogram obtained with reference solution (a) (0.2 per cent);

– *impurities B, C, D*: for each impurity, not more than 0.2 times the area of the principal peak in the chromatogram obtained with reference solution (a) (0.1 per cent);

– *unspecified impurities*: for each impurity, not more than 0.2 times the area of the principal peak in the chromatogram obtained with reference solution (a) (0.10 per cent);

– *total*: not more than the area of the principal peak in the chromatogram obtained with reference solution (a) (0.5 per cent);

– *disregard limit*: the area of the principal peak in the chromatogram obtained with reference solution (b) (0.05 per cent); disregard the peaks due to the blank and maleic acid.

Heavy metals (*2.4.8*): maximum 20 ppm.

1.0 g complies with test C. Prepare the reference solution using 2 ml of *lead standard solution (10 ppm Pb) R.*

Loss on drying (*2.2.32*): maximum 0.5 per cent, determined on 1.000 g by drying in an oven at 105 °C for 4 h.

Sulphated ash (*2.4.14*): maximum 0.1 per cent, determined on 1.0 g.

ASSAY

Dissolve 0.150 g in 25 ml of *anhydrous acetic acid R*. Titrate with *0.1 M perchloric acid*, determining the end-point potentiometrically (*2.2.20*).

1 ml of *0.1 M perchloric acid* is equivalent to 19.54 mg of $C_{20}H_{23}ClN_2O_4$.

STORAGE

Protected from light.

IMPURITIES

Specified impurities: A, B, C, D.

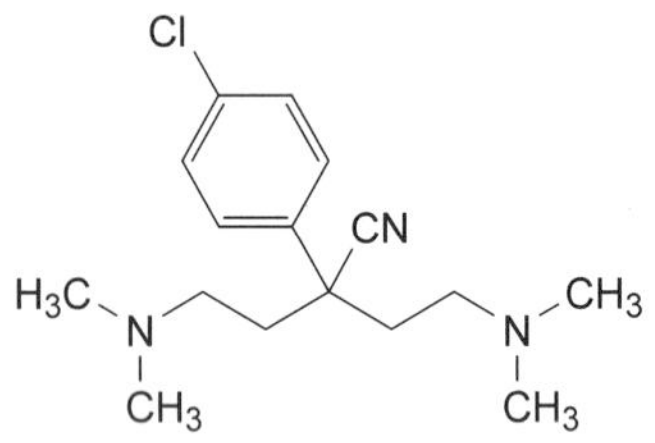

A. 2-(4-chlorophenyl)-4-(dimethylamino)-2-[2-(dimethylamino)ethyl]butanenitrile,

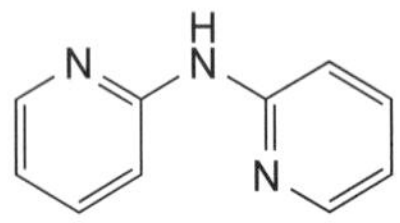

B. *N*-(pyridin-2-yl)pyridin-2-amine (2,2′-dipyridylamine),

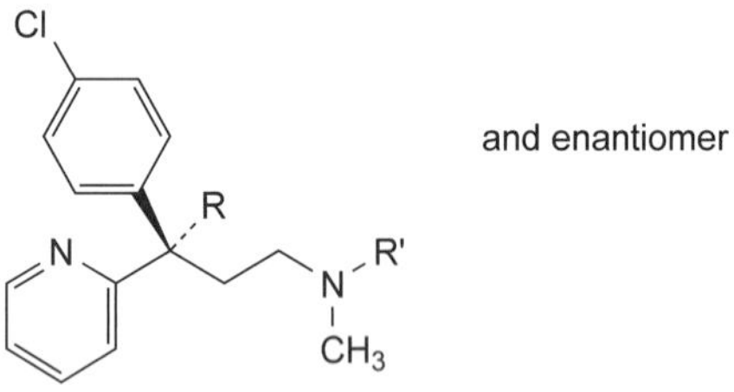

C. R = R′ = H: (3*RS*)-3-(4-chlorophenyl)-*N*-methyl-3-(pyridin-2-yl)propan-1-amine,

D. R = CN, R′ = CH_3: (2*RS*)-2-(4-chlorophenyl)-4-(dimethylamino)-2-(pyridin-2-yl)butanenitrile.

01/2008:1408
corrected 6.1

CILASTATIN SODIUM

Cilastatinum natricum

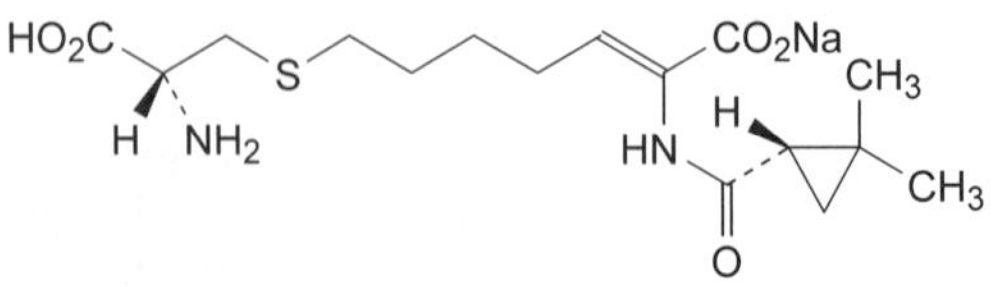

$C_{16}H_{25}N_2NaO_5S$ M_r 380.4
[81129-83-1]

DEFINITION

Sodium (*Z*)-7-[[(*R*)-2-amino-2-carboxyethyl]sulphanyl]-2-[[[(1*S*)-2,2-dimethylcyclopropyl]carbonyl]amino]hept-2-enoate.

Content: 98.0 per cent to 101.5 per cent (anhydrous substance).

CHARACTERS

Appearance: white or light yellow amorphous, hygroscopic powder.

Solubility: very soluble in water and in methanol, slightly soluble in anhydrous ethanol, very slightly soluble in dimethyl sulphoxide, practically insoluble in acetone and in methylene chloride.

IDENTIFICATION

A. Specific optical rotation (see Tests).

B. Infrared absorption spectrophotometry (*2.2.24*).

Comparison: *cilastatin sodium CRS.*

C. It gives reaction (a) of sodium (*2.3.1*).

TESTS

Solution S. Dissolve 1.0 g in *carbon dioxide-free water R* and dilute to 100 ml with the same solvent.

Appearance of solution. Solution S is clear (*2.2.1*) and not more intensely coloured than reference solution Y_6 (*2.2.2, Method II*).

pH (*2.2.3*): 6.5 to 7.5 for solution S.

Specific optical rotation (*2.2.7*): + 41.5 to + 44.5 (anhydrous substance).

Dissolve 0.250 g in a mixture of 1 volume of *hydrochloric acid R* and 120 volumes of *methanol R*, then dilute to 25.0 ml with the same mixture of solvents.

Related substances. Liquid chromatography (*2.2.29*).

Test solution. Dissolve 32.0 mg of the substance to be examined in *water R* and dilute to 20.0 ml with the same solvent.

Reference solution (a). Dilute 2.0 ml of the test solution to 100.0 ml with *water R*. Dilute 5.0 ml of this solution to 100.0 ml with *water R*.

Reference solution (b). Dilute 5.0 ml of the test solution to 100.0 ml with *water R*. Dilute 2.0 ml of this solution to 20.0 ml with *water R*.

Reference solution (c). Dissolve 16 mg of the substance to be examined in *dilute hydrogen peroxide solution R* and dilute to 10.0 ml with the same solution. Allow to stand for 30 min. Dilute 1 ml of this solution to 100 ml with *water R*.

Reference solution (d). Dissolve 32 mg of *mesityl oxide R* (impurity D) in 100 ml of *water R*. Dilute 1 ml of this solution to 50 ml with *water R*.

Column:
- *size*: *l* = 0.25 m, Ø = 4.6 mm;
- *stationary phase*: *octadecylsilyl silica gel for chromatography R* (5 μm);
- *temperature*: 50 °C.

Mobile phase:
- *mobile phase A*: mix 300 volumes of *acetonitrile R1* and 700 volumes of a 0.1 per cent *V/V* solution of *phosphoric acid R* in *water R*;
- *mobile phase B*: 0.1 per cent *V/V* solution of *phosphoric acid R* in *water R*;

Time (min)	Mobile phase A (per cent *V/V*)	Mobile phase B (per cent *V/V*)
0 - 30	15 → 100	85 → 0
30 - 46	100	0
46 - 56	100 → 15	0 → 85

Flow rate: 2.0 ml/min.

Detection: spectrophotometer at 210 nm.

Injection: 20 μl.

System suitability:

- the chromatogram obtained with reference solution (c) shows 3 principal peaks: the first 2 peaks (impurity A) may elute without being completely resolved;
- *mass distribution ratio*: minimum 10 for the peak due to cilastatin (3rd peak) in the chromatogram obtained with reference solution (c);
- *signal-to-noise ratio*: minimum 5.0 for the principal peak in the chromatogram obtained with reference solution (a).

Limits:

- *impurities A, B, C*: for each impurity, not more than the area of the principal peak in the chromatogram obtained with reference solution (b) (0.5 per cent);
- *total*: not more than twice the area of the principal peak in the chromatogram obtained with reference solution (b) (1 per cent);
- *disregard limit*: the area of the principal peak in the chromatogram obtained with reference solution (a) (0.1 per cent); disregard any peak corresponding to the peak due to impurity D in the chromatogram obtained with reference solution (d).

Impurity D, acetone and methanol. Gas chromatography (*2.2.28*).

Internal standard solution. Dissolve 0.5 ml of *propanol R* in *water R* and dilute to 1000 ml with the same solvent.

Test solution. Dissolve 0.200 g of the substance to be examined in *water R*, add 2.0 ml of the internal standard solution and dilute to 10.0 ml with *water R*.

Reference solution. Dissolve 2.0 ml of *acetone R*, 0.5 ml of *methanol R* and 0.5 ml of *mesityl oxide R* (impurity D) in *water R* and dilute to 1000 ml with the same solvent. To 2.0 ml of this solution add 2.0 ml of the internal standard solution and dilute to 10.0 ml with *water R*. This solution contains 316 μg of acetone, 79 μg of methanol and 86 μg of impurity D per millilitre.

Column:

- *material*: fused silica;
- *size*: *l* = 30 m, Ø = 0.53 mm;
- *stationary phase*: *macrogol 20 000 R* (film thickness 1.0 μm).

Carrier gas: *helium for chromatography R*.

Flow rate: 9 ml/min.

Temperature:

	Time (min)	Temperature (°C)
Column	0 - 2.5	50
	2.5 - 5	50 → 70
	5 - 5.5	70
Injection port		160
Detector		220

Detection: flame ionisation.

Injection: 1 μl.

Calculate the percentage contents of acetone, methanol and impurity D using the following expression:

$$\left(\frac{C}{W}\right) \times \left(\frac{R_u}{R_s}\right)$$

C = concentration of the solvent in the reference solution, in μg/ml;

W = quantity of cilastatin sodium in the test solution, in milligrams;

R_u = ratio of the area of the solvent peak to the area of the propanol peak in the chromatogram obtained with the test solution;

R_s = ratio of the area of the solvent peak to the area of the propanol peak in the chromatogram obtained with the reference solution.

Limits:

- *acetone*: maximum 1.0 per cent *m/m*;
- *methanol*: maximum 0.5 per cent *m/m*;
- *impurity D*: maximum 0.4 per cent *m/m*.

Heavy metals (*2.4.8*): maximum 20 ppm.

1.0 g complies with test C. Prepare the reference solution using 2.0 ml of *lead standard solution (10 ppm Pb) R*.

Water (*2.5.12*): maximum 2.0 per cent, determined on 0.50 g.

Bacterial endotoxins (*2.6.14*): less than 0.17 IU/mg, if intended for use in the manufacture of parenteral dosage forms without a further appropriate procedure for the removal of bacterial endotoxins.

ASSAY

Dissolve 0.300 g in 30 ml of *methanol R* and add 5 ml of *water R*. Add *0.1 M hydrochloric acid* to a pH of about 3.0. Carry out a potentiometric titration (*2.2.20*), using *0.1 M sodium hydroxide*. 3 jumps of potential are observed. Titrate to the 3rd equivalence point.

1 ml of *0.1 M sodium hydroxide* is equivalent to 19.02 mg of $C_{16}H_{25}N_2NaO_5S$.

STORAGE

In an airtight container, at a temperature not exceeding 8 °C. If the substance is sterile, store in a sterile, airtight, tamper-proof container.

IMPURITIES

Specified impurities: *A, B, C, D*.

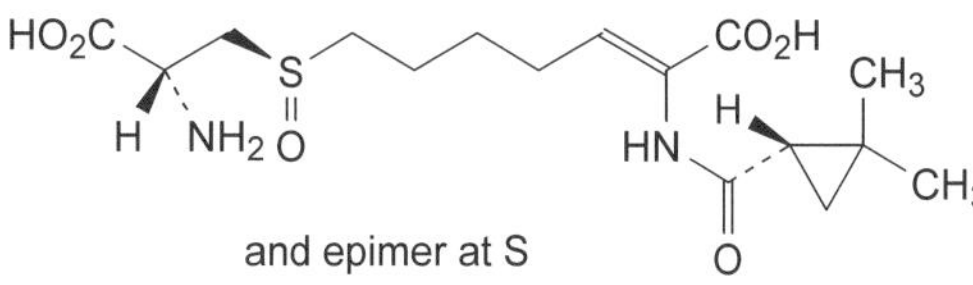

A. (*Z*)-7-[(*RS*)-[(*R*)-2-amino-2-carboxyethyl]sulphinyl]-2-[[[(1*S*)-2,2-dimethylcyclopropyl]carbonyl]amino]hept-2-enoic acid,

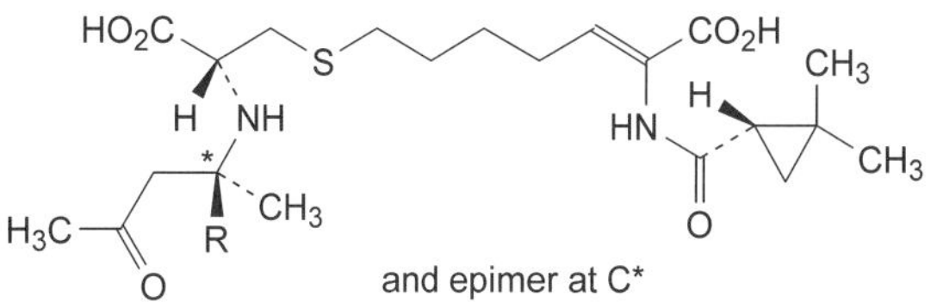

B. R = H: (*Z*)-7-[[(*R*)-2-[[(1*RS*)-1-methyl-3-oxobutyl]amino]-2-carboxyethyl]sulphanyl]-2-[[[(1*S*)-2,2-dimethylcyclopropyl]carbonyl]amino]hept-2-enoic acid,

C. R = CH_3: (*Z*)-7-[[(*R*)-2-[(1,1-dimethyl-3-oxobutyl)amino]-2-carboxyethyl]sulphanyl]-2-[[[(1*S*)-2,2-dimethylcyclopropyl]carbonyl]amino]hept-2-enoic acid,

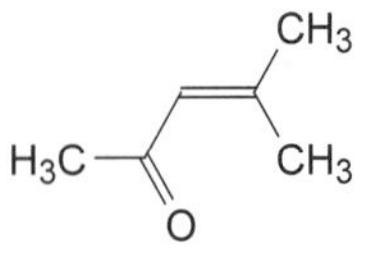

D. 4-methylpent-3-en-2-one (mesityl oxide).

01/2008:1190 corrected 6.1

CLEMASTINE FUMARATE

Clemastini fumaras

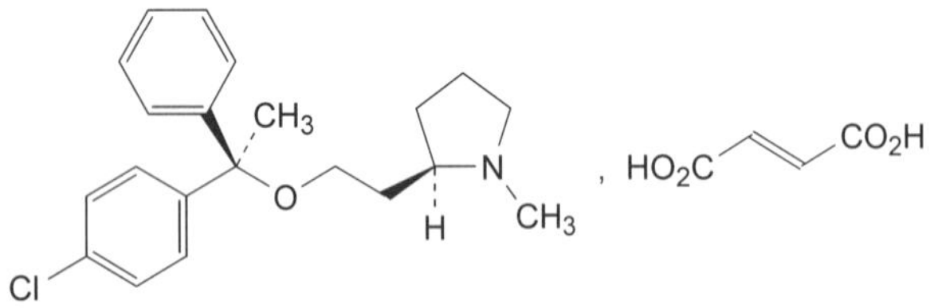

$C_{25}H_{30}ClNO_5$ M_r 460.0
[14976-57-9]

DEFINITION

(2*R*)-2-[2-[(*R*)-1-(4-Chlorophenyl)-1-phenylethoxy]ethyl]-1-methylpyrrolidine (*E*)-butenedioate.

Content: 98.5 per cent to 101.0 per cent (dried substance).

CHARACTERS

Appearance: white or almost white, crystalline powder.

Solubility: very slightly soluble in water, sparingly soluble in ethanol (70 per cent *V/V*), slightly soluble in ethanol (50 per cent *V/V*) and in methanol.

IDENTIFICATION

First identification: A, B.

Second identification: A, C, D.

A. Specific optical rotation (see Tests).

B. Infrared absorption spectrophotometry (*2.2.24*).

Comparison: *clemastine fumarate CRS.*

C. Examine the chromatograms obtained in the test for related substances.

Results: the principal spot in the chromatogram obtained with test solution (b) is similar in position, colour and size to the principal spot in the chromatogram obtained with reference solution (a).

D. Thin-layer chromatography (*2.2.27*).

Test solution. Dissolve 40 mg of the substance to be examined in *methanol R* and dilute to 2 ml with the same solvent.

Reference solution. Dissolve 50 mg of *fumaric acid CRS* in *ethanol (96 per cent) R* and dilute to 10 ml with the same solvent.

Plate: *TLC silica gel G plate R.*

Mobile phase: *water R, anhydrous formic acid R, di-isopropyl ether R* (5:25:70 *V/V/V*).

Application: 5 µl.

Development: over a path of 15 cm.

Drying: at 100-105 °C for 30 min and allow to cool.

Detection: spray with a 16 g/l solution of *potassium permanganate R* and examine in daylight.

Results: the spot with the highest R_F value in the chromatogram obtained with the test solution is similar in position, colour and size to the principal spot in the chromatogram obtained with the reference solution.

TESTS

Solution S. Dissolve 0.500 g in *methanol R* and dilute to 50.0 ml with the same solvent.

Appearance of solution. Solution S is clear (*2.2.1*) and not more intensely coloured than reference solution BY_7 (*2.2.2, Method II*).

pH (*2.2.3*): 3.2 to 4.2.

Suspend 1.0 g in 10 ml of *carbon dioxide-free water R.*

Specific optical rotation (*2.2.7*): + 15.0 to + 18.0 (dried substance), determined on solution S.

Related substances. Thin-layer chromatography (*2.2.27*).

Test solution (a). Dissolve 0.100 g of the substance to be examined in *methanol R* and dilute to 5.0 ml with the same solvent.

Test solution (b). Dilute 1.0 ml of test solution (a) to 10.0 ml with *methanol R.*

Reference solution (a). Dissolve 20.0 mg of *clemastine fumarate CRS* in *methanol R* and dilute to 10.0 ml with the same solvent.

Reference solution (b). Dilute 1.5 ml of test solution (b) to 50.0 ml with *methanol R.*

Reference solution (c). Dilute 0.5 ml of test solution (b) to 50.0 ml with *methanol R.*

Reference solution (d). Dissolve 10.0 mg of *diphenhydramine hydrochloride CRS* in 5.0 ml of reference solution (a).

Plate: *TLC silica gel G plate R.*

Mobile phase: *concentrated ammonia R, methanol R, tetrahydrofuran R* (1:20:80 *V/V/V*).

Application: 5 µl.

Development: over a path of 15 cm.

Drying: in a current of cold air for 5 min.

Detection: spray with a freshly prepared mixture of 1 volume of *potassium iodobismuthate solution R* and 10 volumes of *dilute acetic acid R* and then with *dilute hydrogen peroxide solution R*; cover the plate immediately with a glass plate of the same size and examine the chromatograms after 2 min.

System suitability: reference solution (d):

– the chromatogram shows 2 clearly separated spots.

Limits: test solution (a):

– *any impurity*: any spot, apart from the principal spot, is not more intense than the principal spot in the chromatogram obtained with reference solution (b) (0.3 per cent) and at most 4 such spots are more intense than the principal spot in the chromatogram obtained with reference solution (c) (0.1 per cent);

– *disregard limit*: disregard any spot remaining at the starting point (fumaric acid).

Impurity C. Liquid chromatography (*2.2.29*).

Solvent mixture: *acetonitrile R1*, 10 g/l solution of *ammonium dihydrogen phosphate R* (25:75 *V/V*).

Test solution. Dissolve 20 mg of the substance to be examined in the solvent mixture and dilute to 100 ml with the solvent mixture.

Reference solution (a). Dissolve 6 mg of *1-(4-chlorophenyl)-1-phenylethanol CRS* (impurity C) in the solvent mixture and dilute to 100 ml with the solvent mixture.

Monographs A-C

Reference solution (b). Dilute 1 ml of reference solution (a) to 100 ml with the solvent mixture.

Reference solution (c). Dissolve 10 mg of the substance to be examined in the solvent mixture and dilute to 100 ml with the solvent mixture. To 1 ml of this solution add 1 ml of reference solution (a) and dilute to 100 ml with the solvent mixture.

Column:

- *size*: *l* = 0.1 m, Ø = 4.6 mm;
- *stationary phase*: *octadecylsilyl silica gel for chromatography R* (5 µm).

Mobile phase: *phosphoric acid R, acetonitrile R1,* 10 g/l solution of *ammonium dihydrogen phosphate R* (0.1:45:55 *V/V/V*).

Flow rate: 1 ml/min.

Detection: spectrophotometer at 220 nm.

Injection: 100 µl.

System suitability: reference solution (c):

- *resolution*: minimum 2.2 between the peaks due to clemastine and impurity C.

Limit:

- *impurity C*: not more than the area of the principal peak in the chromatogram obtained with reference solution (b) (0.3 per cent).

Loss on drying (*2.2.32*): maximum 0.5 per cent, determined on 1.000 g by drying in an oven at 105 °C for 6 h.

Sulphated ash (*2.4.14*): maximum 0.1 per cent, determined on 1.0 g.

ASSAY

Dissolve 0.350 g in 60 ml of *anhydrous acetic acid R.* Titrate with *0.1 M perchloric acid,* determining the end-point potentiometrically (*2.2.20*).

1 ml of *0.1 M perchloric acid* is equivalent to 46.00 mg of $C_{25}H_{30}ClNO_5$.

IMPURITIES

Specified impurities: A, B, C.

Other detectable impurities (the following substances would, if present at a sufficient level, be detected by one or other of the tests in the monograph. They are limited by the general acceptance criterion for other/unspecified impurities and/or by the general monograph *Substances for pharmaceutical use (2034).* It is therefore not necessary to identify these impurities for demonstration of compliance. See also *5.10. Control of impurities in substances for pharmaceutical use*): *D.*

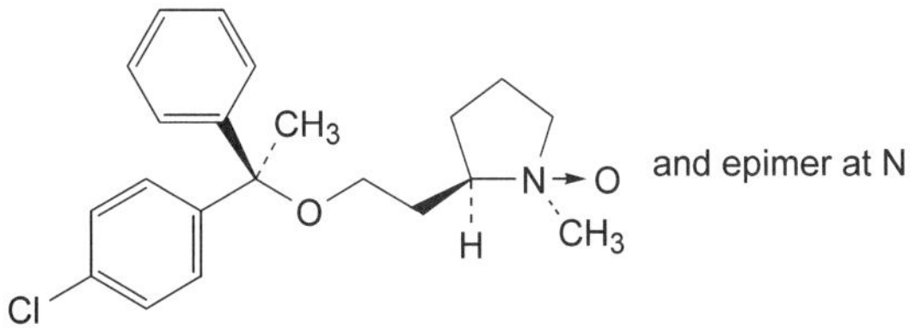

A. (1*RS*,2*R*)-2-[2-[(*R*)-1-(4-chlorophenyl)-1-phenylethoxy]-ethyl]-1-methylpyrrolidine 1-oxide,

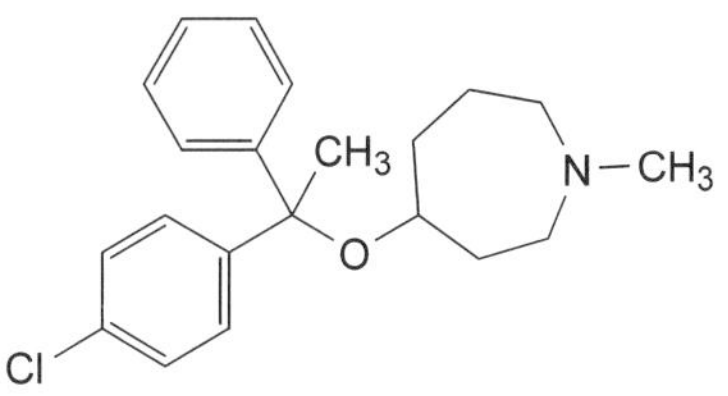

B. 4-[1-(4-chlorophenyl)-1-phenylethoxy]-1-methylazepane,

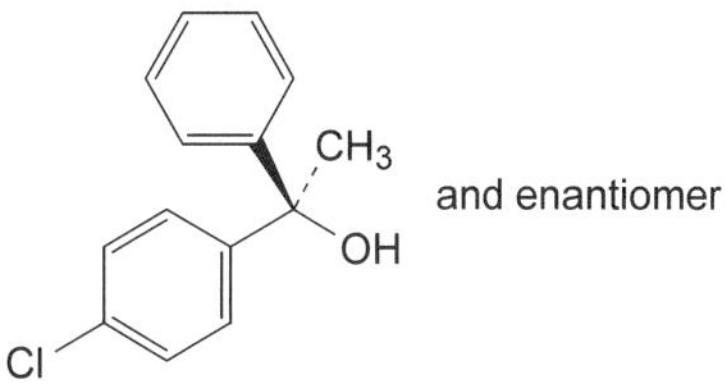

C. (*RS*)-1-(4-chlorophenyl)-1-phenylethanol,

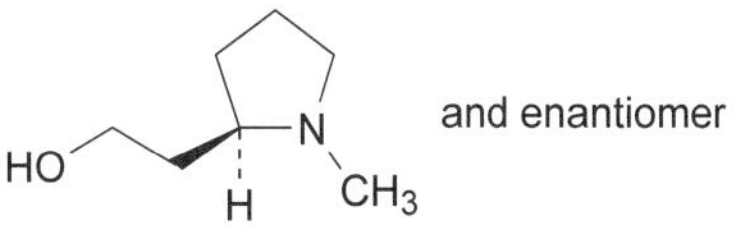

D. 2-[(2*RS*)-1-methylpyrrolidin-2-yl]ethanol.

04/2008:1747

CLOPAMIDE

Clopamidum

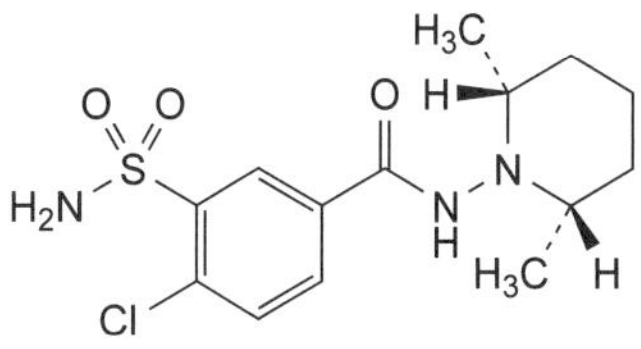

$C_{14}H_{20}ClN_3O_3S$ M_r 345.8

[636-54-4]

DEFINITION

4-Chloro-*N*-[(2*RS*,6*SR*)-2,6-dimethylpiperidin-1-yl]-3-sulfamoylbenzamide.

Content: 99.0 per cent to 101.0 per cent (dried substance).

PRODUCTION

The production method is evaluated to determine the potential for formation of an *N*-nitroso compound (*cis*-2,6-dimethyl-1-nitrosopiperidine). Where necessary, the production method is validated to demonstrate that the *N*-nitroso compound is absent in the final product.

CHARACTERS

Appearance: white or almost white, hygroscopic, crystalline powder.

Solubility: slightly soluble in water and in anhydrous ethanol, sparingly soluble in methanol.

It shows polymorphism (*5.9*).

IDENTIFICATION

Infrared absorption spectrophotometry (*2.2.24*).

Comparison: *clopamide CRS.*

If the spectra obtained in the solid state show differences, dissolve the substance to be examined and the reference substance separately in the minimum volume of *methanol R*, evaporate to dryness on a water-bath and record new spectra using the residues.

TESTS

Related substances. Liquid chromatography (*2.2.29*).

Test solution. Dissolve 100 mg of the substance to be examined in *methanol R* and dilute to 10.0 ml with the same solvent.

Reference solution (a). Dissolve 10 mg of *clopamide for system suitability CRS* (containing impurities B, C and H) in 1.0 ml of *methanol R.*

Reference solution (b). Dilute 2.0 ml of the test solution to 100.0 ml with *methanol R.* Dilute 2.0 ml of this solution to 40.0 ml with *methanol R.*

Column:

- *size*: *l* = 0.15 m, Ø = 4.6 mm;
- *stationary phase*: *end-capped octylsilyl silica gel for chromatography R* (5 μm);

Mobile phase:

- *mobile phase A*: dissolve 1.0 g of *ammonium acetate R* in 950 ml of *water R*, adjust to pH 2.0 with *phosphoric acid R* and dilute to 1000 ml with *water R*;
- *mobile phase B*: *acetonitrile R*;
- *mobile phase C*: *water R*, *tetrahydrofuran for chromatography R* (20:80 *V/V*); this mobile phase allows adequate rinsing of the system;

Time (min)	Mobile phase A (per cent *V/V*)	Mobile phase B (per cent *V/V*)	Mobile phase C (per cent *V/V*)
0 - 35	95 → 75	5 → 25	0
35 - 45	75 → 35	25 → 65	0
45 - 50	35 → 30	65 → 0	0 → 70
50 - 60	30	0	70
60 - 63	30 → 95	0 → 5	70 → 0
63 - 73	95	5	0

Flow rate: 0.4 ml/min.

Detection: spectrophotometer at 235 nm.

Injection: 10 μl.

Identification of impurities: use the chromatogram supplied with *clopamide for system suitability CRS* and the chromatogram obtained with reference solution (a) to identify the peaks due to impurities B, C and H.

Relative retention with reference to clopamide (retention time = about 33 min): impurity C = about 0.8; impurity H = about 1.2; impurity B = about 1.4.

System suitability: reference solution (a):

- *resolution*: minimum 3 between the peaks due to impurity C and clopamide.

Limits:

- *correction factors*: for the calculation of content, multiply the peak areas of the following impurities by the corresponding correction factor: impurity B = 0.5; impurity H = 0.4;
- *impurities B, C, H*: for each impurity, not more than twice the area of the principal peak in the chromatogram obtained with reference solution (b) (0.2 per cent);
- *unspecified impurities*: for each impurity, not more than the area of the principal peak in the chromatogram obtained with reference solution (b) (0.10 per cent);
- *total*: not more than 10 times the area of the principal peak in the chromatogram obtained with reference solution (b) (1.0 per cent);
- *disregard limit*: 0.5 times the area of the principal peak in the chromatogram obtained with reference solution (b) (0.05 per cent).

Heavy metals (*2.4.8*): maximum 20 ppm.

Dissolve 0.25 g in a mixture of 20 volumes of *acetone R* and 85 volumes of *methanol R* and dilute to 20 ml with the same mixture of solvents. 20 ml of the solution complies with modified test B. Prepare the reference solution by diluting 0.5 ml of *lead standard solution (10 ppm Pb) R* to 20 ml with a mixture of 20 volumes of *acetone R* and 85 volumes of *methanol R.* Prepare the blank solution by using 20 ml of a mixture of 20 volumes of *acetone R* and 85 volumes of *methanol R.*

Filter the solutions through a membrane filter (0.45 μm) to evaluate the result.

Loss on drying (*2.2.32*): maximum 2.5 per cent, determined on 1.000 g by drying in an oven at 105 °C.

Sulphated ash (*2.4.14*): maximum 0.1 per cent, determined on 1.0 g.

ASSAY

Dissolve 0.280 g in 70 ml of *anhydrous acetic acid R.* Titrate with *0.1 M perchloric acid*, determining the end-point potentiometrically (*2.2.20*).

1 ml of *0.1 M perchloric acid* is equivalent to 34.58 mg of $C_{14}H_{20}ClN_3O_3S$.

STORAGE

In an airtight container, protected from light.

IMPURITIES

Specified impurities: B, C, H.

Other detectable impurities (the following substances would, if present at a sufficient level, be detected by one or other of the tests in the monograph. They are limited by the general acceptance criterion for other/unspecified impurities and/or by the general monograph *Substances for pharmaceutical use (2034).* It is therefore not necessary to identify these impurities for demonstration of compliance. See also *5.10. Control of impurities in substances for pharmaceutical use*): *A, G.*

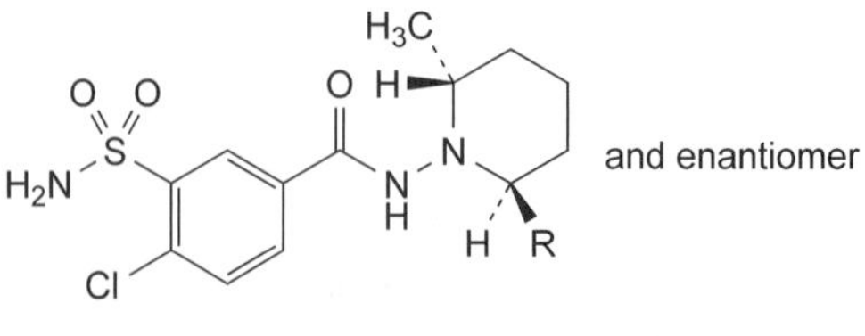

A. R = CH_3: 4-chloro-*N*-[(2*RS*,6*RS*)-2,6-dimethylpiperidin-1-yl]-3-sulfamoylbenzamide (*trans*-clopamide),

G. R = H: 4-chloro-*N*-[(2*RS*)-2-methylpiperidin-1-yl]-3-sulfamoylbenzamide,

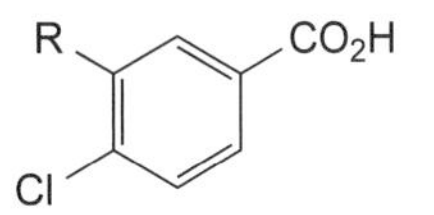

B. R = H: 4-chlorobenzoic acid,

C. R = SO_2-NH_2: 4-chloro-3-sulfamoylbenzoic acid,

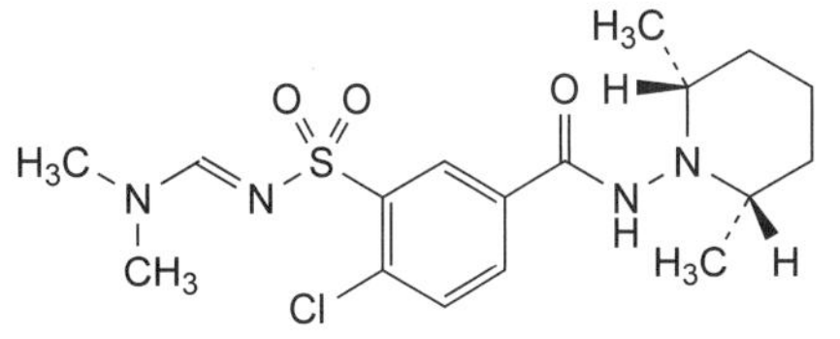

H. 4-chloro-3-[(*E*)-[(dimethylamino)methylene]sulfamoyl]-*N*-[(2*RS*,6*SR*)-2,6-dimethylpiperidin-1-yl]benzamide.

04/2008:0757

CLOTRIMAZOLE

Clotrimazolum

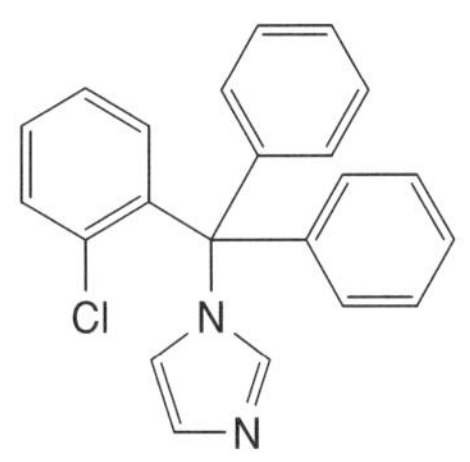

$C_{22}H_{17}ClN_2$ M_r 344.8
[23593-75-1]

DEFINITION

1-[(2-Chlorophenyl)diphenylmethyl]-1*H*-imidazole.

Content: 98.5 per cent to 100.5 per cent (dried substance).

CHARACTERS

Appearance: white or pale yellow, crystalline powder.

Solubility: practically insoluble in water, soluble in ethanol (96 per cent) and in methylene chloride.

IDENTIFICATION

First identification: B.

Second identification: A, C.

A. Melting point (*2.2.14*): 141 °C to 145 °C.

B. Infrared absorption spectrophotometry (*2.2.24*).

Comparison: *clotrimazole CRS.*

C. Thin-layer chromatography (*2.2.27*).

Test solution. Dissolve 50 mg of the substance to be examined in *ethanol (96 per cent) R* and dilute to 5 ml with the same solvent.

Reference solution. Dissolve 50 mg of *clotrimazole CRS* in *ethanol (96 per cent) R* and dilute to 5 ml with the same solvent.

Plate: *TLC silica gel F_{254} plate R.*

Mobile phase: *concentrated ammonia R1, propanol R, toluene R* (0.5:10:90 *V/V/V*).

Application: 10 μl.

Development: over 2/3 of the plate.

Drying: in air.

Detection: examine in ultraviolet light at 254 nm.

Results: the principal spot in the chromatogram obtained with the test solution is similar in position and size to the principal spot in the chromatogram obtained with the reference solution.

TESTS

Related substances. Liquid chromatography (*2.2.29*).

Test solution. Dissolve 50.0 mg of the substance to be examined in *acetonitrile R1* and dilute to 50.0 ml with the same solvent.

Reference solution (a). Dilute 1.0 ml of the test solution to 100.0 ml with *acetonitrile R1.* Dilute 1.0 ml of this solution to 10.0 ml with *acetonitrile R1.*

Reference solution (b). Dissolve the contents of a vial of *clotrimazole for peak identification CRS* (containing impurities A, B and F) in 1.0 ml of *acetonitrile R1.*

Reference solution (c). Dissolve 5.0 mg of *imidazole CRS* (impurity D) and 5.0 mg of *clotrimazole impurity E CRS* in *acetonitrile R1* and dilute to 100.0 ml with the same solvent. Dilute 1.0 ml of this solution to 25.0 ml with *acetonitrile R1.*

Column:

- *size*: *l* = 0.15 m, Ø = 4.6 mm;
- *stationary phase*: spherical *end-capped octylsilyl silica gel for chromatography R* (5 μm);
- *temperature*: 40 °C.

Mobile phase:

- *mobile phase A*: dissolve 1.0 g of *potassium dihydrogen phosphate R* and 0.5 g of *tetrabutylammonium hydrogen sulphate R1* in *water R* and dilute to 1000 ml with the same solvent;
- *mobile phase B*: *acetonitrile R1*;

Time (min)	Mobile phase A (per cent *V/V*)	Mobile phase B (per cent *V/V*)
0 - 3	75	25
3 - 25	75 → 20	25 → 80
25 - 30	20	80

Flow rate: 1.0 ml/min.

Detection: spectrophotometer at 210 nm.

Injection: 10 μl.

Relative retention with reference to clotrimazole (retention time = about 12 min): impurity D = about 0.1; impurity F = about 0.9; impurity B = about 1.1; impurity E = about 1.5; impurity A = about 1.8.

System suitability: reference solution (b):

- *resolution*: minimum 1.5 between the peaks due to impurity F and clotrimazole;
- the chromatogram obtained is similar to the chromatogram supplied with *clotrimazole for peak identification CRS.*

Limits:

- *impurities A, B*: for each impurity, not more than twice the area of the principal peak in the chromatogram obtained with reference solution (a) (0.2 per cent);
- *impurities D, E*: for each impurity, not more than the area of the corresponding peak in the chromatogram obtained with reference solution (c) (0.2 per cent);
- *impurity F*: not more than the area of the principal peak in the chromatogram obtained with reference solution (a) (0.1 per cent);

- *unspecified impurities*: for each impurity, not more than the area of the principal peak in the chromatogram obtained with reference solution (a) (0.10 per cent);
- *total*: not more than 5 times the area of the principal peak in the chromatogram obtained with reference solution (a) (0.5 per cent);
- *disregard limit*: 0.5 times the area of the principal peak in the chromatogram obtained with reference solution (a) (0.05 per cent).

Loss on drying (*2.2.32*): maximum 0.5 per cent, determined on 1.000 g by drying in an oven at 105 °C.

Sulphated ash (*2.4.14*): maximum 0.1 per cent, determined on 1.0 g.

ASSAY

Dissolve 0.300 g in 80 ml of *anhydrous acetic acid R*. Using 0.3 ml of *naphtholbenzein solution R* as indicator, titrate with *0.1 M perchloric acid* until the colour changes from brownish-yellow to green.

1 ml of *0.1 M perchloric acid* is equivalent to 34.48 mg of $C_{22}H_{17}ClN_2$.

STORAGE

Protected from light.

IMPURITIES

Specified impurities: A, B, D, E, F.

Other detectable impurities (the following substances would, if present at a sufficient level, be detected by one or other of the tests in the monograph. They are limited by the general acceptance criterion for other/unspecified impurities and/or by the general monograph *Substances for pharmaceutical use (2034)*. It is therefore not necessary to identify these impurities for demonstration of compliance. See also *5.10. Control of impurities in substances for pharmaceutical use*): *C.*

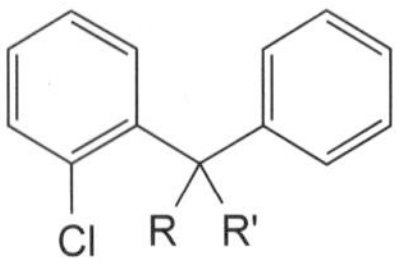

A. R = OH, R′ = C_6H_5: (2-chlorophenyl)diphenylmethanol,

C. R = Cl, R′ = C_6H_5: 1-chloro-2-(chlorodiphenylmethyl)-benzene,

E. R + R′ = O: (2-chlorophenyl)phenylmethanone (2-chlorobenzophenone),

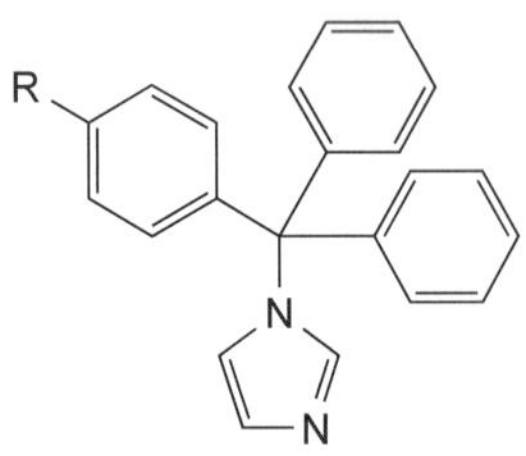

B. R = Cl: 1-[(4-chlorophenyl)diphenylmethyl]-1*H*-imidazole,

F. R = H: 1-(triphenylmethyl)-1*H*-imidazole (deschloroclotrimazole),

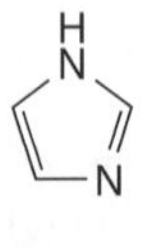

D. imidazole.

04/2008:0076

CODEINE

Codeinum

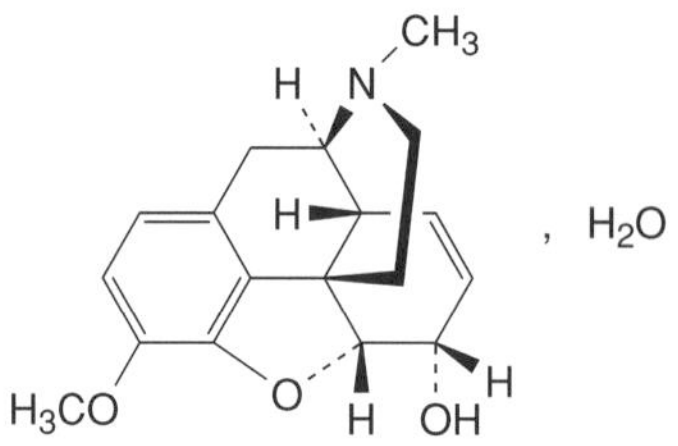

$C_{18}H_{21}NO_3,H_2O$ M_r 317.4

[76-57-3]

DEFINITION

7,8-Didehydro-4,5α-epoxy-3-methoxy-17-methylmorphinan-6α-ol.

Content: 99.0 per cent to 101.0 per cent (dried substance).

CHARACTERS

Appearance: white or almost white, crystalline powder or colourless crystals.

Solubility: soluble in boiling water, freely soluble in ethanol (96 per cent).

IDENTIFICATION

First identification: A, C.

Second identification: A, B, D, E.

A. Melting point (*2.2.14*): 155 °C to 159 °C.

B. To 2.0 ml of solution S (see Tests) add 50 ml of *water R* then 10 ml of *1 M sodium hydroxide* and dilute to 100.0 ml with *water R*. Examined between 250 nm and 350 nm (*2.2.25*), the solution shows only 1 absorption maximum, at 284 nm. The specific absorbance at the absorption maximum is about 50 (dried substance).

C. Infrared absorption spectrophotometry (*2.2.24*).

   Preparation: dried substance prepared as a disc of *potassium bromide R*.

   Comparison: *codeine CRS.*

D. To about 10 mg add 1 ml of *sulphuric acid R* and 0.05 ml of *ferric chloride solution R2* and heat on a water-bath. A blue colour develops. Add 0.05 ml of *nitric acid R*. The colour changes to red.

E. It gives the reaction of alkaloids (*2.3.1*).

TESTS

Solution S. Dissolve 50 mg in *carbon dioxide-free water R* and dilute to 10.0 ml with the same solvent.

Appearance of solution. Solution S is clear (*2.2.1*) and colourless (*2.2.2, Method II*).

Specific optical rotation (*2.2.7*): – 142 to – 146 (dried substance).

Dissolve 0.50 g in *ethanol (96 per cent) R* and dilute to 25.0 ml with the same solvent.

Related substances. Liquid chromatography (*2.2.29*).

Test solution. Dissolve 0.100 g of the substance to be examined and 0.100 g of *sodium octanesulphonate R* in the mobile phase and dilute to 10.0 ml with the mobile phase.

Reference solution (a). Dissolve 5.0 mg of *codeine impurity A CRS* in the mobile phase and dilute to 5.0 ml with the mobile phase.

Reference solution (b). Dilute 1.0 ml of reference solution (a) to 20.0 ml with the mobile phase.

Reference solution (c). Dilute 1.0 ml of the test solution to 50.0 ml with the mobile phase. Dilute 5.0 ml of this solution to 100.0 ml with the mobile phase.

Reference solution (d). To 0.25 ml of the test solution, add 2.5 ml of reference solution (a).

Column:
- *size*: l = 0.25 m, Ø = 4.6 mm;
- *stationary phase*: *end-capped octylsilyl silica gel for chromatography R* (5 µm).

Mobile phase: dissolve 1.08 g of *sodium octanesulphonate R* in a mixture of 20 ml of *glacial acetic acid R* and 250 ml of *acetonitrile R* and dilute to 1000 ml with *water R*.

Flow rate: 2 ml/min.

Detection: spectrophotometer at 245 nm.

Injection: 10 µl.

Run time: 10 times the retention time of codeine.

Relative retention with reference to codeine (retention time = about 6 min): impurity B = about 0.6; impurity E = about 0.7; impurity A = about 2.0; impurity C = about 2.3; impurity D = about 3.6.

System suitability: reference solution (d):
- *resolution*: minimum 3 between the peaks due to codeine and impurity A.

Limits:
- *correction factor*: for the calculation of content, multiply the peak area of impurity C by 0.25;
- *impurity A*: not more than twice the area of the principal peak in the chromatogram obtained with reference solution (b) (1.0 per cent);
- *impurities B, C, D, E*: for each impurity, not more than twice the area of the principal peak in the chromatogram obtained with reference solution (c) (0.2 per cent);
- *any other impurity*: for each impurity, not more than the area of the principal peak in the chromatogram obtained with reference solution (c) (0.1 per cent);
- *sum of impurities other than A*: not more than 10 times the area of the principal peak in the chromatogram obtained with reference solution (c) (1.0 per cent);
- *disregard limit*: 0.5 times the area of the principal peak in the chromatogram obtained with reference solution (c) (0.05 per cent).

Loss on drying (*2.2.32*): 4.0 per cent to 6.0 per cent, determined on 1.000 g by drying in an oven at 105 °C.

Sulphated ash (*2.4.14*): maximum 0.1 per cent, determined on 1.0 g.

ASSAY

Dissolve 0.250 g in 10 ml of *anhydrous acetic acid R*. Add 20 ml of *dioxan R*. Titrate with *0.1 M perchloric acid*, using 0.05 ml of *crystal violet solution R* as indicator.

1 ml of *0.1 M perchloric acid* is equivalent to 29.94 mg of $C_{18}H_{21}NO_3$.

STORAGE

Protected from light.

IMPURITIES

Specified impurities: A, B, C, D, E.

Other detectable impurities (the following substances would, if present at a sufficient level, be detected by one or other of the tests in the monograph. They are limited by the general acceptance criterion for other/unspecified impurities and/or by the general monograph *Substances for pharmaceutical use (2034)*. It is therefore not necessary to identify these impurities for demonstration of compliance. See also *5.10. Control of impurities in substances for pharmaceutical use*): *F, G.*

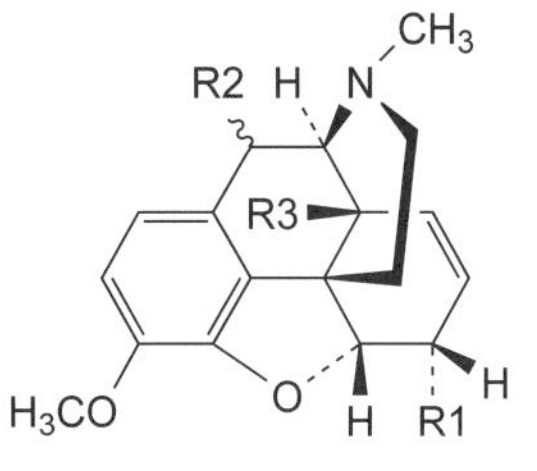

A. R1 = OCH_3, R2 = R3 = H: 7,8-didehydro-4,5α-epoxy-3,6α-dimethoxy-17-methylmorphinan (methylcodeine),

E. R1 = R2 = OH, R3 = H: 7,8-didehydro-4,5α-epoxy-3-methoxy-17-methylmorphinan-6α,10-diol,

F. R1 = R3 = OH, R2 = H: 7,8-didehydro-4,5α-epoxy-3-methoxy-17-methylmorphinan-6α,14-diol,

B. morphine,

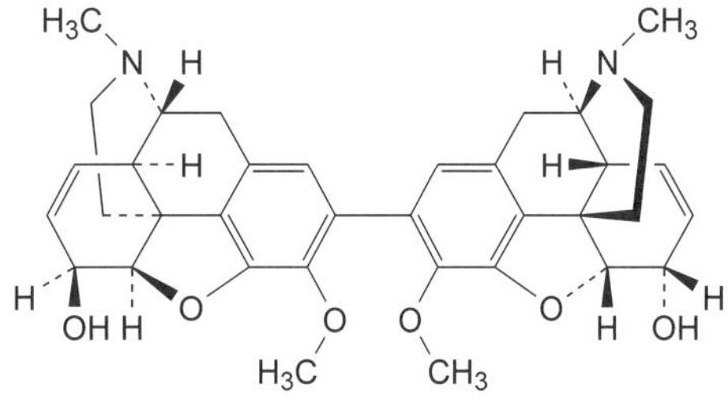

C. 7,7′,8,8′-tetradehydro-4,5α:4′,5′α-diepoxy-3,3′-dimethoxy-17,17′-dimethyl-2,2′-bimorphinanyl-6α,6′α-diol (codeine dimer),

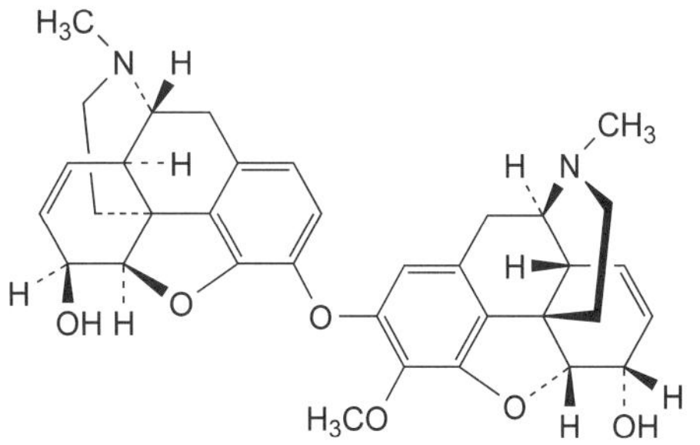

D. 7,8-didehydro-2-[(7,8-didehydro-4,5α-epoxy-6α-hydroxy-17-methylmorphinan-3-yl)oxy]-4,5α-epoxy-3-methoxy-17-methylmorphinan-6α-ol (3-*O*-(codein-2-yl)morphine),

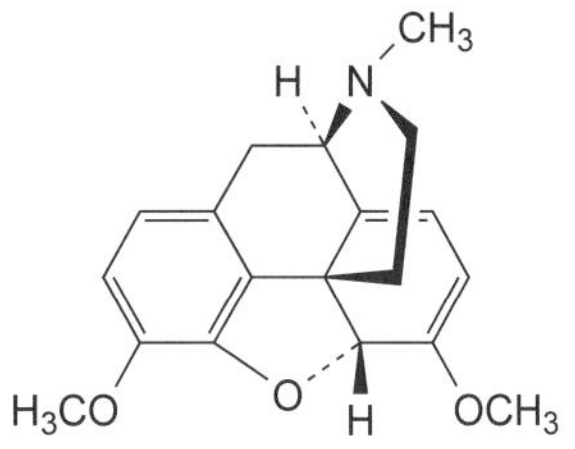

G. 6,7,8,14-tetradehydro-4,5α-epoxy-3,6-dimethoxy-17-methylmorphinan (thebaine).

D

04/2008:1666

DESFLURANE

Desfluranum

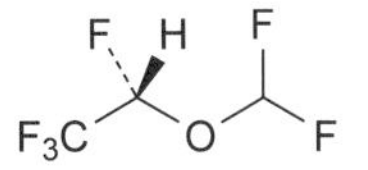

$C_3H_2F_6O$ M_r 168.0

[57041-67-5]

DEFINITION

(2*RS*)-2-(Difluoromethoxy)-1,1,1,2-tetrafluoroethane.

CHARACTERS

Appearance: clear, colourless, mobile, heavy liquid.

Solubility: practically insoluble in water, miscible with anhydrous ethanol.

Relative density: 1.47, determined at 15 °C.

bp: about 22 °C.

IDENTIFICATION

Infrared absorption spectrophotometry (*2.2.24*).

Preparation: examine the substance in the gaseous state.

Comparison: *Ph. Eur. reference spectrum of desflurane.*

TESTS

The substance to be examined must be cooled to a temperature below 10 °C and the tests must be carried out at a temperature below 20 °C.

Acidity or alkalinity. To 20 ml add 20 ml of *carbon dioxide-free water R*, shake for 3 min and allow to stand. Collect the upper layer and add 0.2 ml of *bromocresol purple solution R*. Not more than 0.1 ml of *0.01 M sodium hydroxide* or 0.1 ml of *0.01 M hydrochloric acid* is required to change the colour of the indicator.

Related substances. Gas chromatography (*2.2.28*).

Test solution. The substance to be examined.

Reference solution (a). Introduce 25 ml of the substance to be examined into a 50 ml flask fitted with a septum, and add 0.50 ml of *desflurane impurity A CRS* and 1.0 ml of *isoflurane CRS* (impurity B). Add 50 µl of *acetone R* (impurity H), 10 µl of *chloroform R* (impurity F) and 50 µl of *methylene chloride R* (impurity E) to the solution, using an airtight syringe, and dilute to 50.0 ml with the substance to be examined. Dilute 5.0 ml of this solution to 50.0 ml with the substance to be examined. Store at a temperature below 10 °C.

Reference solution (b). Dilute 5.0 ml of reference solution (a) to 50.0 ml with the substance to be examined. Store at a temperature below 10 °C.

Reference solution (c). Dilute 5.0 ml of reference solution (b) to 25.0 ml with the substance to be examined. Store at a temperature below 10 °C.

Column:
- *material*: fused silica;
- *size*: *l* = 105 m, Ø = 0.32 mm;
- *stationary phase*: *poly[methyl(trifluoropropylmethyl)-siloxane] R* (film thickness 1.5 µm).

Carrier gas: *helium for chromatography R.*

Flow rate: 2.0 ml/min.

Split ratio: 1:25.

Temperature:
- *column*: 30 °C;
- *injection port*: 150 °C;
- *detector*: 200 °C.

Detection: flame ionisation.

Injection: 2.0 µl.

Run time: 35 min.

Relative retention with reference to desflurane (retention time = about 11.5 min): impurity C = about 1.06; impurity D = about 1.09; impurity A = about 1.14; impurity G = about 1.39; impurity E = about 1.5; impurity B = about 1.7; impurity F = about 2.2; impurity H = about 2.6.

System suitability: reference solution (a):
- *number of theoretical plates*: minimum 20 000, calculated for the peak due to impurity A;
- *symmetry factor*: maximum 2.0 for the peak due to impurity B.

Limits:
- *impurity B*: not more than the difference between the area of the corresponding peak in the chromatogram obtained with reference solution (a) and the area of the corresponding peak in the chromatogram obtained with the test solution (0.2 per cent *V/V*);
- *impurity A*: not more than the difference between the area of the corresponding peak in the chromatogram obtained with reference solution (a) and the area of the corresponding peak in the chromatogram obtained with the test solution (0.1 per cent *V/V*);
- *impurities C, D, G*: for each impurity, not more than the difference between the area of the peak due to impurity A in the chromatogram obtained with reference solution (b) and the area of the peak due to impurity A in the chromatogram obtained with the test solution (0.01 per cent *V/V*);
- *impurities E, H*: for each impurity, not more than the difference between the area of the corresponding peak in the chromatogram obtained with reference solution (a) and the area of the corresponding peak in the chromatogram obtained with the test solution (0.01 per cent *V/V*);
- *impurity F*: not more than the difference between the area of the corresponding peak in the chromatogram obtained with reference solution (a) and the area of the corresponding peak in the chromatogram obtained with the test solution (0.002 per cent *V/V*);
- *unspecified impurities*: for each impurity, not more than 0.5 times the difference between the area of the peak due to impurity A in the chromatogram obtained with reference solution (b) and the area of the peak due to impurity A in the chromatogram obtained with the test solution (0.005 per cent *V/V*);
- *sum of impurities other than A, B, C, D, E, F, G and H*: not more than the difference between the area of the peak due to impurity A in the chromatogram obtained with reference solution (b) and the area of the peak due to impurity A in the chromatogram obtained with the test solution (0.01 per cent *V/V*);
- *disregard limit*: the difference between the area of the peak due to impurity A in the chromatogram obtained with reference solution (c) and the area of the peak due to impurity A in the chromatogram obtained with the test solution (0.002 per cent *V/V*).

Fluorides: maximum 10.0 ppm.

Potentiometry (*2.2.36, Method I*).

Test solution. To 10.0 ml in a separating funnel, add 10 ml of a mixture of 30.0 ml of *dilute ammonia R2* and 70.0 ml of *distilled water R*. Shake for 1 min and collect the upper layer. Repeat this extraction procedure twice, collecting the upper layer each time. Adjust the combined upper layers to pH 5.2 with *dilute hydrochloric acid R*. Add 5.0 ml of *fluoride standard solution (1 ppm F) R* and dilute to 50.0 ml with *distilled water R*. To 20.0 ml of this solution add 20.0 ml of *total-ionic-strength-adjustment buffer R* and dilute to 50.0 ml with *distilled water R*.

Reference solutions. To each of 1.0 ml, 2.0 ml, 3.0 ml, 4.0 ml and 5.0 ml of *fluoride standard solution (10 ppm F) R* add 20.0 ml of *total-ionic-strength-adjustment buffer R* and dilute to 50.0 ml with *distilled water R*.

Indicator electrode: fluoride selective.

Reference electrode: silver-silver chloride.

Carry out the measurements on 20 ml of each solution. Calculate the concentration of fluorides using the calibration curve, taking into account the addition of fluoride to the test solution.

Antimony: maximum 3.0 ppm.

Atomic absorption spectrometry (*2.2.23, Method I*).

Solvent mixture: *hydrochloric acid R, nitric acid R* (50:50 *V/V*).

Test solution. Transfer 10 g, cooled to below 10 °C, to a tared flask containing 20 ml of *water R* cooled to below 5 °C. Add 1 ml of the solvent mixture and leave at room temperature until the desflurane has evaporated completely. Subsequently, reduce the volume to about 8 ml on a hot plate. Cool to room temperature and transfer to a volumetric flask. Add 1 ml of the solvent mixture and adjust to 10.0 ml with *water R*.

Reference solutions. To each of 1.0 ml, 2.0 ml, 3.0 ml, 4.0 ml and 5.0 ml of *antimony standard solution (100 ppm Sb) R* add 20 ml of the solvent mixture and dilute to 100.0 ml with *water R*.

Source: antimony hollow-cathode lamp using a transmission band of 0.2 nm and a 75 per cent lamp current.

Wavelength: 217.6 nm.

Atomisation device: air-acetylene flame.

Non-volatile matter: maximum 100 mg/l.

Evaporate 20.0 ml to dryness with the aid of a stream of *nitrogen R*. The residue weighs not more than 2.0 mg.

STORAGE

In a glass bottle fitted with a polyethylene-lined cap. Before opening the bottle, cool the contents to below 10 °C.

IMPURITIES

Specified impurities: A, B, C, D, E, F, G, H.

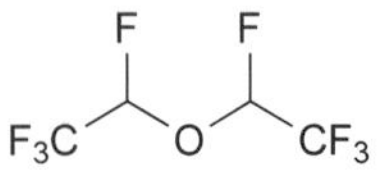

A. 1,1′-oxybis(1,2,2,2-tetrafluoroethane),

B. isoflurane,

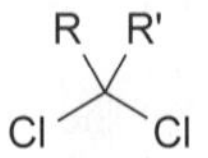

C. R = H, R′ = F: dichlorofluoromethane,

D. R = Cl, R′ = F: trichlorofluoromethane,

E. R = R′ = H: dichloromethane (methylene chloride),

F. R = H, R′ = Cl: trichloromethane (chloroform),

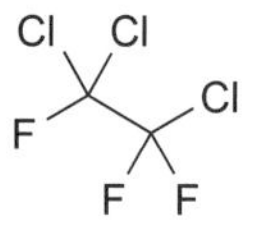

G. 1,1,2-trichloro-1,2,2-trifluoroethane,

H. acetone.

04/2008:1095

DEVIL'S CLAW ROOT

Harpagophyti radix

DEFINITION

Devil's claw root consists of the cut and dried, tuberous secondary roots of *Harpagophytum procumbens* DC. and/or *Harpagophytum zeyheri* Decne.

Content: minimum 1.2 per cent of harpagoside ($C_{24}H_{30}O_{11}$; M_r 494.5) (dried drug).

CHARACTERS

Devil's claw root is greyish-brown to dark brown.

IDENTIFICATION

A. It consists of thick, fan-shaped or rounded slices or of roughly crushed discs. The darker outer surface is traversed by tortuous longitudinal wrinkles. The paler cut surface shows a dark cambial zone and xylem bundles distinctly aligned in radial rows. The central cylinder shows fine concentric striations. Seen under a lens, the cut surface presents yellow to brownish-red granules.

B. Reduce to a powder (355) (*2.9.12*). The powder is brownish-yellow. Examine under a microscope using *chloral hydrate solution R*. The powder shows the following diagnostic characters: fragments of cork layer consisting of yellowish-brown, thin-walled cells; fragments of cortical parenchyma consisting of large, thin-walled cells, sometimes containing reddish-brown granular inclusions and isolated yellow droplets; fragments of reticulately thickened or pitted vessels and fragments of lignified parenchyma, sometimes associated with vessels from the central cylinder; prism crystals and rare small needles of calcium oxalate in the parenchyma. The powder may show rectangular or polygonal sclereids with dark reddish-brown contents. With a solution of phloroglucinol in hydrochloric acid, the parenchyma turns green.

C. Thin-layer chromatography (*2.2.27*).

Test solution. Heat 1.0 g of the powdered drug (355) (*2.9.12*) with 10 ml of *methanol R* on a water-bath at 60 °C for 10 min. Filter and reduce the filtrate to about 2 ml under reduced pressure at a temperature not exceeding 40 °C.

Reference solution. Dissolve 1 mg of *harpagoside R* and 2.5 mg of *fructose R* in 1 ml of *methanol R*.

Plate: *TLC silica gel plate R* (5-40 μm) [or *TLC silica gel plate R* (2-10 μm)].

Mobile phase: *water R, methanol R, ethyl acetate R* (8:15:77 *V/V/V*).

Application: 20 μl [or 5 μl], as bands.

Development: over a path of 10 cm [or 7.5 cm].

Drying: in a current of warm air.

Detection A: examine in ultraviolet light at 254 nm.

Results A: see below the sequence of zones present in the chromatograms obtained with the reference solution and the test solution. The chromatogram obtained with the test solution shows other distinct zones, mainly above the zone due to harpagoside. Furthermore, other faint zones may be present in the chromatogram obtained with the test solution.

Top of the plate	
———	———
Harpagoside: a quenching zone	A quenching zone: harpagoside
———	———
Reference solution	**Test solution**

Detection B: spray with a 10 g/l solution of *phloroglucinol R* in *ethanol (96 per cent) R* and then with *hydrochloric acid R*; heat at 80 °C for 5-10 min and examine in daylight.

Results B: see below the sequence of zones present in the chromatograms obtained with the reference solution and the test solution. The chromatogram obtained with the test solution also shows several yellow to brown zones above the zone due to harpagoside. Furthermore, other faint zones may be present in the chromatogram obtained with the test solution.

Top of the plate	
———	———
Harpagoside: a green zone	A green zone (harpagoside)
———	———
	A yellow zone
	A light green zone
Fructose: a yellowish-grey zone	A yellowish-grey zone may be present (fructose)
	A brown zone
Reference solution	**Test solution**

TESTS

Starch. Examine the powdered drug (355) (*2.9.12*) under a microscope using *water R*. Add *iodine solution R1*. No blue colour develops.

Loss on drying (*2.2.32*): maximum 12.0 per cent, determined on 1.000 g of the powdered drug (355) (*2.9.12*) by drying in an oven at 105 °C.

Total ash (*2.4.16*): maximum 10.0 per cent.

ASSAY

Liquid chromatography (*2.2.29*).

Test solution. To 0.500 g of the powdered drug (355) (*2.9.12*) add 100.0 ml of *methanol R*. Shake for 4 h and filter through a membrane filter (nominal pore size: 0.45 µm).

Reference solution. Dissolve the contents of a vial of *harpagoside CRS* in *methanol R* and dilute to 10.0 ml with the same solvent.

Column:

- *size*: l = 0.10 m, Ø = 4.0 mm;
- *stationary phase*: *octadecylsilyl silica gel for chromatography R* (5 µm).

Mobile phase: *methanol R, water R* (50:50 *V/V*).

Flow rate: 1.5 ml/min.

Detection: spectrophotometer at 278 nm.

Injection: 10 µl.

Run time: 3 times the retention time of harpagoside.

Retention time: harpagoside = about 7 min.

Calculate the percentage content of harpagoside using the following expression:

$$\frac{m_2 \times A_1 \times 1000}{A_2 \times m_1}$$

A_1 = area of the peak due to harpagoside in the chromatogram obtained with the test solution;

A_2 = area of the peak due to harpagoside in the chromatogram obtained with the reference solution;

m_1 = mass of the drug to be examined used to prepare the test solution, in grams;

m_2 = mass of *harpagoside CRS* in the reference solution, in grams.

04/2008:0897

DIETHYL PHTHALATE

Diethylis phthalas

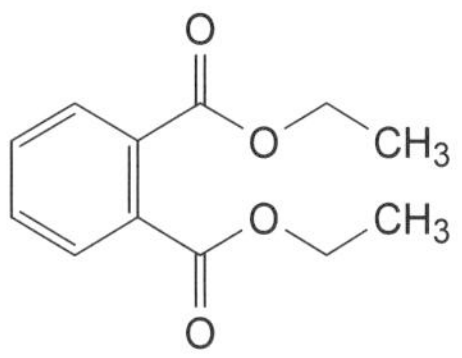

$C_{12}H_{14}O_4$ M_r 222.2

[84-66-2]

DEFINITION

Diethyl benzene-1,2-dicarboxylate.

Content: 99.0 per cent *m/m* to 101.0 per cent *m/m*.

CHARACTERS

Appearance: clear, colourless or very slightly yellow, oily liquid.

Solubility: practically insoluble in water, miscible with ethanol (96 per cent).

IDENTIFICATION

First identification: B, C.

Second identification: A, D, E.

A. Relative density (*2.2.5*): 1.117 to 1.121.

B. Refractive index (*2.2.6*): 1.500 to 1.505.

C. Infrared absorption spectrophotometry (*2.2.24*).

Preparation: thin films.

Comparison: *diethyl phthalate CRS*.

D. Thin-layer chromatography (*2.2.27*).

Test solution. Dissolve 50 mg of the substance to be examined in *ether R* and dilute to 10 ml with the same solvent.

Reference solution. Dissolve 50 mg of *diethyl phthalate CRS* in *ether R* and dilute to 10 ml with the same solvent.

Plate: *TLC silica gel GF_{254} plate R*.

Mobile phase: *heptane R, ether R* (30:70 *V/V*).

Application: 10 µl.

Development: over 2/3 of the plate.

Drying: in air.

Detection: examine in ultraviolet light at 254 nm.

Results: the principal spot in the chromatogram obtained with the test solution is similar in position and size to the principal spot in the chromatogram obtained with the reference solution.

E. To about 0.1 ml add 0.25 ml of *sulphuric acid R* and 50 mg of *resorcinol R*. Heat on a water-bath for 5 min. Allow to cool. Add 10 ml of *water R* and 1 ml of *strong sodium hydroxide solution R*. The solution becomes yellow or brownish-yellow and shows green fluorescence.

TESTS

Appearance. The substance to be examined is clear (*2.2.1*) and not more intensely coloured than reference solution Y_6 (*2.2.2, Method II*).

Acidity. Dissolve 20.0 g in 50 ml of *ethanol (96 per cent) R* previously neutralised to *phenolphthalein solution R1*. Add 0.2 ml of *phenolphthalein solution R1*. Not more than 0.1 ml of *0.1 M sodium hydroxide* is required to change the colour of the indicator to pink.

Related substances. Gas chromatography (*2.2.28*).

Internal standard solution. Dissolve 60 mg of *naphthalene R* in *methylene chloride R* and dilute to 20 ml with the same solvent.

Test solution (a). Dissolve 1.0 g of the substance to be examined in *methylene chloride R* and dilute to 20.0 ml with the same solvent.

Test solution (b). Dissolve 1.0 g of the substance to be examined in *methylene chloride R*, add 2.0 ml of the internal standard solution and dilute to 20.0 ml with *methylene chloride R*.

Reference solution. To 1.0 ml of test solution (a) add 10.0 ml of the internal standard solution and dilute to 100.0 ml with *methylene chloride R*.

Column:
- *material*: glass;
- *size*: *l* = 2 m, Ø = 2 mm;
- *stationary phase*: *silanised diatomaceous earth for gas chromatography R* (150-180 μm) impregnated with 3 per cent *m/m* of *polymethylphenylsiloxane R*.

Carrier gas: *nitrogen for chromatography R*.

Flow rate: 30 ml/min.

Temperature:
- *column*: 150 °C;
- *injection port and detector*: 225 °C.

Detection: flame ionisation.

Injection: 1 μl.

Run time: 3 times the retention time of diethyl phthalate.

Elution order: naphthalene, diethyl phtalate.

System suitability:
- *resolution*: minimum 10 between the peaks due to naphthalene and diethyl phthalate in the chromatogram obtained with the reference solution;
- in the chromatogram obtained with test solution (a), there is no peak with the same retention time as the internal standard.

Limit:
- *total*: calculate the ratio (*R*) of the area of the peak due to diethyl phthalate to the area of the peak due to the internal standard from the chromatogram obtained with the reference solution; from the chromatogram obtained with test solution (b), calculate the ratio of the sum of the areas of any peaks, apart from the principal peak and the peak due to the internal standard, to the area of the peak due to the internal standard: this ratio is not greater than *R* (1.0 per cent).

Water (*2.5.12*): maximum 0.2 per cent, determined on 10.0 g.

Sulphated ash (*2.4.14*): maximum 0.1 per cent, determined on 1.0 g.

ASSAY

Introduce 0.750 g into a 250 ml borosilicate glass flask. Add 25.0 ml of *0.5 M alcoholic potassium hydroxide* and a few glass beads. Boil in a water-bath under a reflux condenser for 1 h. Add 1 ml of *phenolphthalein solution R1* and titrate immediately with *0.5 M hydrochloric acid*. Carry out a blank titration. Calculate the volume of *0.5 M alcoholic potassium hydroxide* used in the saponification.

1 ml of *0.5 M alcoholic potassium hydroxide* is equivalent to 55.56 mg of $C_{12}H_{14}O_4$.

STORAGE

In an airtight container.

01/2008:1310
corrected 6.1

DIHYDRALAZINE SULPHATE, HYDRATED

Dihydralazini sulfas hydricus

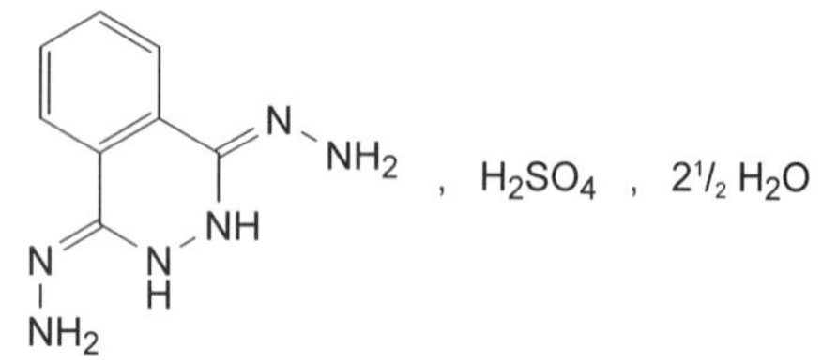

$C_8H_{12}N_6O_4S,2^1/_2H_2O$ — M_r 333.3

[7327-87-9]

DEFINITION

(Phthalazine-1,4(2*H*,3*H*)-diylidene)dihydrazine sulphate 2.5-hydrate.

Content: 98.0 per cent to 102.0 per cent (dried substance).

CHARACTERS

Appearance: white or slightly yellow, crystalline powder.

Solubility: slightly soluble in water, practically insoluble in anhydrous ethanol. It dissolves in dilute mineral acids.

IDENTIFICATION

A. Infrared absorption spectrophotometry (*2.2.24*).

Comparison: *Ph. Eur. reference spectrum of dihydralazine sulphate hydrated.*

B. Dissolve about 50 mg in 5 ml of *dilute hydrochloric acid R*. The solution gives reaction (a) of sulphates (*2.3.1*).

TESTS

Appearance of solution. The solution is clear (*2.2.1*) and not more intensely coloured than reference solution BY_6 (*2.2.2, Method II*).

Dissolve 0.20 g in *dilute nitric acid R* and dilute to 10 ml with the same acid.

Monographs D-K

Related substances. Liquid chromatography (*2.2.29*). *Prepare the solutions immediately before use.*

Test solution. Dissolve 50.0 mg of the substance to be examined in a 6 g/l solution of *glacial acetic acid R* and dilute to 50.0 ml with the same solution.

Reference solution (a). Dilute 1.0 ml of the test solution to 100.0 ml with the mobile phase containing 0.5 g/l of *sodium edetate R*. Dilute 1.0 ml of this solution to 10.0 ml with the mobile phase containing 0.5 g/l of *sodium edetate R*.

Reference solution (b). Dilute 1.0 ml of the test solution to 50.0 ml with the mobile phase containing 0.5 g/l of *sodium edetate R*.

Reference solution (c). Dissolve 5 mg of *dihydralazine for system suitability CRS* in a 6 g/l solution of *glacial acetic acid R* and dilute to 5.0 ml with the same solution.

Column:

- *size*: *l* = 0.25 m, Ø = 4.6 mm;
- *stationary phase*: *nitrile silica gel for chromatography R* (5 µm).

Mobile phase: mix 22 volumes of *acetonitrile R1* and 78 volumes of a solution containing 1.44 g/l of *sodium laurilsulfate R* and 0.75 g/l of *tetrabutylammonium bromide R*, then adjust to pH 3.0 with *0.05 M sulphuric acid.*

Flow rate: 1.5 ml/min.

Detection: spectrophotometer at 230 nm.

Injection: 20 µl.

Run time: twice the retention time of dihydralazine.

Relative retention with reference to dihydralazine: impurity A = about 0.8.

System suitability: reference solution (c):

- the peaks due to impurity A and dihydralazine are baseline separated as in the chromatogram supplied with *dihydralazine for system suitability CRS*.

Limits:

- *impurity A*: not more than the area of the principal peak in the chromatogram obtained with reference solution (b) (2 per cent);
- *impurity C*: not more than the area of the principal peak in the chromatogram obtained with reference solution (a) (0.1 per cent);
- *unspecified impurities*: for each impurity, not more than the area of the principal peak in the chromatogram obtained with reference solution (a) (0.10 per cent);
- *sum of impurities other than A*: not more than 5 times the area of the principal peak in the chromatogram obtained with reference solution (a) (0.5 per cent);
- *disregard limit*: 0.1 times the area of the principal peak in the chromatogram obtained with reference solution (a) (0.01 per cent).

Impurity B. Liquid chromatography (*2.2.29*). *Prepare the solutions immediately before use.*

Test solution. Dissolve 40.0 mg of *hydrazine sulphate R* (impurity B) in *water R* and dilute to 100.0 ml with the same solvent. Dilute 1.0 ml of the solution to 25.0 ml with *water R*. To 0.50 ml of this solution, add 0.200 g of the substance to be examined and dissolve in 6 ml of *dilute hydrochloric acid R*, then dilute to 10.0 ml with *water R*. In a centrifuge tube with a ground-glass stopper, place immediately 0.50 ml of this solution and 2.0 ml of a 60 g/l solution of *benzaldehyde R* in a mixture of equal volumes of *methanol R* and *water R*. Shake for 90 s. Add 1.0 ml of *water R* and 5.0 ml of *heptane R*. Shake for 1 min and centrifuge. Use the upper layer.

Reference solution. Dissolve 40.0 mg of *hydrazine sulphate R* (impurity B) in *water R* and dilute to 100.0 ml with the same solvent. Dilute 1.0 ml of the solution to 25.0 ml with *water R*. To 0.50 ml of this solution, add 6 ml of *dilute hydrochloric acid R* and dilute to 10.0 ml with *water R*. In a centrifuge tube with a ground-glass stopper, place 0.50 ml of this solution and 2.0 ml of a 60 g/l solution of *benzaldehyde R* in a mixture of equal volumes of *methanol R* and *water R*. Shake for 90 s. Add 1.0 ml of *water R* and 5.0 ml of *heptane R*. Shake for 1 min and centrifuge. Use the upper layer.

Blank solution. Prepare in the same manner as for the reference solution but replacing the 0.50 ml of hydrazine sulphate solution by 0.50 ml of *water R*.

Column:

- *size*: *l* = 0.25 m, Ø = 4.6 mm;
- *stationary phase*: *octadecylsilyl silica gel for chromatography R* (5 µm).

Mobile phase: 0.3 g/l solution of *sodium edetate R*, *acetonitrile R* (30:70 *V/V*).

Flow rate: 1 ml/min.

Detection: spectrophotometer at 305 nm.

Injection: 20 µl.

Relative retention with reference to benzaldehyde: benzaldehyde azine (benzalazine) corresponding to impurity B = about 1.8.

Limit:

- *impurity B*: the area of the peak due to benzaldehyde azine is not greater than twice the area of the corresponding peak in the chromatogram obtained with the reference solution (10 ppm).

Iron (*2.4.9*): maximum 20 ppm.

To the residue obtained in the test for sulphated ash add 0.2 ml of *sulphuric acid R* and heat carefully until the acid is almost completely eliminated. Allow to cool and dissolve the residue with heating in 5.5 ml of *hydrochloric acid R1*. Filter the hot solution through a filter previously washed 3 times with *dilute hydrochloric acid R*. Wash the crucible and the filter with 5 ml of *water R*. Combine the filtrate and the washings and neutralise with about 3.5 ml of *strong sodium hydroxide solution R*. Adjust to pH 3-4 with *acetic acid R* and dilute to 20 ml with *water R*. Prepare the standard with 5 ml of *iron standard solution (2 ppm Fe) R* and 5 ml of *water R*.

Loss on drying (*2.2.32*): 13.0 per cent to 15.0 per cent, determined on 1.000 g by drying in an oven at 50 °C at a pressure not exceeding 0.7 kPa for 5 h.

Sulphated ash (*2.4.14*): maximum 0.1 per cent, determined on 1.0 g.

ASSAY

Dissolve 60.0 mg in 25 ml of *water R*. Add 35 ml of *hydrochloric acid R* and titrate slowly with *0.05 M potassium iodate*, determining the end-point potentiometrically (*2.2.20*), using a calomel reference electrode and a platinum indicator electrode.

1 ml of *0.05 M potassium iodate* is equivalent to 7.208 mg of $C_8H_{12}N_6O_4S$.

IMPURITIES

Specified impurities: A, B, C.

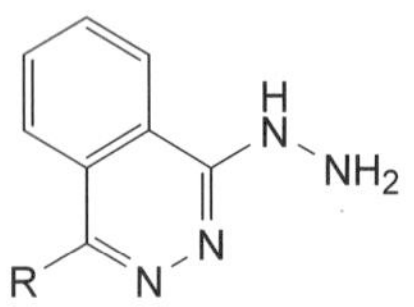

A. R = NH_2: 4-hydrazinophthalazin-1-amine,

C. R = H: (phthalazin-1-yl)hydrazine (hydralazine),

B. H_2N-NH_2: hydrazine.

04/2008:0551

DIHYDROERGOTAMINE MESILATE

Dihydroergotamini mesilas

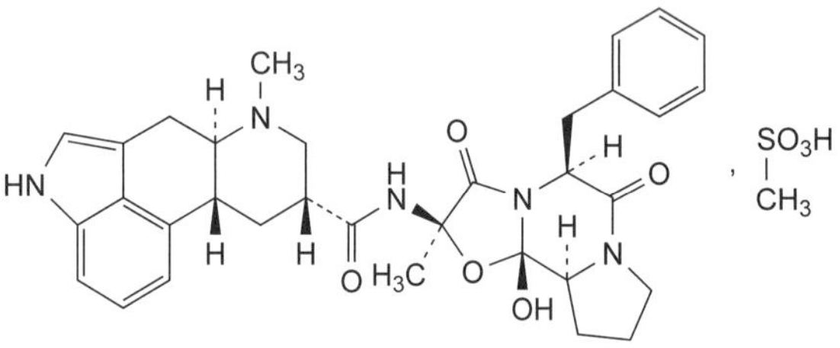

$C_{34}H_{41}N_5O_8S$ M_r 680

[6190-39-2]

DEFINITION

(6a*R*,9*R*,10a*R*)-*N*-[(2*R*,5*S*,10a*S*,10b*S*)-5-Benzyl-10b-hydroxy-2-methyl-3,6-dioxooctahydro-8*H*-oxazolo[3,2-*a*]pyrrolo[2,1-*c*]pyrazin-2-yl]-7-methyl-4,6,6a,7,8,9,10,10a-octahydroindolo[4,3-*fg*]quinoline-9-carboxamide methanesulphonate.

Content: 98.0 per cent to 101.0 per cent (dried substance).

PRODUCTION

The production method must be evaluated to determine the potential for formation of alkyl mesilates, which is particularly likely to occur if the reaction medium contains lower alcohols. Where necessary, the production method is validated to demonstrate that alkyl mesilates are not detectable in the final product.

CHARACTERS

Appearance: white or almost white, crystalline powder or colourless crystals.

Solubility: slightly soluble in water, sparingly soluble in methanol, slightly soluble in ethanol (96 per cent).

IDENTIFICATION

First identification: B, C.

Second identification: A, C, D.

A. Ultraviolet and visible absorption spectrophotometry (*2.2.25*).

Test solution. Dissolve 5.0 mg in *methanol R* and dilute to 100.0 ml with the same solvent.

Spectral range: 250-350 nm.

Absorption maxima: at 281 nm and 291 nm.

Shoulder: at 275 nm.

Absorbance: negligible above 320 nm.

Specific absorbance at the absorption maximum at 281 nm: 95 to 105 (dried substance).

B. Infrared absorption spectrophotometry (*2.2.24*).

Comparison: *dihydroergotamine mesilate CRS.*

C. Thin-layer chromatography (*2.2.27*). *Prepare the reference solution and the test solution immediately before use.*

Solvent mixture: *methanol R, methylene chloride R* (10:90 *V/V*).

Test solution. Dissolve 5 mg of the substance to be examined in the solvent mixture and dilute to 2.5 ml with the solvent mixture.

Reference solution. Dissolve 5 mg of *dihydroergotamine mesilate CRS* in the solvent mixture and dilute to 2.5 ml with the solvent mixture.

Plate: *TLC silica gel G plate R.*

Mobile phase: *concentrated ammonia R, methanol R, ethyl acetate R, methylene chloride R* (1:6:50:50 *V/V/V/V*).

Application: 5 μl.

Development: protected from light, over a path of 15 cm; dry in a current of cold air for not longer than 1 min and repeat the development protected from light over a path of 15 cm using a freshly prepared amount of the mobile phase.

Drying: in a current of cold air.

Detection: spray abundantly with *dimethylaminobenzaldehyde solution R7* and dry in a current of hot air for about 2 min.

Results: the principal spot in the chromatogram obtained with the test solution is similar in position, colour and size to the principal spot in the chromatogram obtained with the reference solution.

D. To 0.1 g of the substance to be examined, add 5 ml of *dilute hydrochloric acid R* and shake for about 5 min. Filter, then add 1 ml of *barium chloride solution R1*. The filtrate remains clear. Mix 0.1 g of the substance to be examined with 0.4 g of powdered *sodium hydroxide R*, heat to fusion and continue to heat for 1 min. Cool, add 5 ml of *water R*, boil and filter. Acidify the filtrate with *hydrochloric acid R1* and filter again. The filtrate gives reaction (a) of sulphates (*2.3.1*).

TESTS

Appearance of solution. The solution is clear (*2.2.1*) and not more intensely coloured than reference solution Y_7 or BY_7 (*2.2.2, Method II*).

Dissolve 0.10 g in a mixture of 0.1 ml of a 70 g/l solution of *methanesulphonic acid R* and 50 ml of *water R*.

pH (*2.2.3*): 4.4 to 5.4.

Dissolve 0.10 g in *carbon dioxide-free water R* and dilute to 100 ml with the same solvent.

Specific optical rotation (*2.2.7*): − 42 to − 47 (dried substance).

Dissolve 0.250 g in *anhydrous pyridine R* and dilute to 25.0 ml with the same solvent.

Related substances. Liquid chromatography (*2.2.29*). *Carry out the test protected from light.*

Solvent mixture: *acetonitrile R, water R* (50:50 *V/V*).

Test solution. Dissolve 70 mg of the substance to be examined in the solvent mixture and dilute to 100.0 ml with the solvent mixture.

Monographs D-K

Reference solution (a). Dilute 1.0 ml of the test solution to 10.0 ml with the solvent mixture. Dilute 1.0 ml of this solution to 100.0 ml with the solvent mixture.

Reference solution (b). Dissolve 7 mg of the substance to be examined and 6.8 mg of *ergotamine tartrate CRS* (impurity A) (equivalent to 7 mg of ergotamine mesilate) in the solvent mixture and dilute to 100 ml with the solvent mixture. Dilute 5 ml of this solution to 10 ml with the solvent mixture.

Reference solution (c). Dissolve 5 mg of *dihydroergotamine for peak identification CRS* (containing impurities A, B, C and D) in the solvent mixture, add 100 µl of *dilute sulphuric acid R* and dilute to 5 ml with the solvent mixture.

Column:

- *size*: *l* = 0.15 m, Ø = 4.6 mm;
- *stationary phase*: spherical *end-capped octadecylsilyl silica gel for chromatography R* (3 µm);
- *temperature*: 25 °C.

Mobile phase:

- *mobile phase A*: 3 g/l solution of *sodium heptanesulphonate monohydrate R* adjusted to pH 2.0 with *phosphoric acid R*;
- *mobile phase B*: mobile phase A, *acetonitrile for chromatography R* (20:80 *V/V*);

Time (min)	Mobile phase A (per cent *V/V*)	Mobile phase B (per cent *V/V*)
0 - 15	58 → 40	42 → 60

Flow rate: 1.5 ml/min.

Detection: spectrophotometer at 220 nm.

Injection: 5 µl.

Identification of impurities: use the chromatogram supplied with *dihydroergotamine for peak identification CRS* and the chromatogram obtained with reference solution (c) to identify the peaks due to impurities A, B, C and D.

Relative retention with reference to dihydroergotamine (retention time = about 6.5 min): impurity D = about 0.7; impurity C = about 0.86; impurity A = about 0.95; impurity B = about 1.2.

System suitability: reference solution (b):

- *resolution*: minimum 1.5 between the peaks due to impurity A and dihydroergotamine.

Limits:

- *correction factors*: for the calculation of content, multiply the peak areas of the following impurities by the corresponding correction factor: impurity A = 1.3; impurity C = 1.3;
- *impurity B*: not more than 5 times the area of the principal peak in the chromatogram obtained with reference solution (a) (0.5 per cent);
- *impurity C*: not more than 3 times the area of the principal peak in the chromatogram obtained with reference solution (a) (0.3 per cent);
- *impurities A and D*: for each impurity, not more than 1.5 times the area of the principal peak in the chromatogram obtained with reference solution (a) (0.15 per cent);
- *unspecified impurities*: for each impurity, not more than the area of the principal peak in the chromatogram obtained with reference solution (a) (0.10 per cent);
- *total*: not more than 10 times the area of the principal peak in the chromatogram obtained with reference solution (a) (1.0 per cent);
- *disregard limit*: 0.5 times the area of the principal peak in the chromatogram obtained with reference solution (a) (0.05 per cent).

Loss on drying (*2.2.32*): maximum 4.0 per cent, determined on 0.500 g by drying at 105 °C at a pressure not exceeding 0.1 kPa for 5 h.

ASSAY

Dissolve 0.500 g in a mixture of 10 ml of *anhydrous acetic acid R* and 70 ml of *acetic anhydride R*. Titrate with *0.1 M perchloric acid*, determining the end-point potentiometrically (*2.2.20*).

1 ml of *0.1 M perchloric acid* is equivalent to 68.00 mg of $C_{34}H_{41}N_5O_8S$.

STORAGE

Protected from light.

IMPURITIES

Specified impurities: A, B, C, D.

Other detectable impurities (the following substances would, if present at a sufficient level, be detected by one or other of the tests in the monograph. They are limited by the general acceptance criterion for other/unspecified impurities and/or by the general monograph *Substances for pharmaceutical use (2034)*. It is therefore not necessary to identify these impurities for demonstration of compliance. See also *5.10. Control of impurities in substances for pharmaceutical use*): *E.*

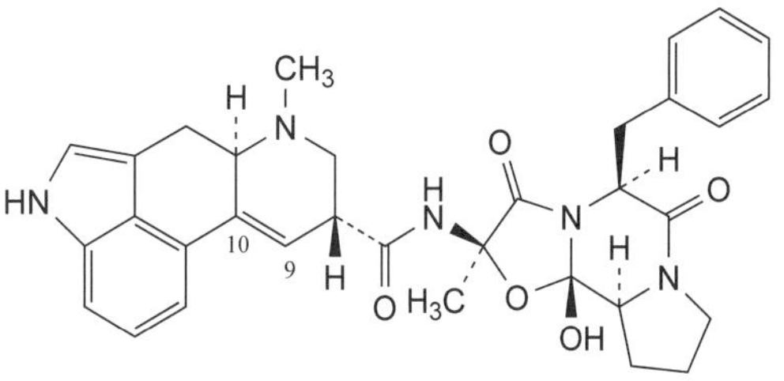

A. (6a*R*,9*R*)-*N*-[(2*R*,5*S*,10a*S*,10b*S*)-5-benzyl-10b-hydroxy-2-methyl-3,6-dioxooctahydro-8*H*-oxazolo[3,2-*a*]pyrrolo[2,1-*c*]pyrazin-2-yl]-7-methyl-4,6,6a,7,8,9-hexahydroindolo[4,3-*fg*]quinoline-9-carboxamide (ergotamine),

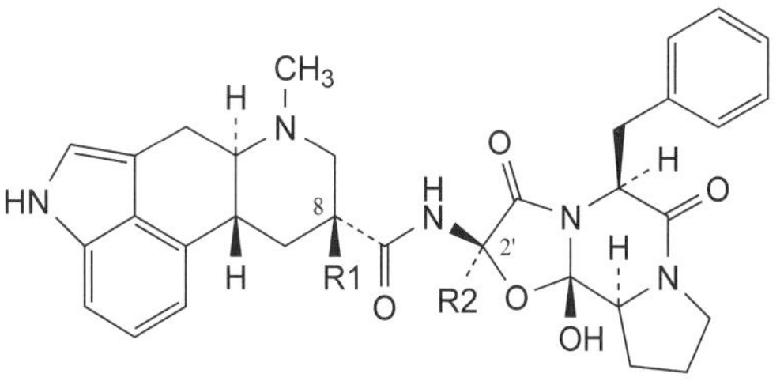

B. R1 = H, R2 = C_2H_5: (6a*R*,9*R*,10a*R*)-*N*-[(2*R*,5*S*,10a*S*,10b*S*)-5-benzyl-2-ethyl-10b-hydroxy-3,6-dioxooctahydro-8*H*-oxazolo[3,2-*a*]pyrrolo[2,1-*c*]pyrazin-2-yl]-7-methyl-4,6,6a,7,8,9,10,10a-octahydroindolo[4,3-*fg*]quinoline-9-carboxamide (9,10-dihydroergostine),

C. R1 = OH, R2 = CH_3: (6a*R*,9*S*,10a*R*)-*N*-[(2*R*,5*S*,10a*S*,10b*S*)-5-benzyl-10b-hydroxy-2-methyl-3,6-dioxooctahydro-8*H*-oxazolo[3,2-*a*]pyrrolo[2,1-*c*]pyrazin-2-yl]-9-hydroxy-7-methyl-4,6,6a,7,8,9,10,10a-octahydroindolo[4,3-*fg*]quinoline-9-carboxamide (8-hydroxy-9,10-dihydroergotamine),

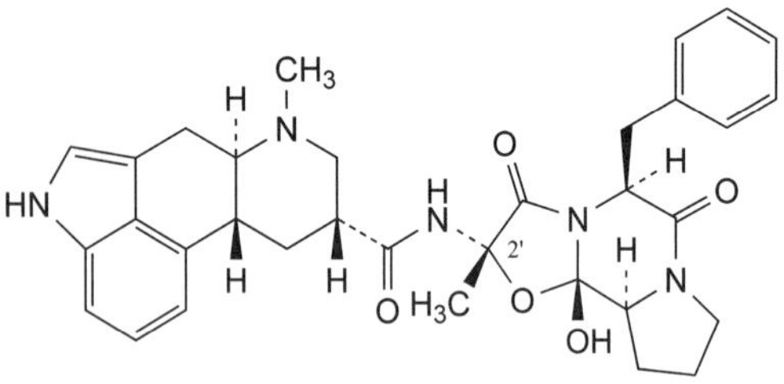

D. (6a*R*,9*R*,10a*R*)-*N*-[(2*S*,5*S*,10a*S*,10b*S*)-5-benzyl-10b-hydroxy-2-methyl-3,6-dioxooctahydro-8*H*-oxazolo[3,2-*a*]pyrrolo[2,1-*c*]pyrazin-2-yl]-7-methyl-4,6,6a,7,8,9,10,10a-octahydroindolo[4,3-*fg*]quinoline-9-carboxamide (2′-*epi*-9,10-dihydroergotamine),

E. dihydroergocristine.

04/2008:1004

DILTIAZEM HYDROCHLORIDE

Diltiazemi hydrochloridum

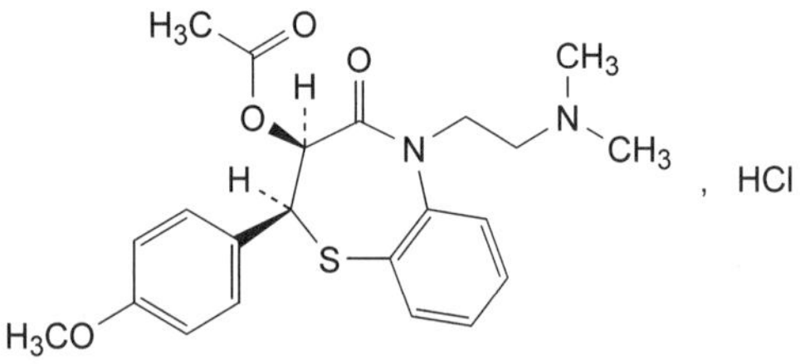

$C_{22}H_{27}ClN_2O_4S$ M_r 451.0

[33286-22-5]

DEFINITION

Hydrochloride of (2*S*,3*S*)-5-[2-(dimethylamino)ethyl]-2-(4-methoxyphenyl)-4-oxo-2,3,4,5-tetrahydro-1,5-benzothiazepin-3-yl acetate.

Content: 98.5 per cent to 101.0 per cent (dried substance).

CHARACTERS

Appearance: white or almost white, crystalline powder.

Solubility: freely soluble in water, in methanol and in methylene chloride, slightly soluble in anhydrous ethanol.

mp: about 213 °C, with decomposition.

IDENTIFICATION

First identification: A, D.

Second identification: B, C, D.

A. Infrared absorption spectrophotometry (*2.2.24*).

Comparison: *diltiazem hydrochloride CRS.*

B. Thin-layer chromatography (*2.2.27*).

Test solution. Dissolve 0.10 g of the substance to be examined in *methylene chloride R* and dilute to 10 ml with the same solvent.

Reference solution. Dissolve 0.10 g of *diltiazem hydrochloride CRS* in *methylene chloride R* and dilute to 10 ml with the same solvent.

Plate: *TLC silica gel F_{254} plate R.*

Mobile phase: *acetic acid R, water R, methylene chloride R, anhydrous ethanol R* (1:3:10:12 *V/V/V/V*).

Application: 10 µl.

Development: over 2/3 of the plate.

Drying: in air.

Detection: examine in ultraviolet light at 254 nm.

Results: the principal spot in the chromatogram obtained with the test solution is similar in position and size to the principal spot in the chromatogram obtained with the reference solution.

C. Dissolve 50 mg in 5 ml of *water R*. Add 1 ml of *ammonium reineckate solution R*. A pink precipitate is produced.

D. It gives reaction (a) of chlorides (*2.3.1*).

TESTS

Solution S. Dissolve 1.00 g in *carbon-dioxide free water R* and dilute to 20.0 ml with the same solvent.

Appearance of solution. Solution S is clear (*2.2.1*) and colourless (*2.2.2, Method II*).

pH (*2.2.3*): 4.3 to 5.3.

Dilute 2.0 ml of solution S to 10.0 ml with *carbon dioxide-free water R*.

Specific optical rotation (*2.2.7*): + 115 to + 120 (dried substance).

Dilute 5.0 ml of solution S to 25.0 ml with *water R*.

Related substances. Liquid chromatography (*2.2.29*).

Test solution. Dissolve 50.0 mg of the substance to be examined in the mobile phase and dilute to 200.0 ml with the mobile phase.

Reference solution (a). Dissolve 50.0 mg of *diltiazem hydrochloride CRS* in the mobile phase and dilute to 200.0 ml with the mobile phase. Dilute 1.2 ml of this solution to 100.0 ml with the mobile phase.

Reference solution (b). Dissolve the contents of a vial of *diltiazem impurity A CRS* in 1.0 ml of reference solution (a).

Reference solution (c). Dilute 0.3 ml of the test solution to 100.0 ml with the mobile phase.

Column:
- *size*: *l* = 0.10 m, Ø = 4.6 mm;
- *stationary phase*: *octadecylsilyl silica gel for chromatography R* (3 µm).

Mobile phase: mix 5 volumes of *anhydrous ethanol R*, 25 volumes of *acetonitrile R* and 70 volumes of a solution containing 6.8 g/l of *potassium dihydrogen phosphate R* and 0.1 ml/l of *N,N-dimethyloctylamine R*, adjusted to pH 4.5 with *dilute phosphoric acid R*.

Flow rate: 1.5 ml/min.

Detection: spectrophotometer at 240 nm.

Injection: 20 µl.

Run time: 5 times the retention time of diltiazem.

System suitability: reference solution (b):
- *resolution*: minimum 4.0 between the peaks due to impurity A and diltiazem; if necessary, adjust the concentration of *N,N*-dimethyloctylamine in the mobile phase;
- *symmetry factor*: maximum 2.0 for the peaks due to impurity A and diltiazem; if necessary, adjust the concentration of *N,N*-dimethyloctylamine in the mobile phase.

Limits:
- *total*: not more than the area of the principal peak in the chromatogram obtained with reference solution (c) (0.3 per cent);
- *disregard limit*: 0.025 times the area of the principal peak in the chromatogram obtained with reference solution (c).

Heavy metals (*2.4.8*): maximum 10 ppm.

Dissolve 2.0 g in *water R* and dilute to 20.0 ml with the same solvent. 12 ml of the solution complies with test A. Prepare the reference solution using *lead standard solution (1 ppm Pb) R*.

Loss on drying (*2.2.32*): maximum 0.5 per cent, determined on 1.000 g by drying in an oven at 105 °C for 2 h.

Sulphated ash (*2.4.14*): maximum 0.1 per cent, determined on 1.0 g.

ASSAY

Dissolve 0.400 g in a mixture of 2 ml of *anhydrous formic acid R* and 60 ml of *acetic anhydride R* and titrate with *0.1 M perchloric acid*, determining the end-point potentiometrically (*2.2.20*).

1 ml of *0.1 M perchloric acid* is equivalent to 45.1 mg of $C_{22}H_{27}ClN_2O_4S$.

STORAGE

In an airtight container, protected from light.

IMPURITIES

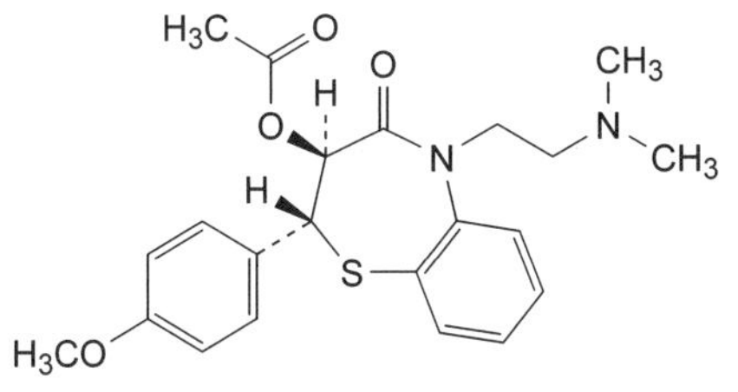

A. (2*R*,3*S*)-5-[2-(dimethylamino)ethyl]-2-(4-methoxyphenyl)-4-oxo-2,3,4,5-tetrahydro-1,5-benzothiazepin-3-yl acetate,

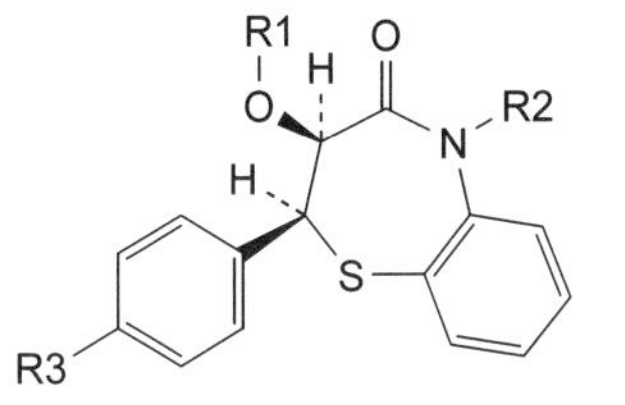

B. R1 = CO-CH_3, R2 = H, R3 = OCH_3: (2*S*,3*S*)-2-(4-methoxyphenyl)-4-oxo-2,3,4,5-tetrahydro-1,5-benzothiazepin-3-yl acetate,

C. R1 = CO-CH_3, R2 = CH_2-CH_2-$N(CH_3)_2$, R3 = OH: (2*S*,3*S*)-5-[2-(dimethylamino)ethyl]-2-(4-hydroxyphenyl)-4-oxo-2,3,4,5-tetrahydro-1,5-benzothiazepin-3-yl acetate,

D. R1 = CO-CH_3, R2 = CH_2-CH_2-NH-CH_3, R3 = OCH_3: (2*S*,3*S*)-2-(4-methoxyphenyl)-5-[2-(methylamino)ethyl]-4-oxo-2,3,4,5-tetrahydro-1,5-benzothiazepin-3-yl acetate,

E. R1 = R2 = H, R3 = OCH_3: (2*S*,3*S*)-3-hydroxy-2-(4-methoxyphenyl)-2,3-dihydro-1,5-benzothiazepin-4(5*H*)-one,

F. R1 = H, R2 = CH_2-CH_2-$N(CH_3)_2$, R3 = OCH_3: (2*S*,3*S*)-5-[2-(dimethylamino)ethyl]-3-hydroxy-2-(4-methoxyphenyl)-2,3-dihydro-1,5-benzothiazepin-4(5*H*)-one.

01/2008:1313
corrected 6.1

DIRITHROMYCIN

Dirithromycinum

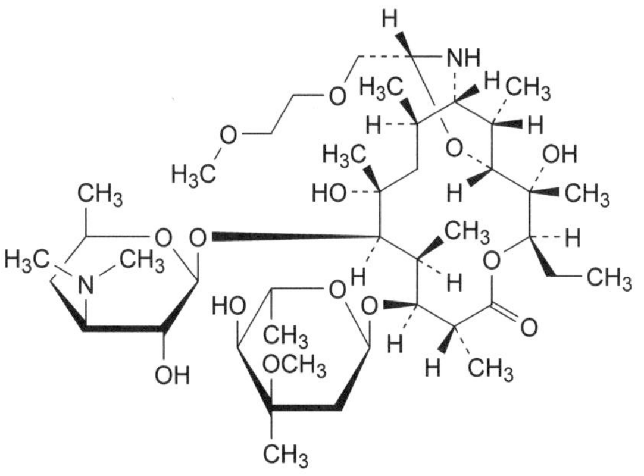

$C_{42}H_{78}N_2O_{14}$ M_r 835
[62013-04-1]

DEFINITION

(1*R*,2*S*,3*R*,6*R*,7*S*,8*S*,9*R*,10*R*,12*R*,13*S*,15*R*,17*S*)-9-[[3-(Dimethylamino)-3,4,6-trideoxy-β-D-*xylo*-hexopyranosyl]oxy]-3-ethyl-2,10-dihydroxy-15-[(2-methoxyethoxy)methyl]-2,6,8,10,12,17-hexamethyl-7-[(3-*C*-methyl-3-*O*-methyl-2,6-dideoxy-α-L-*ribo*-hexopyranosyl)oxy]-4,16-dioxa-14-azabicyclo[11.3.1]heptadecan-5-one (or (9*S*)-9,11-[imino[(1*R*)-2-(2-methoxyethoxy)ethylidene]oxy]-9-deoxo-11-deoxyerythromycin).

Semi-synthetic product derived from a fermentation product.

Content: 96.0 per cent to 102.0 per cent for the sum of the percentage contents of $C_{42}H_{78}N_2O_{14}$ and dirithromycin 15*S*-epimer (anhydrous substance).

CHARACTERS

Appearance: white or almost white powder.

Solubility: very slightly soluble in water, very soluble in methanol and in methylene chloride.

It shows polymorphism (*5.9*).

IDENTIFICATION

A. Infrared absorption spectrophotometry (*2.2.24*).

Comparison: *dirithromycin CRS*.

B. Examine the chromatograms obtained in the assay.

Results: the principal peak in the chromatogram obtained with test solution (a) is similar in retention time and size to the principal peak in the chromatogram obtained with reference solution (a).

TESTS

Related substances. Liquid chromatography (*2.2.29*).

Solvent mixture: *methanol R, acetonitrile R1* (30:70 *V/V*).

Test solution (a). Dissolve 20.0 mg of the substance to be examined in the solvent mixture and dilute to 10.0 ml with the solvent mixture.

Test solution (b). Dissolve 0.10 g of the substance to be examined in the solvent mixture and dilute to 10.0 ml with the solvent mixture.

Reference solution (a). Dissolve 20.0 mg of *dirithromycin CRS* in the solvent mixture and dilute to 10.0 ml with the solvent mixture.

Reference solution (b). Dilute 5.0 ml of reference solution (a) to 50.0 ml with the solvent mixture.

Reference solution (c). Dissolve 20 mg of *dirithromycin CRS* in the mobile phase and dilute to 10 ml with the mobile phase. Allow to stand for 24 h before use.

Column:

- *size*: *l* = 0.25 m, Ø = 4.6 mm;
- *stationary phase*: *octadecylsilyl silica gel for chromatography R* (5 µm);
- *temperature*: 40 °C.

Mobile phase: mix 9 volumes of *water R*, 19 volumes of *methanol R*, 28 volumes of a solution containing 1.9 g/l of *potassium dihydrogen phosphate R* and 9.1 g/l of *dipotassium hydrogen phosphate R* adjusted to pH 7.5 if necessary with a 100 g/l solution of *potassium hydroxide R*, and 44 volumes of *acetonitrile R1*.

Flow rate: 2.0 ml/min.

Detection: spectrophotometer at 205 nm.

Injection: 10 µl of test solution (b) and reference solutions (b) and (c).

Run time: 3 times the retention time of dirithromycin.

Relative retention with reference to dirithromycin: impurity A = about 0.7; 15*S*-epimer = about 1.1.

System suitability: reference solution (c):

- *resolution*: minimum 2.0 between the peaks due to dirithromycin and its 15*S*-epimer; if necessary, adjust the concentration of the organic modifiers in the mobile phase.

Limits:

- *impurity A*: not more than 0.75 times the area of the principal peak in the chromatogram obtained with reference solution (b) (1.5 per cent);
- *any other impurity*: for each impurity, not more than 0.5 times the area of the principal peak in the chromatogram obtained with reference solution (b) (1 per cent);
- *disregard limit*: disregard the peak due to the 15*S*-epimer.

Dirithromycin 15S-epimer. Liquid chromatography (*2.2.29*) as described in the test for related substances with the following modifications.

Injection: test solution (b) and reference solution (b).

System suitability: reference solution (b):

- *repeatability*: maximum relative standard deviation of 5.0 per cent after 6 injections.

Limit:

- *15S-epimer*: maximum 1.5 per cent.

Acetonitrile (*2.4.24, System A*): maximum 0.1 per cent.

Prepare the solutions using *dimethylformamide R* instead of *water R*.

Sample solution. Dissolve 0.200 g of the substance to be examined in *dimethylformamide R* and dilute to 20.0 ml with the same solvent.

Static head-space injection conditions that may be used:

- *equilibration temperature*: 120 °C;
- *equilibration time*: 60 min;
- *transfer-line temperature*: 125 °C.

Heavy metals (*2.4.8*): maximum 20 ppm.

Dissolve 1.0 g in 20 ml of a mixture of equal volumes of *methanol R* and *water R*. 12 ml of the solution complies with test B. Prepare the reference solution using lead standard solution (1 ppm Pb) obtained by diluting *lead standard solution (100 ppm Pb) R* with a mixture of equal volumes of *methanol R* and *water R*.

Water (*2.5.12*): maximum 1.0 per cent, determined on 1.00 g.

Sulphated ash (*2.4.14*): maximum 0.1 per cent, determined on 1.0 g.

ASSAY

Liquid chromatography (*2.2.29*) as described in the test for related substances with the following modifications.

Injection: test solution (a) and reference solution (a).

System suitability: reference solution (a):

- *repeatability*: maximum relative standard deviation of 1.0 per cent after 6 injections.

IMPURITIES

Specified impurities: A.

Other detectable impurities (the following substances would, if present at a sufficient level, be detected by one or other of the tests in the monograph. They are limited by the general acceptance criterion for other/unspecified impurities and/or by the general monograph *Substances for pharmaceutical use (2034)*. It is therefore not necessary to identify these impurities for demonstration of compliance. See also *5.10. Control of impurities in substances for pharmaceutical use*)*: B, C, D, E.*

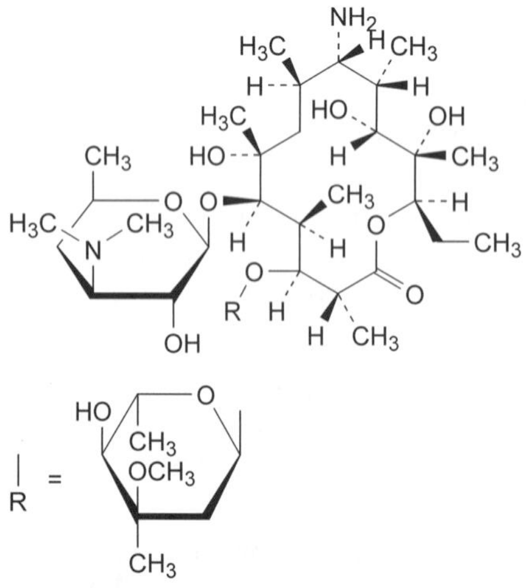

A. (9*S*)-9-amino-9-deoxoerythromycin,

B. R = H: (9*S*)-9-amino-3-de(2,6-dideoxy-3-*C*-methyl-3-*O*-methyl-α-L-*ribo*-hexopyranosyl)-9-deoxoerythromycin,

Monographs D-K

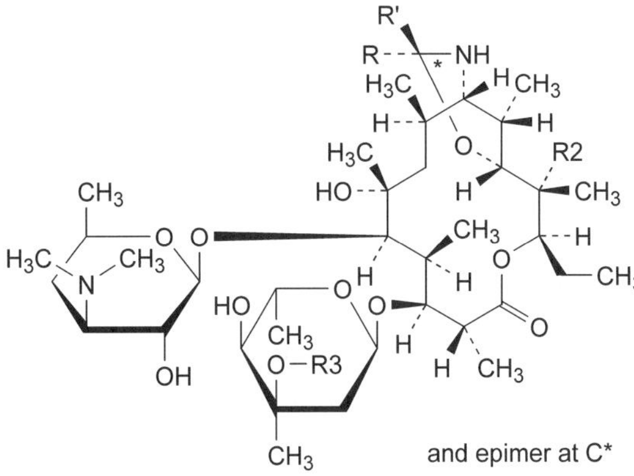

C. R = CH_2-O-CH_2-CH_2-O-CH_3, R′ = H, R2 = H, R3 = CH_3: (9*S*)-9,11-[imino[(1*RS*)-2-(2-methoxyethoxy)ethylidene]oxy]-9-deoxo-11,12-dideoxyerythromycin (dirithromycin B),

D. R = CH_2-O-CH_2-CH_2-O-CH_3, R′ = H, R2 = OH, R3 = H: (9*S*)-9,11-[imino[(1*RS*)-2-(2-methoxyethoxy)ethylidene]oxy]-3′-*O*-demethyl-9-deoxo-11-deoxyerythromycin (dirithromycin C),

E. R = CH_3, R′ = CH_3, R2 = OH, R3 = CH_3: 9,11-[imino(1-methylethylidene)oxy]-9-deoxo-11-deoxyerythromycin.

04/2008:0118

DISODIUM PHOSPHATE DODECAHYDRATE

Dinatrii phosphas dodecahydricus

$Na_2HPO_4,12H_2O$ M_r 358.1
[10039-32-4]

DEFINITION

Content: 98.5 per cent to 102.5 per cent.

CHARACTERS

Appearance: colourless, transparent crystals, very efflorescent.

Solubility: very soluble in water, practically insoluble in ethanol (96 per cent).

IDENTIFICATION

A. Solution S (see Tests) is slightly alkaline (*2.2.4*).

B. Water (see Tests).

C. Solution S gives reaction (b) of phosphates (*2.3.1*).

D. Solution S gives reaction (a) of sodium (*2.3.1*).

TESTS

Solution S. Dissolve 5.0 g in *distilled water R* and dilute to 50 ml with the same solvent.

Appearance of solution. Solution S is clear (*2.2.1*) and colourless (*2.2.2, Method II*).

Reducing substances. To 5 ml of solution S add 5 ml of *dilute sulphuric acid R* and 0.25 ml of *0.02 M potassium permanganate* and heat on a water-bath for 5 min. The solution retains a slight red colour.

Monosodium phosphate: maximum 2.5 per cent.

From the volume of *1 M hydrochloric acid* (25 ml) and of *1 M sodium hydroxide* (n_1 ml and n_2 ml) used in the assay, calculate the following ratio:

$$\frac{n_2 - 25}{25 - n_1}$$

This ratio is not greater than 0.025.

Chlorides (*2.4.4*): maximum 200 ppm.

To 2.5 ml of solution S add 10 ml of *dilute nitric acid R* and dilute to 15 ml with *water R*.

Sulphates (*2.4.13*): maximum 500 ppm.

To 3 ml of solution S add 2 ml of *dilute hydrochloric acid R* and dilute to 15 ml with *distilled water R*.

Arsenic (*2.4.2, Method A*): maximum 2 ppm, determined on 5 ml of solution S.

Iron (*2.4.9*): maximum 20 ppm.

Dilute 5 ml of solution S to 10 ml with *water R*.

Heavy metals (*2.4.8*): maximum 10 ppm.

12 ml of solution S complies with test A. Prepare the reference solution using *lead standard solution (1 ppm Pb) R*.

Water (*2.5.12*): 57.0 per cent to 61.0 per cent, determined on 50.0 mg. Use a mixture of 10 volumes of *anhydrous methanol R* and 40 volumes of *formamide R1* as solvent.

ASSAY

Dissolve 4.00 g (*m*) in 25 ml of *water R* and add 25.0 ml of *1 M hydrochloric acid*. Carry out a potentiometric titration (*2.2.20*) using *1 M sodium hydroxide*. Read the volume added at the 1st inflexion point (n_1 ml). Continue the titration to the 2nd inflexion point (total volume of *1 M sodium hydroxide* required, n_2 ml).

Calculate the percentage content of $Na_2HPO_4,12H_2O$ from the following expression:

$$\frac{3581\,(25 - n_1)}{m \times 100}$$

04/2008:1096

DOXEPIN HYDROCHLORIDE

Doxepini hydrochloridum

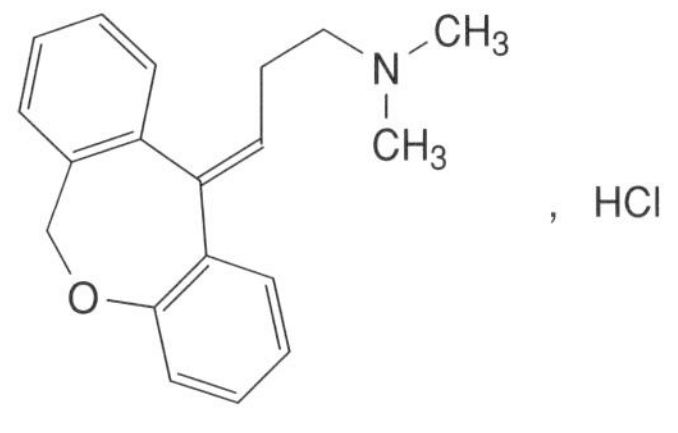

$C_{19}H_{22}ClNO$ M_r 315.8
[1229-29-4]

DEFINITION

(*E*)-3-(Dibenzo[*b,e*]oxepin-11(6*H*)-ylidene)-*N,N*-dimethylpropan-1-amine hydrochloride.

Content: 98.0 per cent to 101.0 per cent of $C_{19}H_{22}ClNO$ (dried substance).

CHARACTERS

Appearance: white or almost white, crystalline powder.

Solubility: freely soluble in water, in ethanol (96 per cent) and in methylene chloride.

IDENTIFICATION

First identification: C, E.

Second identification: A, B, D, E.

A. Melting point (*2.2.14*): 185 °C to 191 °C.

B. Ultraviolet and visible absorption spectrophotometry (*2.2.25*).

Test solution. Dissolve 50.0 mg in a 1 g/l solution of *hydrochloric acid R* in *methanol R* and dilute to 100.0 ml with the same acid solution. Dilute 5.0 ml to 50.0 ml with a 1 g/l solution of *hydrochloric acid R* in *methanol R.*

Spectral range: 230-350 nm.

Absorption maximum: at 297 nm.

Specific absorbance at the absorption maximum: 128 to 142.

C. Infrared absorption spectrophotometry (*2.2.24*).

Comparison: *doxepin hydrochloride CRS.*

D. Dissolve about 5 mg in 2 ml of *sulphuric acid R.* A dark red colour is produced.

E. Solution S (see Tests) gives reaction (a) of chlorides (*2.3.1*).

TESTS

Solution S. Dissolve 1.5 g in *carbon dioxide-free water R* and dilute to 30 ml with the same solvent.

Appearance of solution. Dilute 10 ml of solution S to 25 ml with *water R.* The solution is clear (*2.2.1*) and colourless (*2.2.2, Method II*).

Acidity. To 10 ml of solution S add 0.1 ml of *methyl red solution R.* Not more than 0.1 ml of *0.1 M sodium hydroxide* is required to change the colour of the indicator to yellow.

Related substances. Liquid chromatography (*2.2.29*). *Prepare the solutions immediately before use and protect them from light.*

Phosphate buffer solution. Dissolve 1.42 g of *anhydrous disodium hydrogen phosphate R* in *water R,* adjust to pH 7.7 with *dilute phosphoric acid R* and dilute to 1000 ml with *water R.*

Solvent mixture. Mix 1 volume of *1 M sodium hydroxide* and 250 volumes of the mobile phase.

Test solution. Dissolve 50 mg of the substance to be examined in the solvent mixture and dilute to 50.0 ml with the solvent mixture.

Reference solution (a). Dilute 1.0 ml of the test solution to 100.0 ml with the solvent mixture. Dilute 1.0 ml of this solution to 10.0 ml with the solvent mixture.

Reference solution (b). Dissolve the contents of a vial of *doxepin for system suitability CRS* (containing impurities A, B and C) in 1.0 ml of mobile phase.

Column:

- *size*: l = 0.25 m, Ø = 4.6 mm;
- *stationary phase*: *end-capped octadecylsilyl silica gel for chromatography R* (5 µm);
- *temperature*: 30 °C.

Mobile phase: *acetonitrile R1,* phosphate buffer solution, *methanol R1* (20:30:50 *V/V/V*).

Flow rate: 1.0 ml/min.

Detection: spectrophotometer at 215 nm.

Injection: 20 µl.

Run time: 1.5 times the retention time of doxepin.

Identification of impurities: use the chromatogram supplied with *doxepin for system suitability CRS* and the chromatogram obtained with reference solution (b) to identify the peaks due to impurities A, B and C.

Relative retention with reference to doxepin (retention time = about 18 min): impurity A = about 0.5; impurity C = about 0.6; impurity B = about 0.7; the peak due to doxepin might show a shoulder caused by the (*Z*)-isomer (impurity D).

System suitability: reference solution (b):

- *resolution*: minimum 1.5 between the peaks due to impurities A and C, and minimum 1.5 between the peaks due to impurities C and B;
- the chromatogram obtained is similar to the chromatogram supplied with *doxepin for system suitability CRS.*

Limits:

- *correction factor*: for the calculation of content, multiply the peak area of impurity B by 1.7;
- *impurities A, B*: for each impurity, not more than the area of the principal peak in the chromatogram obtained with reference solution (a) (0.1 per cent);
- *impurity C*: not more than twice the area of the principal peak in the chromatogram obtained with reference solution (a) (0.2 per cent);
- *unspecified impurities*: for each impurity, not more than the area of the principal peak in the chromatogram obtained with reference solution (a) (0.10 per cent);
- *total*: not more than 3 times the area of the principal peak in the chromatogram obtained with reference solution (a) (0.3 per cent);
- *disregard limit*: 0.5 times the area of the principal peak in the chromatogram obtained with reference solution (a) (0.05 per cent).

(*Z*)-Isomer. Liquid chromatography (*2.2.29*).

Test solution. Dissolve 20.0 mg of the substance to be examined in the mobile phase and dilute to 20.0 ml with the mobile phase. Dilute 1.0 ml of this solution to 10.0 ml with the mobile phase.

Column:

- *size*: l = 0.12 m, Ø = 4 mm;
- *stationary phase*: spherical *octylsilyl silica gel for chromatography R* (5 µm) with a specific surface area of 220 m^2/g and a pore size of 80 nm;
- *temperature*: 50 °C.

Mobile phase: mix 30 volumes of *methanol R* and 70 volumes of a 30 g/l solution of *sodium dihydrogen phosphate R* previously adjusted to pH 2.5 with *phosphoric acid R.*

Flow rate: 1 ml/min.

Detection: spectrophotometer at 254 nm.

Injection: 20 µl.

System suitability:

- *resolution*: minimum 1.5 between the peaks due to the (*E*)-isomer (1st peak) and to the (*Z*)-isomer (2nd peak).

Results:

- calculate the ratio of the area of the peak due to the (*E*)-isomer to the area of the peak due to the (*Z*)-isomer: this ratio is 4.4 to 6.7 (13.0 per cent to 18.5 per cent of the (*Z*)-isomer).

Monographs D-K

Heavy metals (*2.4.8*): maximum 20 ppm.

1.0 g complies with test D. Prepare the reference solution using 2 ml of *lead standard solution (10 ppm Pb) R*.

Loss on drying (*2.2.32*): maximum 0.5 per cent, determined on 1.000 g by drying in an oven at 105 °C.

Sulphated ash (*2.4.14*): maximum 0.1 per cent, determined on 1.0 g.

ASSAY

Dissolve 0.250 g in a mixture of 5 ml of *anhydrous acetic acid R* and 35 ml of *acetic anhydride R*. Using 0.2 ml of *crystal violet solution R* as indicator, titrate with *0.1 M perchloric acid* until the colour changes from blue to green.

1 ml of *0.1 M perchloric acid* is equivalent to 31.58 mg of $C_{19}H_{22}ClNO$.

STORAGE

Protected from light.

IMPURITIES

Specified impurities: A, B, C, D.

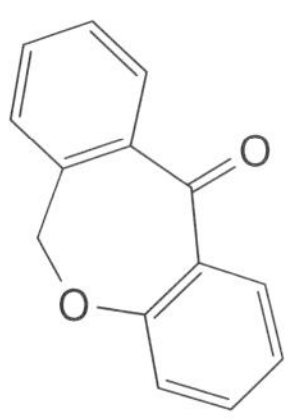

A. dibenzo[*b,e*]oxepin-11(6*H*)-one (doxepinone),

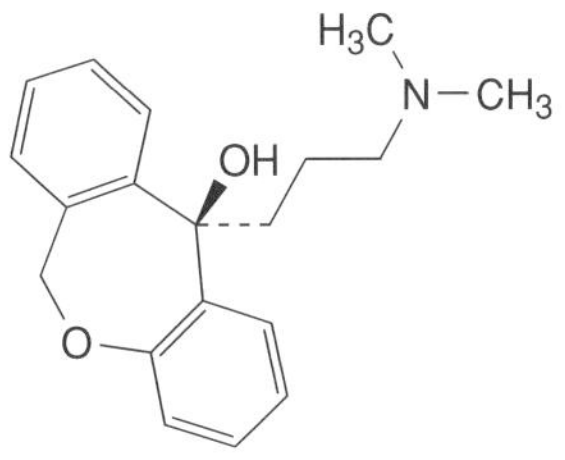

and enantiomer

B. (11*RS*)-11-[3-(dimethylamino)propyl]-6,11-dihydrodibenzo[*b,e*]oxepin-11-ol (doxepinol),

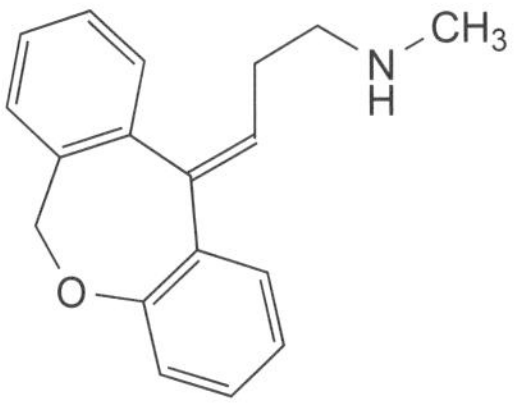

C. (*E*)-3-(dibenzo[*b,e*]oxepin-11(6*H*)-ylidene)-*N*-methylpropan-1-amine (desmethyldoxepin),

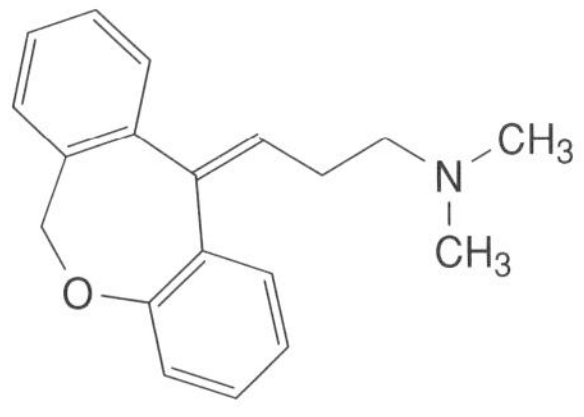

D. (*Z*)-3-(dibenzo[*b,e*]oxepin-11(6*H*)-ylidene)-*N,N*-dimethylpropan-1-amine.

01/2008:1589
corrected 6.1

DOXYLAMINE HYDROGEN SUCCINATE

Doxylamini hydrogenosuccinas

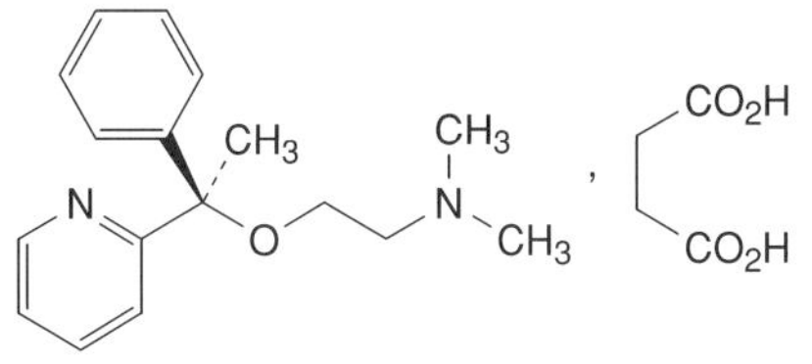

and enantiomer

$C_{21}H_{28}N_2O_5$ M_r 388.5
[562-10-7]

DEFINITION

N,N-dimethyl-2-[(1*RS*)-1-phenyl-1-(pyridin-2-yl)ethoxy(ethanamine hydrogen butanedioate.

Content: 99.0 per cent to 101.0 per cent (anhydrous substance).

CHARACTERS

Appearance: a white or almost white powder.

Solubility: very soluble in water, freely soluble in ethanol (96 per cent).

IDENTIFICATION

First identification: C.

Second identification: A, B.

A. Melting point (*2.2.14*): 103 °C to 108 °C.

B. Dissolve 0.200 g in *0.1 M hydrochloric acid* and dilute to 100.0 ml with the same solvent. Dilute 1.0 ml of this solution to 100.0 ml with *0.1 M hydrochloric acid*. Examined between 230 nm and 350 nm (*2.2.25*), the solution shows an absorption maximum at 262 nm. The specific absorbance at the maximum is 229 to 243 (anhydrous substance).

C. Infrared absorption spectrophotometry (*2.2.24*).

Comparison: Ph. Eur. reference spectrum of doxylamine hydrogen succinate.

TESTS

Appearance of solution. The solution is clear (*2.2.1*) and colourless (*2.2.2, Method II*).

Dissolve 0.4 g of the substance to be examined in *water R* and dilute to 20 ml with the same solvent.

Optical rotation (*2.2.7*): - 0.10° to + 0.10°.

Dissolve 2.50 g of the substance to be examined in *water R* and dilute to 25.0 ml with the same solvent.

Related substances. Gas chromatography (*2.2.28*).

Test solution. Dissolve 0.650 g of the substance to be examined in 20 ml of *0.1 M hydrochloric acid*. Add 3 ml of a 100 g/l solution of *sodium hydroxide R* and extract with 3 quantities, each of 25 ml, of *methylene chloride R*. Combine the methylene chloride extracts and filter using hydrophobic phase-separation filter paper. Rinse the filter with 10 ml of *methylene chloride R* and combine the rinsings with the methylene chloride extracts. Evaporate the solvent under reduced pressure at a temperature not exceeding 40 °C. Dissolve the residue in 20.0 ml of *anhydrous ethanol R*.

Reference solution (a). Dilute 1.0 ml of the test solution to 200.0 ml with *anhydrous ethanol R.*

Reference solution (b). Dissolve 4 mg of *doxylamine impurity A CRS* and 4 mg of *2-benzoylpyridine R* in *anhydrous ethanol R* and dilute to 40 ml with the same solvent.

Column:

- *material*: fused silica;
- *size*: l = 30 m, Ø = 0.53 mm;
- *stationary phase*: *poly(dimethyl)(diphenyl)siloxane R* (film thickness 1.5 μm).

Carrier gas: *helium for chromatography R.*

Flow rate: 7 ml/min.

Temperature:

	Time (min)	Temperature (°C)
Column	0 - 12	160 → 220
	12 - 27	220
Injection port		250
Detector		250

Detection: flame ionisation.

Injection: 1 μl.

System suitability: reference solution (b):

- *resolution*: minimum 1.5 between the peaks due to impurities A and D.

Limits:

- *any impurity*: not more than the area of the principal peak in the chromatogram obtained with reference solution (a) (0.5 per cent);
- *total*: not more than twice the area of the principal peak in the chromatogram obtained with reference solution (a) (1 per cent);
- *disregard limit*: 0.1 times the area of the principal peak in the chromatogram obtained with reference solution (a) (0.05 per cent).

Water (*2.5.12*): maximum 0.5 per cent, determined on 2.00 g.

Sulphated ash (*2.4.14*): maximum 0.1 per cent, determined on 1.0 g.

ASSAY

Dissolve 0.150 g in 50 ml of *anhydrous acetic acid R.* Titrate with *0.1 M perchloric acid,* determining the end-point potentiometrically (*2.2.20*).

1 ml of *0.1 M perchloric acid* is equivalent to 19.43 mg of $C_{21}H_{28}N_2O_5$.

IMPURITIES

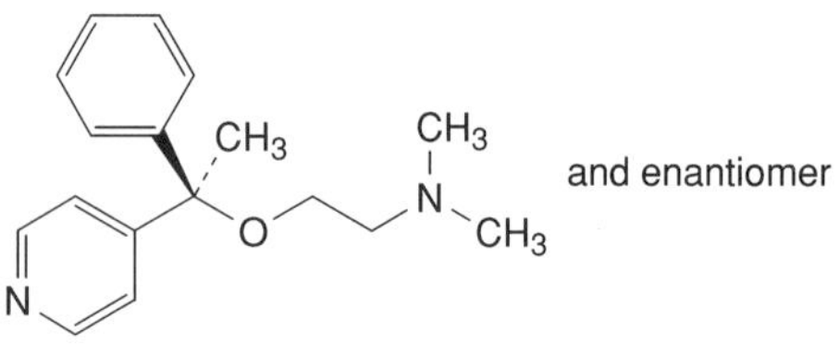

A. *N,N*-dimethyl-2-[1(*RS*)-1-phenyl-1-(pyridin-4-yl)ethoxy]ethanamine,

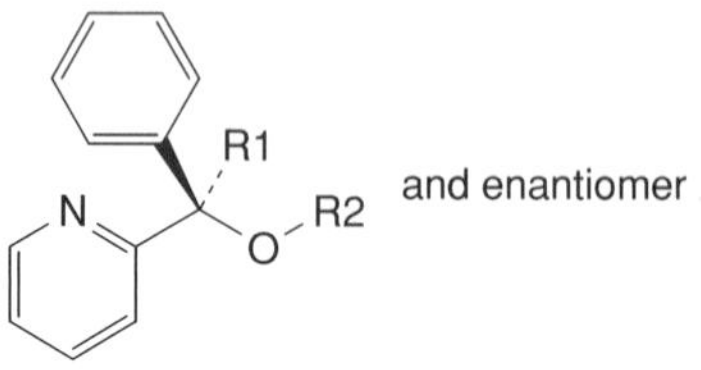

B. R1 = CH_3, R2 = H: (1*RS*)-1-phenyl-1-(pyridin-2-yl)ethanol,

C. R1 = H, R2 = CH_2-CH_2-N$(CH_3)_2$: *N,N*-dimethyl-2-[(*RS*)-1-phenyl(pyridin-2-yl)methoxy]ethanamine,

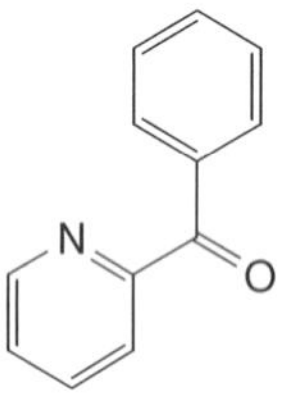

D. phenyl(pyridin-2-yl)methanone (2-benzoylpyridine).

Monographs D-K

E

04/2008:0139

ESTRADIOL BENZOATE

Estradioli benzoas

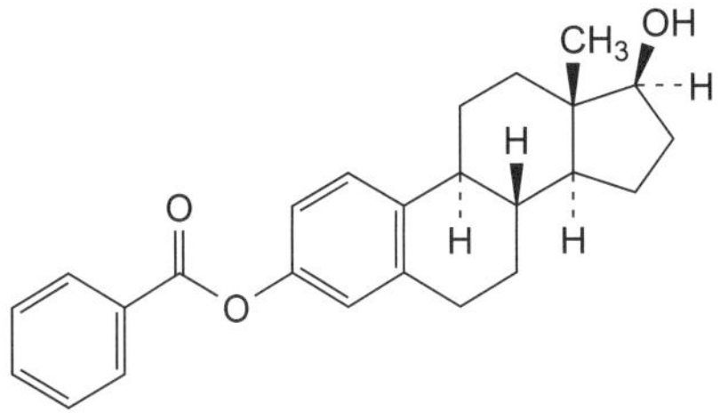

$C_{25}H_{28}O_3$ M_r 376.5
[50-50-0]

DEFINITION

17β-Hydroxyestra-1,3,5(10)-trien-3-yl benzoate.

Content: 97.0 per cent to 103.0 per cent (dried substance).

CHARACTERS

Appearance: almost white, crystalline powder or colourless crystals.

Solubility: practically insoluble in water, freely soluble in methylene chloride, sparingly soluble in acetone, slightly soluble in methanol.

It shows polymorphism (*5.9*).

IDENTIFICATION

Infrared absorption spectrophotometry (*2.2.24*).

Comparison: *estradiol benzoate CRS.*

If the spectra obtained in the solid state show differences, dissolve the substance to be examined and the reference substance separately in *acetone R*, evaporate to dryness and record new spectra using the residues.

TESTS

Specific optical rotation (*2.2.7*): + 55.0 to + 59.0 (dried substance).

Dissolve 0.250 g in *acetone R* and dilute to 25.0 ml with the same solvent.

Related substances. Liquid chromatography (*2.2.29*).

Test solution. Dissolve 20 mg of the substance to be examined in *acetonitrile R1* and dilute to 10.0 ml with the same solvent.

Reference solution (a). Dissolve 5 mg of *estradiol benzoate for system suitability CRS* (containing impurities A, B, C, E and G) in *acetonitrile R1* and dilute to 2.5 ml with the same solvent.

Reference solution (b). Dilute 0.5 ml of the test solution to 100.0 ml with *acetonitrile R1.*

Column:

- *size*: l = 0.25 m, Ø = 4.6 mm;
- *stationary phase*: *end-capped octylsilyl silica gel for chromatography R* (5 μm).

Mobile phase:

- *mobile phase A*: *water R, acetonitrile R1* (40:60 *V/V*);
- *mobile phase B*: *acetonitrile R1*;

Time (min)	Mobile phase A (per cent *V/V*)	Mobile phase B (per cent *V/V*)
0 - 20	100	0
20 - 21	100 → 10	0 → 90
21 - 31	10	90

Flow rate: 1.0 ml/min.

Detection: spectrophotometer at 230 nm.

Injection: 10 μl.

Identification of impurities: use the chromatogram supplied with *estradiol benzoate for system suitability CRS* and the chromatogram obtained with reference solution (a) to identify the peaks due to impurities A, B, C, E and G.

Relative retention with reference to estradiol benzoate (retention time = about 19 min): impurity A = about 0.3; impurity E = about 1.1; impurity B = about 1.2; impurity G = about 1.3; impurity C = about 1.5.

System suitability: reference solution (a):

- *peak-to-valley ratio*: minimum 2.0, where H_p = height above the baseline of the peak due to impurity E and H_v = height above the baseline of the lowest point of the curve separating this peak from the peak due to estradiol benzoate.

Limits:

- *correction factors*: for the calculation of content, multiply the peak areas of the following impurities by the corresponding correction factor: impurity A = 3.3; impurity C = 0.7;
- *impurity C*: not more than the area of the principal peak in the chromatogram obtained with reference solution (b) (0.5 per cent);
- *impurities B, E, G*: for each impurity, not more than 0.6 times the area of the principal peak in the chromatogram obtained with reference solution (b) (0.3 per cent);
- *impurity A*: not more than 0.4 times the area of the principal peak in the chromatogram obtained with reference solution (b) (0.2 per cent);
- *unspecified impurities*: for each impurity, not more than 0.2 times the area of the principal peak in the chromatogram obtained with reference solution (b) (0.10 per cent);
- *total*: not more than twice the area of the principal peak in the chromatogram obtained with reference solution (b) (1.0 per cent);
- *disregard limit*: 0.1 times the area of the principal peak in the chromatogram obtained with reference solution (b) (0.05 per cent).

Loss on drying (*2.2.32*): maximum 0.5 per cent, determined on 1.000 g by drying in an oven at 105 °C for 3 h.

ASSAY

Dissolve 25.0 mg in *anhydrous ethanol R* and dilute to 250.0 ml with the same solvent. Dilute 10.0 ml of this solution to 100.0 ml with *anhydrous ethanol R*. Measure the absorbance (*2.2.25*) at the absorption maximum at 231 nm.

Calculate the content of $C_{25}H_{28}O_3$ taking the specific absorbance to be 500.

IMPURITIES

Specified impurities: A, B, C, E, G.

Other detectable impurities (the following substances would, if present at a sufficient level, be detected by one or other of the tests in the monograph. They are limited by the general acceptance criterion for other/unspecified impurities and/or by the general monograph *Substances for pharmaceutical use (2034)*. It is therefore not necessary to identify these impurities for demonstration of compliance. See also *5.10. Control of impurities in substances for pharmaceutical use*): *D, F, H.*

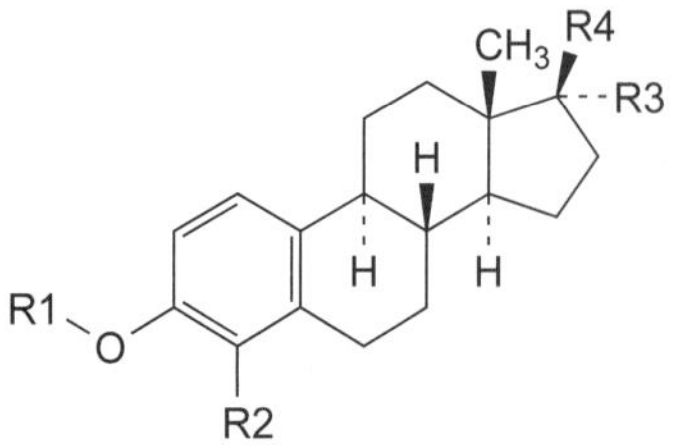

A. R1 = R2 = R3 = H, R4 = OH: estradiol,

B. R1 = CO-C_6H_5, R2 = CH_3, R3 = H, R4 = OH: 17β-hydroxy-4-methylestra-1,3,5(10)-trien-3-yl benzoate,

C. R1 = CO-C_6H_5, R2 = R3 = H, R4 = O-CO-C_6H_5: estra-1,3,5(10)-triene-3,17β-diyl dibenzoate,

E. R1 = CO-C_6H_5, R2 = R4 = H, R3 = OH: 17α-hydroxyestra-1,3,5(10)-trien-3-yl benzoate,

G. R1 = CO-C_6H_5, R2 = H, R3 + R4 = O: 17-oxoestra-1,3,5(10)-trien-3-yl benzoate (estrone benzoate),

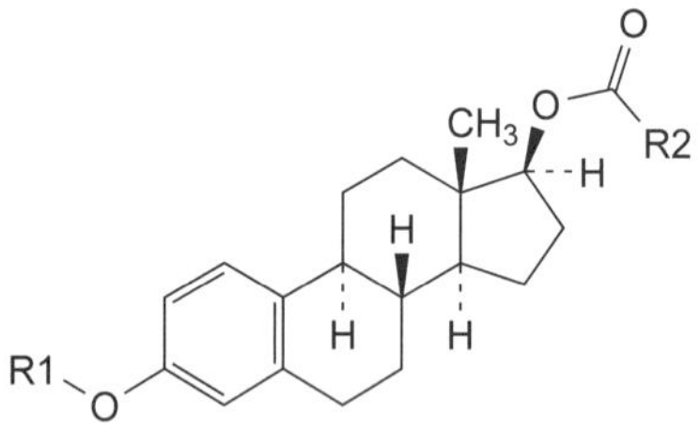

D. R1 = H, R2 = C_6H_5: 3-hydroxyestra-1,3,5(10)-trien-17β-yl benzoate,

H. R1 = CO-C_6H_5, R2 = CH_3: estra-1,3,5(10)-triene-3,17β-diyl 17-acetate 3-benzoate,

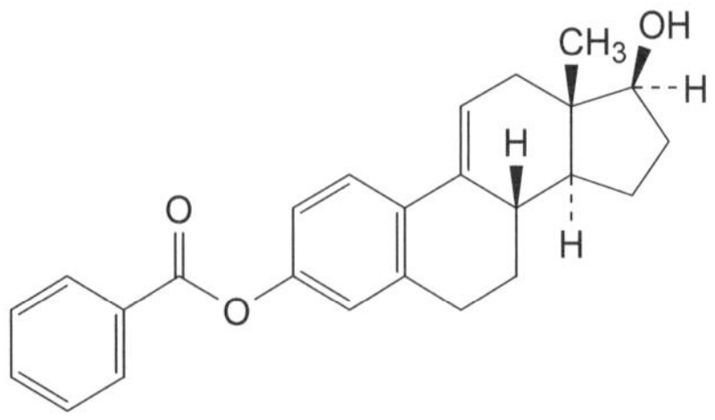

F. 17β-hydroxyestra-1,3,5(10),9(11)-tetraen-3-yl benzoate.

04/2008:0553

ETHAMBUTOL HYDROCHLORIDE

Ethambutoli hydrochloridum

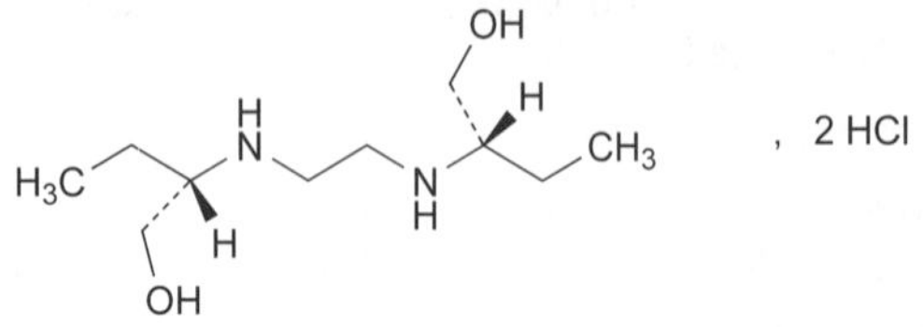

$C_{10}H_{26}Cl_2N_2O_2$ — M_r 277.2

[1070-11-7]

DEFINITION

(2*S*,2′*S*)-2,2′-(ethylenediimino)dibutan-1-ol dihydrochloride.

Content: 99.0 per cent to 101.0 per cent (dried substance).

CHARACTERS

Appearance: white or almost white, crystalline powder, hygroscopic.

Solubility: freely soluble in water, soluble in ethanol (96 per cent).

IDENTIFICATION

First identification: A, D, E.

Second identification: B, C, D.

A. Infrared absorption spectrophotometry (*2.2.24*).

Comparison: *ethambutol hydrochloride CRS.*

B. Examine the chromatograms obtained in the test for impurity A.

Results: the principal spot in the chromatogram obtained with test solution (b) is similar in position, colour and size to the principal spot in the chromatogram obtained with reference solution (b).

C. Dissolve 0.1 g in 10 ml of *water R*. Add 0.2 ml of *copper sulphate solution R* and 0.5 ml of *dilute sodium hydroxide solution R*; a blue colour is produced.

D. It gives reaction (a) of chlorides (*2.3.1*).

E. Related substances (see Tests).

TESTS

pH (*2.2.3*): 3.7 to 4.0.

Dissolve 0.2 g in 10 ml of *carbon dioxide-free water R.*

Impurity A. Thin-layer chromatography (*2.2.27*).

Test solution (a). Dissolve 0.50 g of the substance to be examined in *methanol R* and dilute to 10 ml with the same solvent.

Test solution (b). Dilute 1 ml of test solution (a) to 10 ml with *methanol R.*

Reference solution (a). Dissolve 50.0 mg of *2-aminobutanol R* (impurity A) in *methanol R* and dilute to 10.0 ml with the same solvent. Dilute 1.0 ml of this solution to 10.0 ml with *methanol R.*

Reference solution (b). Dissolve 50 mg of *ethambutol hydrochloride CRS* and 5 mg of *2-aminobutanol R* in *methanol R* and dilute to 10 ml with the same solvent.

Plate: *TLC silica gel plate R.*

Mobile phase: *concentrated ammonia R, water R, methanol R* (10:15:75 *V/V/V*).

Application: 2 µl.

Development: over 2/3 of the plate.

Drying: in air; heat at 110 °C for 10 min.

Detection: cool then spray with *ninhydrin solution R1*; heat at 110 °C for 5 min.

System suitability: reference solution (b):

– the chromatogram shows 2 clearly separated spots.

Limit:

– *impurity A*: any spot due to impurity A in the chromatogram obtained with test solution (a) is not more intense than the spot in the chromatogram obtained with reference solution (a) (1.0 per cent).

Related substances. Liquid chromatography (*2.2.29*). *Prepare the solutions immediately before use.*

Test solution. Suspend 4.0 mg of the substance to be examined in 4.0 ml of *acetonitrile R1* and add 100 µl of *triethylamine R.* Sonicate the mixture for 5 min. Add 15 µl of *(R)-(+)-α-methylbenzyl isocyanate R* and heat at 70 °C for 20 min.

Reference solution (a). Dilute 0.50 ml of the test solution to 100.0 ml with *acetonitrile R1.*

Reference solution (b). Treat 4.0 mg of *ethambutol for system suitability CRS* (containing impurity B) as described for the test solution.

Column:
- *size*: *l* = 0.10 m, Ø = 4.6 mm;
- *stationary phase*: *end-capped octadecylsilyl silica gel for chromatography R* (3 µm);
- *temperature*: 40 °C.

Mobile phase:
- *mobile phase A*: *methanol R, water R* (50:50 *V/V*);
- *mobile phase B*: *methanol R*;

Time (min)	Mobile phase A (per cent *V/V*)	Mobile phase B (per cent *V/V*)
0 - 30	71	29
30 - 35	71 → 0	29 → 100
35 - 37	0	100
37 - 38	0 → 71	100 → 29

Flow rate: 1.0 ml/min.

Detection: spectrophotometer at 215 nm.

Injection: 10 µl.

Relative retention with reference to ethambutol (retention time = about 14 min): impurity B = about 1.3.

System suitability: reference solution (b):
- *resolution*: minimum 4.0 between the peaks due to ethambutol and impurity B.

Limits:
- *impurity B*: not more than twice the area of the principal peak in the chromatogram obtained with reference solution (a) (1.0 per cent);
- *unspecified impurities with a relative retention of 0.75 to 1.5 with reference to ethambutol*: for each impurity, not more than 0.2 times the area of the peak due to ethambutol in the chromatogram obtained with reference solution (a) (0.10 per cent);
- *total (impurity B and unspecified impurities with a relative retention of 0.75 to 1.5 with reference to ethambutol)*: not more than twice the area of the principal peak in the chromatogram obtained with reference solution (a) (1.0 per cent);
- *disregard limit*: 0.1 times the area of the peak due to ethambutol in the chromatogram obtained with reference solution (a) (0.05 per cent).

Impurity D (1,2-dichloroethane) (*2.4.24*): maximum 5 ppm.

Heavy metals (*2.4.8*): maximum 10 ppm.

Dissolve 2.0 g in *water R* and dilute to 20 ml with the same solvent. 12 ml of the solution complies with test A. Prepare the reference solution using 10 ml of *lead standard solution (1 ppm Pb) R.*

Loss on drying (*2.2.32*): maximum 0.5 per cent, determined on 0.500 g by drying in an oven at 105 °C for 3 h.

Sulphated ash (*2.4.14*): maximum 0.1 per cent, determined on 1.0 g.

ASSAY

Dissolve 0.200 g in 50 ml of *water R* and add 1.0 ml of *0.1 M hydrochloric acid.* Carry out a potentiometric titration (*2.2.20*), using *0.1 M sodium hydroxide.* Read the volume added between the 2 points of inflexion.

1 ml of *0.1 M sodium hydroxide* is equivalent to 27.72 mg of $C_{10}H_{26}Cl_2N_2O_2$.

STORAGE

In an airtight container.

IMPURITIES

Specified impurities: A, B, D.

Other detectable impurities (the following substances would, if present at a sufficient level, be detected by one or other of the tests in the monograph. They are limited by the general acceptance criterion for other/unspecified impurities and/or by the general monograph *Substances for pharmaceutical use (2034).* It is therefore not necessary to identify these impurities for demonstration of compliance. See also *5.10. Control of impurities in substances for pharmaceutical use*): *C.*

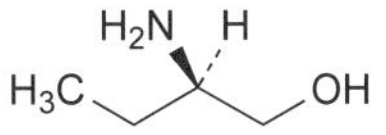

A. 2-aminobutan-1-ol,

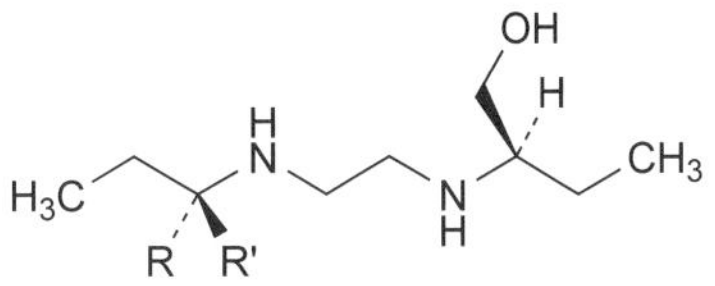

B. R = CH_2-OH, R′ = H: (2*R*,2′*S*)-2,2′-(ethylenediimino)-dibutan-1-ol (meso-ethambutol),

C. R = H, R′ = CH_2-OH: (2*R*,2′*R*)-2,2′-(ethylenediimino)dibutan-1-ol ((*R*,*R*)-ethambutol),

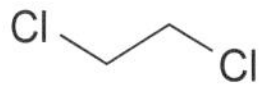

D. 1,2-dichloroethane (ethylene chloride).

Monographs D-K

G

04/2008:1827

GINKGO DRY EXTRACT, REFINED AND QUANTIFIED

Ginkgonis extractum siccum raffinatum et quantificatum

DEFINITION

Refined and quantified dry extract produced from *Ginkgo leaf (1828)*.

Content:

- *flavonoids, expressed as flavone glycosides* (M_r 756.7): 22.0 per cent to 27.0 per cent (dried extract);
- *bilobalide*: 2.6 per cent to 3.2 per cent (dried extract);
- *ginkgolides A, B and C*: 2.8 per cent to 3.4 per cent (dried extract);
- *ginkgolic acids*: maximum 5 ppm (dried extract).

PRODUCTION

The extract is produced from the herbal drug by an appropriate procedure using organic solvents and their mixtures with water, physical separation steps as well as other suitable processes.

CHARACTERS

Appearance: bright yellow-brown, powder or friable mass.

IDENTIFICATION

Thin-layer chromatography (*2.2.27*).

Test solution. Dissolve 20.0 mg of the extract to be examined in 10 ml of a mixture of 2 volumes of *water R* and 8 volumes of *methanol R*.

Reference solution. Dissolve 1.0 mg of *chlorogenic acid R* and 3.0 mg of *rutin R* in 20 ml of *methanol R*.

Plate: *TLC silica gel plate R* (5-40 µm) or [*TLC silica gel plate R* (2-10 µm)].

Mobile phase: *anhydrous formic acid R, glacial acetic acid R, water R, ethyl acetate R* (7.5:7.5:17.5:67.5 *V/V/V/V*).

Application: 20 µl [or 5 µl], as bands.

Development: over a path of 17 cm [or 6 cm].

Drying: at 100-105 °C.

Detection: spray the plate whilst still hot with a 10 g/l solution of *diphenylboric acid aminoethyl ester R* in *methanol R*, then spray with a 50 g/l solution of *macrogol 400 R* in *methanol R*; allow to dry in air for about 30 min and examine in ultraviolet light at 365 nm.

Results: see below the sequence of zones present in the chromatograms obtained with the reference solution and the test solution. Furthermore, other, weaker fluorescent zones may be present in the chromatogram obtained with the test solution.

Top of the plate	
	A blue fluorescent zone
	Several faint coloured zones
_______	_______
	A brown fluorescent zone
	A green fluorescent zone
	An intense light blue fluorescent zone sometimes overlapped by a greenish-brown fluorescent zone
Chlorogenic acid: a light blue fluorescent zone	
	One or two green fluorescent zones
Rutin: a yellowish-brown fluorescent zone	One or two yellowish-brown fluorescent zones
_______	_______
	Several green and yellowish-brown fluorescent zones
Reference solution	**Test solution**

ASSAY

Flavonoids. Liquid chromatography (*2.2.29*).

Test solution. Dissolve 0.200 g of the extract to be examined in 20 ml of *methanol R*. Add 15.0 ml of *dilute hydrochloric acid R* and 5 ml of *water R* and dilute to 50.0 ml with *methanol R*. Transfer 10.0 ml of this solution into a 10 ml brown-glass vial. Close the vial with a tight rubber membrane stopper and secure with an aluminium crimped cap. Heat on a water-bath for 25 min. Allow to cool to 20 °C.

Reference solution. Dissolve 10.0 mg of *quercetin dihydrate CRS* in 20 ml of *methanol R*. Add 15.0 ml of *dilute hydrochloric acid R* and 5 ml of *water R* and dilute to 50.0 ml with *methanol R*.

Column:

- *size*: l = 0.125 m, Ø = 4 mm;
- *stationary phase*: *octadecylsilyl silica gel for chromatography R* (5 µm);
- *temperature*: 25 °C.

Mobile phase:

- *mobile phase A*: 0.3 g/l solution of *phosphoric acid R* adjusted to pH 2.0;
- *mobile phase B*: *methanol R*;

Time (min)	Mobile phase A (per cent *V/V*)	Mobile phase B (per cent *V/V*)
0 - 1	60	40
1 - 20	60 → 45	40 → 55
20 - 21	45 → 0	55 → 100
21 - 25	0	100

Flow rate: 1.0 ml/min.

Detector: spectrophotometer at 370 nm.

Injection: 10 µl.

Relative retention with reference to quercetin (retention time = about 12.5 min): kaempferol = about 1.4; isorhamnetin = about 1.5.

System suitability: test solution:

- *resolution*: minimum 1.5 between the peaks due to kaempferol and isorhamnetin.

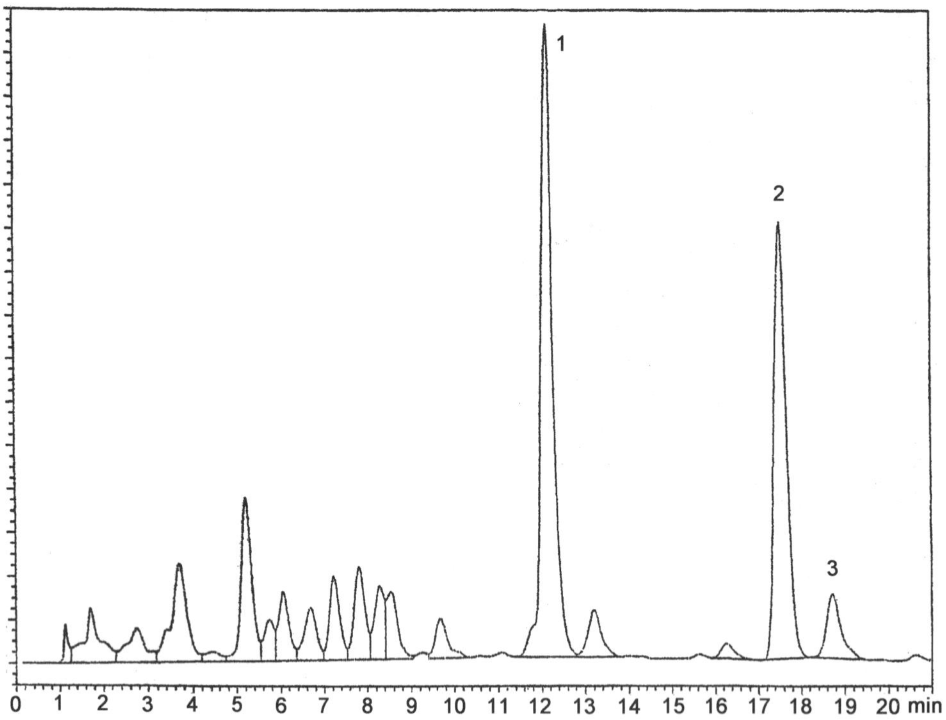

1. quercetin 2. kaempferol 3. isorhamnetin

Figure 1827.-1. – *Chromatogram for the assay of flavonoids in refined and quantified ginkgo dry extract*

Determine the sum of the areas including all the peaks from the peak due to quercetin to the peak due to isorhamnetin in the chromatogram obtained with the test solution (see Figure 1827.-1).

Calculate the percentage content of flavonoids, expressed as flavone glycosides, using the following expression:

$$\frac{F_1 \times m_1 \times 2.514 \times p}{F_2 \times m_2}$$

F_1 = sum of the areas of all the peaks from the peak due to quercetin to the peak due to isorhamnetin in the chromatogram obtained with the test solution;

F_2 = area of the peak due to quercetin in the chromatogram obtained with the reference solution;

m_1 = mass of *quercetin dihydrate CRS* in the reference solution, in grams;

m_2 = mass of the extract to be examined used to prepare the test solution, in grams;

p = percentage content of anhydrous quercetin in *quercetin dihydrate CRS*.

Terpene lactones. Liquid chromatography (*2.2.29*).

Test solution. Place 0.120 g of the extract to be examined in a 25 ml beaker and dissolve it in 10 ml of *phosphate buffer solution pH 5.8 R* by stirring. Transfer the solution into a chromatography column, about 0.15 m long and about 30 mm in internal diameter, containing 15 g of *kieselguhr for chromatography R*. Wash the beaker with 2 quantities, each of 5 ml, of *phosphate buffer solution pH 5.8 R* and transfer the washings to the chromatography column. Allow to stand for 15 min. Elute with 100 ml of *ethyl acetate R*. Evaporate the eluate to dryness at a pressure not exceeding 4 kPa in a water-bath at 50 °C. The residue of solvent is eliminated by an air-current. Take up the residue in 2.5 ml of the mobile phase.

Reference solution (a). Dissolve 30.0 mg of *benzyl alcohol CRS* in the mobile phase and dilute to 100.0 ml with the mobile phase.

Reference solution (b). Place 0.120 g of the *ginkgo dry extract for peak identification CRS* in a 25 ml beaker and dissolve it in 10 ml of *phosphate buffer solution pH 5.8 R* by stirring, then proceed as described for the test solution.

Column:

– *size*: *l* = 0.25 m, Ø = 4 mm;
– *stationary phase*: *octylsilyl silica gel for chromatography R* (5 µm);
– *temperature*: 25 °C.

Mobile phase: *tetrahydrofuran R, methanol R, water R* (10:20:75 *V/V/V*).

Flow rate: 1.0 ml/min.

Detection: refractometer maintained at 35 °C.

Injection: 100 µl.

Identification of peaks: use the chromatogram supplied with *ginkgo dry extract for peak identification CRS* and the chromatogram obtained with the reference solution (b) to identify the peaks due to bilobalide and ginkgolides A, B and C.

System suitability:

– the chromatogram obtained with reference solution (b) is similar to the chromatogram supplied with *ginkgo dry extract for peak identification CRS*.

Calculate the percentage content of bilobalide, using the following expression:

$$\frac{F_1 \times m_1 \times p \times 0.025 \times 1.20}{F_5 \times m_2}$$

Calculate the percentage content of ginkgolide A, using the following expression:

$$\frac{F_2 \times m_1 \times p \times 0.025 \times 1.22}{F_5 \times m_2}$$

Monographs D-K

Calculate the percentage content of ginkgolide B, using the following expression:

$$\frac{F_3 \times m_1 \times p \times 0.025 \times 1.19}{F_5 \times m_2}$$

Calculate the percentage content of ginkgolide C, using the following expression:

$$\frac{F_4 \times m_1 \times p \times 0.025 \times 1.27}{F_5 \times m_2}$$

F_1 = area of the peak due to bilobalide in the chromatogram obtained with the test solution;

F_2 = area of the peak due to ginkgolide A in the chromatogram obtained with the test solution;

F_3 = area of the peak due to ginkgolide B in the chromatogram obtained with the test solution;

F_4 = area of the peak due to ginkgolide C in the chromatogram obtained with the test solution;

F_5 = area of the peak due to benzyl alcohol in the chromatogram obtained with reference solution (a);

m_1 = mass of *benzyl alcohol CRS* in reference solution (a), in grams;

m_2 = mass of the extract to be examined used to prepare the test solution, in grams;

p = percentage content of benzyl alcohol in *benzyl alcohol CRS*.

Calculate the percentage content of the sum of ginkgolides A, B and C, using the following expression:

$$G_A + G_B + G_C$$

G_A = percentage content of ginkgolide A;

G_B = percentage content of ginkgolide B;

G_C = percentage content of ginkgolide C.

Ginkgolic acids. Liquid chromatography (*2.2.29*).

Test solution. Dissolve 0.500 g of the powdered extract to be examined in 8 ml of *methanol R*, sonicating if necessary, and dilute to 10.0 ml with the same solvent. Centrifuge if necessary.

Reference solution. Dissolve 10.0 mg of *ginkgolic acids CRS* in 8 ml of *methanol R*, sonicating if necessary, and dilute to 10.0 ml with the same solvent. Dilute 2.0 ml of this solution to 10.0 ml with *methanol R*.

Column:
- *size*: *l* = 0.25 m, Ø = 4.6 mm;
- *stationary phase*: *octylsilyl silica gel for chromatography R* (5 µm);
- *temperature*: 35 °C.

Mobile phase:
- *mobile phase A*: dilute 0.1 ml of *trifluoroacetic acid R* to 1000 ml with *water R*;
- *mobile phase B*: dilute 0.1 ml of *trifluoroacetic acid R* to 1000 ml with *acetonitrile R*;

Time (min)	Mobile phase A (per cent *V/V*)	Mobile phase B (per cent *V/V*)
0 - 30	25 → 10	75 → 90
30 - 35	10	90
35 - 36	10 → 25	90 → 75
36 - 45	25	75

Flow rate: 1.0 ml/min.

Detection: spectrophotometer at 210 nm.

Injection: 50 µl.

Identification of components: use the chromatogram supplied with *ginkgolic acids CRS* and the chromatogram obtained with the test solution to identify the peaks due to ginkgolic acids C13, C15 and C17.

System suitability: reference solution:
- *resolution*: minimum 2.0 between the peaks due to ginkgolic acids C13 and C15;
- *symmetry factor*: 0.8 to 2.0 for the peaks due to ginkgolic acids C13, C15 and C17.

Calculate the content in ppm of ginkgolic acids expressed as ginkgolic acid C17, using the following expression:

$$\frac{A_1 \times m_2 \times p \times 2000}{A_2 \times m_1}$$

A_1 = sum of the areas of the peaks due to the ginkgolic acids C13, C15 and C17 in the chromatogram obtained with the test solution;

A_2 = area of the peak due to ginkgolic acid C17 in the chromatogram obtained with the reference solution;

m_1 = mass of the extract to be examined used to prepare the test solution, in grams;

m_2 = mass of *ginkgolic acids CRS* used to prepare the reference solution, in grams;

p = percentage content of ginkgolic acid C17 in *ginkgolic acids CRS*.

04/2008:1670

GLUTATHIONE

Glutathionum

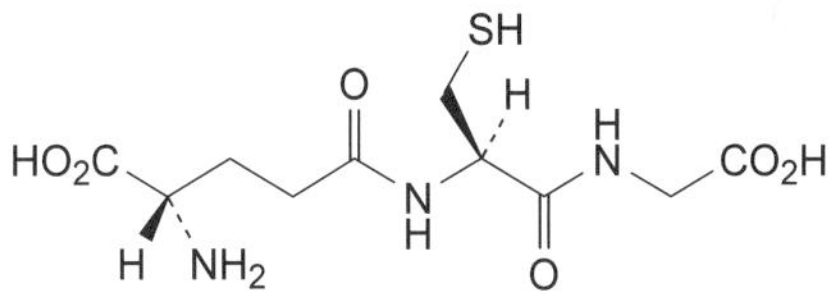

$C_{10}H_{17}N_3O_6S$ M_r 307.3

[70-18-8]

DEFINITION

L-γ-Glutamyl-L-cysteinylglycine.

Fermentation product.

Content: 98.0 per cent to 101.0 per cent (dried substance).

CHARACTERS

Appearance: white or almost white, crystalline powder or colourless crystals.

Solubility: freely soluble in water, very slightly soluble in ethanol (96 per cent) and in methylene chloride.

IDENTIFICATION

A. Specific optical rotation (see Tests).

B. Infrared absorption spectrophotometry (*2.2.24*).

Comparison: *glutathione CRS*.

TESTS

Solution S. Dissolve 5.0 g in *distilled water R* and dilute to 50 ml with the same solvent.

Monographs D-K

Appearance of solution. Solution S is clear (*2.2.1*) and colourless (*2.2.2, Method II*).

Specific optical rotation (*2.2.7*): – 15.5 to – 17.5 (dried substance).

Dissolve 1.0 g in *water R* and dilute to 25.0 ml with the same solvent.

Related substances. Capillary electrophoresis (*2.2.47*). *Prepare the solutions immediately before use.*

Internal standard solution (a). Dissolve 0.100 g of *phenylalanine R* in the electrolyte solution and dilute to 50.0 ml with the same solution.

Internal standard solution (b). Dilute 10.0 ml of internal standard solution (a) to 100.0 ml with the electrolyte solution.

Test solution (a). Dissolve 0.200 g of the substance to be examined in the electrolyte solution and dilute to 10.0 ml with the same solution.

Test solution (b). Dissolve 0.200 g of the substance to be examined in internal standard solution (b) and dilute to 10.0 ml with the same solution.

Reference solution (a). Dissolve 20.0 mg of the substance to be examined in internal standard solution (a) and dilute to 10.0 ml with the same solution.

Reference solution (b). Dilute 5.0 ml of reference solution (a) to 50.0 ml with the electrolyte solution.

Reference solution (c). Dissolve 0.200 g of the substance to be examined in 5 ml of the electrolyte solution. Add 1.0 ml of internal standard solution (a), 0.5 ml of a 2 mg/ml solution of *L-cysteine R* (impurity B) in the electrolyte solution, 0.5 ml of a 2 mg/ml solution of *oxidised L-glutathione R* (impurity C) in the electrolyte solution and 0.5 ml of a 2 mg/ml solution of *L-γ-glutamyl-L-cysteine R* (impurity D) in the electrolyte solution. Dilute to 10.0 ml with the electrolyte solution.

Capillary:

- *material*: uncoated fused silica;
- *size*: length to the detector cell = 0.5 m; total length = 0.6 m; Ø = 75 µm.

Temperature: 25 °C.

Electrolyte solution. Dissolve 1.50 g of *anhydrous sodium dihydrogen phosphate R* in 230 ml of *water R* and adjust to pH 1.80 with *phosphoric acid R*. Dilute to 250.0 ml with *water R*. Check the pH and, if necessary, adjust with *phosphoric acid R* or *dilute sodium hydroxide solution R*.

Detection: spectrophotometer at 200 nm.

Preconditioning of a new capillary: rinse the new capillary before the first injection with *0.1 M hydrochloric acid* at 138 kPa for 20 min and with *water R* at 138 kPa for 10 min; for complete equilibration, condition the capillary with the electrolyte solution at 350 kPa for 40 min, and subsequently at a voltage of 20 kV for 60 min.

Preconditioning of the capillary: rinse the capillary with the electrolyte solution at 138 kPa for 40 min.

Between-run rinsing: rinse the capillary with *water R* at 138 kPa for 1 min, with *0.1 M sodium hydroxide* at 138 kPa for 2 min, with *water R* at 138 kPa for 1 min, with *0.1 M hydrochloric acid* at 138 kPa for 3 min and with the electrolyte solution at 138 kPa for 10 min.

Injection: test solutions (a) and (b), reference solutions (b) and (c) and the electrolyte solution (blank): under pressure (3.45 kPa) for 5 s.

Migration: apply a voltage of 20 kV.

Run time: 45 min.

Relative migration with reference to the internal standard (about 14 min): impurity A = about 0.77; impurity B = about 1.04; impurity E = about 1.2; impurity C = about 1.26; impurity D = about 1.3.

System suitability:

- *resolution*: minimum 1.5 between the peaks due to the internal standard and impurity B in the chromatogram obtained with reference solution (c); if necessary, increase the pH with *dilute sodium hydroxide solution R*;
- *peak-to-valley ratio*: minimum 2.5, where H_p = height above the baseline of the peak due to impurity D and H_v = height above the baseline of the lowest point of the curve separating this peak from the peak due to glutathione in the chromatogram obtained with reference solution (c); if necessary, lower the pH with *phosphoric acid R*;
- check that in the electropherogram obtained with test solution (a) there is no peak with the same migration time as the internal standard (in such case correct the area of the phenylalanine peak).

Limits: test solution (b):

- *corrected areas*: divide all the peak areas by the corresponding migration times;
- *correction factors*: for the calculation of content, multiply the ratio of time-corrected peak areas of impurity and the internal standard by the corresponding correction factor: impurity B = 3.0; impurity D = 1.4;
- *impurity C*: not more than 1.5 times the ratio of the area of the peak due to glutathione to the area of the peak due to the internal standard in the electropherogram obtained with reference solution (b) (1.5 per cent);
- *impurity D*: not more than the ratio of the area of the peak due to glutathione to the area of the peak due to the internal standard in the electropherogram obtained with reference solution (b) (1.0 per cent);
- *impurities A, B, E*: for each impurity, not more than 0.5 times the ratio of the area of the peak due to glutathione to the area of the peak due to the internal standard in the electropherogram obtained with reference solution (b) (0.5 per cent);
- *any other impurity*: for each impurity, not more than 0.2 times the ratio of the area of the peak due to glutathione to the area of the peak due to the internal standard in the electropherogram obtained with reference solution (b) (0.2 per cent);
- *total*: not more than 2.5 times the ratio of the area of the peak due to glutathione to the area of the peak due to the internal standard in the electropherogram obtained with reference solution (b) (2.5 per cent);
- *disregard limit*: 0.05 times the ratio of the area of the peak due to glutathione to the area of the peak due to the internal standard in the electropherogram obtained with reference solution (b) (0.05 per cent).

Chlorides (*2.4.4*): maximum 200 ppm.

Dilute 2.5 ml of solution S to 15 ml with *water R*.

Sulphates (*2.4.13*): maximum 300 ppm.

Dilute 5 ml of solution S to 15 ml with *distilled water R*.

Ammonium (*2.4.1, Method B*): maximum 200 ppm, determined on 50 mg.

Prepare the standard using 0.1 ml of *ammonium standard solution (100 ppm NH_4) R*.

Iron (*2.4.9*): maximum 10 ppm.

In a separating funnel, dissolve 1.0 g in 10 ml of *dilute hydrochloric acid R*. Shake with 3 quantities, each of 10 ml,

Monographs D-K

of *methyl isobutyl ketone R1*, shaking for 3 min each time. To the combined organic layers, add 10 ml of *water R* and shake for 3 min. The aqueous layer complies with the test.

Heavy metals (*2.4.8*): maximum 10 ppm.

12 ml of solution S complies with test A. Prepare the reference solution using *lead standard solution (1 ppm Pb) R*.

Loss on drying (*2.2.32*): maximum 0.5 per cent, determined on 1.000 g by drying in an oven at 105 °C for 3 h.

Sulphated ash (*2.4.14*): maximum 0.1 per cent, determined on 1.0 g.

ASSAY

In a ground-glass-stoppered flask, dissolve 0.500 g of the substance to be examined and 2 g of *potassium iodide R* in 50 ml of *water R*. Cool the solution in iced water and add 10 ml of *hydrochloric acid R1* and 20.0 ml of *0.05 M iodine*. Stopper the flask and allow to stand in the dark for 15 min. Titrate with *0.1 M sodium thiosulphate* using 1 ml of *starch solution R*, added towards the end of the titration, as indicator. Carry out a blank titration.

1 ml of *0.05 M iodine* is equivalent to 30.73 mg of $C_{10}H_{17}N_3O_6S$.

STORAGE

Protected from light.

IMPURITIES

Specified impurities: A, B, C, D, E.

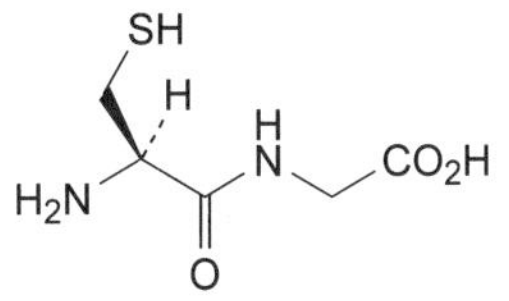

A. L-cysteinylglycine,

B. cysteine,

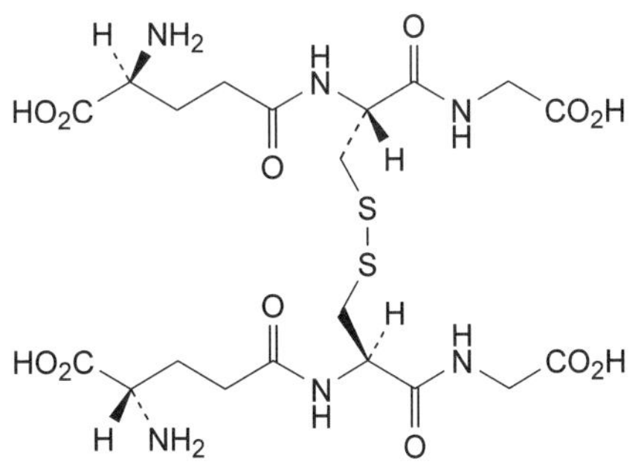

C. bis(L-γ-glutamyl-L-cysteinylglycine) disulfide (L-glutathione oxidised),

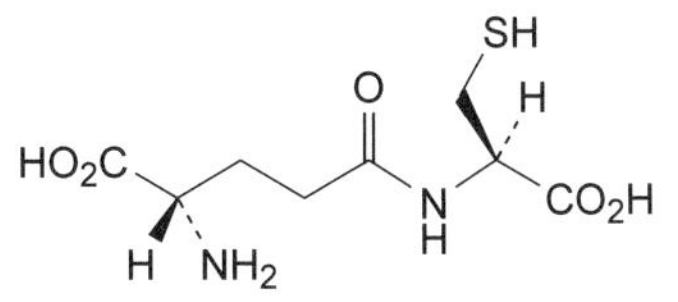

D. L-γ-glutamyl-L-cysteine,

E. unknown structure (product of degradation).

01/2008:1331
corrected 6.1

GLYCERYL TRINITRATE SOLUTION

Glyceroli trinitratis solutio

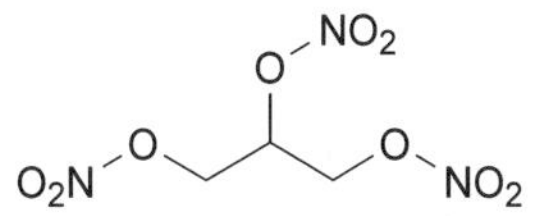

$C_3H_5N_3O_9$ M_r 227.1

DEFINITION

Ethanolic solution of glyceryl trinitrate.

Content: 1 per cent *m/m* to 10 per cent *m/m* of propane-1,2,3-triyl trinitrate and 96.5 per cent to 102.5 per cent of the declared content of glyceryl trinitrate stated on the label.

CHARACTERS

Appearance: clear, colourless or slightly yellow solution.

Solubility: miscible with acetone and with anhydrous ethanol.

Solubility of pure glyceryl trinitrate: practically insoluble in water, freely soluble in anhydrous ethanol, miscible with acetone.

IDENTIFICATION

First identification: A, C.

Second identification: B, C.

Upon diluting glyceryl trinitrate solution, care must be taken to always use anhydrous ethanol, otherwise droplets of pure glyceryl trinitrate may precipitate from the solution.

After examination, the residues and the solutions obtained in both the identification and the test sections must be heated on a water-bath for 5 min with dilute sodium hydroxide solution R.

A. Infrared absorption spectrophotometry (*2.2.24*).

Preparation: place 50 µl of a solution diluted, if necessary, with *anhydrous ethanol R*, to contain 10 g/l of glyceryl trinitrate, on a disc of *potassium bromide R* and evaporate the solvent *in vacuo*.

Comparison: *Ph. Eur. reference spectrum of glyceryl trinitrate.*

B. Thin-layer chromatography (*2.2.27*).

Test solution. Dilute a quantity of the substance to be examined corresponding to 50 mg of glyceryl trinitrate in *acetone R* and dilute to 100 ml with the same solvent.

Reference solution. Dilute 0.05 ml of *glyceryl trinitrate solution CRS* to 1 ml with *acetone R*.

Plate: *TLC silica gel G plate R.*

Mobile phase: *ethyl acetate R, toluene R* (20:80 *V/V*).

Application: 5 µl.

Development: over 2/3 of the plate.

Drying: in air.

Detection: spray with freshly prepared *potassium iodide and starch solution R*; expose to ultraviolet light at 254 nm for 15 min and examine in daylight.

Results: the principal spot in the chromatogram obtained with the test solution is similar in position, colour and size to the principal spot in the chromatogram obtained with the reference solution.

C. It complies with the limits of the assay.

TESTS

Upon diluting glyceryl trinitrate solution, care must be taken always to use anhydrous ethanol, otherwise droplets of pure glyceryl trinitrate may precipitate from the solution.

After examination, the residues and the solutions obtained in both the identification and the test sections must be heated on a water-bath for 5 min with dilute sodium hydroxide solution R.

Appearance of solution. If necessary dilute the solution to be examined to a concentration of 10 g/l with *anhydrous ethanol R*. The solution is not more intensely coloured than reference solution Y_7 (*2.2.2, Method II*).

Inorganic nitrates. Thin-layer chromatography (*2.2.27*).

Test solution. If necessary dilute the solution to be examined to a concentration of 10 g/l with *anhydrous ethanol R*.

Reference solution. Dissolve 5 mg of *potassium nitrate R* in 1 ml of *water R* and dilute to 100 ml with *ethanol (96 per cent) R*.

Plate: *TLC silica gel plate R*.

Mobile phase: *glacial acetic acid R, acetone R, toluene R* (15:30:60 *V/V/V*).

Application: 10 µl.

Development: over 2/3 of the plate.

Drying: in a current of air until the acetic acid is completely removed.

Detection: spray intensively with freshly prepared *potassium iodide and starch solution R*; expose to ultraviolet light at 254 nm for 15 min and examine in daylight.

Limit:

- *nitrate ion*: any spot due to the nitrate ion in the chromatogram obtained with the test solution is not more intense than the spot in the chromatogram obtained with the reference solution (0.5 per cent of the content of glyceryl trinitrate calculated as potassium nitrate).

Related substances. Liquid chromatography (*2.2.29*).

Test solution. Dissolve a quantity of the substance to be examined equivalent to 2 mg of glyceryl trinitrate in the mobile phase and dilute to 20.0 ml with the mobile phase.

Reference solution (a). Dissolve 0.10 g of *glyceryl trinitrate solution CRS* and a quantity of *diluted pentaerythrityl tetranitrate CRS* equivalent to 1.0 mg of pentaerythrityl tetranitrate in the mobile phase and dilute to 100.0 ml with the mobile phase. Sonicate and filter if necessary.

Reference solution (b). Dilute 1.0 ml of the test solution to 100.0 ml with the mobile phase.

Column:

- *size*: *l* = 0.25 m, Ø = 4.6 mm;
- *stationary phase*: *octadecylsilyl silica gel for chromatography R* (5 µm).

Mobile phase: *acetonitrile R, water R* (50:50 *V/V*).

Flow rate: 1 ml/min.

Detection: spectrophotometer at 210 nm.

Injection: 20 µl.

Run time: 3 times the retention time of the principal peak.

System suitability: reference solution (a):

- *resolution*: minimum 2.0 between the peaks due to glyceryl trinitrate and to pentaerythrityl tetranitrate.

Limits:

- *any impurity*: not more than the area of the principal peak in the chromatogram obtained with reference solution (b) (1 per cent, expressed as glyceryl trinitrate),
- *total*: not more than 3 times the area of the principal peak in the chromatogram obtained with reference solution (b) (3 per cent, expressed as glyceryl trinitrate),
- *disregard limit*: 0.1 times the area of the principal peak in the chromatogram obtained with reference solution (b) (0.1 per cent).

ASSAY

Test solution. Prepare a solution containing 1.0 mg of glyceryl trinitrate in 250.0 ml of *methanol R*.

Reference solution. Dissolve 70.0 mg of *sodium nitrite R* in *methanol R* and dilute to 250.0 ml with the same solvent. Dilute 5.0 ml of the solution to 500.0 ml with *methanol R*.

Into three 50 ml volumetric flasks introduce 10.0 ml of the test solution, 10.0 ml of the reference solution and 10 ml of *methanol R* as a blank. To each flask add 5 ml of *dilute sodium hydroxide solution R*, close the flask, mix and allow to stand at room temperature for 30 min. Add 10 ml of *sulphanilic acid solution R* and 10 ml of *dilute hydrochloric acid R* and mix. After exactly 4 min, add 10 ml of *naphthylethylenediamine dihydrochloride solution R*, dilute to volume with *water R* and mix. After 10 min read the absorbance (*2.2.25*) of the test solution and the reference solution at 540 nm using the blank solution as the compensation liquid.

Calculate the amount of glyceryl trinitrate in milligrams in the test solution using the following expression:

$$\frac{A_T \times m_S \times C}{A_R \times m_T \times 60.8}$$

A_T = absorption of the test solution,

m_T = mass of the substance to be examined, in milligrams,

C = percentage content of sodium nitrite used as reference,

A_R = absorption of the reference solution,

m_S = mass of sodium nitrite, in milligrams.

STORAGE

Store the diluted solutions (10 g/l) protected from light, at a temperature of 2 °C to 15 °C.

Store more concentrated solutions protected from light, at a temperature of 15 °C to 20 °C.

LABELLING

The label states the declared content of glyceryl trinitrate.

IMPURITIES

A. inorganic nitrates,

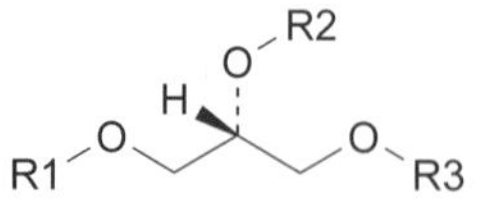

and enantiomer

B. R1 = NO_2, R2 = R3 = H: (2*RS*)-2,3-dihydroxypropyl nitrate,

C. R1 = R3 = H, R2 = NO_2: 2-hydroxy-1-(hydroxymethyl)ethyl nitrate,

D. R1 = R2 = NO_2, R3 = H: (2*RS*)-3-hydroxypropane-1,2-diyl dinitrate,

E. R1 = R3 = NO_2, R2 = H: 2-hydroxypropane-1,3-diyl dinitrate.

04/2008:1831

GOLDENSEAL RHIZOME

Hydrastis rhizoma

DEFINITION

Whole or cut, dried rhizome and root of *Hydrastis canadensis* L.

Content:

- *hydrastine* ($C_{21}H_{21}NO_6$; M_r 383.4): minimum 2.5 per cent (dried drug);
- *berberine* ($C_{20}H_{19}NO_5$; M_r 353.4): minimum 3.0 per cent (dried drug).

IDENTIFICATION

A. The rhizome is tortuous and knotty, about 5 cm long and 5-10 mm thick. The surface is yellowish or brownish-grey, irregularly wrinkled, and bears the remains of numerous slender, wiry roots; stem bases and scale leaves occur on the upper surface. The fracture is short and resinous. The transversely-cut surface is yellowish-brown and shows a fairly wide bark, a ring of from about 12 to 20 widely separated xylem bundles and a large, central pith.

B. Reduce to a powder (180) (*2.9.12*). The powder is greenish-yellow. Examine under a microscope using *chloral hydrate solution R*. The powder shows the following diagnostic characters: abundant thin-walled fragments of parenchyma; occasional fragments of yellowish-brown cork from the rhizome and roots; groups of small vessels with conspicuous perforations in the oblique end walls and with simple or bordered, slit-shaped pits; infrequent groups of thin-walled, pitted fibres, usually found associated with the vessels; numerous ovoid or spherical, orange-brown granular masses. Examine under a microscope using a 50 per cent *V/V* solution of *glycerol R*. The powder shows abundant starch granules, mostly simple but sometimes compound with up to 4 components; the granules are small, spherical or ovoid, up to about 10 µm in diameter, occasionally with a small, rounded or slit-shaped hilum.

C. Thin-layer chromatography (*2.2.27*).

Test solution. To 250 mg of powdered drug (180) (*2.9.12*) add 4 ml of a mixture of 20 ml of *water R* and 80 ml of *methanol R*. Sonicate for 10 min and filter. Wash the residue with 2 quantities, each of 2 ml, of *methanol R*. Combine the solutions and dilute to 20 ml with *methanol R*.

Reference solution. Dissolve 5 mg of *hydrastine hydrochloride R* and 5 mg of *berberine chloride R* in 20 ml of *methanol R*.

Plate: *TLC silica gel plate R*.

Mobile phase: *anhydrous formic acid R, water R, ethyl acetate R* (10:10:80 *V/V/V*).

Application: 20 µl, as bands.

Development: over a path of 15 cm.

Drying: in air.

Detection: examine in ultraviolet light at 365 nm.

Results: see below the sequence of zones present in the chromatograms obtained with the reference solution and the test solution. Furthermore, other fluorescent zones may be present in the chromatogram obtained with the test solution.

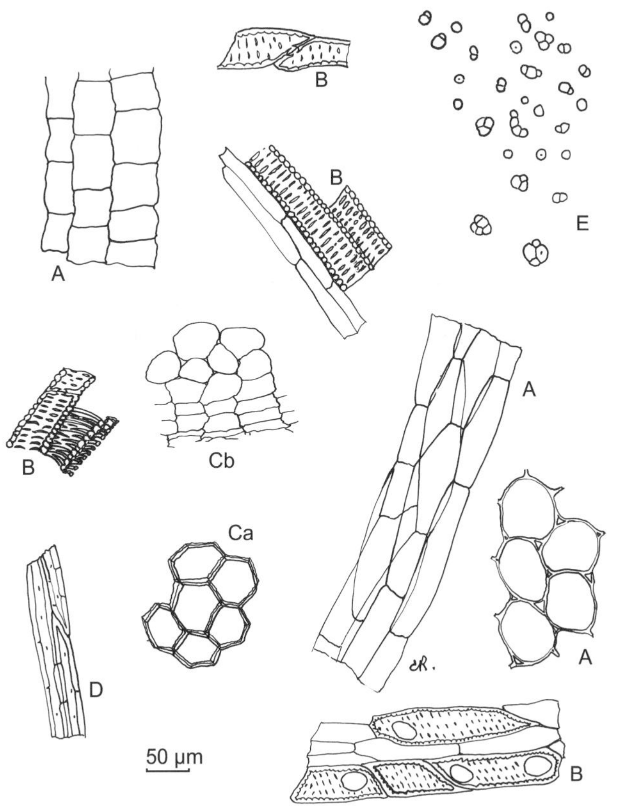

A. Thin-walled parenchyma cells
B. Vessels
C. Fragment of cork from the rhizome and roots in surface view (Ca) and in side view (Cb)
D. Pitted fibres
E. Starch granules

Figure 1831.-1. – *Illustration of powdered herbal drug of goldenseal rhizome (see Identification B)*

Top of the plate	
_______	_______
Berberine: a bright yellow fluorescent zone	A bright yellow fluorescent zone (berberine)
Hydrastine: a deep blue fluorescent zone	A deep blue fluorescent zone (hydrastine)
_______	_______
	A bright light blue fluorescent zone (hydrastinine)
	A deep blue fluorescent zone
Reference solution	**Test solution**

TESTS

Loss on drying (*2.2.32*): maximum 10.0 per cent, determined on 1.000 g of the powdered drug (180) (*2.9.12*) by drying in an oven at 105 °C for 2 h.

Total ash (*2.4.16*): maximum 8.0 per cent.

Ash insoluble in hydrochloric acid (*2.8.1*): maximum 4.0 per cent.

ASSAY

Liquid chromatography (*2.2.29*).

Test solution. To 1.000 g of the powdered drug (355) (*2.9.12*) in a 100 ml round-bottomed flask, add 50 ml of a 1 per cent *V/V* solution of *concentrated ammonia R* in *ethanol (96 per cent) R* and boil the mixture under a reflux condenser for 30 min. Allow to cool to room temperature and filter the liquid through a plug of absorbent cotton into a flask. Add the plug of absorbent cotton to the residue in

Monographs D-K

the round-bottomed flask and repeat the extraction with a further 2 quantities, each of 30 ml, of a 1 per cent *V/V* solution of *concentrated ammonia R* in *ethanol (96 per cent) R*, each time boiling under a reflux condenser for 10 min and filtering through a plug of absorbent cotton in the same flask as previously. Filter the combined filtrates through a filter paper into a 250 ml round-bottomed flask, and rinse flask and filter with 20 ml of a 1 per cent *V/V* solution of *concentrated ammonia R* in *ethanol (96 per cent) R*. Evaporate the filtrate to dryness *in vacuo* in a water-bath at 55 °C. Dissolve the residue in 50.0 ml of the mobile phase. Dilute 10.0 ml of this solution to 250.0 ml with the mobile phase.

Reference solution. Dissolve 10 mg of *hydrastine hydrochloride R* and 10 mg of *berberine chloride R* in *methanol R* and dilute to 100.0 ml with the same solvent.

Column:

– *size*: *l* = 0.125 m, Ø = 4 mm;
– *stationary phase*: *end-capped octadecylsilyl silica gel for chromatography R* (5 μm).

Mobile phase: dissolve 9.93 g of *potassium dihydrogen phosphate R* in 730 ml of *water R*, add 270 ml of *acetonitrile R* and mix.

Flow rate: 1.2 ml/min.

Detection: spectrophotometer at 235 nm.

Injection: 10 μl.

System suitability: reference solution:

– *elution order*: order indicated in the composition of the reference solution; record the retention times of these substances;
– *resolution*: minimum 1.5 between the peaks due to hydrastine and berberine.

Using the retention times determined from the chromatogram obtained with the reference solution, locate in the chromatogram obtained with the test solution the components of the reference solution.

Calculate the percentage content of each alkaloid (hydrastine and berberine) using the following expression:

$$\frac{A_1 \times m_2 \times p}{A_2 \times m_1} \times 12.5$$

A_1 = area of the peak due to hydrastine or berberine in the chromatogram obtained with the test solution;

A_2 = area of the peak due to hydrastine or berberine in the chromatogram obtained with the reference solution;

m_1 = mass of the drug to be examined, in grams;

m_2 = mass of hydrastine hydrochloride or berberine chloride in the reference solution, in grams;

p = percentage content of hydrastine in *hydrastine hydrochloride R* or berberine in *berberine chloride R*.

Monographs D-K

H

04/2008:0909

HAMAMELIS LEAF

Hamamelidis folium

DEFINITION

Whole or cut, dried leaf of *Hamamelis virginiana* L.

Content: minimum 3 per cent of tannins, expressed as pyrogallol ($C_6H_6O_3$; M_r 126.1) (dried drug).

IDENTIFICATION

A. The leaf is green or greenish-brown, often broken, crumpled and compressed into more or less compact masses. The lamina is broadly ovate or obovate; the base is oblique and asymmetric and the apex is acute or, rarely, obtuse. The margins of the lamina are roughly crenate or dentate. The venation is pinnate and prominent on the abaxial surface. Usually, 4-6 pairs of secondary veins are attached to the main vein, emerging at an acute angle and curving gently to the marginal points where there are fine veins often at right angles to the secondary veins.

B. Reduce to a powder (355) (*2.9.12*). The powder is brownish-green. Examine under a microscope using *chloral hydrate solution R*. The powder shows the following diagnostic characters: fragments of adaxial epidermis with wavy anticlinal walls; abaxial epidermis with stomata mainly paracytic (*2.8.3*); star-shaped covering trichomes, either entire or broken, composed of 4-12 unicellular branches that are united by their bases, elongated, conical and curved, usually up to 250 µm long, thick-walled and with a clearly visible lumen whose contents are often brown; fibres are lignified and thick-walled, isolated or in groups, and accompanied by a sheath of prismatic calcium oxalate crystals; small, cylindrical parenchymatous cells of palisade; irregular-shaped cells of spongy mesophyll; sclereids, frequently enlarged at 1 or both ends, 150-180 µm long, whole or fragmented; fragments of annular or spiral vessels; isolated prisms of calcium oxalate.

C. Thin-layer chromatography (*2.2.27*).

Test solution. To 1.0 g of the powdered drug (355) (*2.9.12*) add 10 ml of *ethanol (60 per cent V/V) R*, shake for 15 min and filter.

Reference solution (a). Dissolve 30 mg of *tannic acid R* in 5 ml of *ethanol (60 per cent V/V) R*.

Reference solution (b). Dissolve 5 mg of *gallic acid R* in 5 ml of *ethanol (60 per cent V/V) R*.

Plate: *TLC silica gel G plate R*.

Mobile phase: *anhydrous formic acid R, water R, ethyl formate R* (10:10:80 *V/V/V*).

Application: 10 µl, as bands.

Development: over a path of 10 cm.

Drying: at 100-105 °C for 10 min, then allow to cool.

Detection: spray with *ferric chloride solution R2* until bluish-grey zones (phenolic compounds) appear.

Results: the chromatogram obtained with the test solution shows in its lower third a principal zone similar in position to the principal zone in the chromatogram obtained with reference solution (a) and, in its upper part, a narrow zone similar in position to the principal zone in the chromatogram obtained with reference solution (b). The chromatogram obtained with the test solution shows, in addition, several slightly coloured zones in the central part.

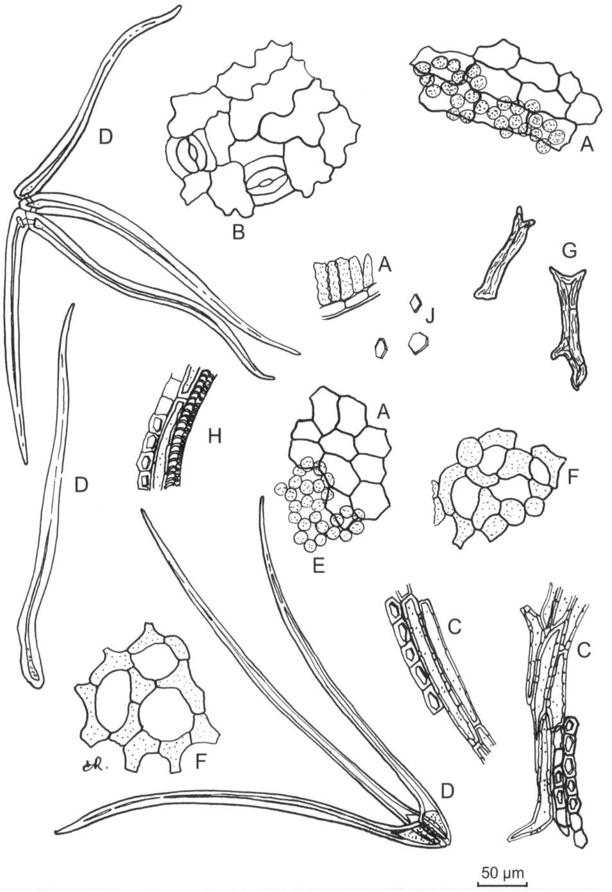

A. Adaxial epidermis and palisade parenchyma

B. Abaxial epidermis

C. Lignified fibres with sheath of prismatic calcium oxalate crystals

D. Star-shaped covering trichomes and free covering trichome

E. Palisade parenchyma

F. Spongy mesophyll

G. Sclereid

H. Vessels accompanied by fibres and by sheaths made up of calcium oxalate tubes

J. Isolated prisms of calcium oxalate

Figure 0909.-1. – *Illustration of powdered herbal drug of hamamelis leaf (see Identification B)*

TESTS

Foreign matter (*2.8.2*): maximum 7 per cent of stems and maximum 2 per cent of other foreign matter, determined on 50 g.

Loss on drying (*2.2.32*): maximum 10.0 per cent, determined on 2.000 g of powdered drug (355) (*2.9.12*) by drying in an oven at 105 °C for 4 h.

Total ash (*2.4.16*): maximum 7.0 per cent.

Ash insoluble in hydrochloric acid (*2.8.1*): maximum 2.0 per cent.

ASSAY

Carry out the determination of tannins in herbal drugs (*2.8.14*). Use 0.750 g of the powdered drug (180) (*2.9.12*).

04/2008:1222

HOP STROBILE

Lupuli flos

DEFINITION

Dried, generally whole, female inflorescence of *Humulus lupulus* L.

CHARACTERS

Characteristic, aromatic odour.

IDENTIFICATION

A. Hop strobiles are generally isolated and 2-5 cm long, petiolate, ovoid, made up of many oval, greenish-yellow, sessile, membranous, overlapping bracts. The external bracts are flattened and symmetrical. The internal bracts are longer and asymmetrical at the base because of a fold generally encircling an induviate fruit (achene). The ovary or rarely the fruit, the base of the bracts and especially the induvial fold, are covered with small orange-yellow glands.

B. Reduce to a powder (355) (*2.9.12*). The powder is greenish-yellow. Examine under a microscope using *chloral hydrate solution R*. The powder shows the following diagnostic characters: fragments of bracts and bracteoles covered by polygonal, irregular epidermal cells with wavy walls; unicellular, conical, straight or curved covering trichomes with thin, smooth walls; rare anomocytic stomata (*2.8.3*); glandular trichomes, usually free, with bicellular biseriate stalks and heads consisting of 8 small cells; fragments of mesophyll containing small calcium oxalate cluster crystals; many characteristic orange-yellow glandular trichomes with short, bicellular biseriate stalks, bearing a part widening into a cup, 150-250 μm in diameter, made up of a hemispherical layer of secretory cells with a cuticle that has been detached and distended by the accumulation of oleoresinous secretions; fragments of elongated sclerenchymatous cells of the testa with thick walls showing striations and numerous pits.

C. Thin-layer chromatography (*2.2.27*).

Test solution. To 1.0 g of the freshly powdered drug (355) (*2.9.12*) add 10 ml of a mixture of 3 volumes of *water R* and 7 volumes of *methanol R*; shake for 15 min and filter.

Reference solution. Dissolve 1.0 mg of *Sudan orange R*, 2.0 mg of *curcumin R* and 2.0 mg of *dimethylaminobenzaldehyde R* in 20 ml of *methanol R*.

Plate: *TLC silica gel F_{254} plate R.*

Mobile phase: *anhydrous acetic acid R, ethyl acetate R, cyclohexane R* (2:38:60 *V/V/V*).

Application: 20 μl, as bands.

Development: over a path of 15 cm.

Drying: in air.

Detection A: examine in ultraviolet light at 254 nm.

Results A: the chromatogram obtained with the reference solution shows 3 quenching zones; in the lower quarter is the faint zone due to curcumin, somewhat below the middle is the zone due to dimethylaminobenzaldehyde and above the zone due to Sudan orange. The chromatogram obtained with the test solution shows a number of quenching zones similar in position to the zones in the chromatogram obtained with the reference solution: at about the level of the zone due to curcumin is a faint zone due to xanthohumol, near the level of the zone due to dimethylaminobenzaldehyde are zones due to humulones, and near the level of the zone due to Sudan orange are zones due to lupulones.

Detection B: examine in ultraviolet light at 365 nm.

Results B: in the chromatogram obtained with the test solution the zones due to lupulones show blue fluorescence, the zones due to humulones show brown fluorescence and the zone due to xanthohumol shows dark brown fluorescence.

Detection C: spray with *dilute phosphomolybdotungstic reagent R*; expose to ammonia vapour and examine in daylight.

Results C: in the chromatogram obtained with the test solution, the zones due to humulones and to lupulones are bluish-grey and the zone due to xanthohumol is greenish-grey. In the chromatogram obtained with the reference solution, the zones are bluish-grey or brownish-grey.

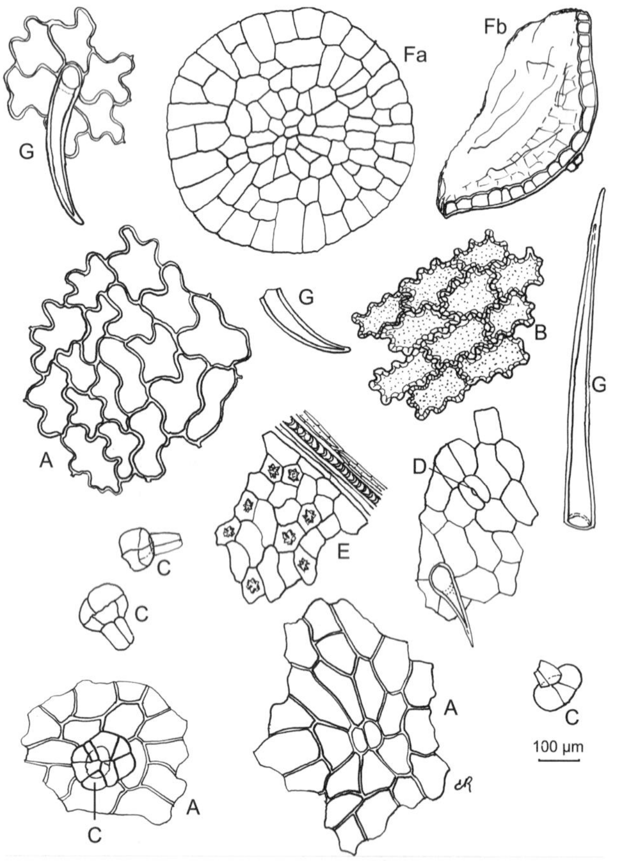

A. Epidermis of bracts and bracteoles

B. Sclerenchymatous cells of the testa

C. Multicellular glandular trichome

D. Anomocytic stoma

E. Mesophyll containing calcium oxalate cluster crystals and vessels

F. Glandular trichome in surface view (Fa) and in side view (Fb)

G. Covering trichome

Figure 1222.-1. – *Illustration of powdered herbal drug of hop strobile (see Identification B)*

TESTS

Matter extractable by ethanol (70 per cent *V/V*): minimum 25.0 per cent.

To 10.0 g of the powdered drug (355) (*2.9.12*) add 300 ml of *ethanol (70 per cent V/V) R* and heat for 10 min on a water bath under a reflux condenser. Allow to cool, filter and discard the first 10 ml of the filtrate. Evaporate 30.0 ml of the filtrate to dryness on a water-bath and dry in an oven at 100-105 °C for 2 h. The residue weighs a minimum of 0.250 g.

Loss on drying (*2.2.32*): maximum 10.0 per cent, determined on 1.000 g of the powdered drug (355) (*2.9.12*) by drying in an oven at 105 °C for 2 h.

Total ash (*2.4.16*): maximum 12.0 per cent.

01/2008:0348
corrected 6.1

HYPROMELLOSE

Hypromellosum

[9004-65-3]

DEFINITION

Hydroxypropylmethylcellulose.

Partly *O*-methylated and *O*-(2-hydroxypropylated) cellulose.

CHARACTERS

Appearance: white, yellowish-white or greyish-white powder or granules, hygroscopic after drying.

Solubility: practically insoluble in hot water, in acetone, in anhydrous ethanol and in toluene. It dissolves in cold water giving a colloidal solution.

IDENTIFICATION

A. Evenly distribute 1.0 g on the surface of 100 ml of *water R* in a beaker, tapping the top of the beaker, gently if necessary to ensure a uniform layer on the surface. Allow to stand for 1-2 min: the powdered material aggregates on the surface.

B. Evenly distribute 1.0 g into 100 ml of boiling *water R*, and stir the mixture using a magnetic stirrer with a bar 25 mm long: a slurry is formed and the particles do not dissolve. Allow the slurry to cool to 10 °C and stir using a magnetic stirrer: a clear or slightly turbid solution occurs with its thickness dependent on the viscosity grade.

C. To 0.1 ml of the solution obtained in identification B add 9 ml of a 90 per cent *V/V* solution of *sulphuric acid R*, shake, heat on a water-bath for exactly 3 min, immediately cool in an ice-bath, carefully add 0.6 ml of a 20 g/l solution of *ninhydrin R*, shake and allow to stand at 25 °C: a red colour develops at first and changes to purple within 100 min.

D. Place 2-3 ml of the solution obtained in identification B onto a glass slide as a thin film and allow the water to evaporate: a coherent, clear film forms on the glass slide.

E. Add exactly 50 ml of the solution obtained in identification B to exactly 50 ml of *water R* in a beaker. Insert a thermometer into the solution. Stir the solution on a magnetic stirrer/hot plate and begin heating, increasing the temperature at a rate of 2-5 °C per minute. Determine the temperature at which a turbidity increase begins to occur and designate the temperature as the flocculation temperature: the flocculation temperature is higher than 50 °C.

TESTS

Solution S. While stirring, introduce a quantity of the substance to be examined equivalent to 1.0 g of the dried substance into 50 g of *carbon dioxide-free water R* heated to 90 °C. Allow to cool, adjust the mass of the solution to 100 g with *carbon dioxide-free water R* and stir until dissolution is complete.

Appearance of solution. Solution S is not more opalescent than reference suspension III (*2.2.1*) and not more intensely coloured than reference solution Y_6 (*2.2.2, Method II*).

pH (*2.2.3*): 5.0 to 8.0 for the solution prepared as described under Apparent viscosity.

Carry out the test at 20 ± 2 °C and read the indicated pH value after the probe has been immersed for 5 ± 0.5 min.

Heavy metals (*2.4.8*): maximum 20 ppm.

1.0 g complies with test F. Prepare the reference solution using 2 ml of *lead standard solution (10 ppm Pb) R*.

Loss on drying (*2.2.32*): maximum 5.0 per cent, determined on 1.000 g by drying in an oven at 105 °C for 1 h.

Sulphated ash (*2.4.14*): maximum 1.5 per cent, determined on 1.0 g.

FUNCTIONALITY-RELATED CHARACTERISTICS

This section provides information on characteristics that are recognised as being relevant control parameters for one or more functions of the substance when used as an excipient. This section is a non-mandatory part of the monograph and it is not necessary to verify the characteristics to demonstrate compliance. Control of these characteristics can however contribute to the quality of a medicinal product by improving the consistency of the manufacturing process and the performance of the medicinal product during use. Where control methods are cited, they are recognised as being suitable for the purpose, but other methods can also be used. Wherever results for a particular characteristic are reported, the control method must be indicated.

The following characteristics may be relevant for hypromellose used as binder, viscosity-increasing agent or film former.

Apparent viscosity: minimum 80 per cent and maximum 120 per cent of the nominal value for samples with a viscosity less than 600 mPa·s (Method 1); minimum 75 per cent and maximum 140 per cent of the nominal value for samples with a viscosity of 600 mPa·s or higher (Method 2).

Method 1, to be applied to samples with a viscosity of less than 600 mPa·s. Weigh accurately a quantity of the substance to be examined equivalent to 4.000 g of the dried substance. Transfer into a wide-mouthed bottle, and adjust the mass to 200.0 g with hot *water R*. Capping the bottle, stir by mechanical means at 400 ± 50 r/min for 10-20 min until the particles are thoroughly dispersed and wetted. Scrape down the insides of the bottle with a spatula if necessary, to ensure that there is no undissolved material on the sides of the bottle, and continue the stirring in a cooling water-bath maintained at a temperature below 10 °C for another 20-40 min. Adjust the solution mass if necessary to 200.0 g using cold *water R*. Centrifuge the solution if necessary to expel any entrapped air bubbles. Using a spatula, remove any foam, if present. Determine the viscosity of this solution using the capillary viscometer method (*2.2.9*) to obtain the kinematic viscosity (ν). Separately, determine the density (ρ) (*2.2.5*) of the solution and calculate the dynamic viscosity (η), as $\eta = \rho\nu$.

Method 2, to be applied to samples with a viscosity of 600 mPa·s or higher. Weigh accurately a quantity of the substance to be examined equivalent to 10.00 g of the dried substance. Transfer into a wide-mouthed bottle, and adjust

Monographs D-K

the mass to 500.0 g with hot *water R*. Capping the bottle, stir by mechanical means at 400 ± 50 r/min for 10-20 min until the particles are thoroughly dispersed and wetted. Scrape down the insides of the bottle with a spatula if necessary, to ensure that there is no undissolved material on the sides of the bottle, and continue the stirring in a cooling water-bath maintained at a temperature below 10 °C for another 20-40 min. Adjust the solution mass if necessary to 500.0 g using cold *water R*. Centrifuge the solution if necessary to expel any entrapped air bubbles. Using a spatula, remove any foam, if present. Determine the viscosity (*2.2.10*) of this solution at 20 ± 0.1 °C using a rotating viscometer.

Apparatus: single-cylinder type spindle viscometer.

Rotor number, revolution and calculation multiplier: apply the conditions specified in Table 0348.-1.

Allow the spindle to rotate for 2 min before taking the measurement. Allow a rest period of 2 min between subsequent measurements. Repeat the measurement twice and determine the mean of the 3 readings.

Table 0348.-1.

Labelled viscosity* (mPa·s)	Rotor number	Revolution (r/min)	Calculation multiplier
600 to less than 1400	3	60	20
1400 to less than 3500	3	12	100
3500 to less than 9500	4	60	100
9500 to less than 99 500	4	6	1000
99 500 or more	4	3	2000

* the nominal viscosity is based on the manufacturer's specifications.

Degree of substitution. Gas chromatography (*2.2.28*).

Apparatus:

- *reaction vial*: a 5 ml pressure-tight vial, 50 mm in height, 20 mm in external diameter and 13 mm in internal diameter at the mouth, equipped with a pressure-tight butyl rubber membrane stopper coated with polytetrafluoroethylene and secured with an aluminium crimped cap or another sealing system providing a sufficient air-tightness;
- *heater*: a heating module with a square aluminium block having holes 20 mm in diameter and 32 mm in depth, so that the reaction vials fit; mixing of the contents of the vial is effected using a magnetic stirrer equipped in the heating module or using a reciprocal shaker that performs approximately 100 cycles/min.

Internal standard solution: 30 g/l solution of *octane R* in *xylene R*.

Test solution. Weigh 65.0 mg of the substance to be examined, place in a reaction vial, add 0.06-0.10 g of *adipic acid R*, 2.0 ml of the internal standard solution and 2.0 ml of a 570 g/l solution of *hydriodic acid R*, immediately cap and seal the vial, and weigh accurately. Mix the contents of the vial continuously for 60 min while heating the block so that the temperature of the contents is maintained at 130 ± 2 °C. If a reciprocal shaker or magnetic stirrer cannot be used, shake the vial well by hand at 5-minute intervals during the initial 30 min of the heating time. Allow the vial to cool, and again weigh accurately. If the loss of mass is less than 0.50 per cent of the contents and there is no evidence of a leak, use the upper layer of the mixture as the test solution.

Reference solution. Place 0.06-0.10 g of *adipic acid R*, 2.0 ml of the internal standard solution and 2.0 ml of *hydroiodic acid R* in another reaction vial, cap and seal the vial, and weigh accurately. Add 15-22 µl of *isopropyl iodide R* through the septum with a syringe, weigh accurately, add 45 µl of *methyl iodide R* in the same manner, and weigh accurately. Shake the reaction vial well, and use the upper layer as the reference solution.

Column:

- *size*: l = 1.8-3 m, Ø = 3-4 mm;
- *stationary phase*: *diatomaceous earth for gas chromatography R* impregnated with 10-20 per cent of *poly(dimethyl)(75)(diphenyl)(25)siloxane R* (film thickness 125-150 µm);
- *temperature*: 100 °C.

Carrier gas: *helium for chromatography R* (thermal conductivity); *helium for chromatography R* or *nitrogen for chromatography R* (flame ionisation).

Flow rate: adjusted so that the retention time of the internal standard is about 10 min.

Detection: flame ionisation or thermal conductivity.

Injection: 1-2 µl.

System suitability: reference solution:

- *resolution*: well resolved peaks of methyl iodide (1st peak), isopropyl iodide (2nd peak) and internal standard (3rd peak).

Calculation:

- *methoxy and hydroxypropoxy groups*: calculate the ratios (Q_1 and Q_2) of the areas of the peaks due to methyl iodide and isopropyl iodide to the area of the peak due to the internal standard in the chromatogram obtained with the test solution, and the ratios (Q_3 and Q_4) of the areas of the peaks due to methyl iodide and isopropyl iodide to the area of the peak due to the internal standard in the chromatogram obtained with the reference solution.

Calculate the percentage content of methoxy groups using the following expression:

$$\frac{Q_1}{Q_3} \times \frac{m_1}{m} \times 21.864$$

Calculate the percentage content of hydroxypropoxy groups using the following expression:

$$\frac{Q_2}{Q_4} \times \frac{m_2}{m} \times 44.17$$

m_1 = mass of methyl iodide in the reference solution, in milligrams;

m_2 = mass of isopropyl iodide in the reference solution, in milligrams;

m = mass of the sample (dried substance), in milligrams.

Substitution type	Methoxy (per cent)	Hydroxypropoxy (per cent)
1828	16.5 to 20.0	23.0 to 32.0
2208	19.0 to 24.0	4.0 to 12.0
2906	27.0 to 30.0	4.0 to 7.5
2910	28.0 to 30.0	7.0 to 12.0

Monographs D-K

The following characteristics may be relevant for hypromellose used as matrix former in prolonged-release tablets.

Apparent viscosity: see test above.

Degree of substitution: see test above.

Molecular mass distribution (*2.2.30*).

Particle-size distribution (*2.9.31* or *2.9.38*).

Powder flow (*2.9.36*).

04/2008:0347

HYPROMELLOSE PHTHALATE

Hypromellosi phthalas

DEFINITION

Hydroxypropylmethylcellulose phtalate.

Monophthalic acid ester of hypromellose, containing methoxy (-OCH_3), 2-hydroxypropoxy (-$OCH_2CHOHCH_3$) and phthaloyl (*o*-carboxybenzoyl $C_8H_5O_3$) groups.

CHARACTERS

Appearance: white or almost white, free-flowing flakes or granular powder.

Solubility: practically insoluble in water, soluble in a mixture of equal volumes of acetone and methanol and in a mixture of equal volumes of methanol and methylene chloride, very slightly soluble in acetone and in toluene, practically insoluble in anhydrous ethanol.

IDENTIFICATION

Infrared absorption spectrophotometry (*2.2.24*).

Comparison: *hypromellose phthalate CRS*.

TESTS

Free phthalic acid. Liquid chromatography (*2.2.29*).

Test solution. Dissolve 0.20 g of the substance to be examined in about 50 ml of *acetonitrile R* with the aid of ultrasound. Add 10 ml of *water R*, cool to room temperature, dilute to 100.0 ml with *acetonitrile R* and mix.

Reference solution. Dissolve 12.5 mg of *phthalic acid R* in 125 ml of *acetonitrile R*. Add 25 ml of *water R*, dilute to 250.0 ml with *acetonitrile R* and mix.

Column:

- *size*: *l* = 0.25 m, Ø = 4.6 mm;
- *stationary phase*: *octadecylsilyl silica gel for chromatography R* (5-10 µm).

Mobile phase: *acetonitrile R*, 1 g/l solution of *trifluoroacetic acid R* (1:9 *V/V*).

Flow rate: 2.0 ml/min.

Detection: spectrophotometer at 235 nm.

Injection: 10 µl.

System suitability: reference solution:

- *repeatability*: maximum relative standard deviation of 1.0 per cent after 2 injections.

Limit:

- *phthalic acid*: not more than 0.4 times the area of the corresponding peak in the chromatogram obtained with the reference solution (1.0 per cent).

Chlorides: maximum 0.07 per cent.

Dissolve 1.0 g in 40 ml of *0.2 M sodium hydroxide*, add 0.05 ml of *phenolphthalein solution R* and add *dilute nitric acid R* dropwise, with stirring, until the red colour disappears. Add an additional 20 ml of *dilute nitric acid R* with stirring. Heat on a water-bath with stirring until the gel-like precipitate formed becomes granular. Cool and centrifuge. Separate the liquid phase and wash the residue with 3 quantities, each of 20 ml, of *water R*, separating the washings by centrifugation. Combine the liquid phases, dilute to 200 ml with *water R*, mix and filter. To 50 ml of this solution, add 1 ml of *0.1 M silver nitrate*. The solution is not more opalescent than a standard prepared by mixing 0.5 ml of *0.01 M hydrochloric acid* with 10 ml of *0.2 M sodium hydroxide*, adding 7 ml of *dilute nitric acid R* and 1 ml of *0.1 M silver nitrate*, and diluting to 50 ml with *water R*.

Heavy metals (*2.4.8*): maximum 10 ppm.

2.0 g complies with test C. Prepare the reference solution using 2 ml of *lead standard solution (10 ppm Pb) R*.

Water (*2.5.12*): maximum 5.0 per cent, determined on 0.500 g.

Sulphated ash (*2.4.14*): maximum 0.2 per cent, determined on 1.0 g.

STORAGE

In an airtight container.

FUNCTIONALITY-RELATED CHARACTERISTICS

This section provides information on characteristics that are recognised as being relevant control parameters for one or more functions of the substance when used as an excipient. This section is a non-mandatory part of the monograph and it is not necessary to verify the characteristics to demonstrate compliance. Control of these characteristics can however contribute to the quality of a medicinal product by improving the consistency of the manufacturing process and the performance of the medicinal product during use. Where control methods are cited, they are recognised as being suitable for the purpose, but other methods can also be used. Wherever results for a particular characteristic are reported, the control method must be indicated.

The following characteristics may be relevant for hypromellose phthalate used as a gastro-resistant coating agent.

Apparent viscosity (*2.2.9*): 80 per cent to 120 per cent of the nominal value.

Dissolve 10 g, previously dried at 105 °C for 1 h, in 90 g of a mixture of equal masses of *methanol R* and *methylene chloride R* by mixing and shaking.

Solubility. 0.2 g does not dissolve in *0.1 M hydrochloric acid* but dissolves quickly and completely in 100 ml of *phosphate buffer solution pH 6.8 R* with stirring.

Phthaloyl groups: typically 21.0 per cent to 35.0 per cent (anhydrous substance).

Dissolve 1.000 g in 50 ml of a mixture of 1 volume of *water R*, 2 volumes of *acetone R* and 2 volumes of *ethanol (96 per cent) R*. Add 0.1 ml of *phenolphthalein solution R* and titrate with *0.1 M sodium hydroxide* until a faint pink colour is obtained. Carry out a blank titration.

Calculate the percentage content of phthaloyl groups using the following expression:

$$\frac{149n}{(100 - a)\,m} - 1.795S$$

a = percentage content of water;

m = mass of the substance to be examined, in grams;

n = volume of *0.1 M sodium hydroxide* used, in millilitres;

S = percentage content of free phthalic acid (see Tests).

I

04/2008:0721

IBUPROFEN

Ibuprofenum

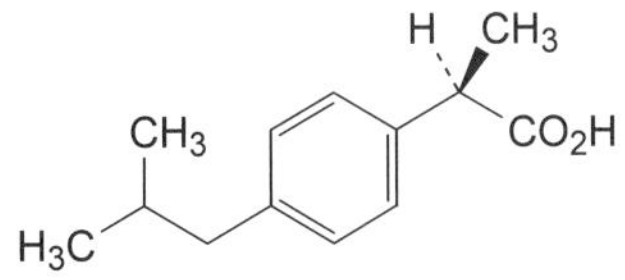

and enantiomer

$C_{13}H_{18}O_2$ M_r 206.3
[15687-27-1]

DEFINITION

(2*RS*)-2-[4-(2-Methylpropyl)phenyl]propanoic acid.

Content: 98.5 per cent to 101.0 per cent (dried substance).

CHARACTERS

Appearance: white or almost white, crystalline powder or colourless crystals.

Solubility: practically insoluble in water, freely soluble in acetone, in methanol and in methylene chloride. It dissolves in dilute solutions of alkali hydroxides and carbonates.

IDENTIFICATION

First identification: A, C.

Second identification: A, B, D.

A. Melting point (*2.2.14*): 75 °C to 78 °C.

B. Ultraviolet and visible absorption spectrophotometry (*2.2.25*).

Test solution. Dissolve 50.0 mg in a 4 g/l solution of *sodium hydroxide R* and dilute to 100.0 ml with the same alkaline solution.

Spectral range: 240-300 nm, using a spectrophotometer with a band width of 1.0 nm and a scan speed of not more than 50 nm/min.

Absorption maxima: at 264 nm and 272 nm.

Shoulder: at 258 nm.

Absorbance ratio:

– A_{264} / A_{258} = 1.20 to 1.30;

– A_{272} / A_{258} = 1.00 to 1.10.

C. Infrared absorption spectrophotometry (*2.2.24*).

Comparison: *ibuprofen CRS.*

D. Thin-layer chromatography (*2.2.27*).

Test solution. Dissolve 50 mg of the substance to be examined in *methylene chloride R* and dilute to 10 ml with the same solvent.

Reference solution. Dissolve 50 mg of *ibuprofen CRS* in *methylene chloride R* and dilute to 10 ml with the same solvent.

Plate: *TLC silica gel plate R.*

Mobile phase: *anhydrous acetic acid R, ethyl acetate R, hexane R* (5:24:71 *V/V/V*).

Application: 5 µl.

Development: over a path of 10 cm.

Drying: at 120 °C for 30 min.

Detection: lightly spray with a 10 g/l solution of *potassium permanganate R* in *dilute sulphuric acid R* and heat at 120 °C for 20 min; examine in ultraviolet light at 365 nm.

Results: the principal spot in the chromatogram obtained with the test solution is similar in position, colour and size to the principal spot in the chromatogram obtained with the reference solution.

TESTS

Solution S. Dissolve 2.0 g in *methanol R* and dilute to 20 ml with the same solvent.

Appearance of solution. Solution S is clear (*2.2.1*) and colourless (*2.2.2, Method II*).

Optical rotation (*2.2.7*): – 0.05° to + 0.05°.

Dissolve 0.50 g in *methanol R* and dilute to 20.0 ml with the same solvent.

Related substances. Liquid chromatography (*2.2.29*).

Test solution. Dissolve 20 mg of the substance to be examined in 2 ml of *acetonitrile R1* and dilute to 10.0 ml with mobile phase A.

Reference solution (a). Dilute 1.0 ml of the test solution to 100.0 ml with mobile phase A. Dilute 1.0 ml of this solution to 10.0 ml with mobile phase A.

Reference solution (b). Dilute 1.0 ml of *ibuprofen impurity B CRS* to 10.0 ml with *acetonitrile R1* (solution A). Dissolve 20 mg of *ibuprofen CRS* in 2 ml of *acetonitrile R1*, add 1.0 ml of solution A and dilute to 10.0 ml with mobile phase A.

Reference solution (c). Dissolve the contents of a vial of *ibuprofen for peak identification CRS* (mixture of impurities A, J and N) in 1 ml of *acetonitrile R1* and dilute to 5 ml with mobile phase A.

Column:

– *size*: l = 0.15 m, Ø = 4.6 mm;

– *stationary phase*: *octadecylsilyl silica gel for chromatography R* (5 µm).

Mobile phase:

– *mobile phase A*: mix 0.5 volumes of *phosphoric acid R*, 340 volumes of *acetonitrile R1* and 600 volumes of *water R*; allow to equilibrate and dilute to 1000 volumes with *water R*;

– *mobile phase B*: *acetonitrile R1*;

Time (min)	Mobile phase A (per cent *V/V*)	Mobile phase B (per cent *V/V*)
0 - 25	100	0
25 - 55	100 → 15	0 → 85
55 - 70	15	85

Flow rate: 2 ml/min.

Detection: spectrophotometer at 214 nm.

Injection: 20 µl.

Identification of impurities: use the chromatogram supplied with *ibuprofen for peak identification CRS* and the chromatogram obtained with reference solution (c) to identify the peaks due to impurities A, J and N.

Relative retention with reference to ibuprofen (retention time = about 16 min): impurity J = about 0.2; impurity N = about 0.3; impurity A = about 0.9; impurity B = about 1.1.

System suitability: reference solution (b):

– *peak-to-valley ratio*: minimum 1.5, where H_p = height above the baseline of the peak due to impurity B, and H_v = height above the baseline of the lowest point of the curve separating this peak from the peak due to ibuprofen. If necessary, adjust the concentration of acetonitrile in mobile phase A.

Limits:

- *impurities A, J, N*: for each impurity, not more than 1.5 times the area of the principal peak in the chromatogram obtained with reference solution (a) (0.15 per cent);
- *unspecified impurities*: for each impurity, not more than 0.5 times the area of the principal peak in the chromatogram obtained with reference solution (a) (0.05 per cent);
- *total*: not more than twice the area of the principal peak in the chromatogram obtained with reference solution (a) (0.2 per cent);
- *disregard limit*: 0.3 times the area of the principal peak in the chromatogram obtained with reference solution (a) (0.03 per cent).

Impurity F. Gas chromatography (*2.2.28*): use the normalisation procedure.

Methylating solution. Dilute 1 ml of *N,N-dimethylformamide dimethyl acetal R* and 1 ml of *pyridine R* to 10 ml with *ethyl acetate R*.

Test solution. Weigh about 50.0 mg of the substance to be examined into a sealable vial, dissolve in 1.0 ml of *ethyl acetate R*, add 1 ml of the methylating solution, seal and heat at 100 °C in a block heater for 20 min. Allow to cool. Remove the reagents under a stream of nitrogen at room temperature. Dissolve the residue in 5 ml of *ethyl acetate R*.

Reference solution (a). Dissolve 0.5 mg of *ibuprofen impurity F CRS* in *ethyl acetate R* and dilute to 10.0 ml with the same solvent.

Reference solution (b). Weigh about 50.0 mg of *ibuprofen CRS* into a sealable vial, dissolve in 1.0 ml of reference solution (a), add 1 ml of the methylating solution, seal and heat at 100 °C in a block heater for 20 min. Allow to cool. Remove the reagents under a stream of nitrogen at room temperature. Dissolve the residue in 5 ml of *ethyl acetate R*.

Column:

- *material*: fused silica;
- *size*: l = 25 m, Ø = 0.53 mm;
- *stationary phase*: *macrogol 20 000 R* (film thickness 2 µm).

Carrier gas: *helium for chromatography R*.

Flow rate: 5.0 ml/min.

Temperature:

- *column*: 150 °C;
- *injection port*: 200 °C;
- *detector*: 250 °C.

Detection: flame ionisation.

Injection: 1 µl of the test solution and reference solution (b).

Run time: twice the retention time of ibuprofen.

System suitability:

- *relative retention* with reference to ibuprofen (retention time = about 17 min): impurity F = about 1.5.

Limit:

- *impurity F*: maximum 0.1 per cent.

Heavy metals (*2.4.8*): maximum 10 ppm.

12 ml of solution S complies with test B. Prepare the reference solution using lead standard solution (1 ppm Pb) obtained by diluting *lead standard solution (100 ppm Pb) R* with *methanol R*.

Loss on drying (*2.2.32*): maximum 0.5 per cent, determined on 1.000 g by drying *in vacuo*.

Sulphated ash (*2.4.14*): maximum 0.1 per cent, determined on 1.0 g.

ASSAY

Dissolve 0.450 g in 50 ml of *methanol R*. Add 0.4 ml of *phenolphthalein solution R1*. Titrate with *0.1 M sodium hydroxide* until a red colour is obtained. Carry out a blank titration.

1 ml of *0.1 M sodium hydroxide* is equivalent to 20.63 mg of $C_{13}H_{18}O_2$.

IMPURITIES

Specified impurities: A, F, J, N.

Other detectable impurities (the following substances would, if present at a sufficient level, be detected by one or other of the tests in the monograph. They are limited by the general acceptance criterion for other/unspecified impurities and/or by the general monograph *Substances for pharmaceutical use (2034)*. It is therefore not necessary to identify these impurities for demonstration of compliance. See also *5.10. Control of impurities in substances for pharmaceutical use*): *B, C, D, E, G, H, I, K, L, M, O, P, Q, R.*

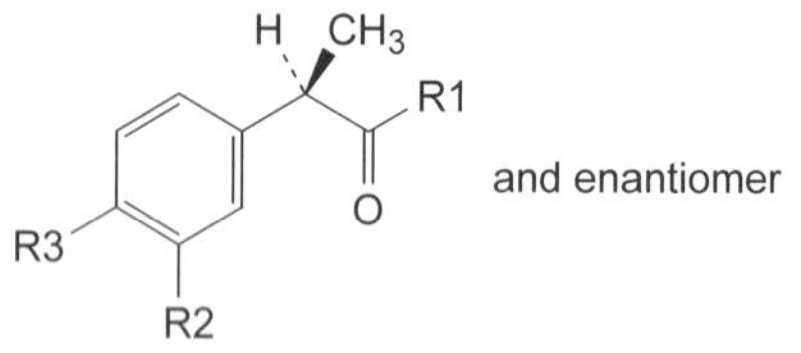

A. R1 = OH, R2 = CH_2-$CH(CH_3)_2$, R3 = H: (2*RS*)-2-[3-(2-methylpropyl)phenyl]propanoic acid,

B. R1 = OH, R2 = H, R3 = $[CH_2]_3$-CH_3: (2*RS*)-2-(4-butylphenyl)propanoic acid,

C. R1 = NH_2, R2 = H, R3 = CH_2-$CH(CH_3)_2$: (2*RS*)-2-[4-(2-methylpropyl)phenyl]propanamide,

D. R1 = OH, R2 = H, R3 = CH_3: (2*RS*)-2-(4-methylphenyl)propanoic acid,

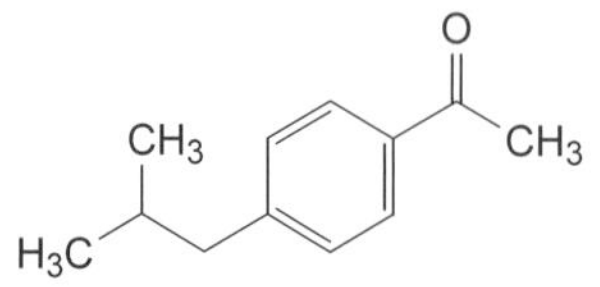

E. 1-[4-(2-methylpropyl)phenyl]ethanone,

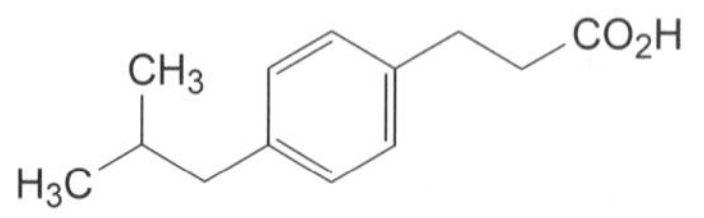

F. 3-[4-(2-methylpropyl)phenyl]propanoic acid,

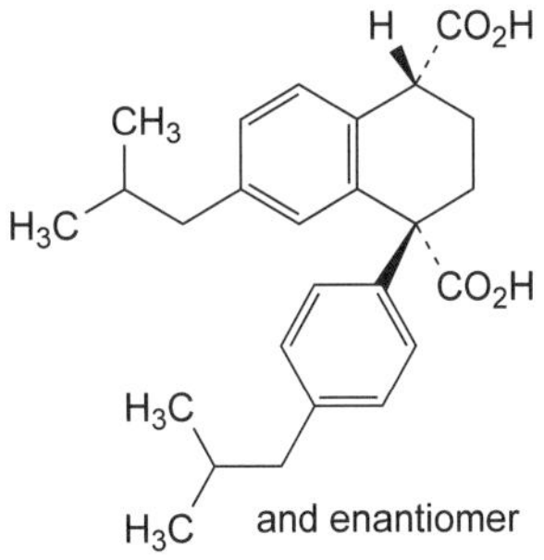

G. (1*RS*,4*RS*)-7-(2-methylpropyl)-1-[4-(2-methylpropyl)-phenyl]-1,2,3,4-tetrahydronaphthalene-1,4-dicarboxylic acid,

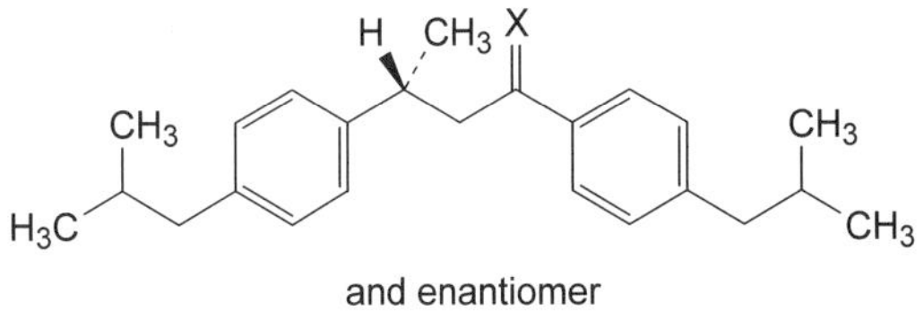

H. X = O : (3*RS*)-1,3-bis[4-(2-methylpropyl)phenyl]butan-1-one,

I. X = H_2 : 1-(2-methylpropyl)-4-[(3*RS*)-3-[4-(2-methylpropyl)-phenyl]butyl]benzene,

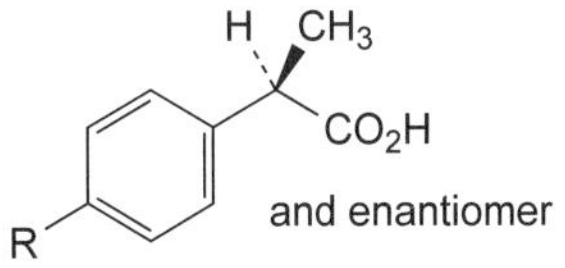

J. R = CO-CH$(CH_3)_2$: (2*RS*)-2-[4-(2-methylpropanoyl)-phenyl]propanoic acid,

N. R = C_2H_5 : (2*RS*)-2-(4-ethylphenyl)propanoic acid,

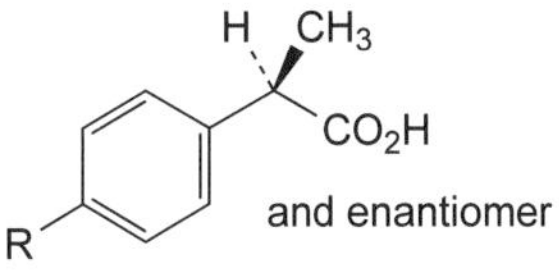

K. R = CHO : (2*RS*)-2-(4-formylphenyl)propanoic acid,

L. R = CHOH-CH$(CH_3)_2$: 2-[4-(1-hydroxy-2-methylpropyl)-phenyl]propanoic acid,

O. R = CH(CH_3)-C_2H_5 : 2-[4-(1-methylpropyl)phenyl]propanoic acid,

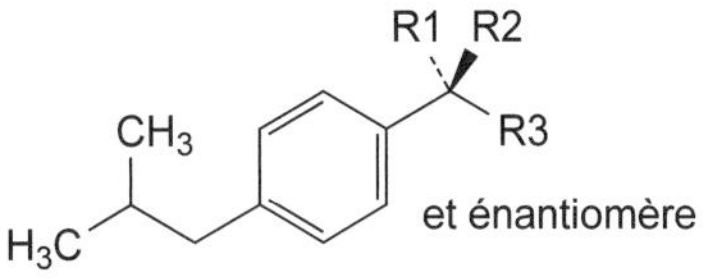

M. R1 = OH, R2 = CH_3, R3 = CO_2H : (2*RS*)-2-hydroxy-2-[4-(2-methylpropyl)phenyl]propanoic acid,

P. R1 = H, R2 = CH_3, R3 = CH_2OH : (2*RS*)-2-[4-(2-methylpropyl)phenyl]propan-1-ol,

Q. R1 = R2 = H, R3 = CH_2OH : 2-[4-(2-methylpropyl)-phenyl]ethanol,

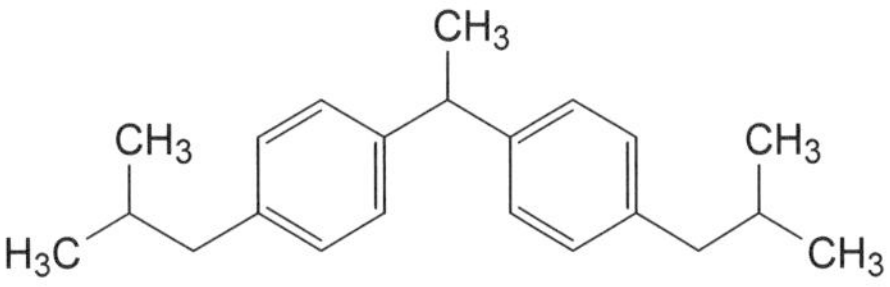

R. 1,1′-(ethane-1,1-diyl)-4,4′-(2-methylpropyl)dibenzene.

L

04/2008:0727

LIDOCAINE

Lidocainum

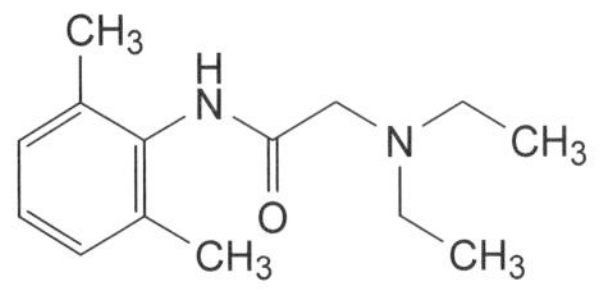

$C_{14}H_{22}N_2O$ M_r 234.3
[137-58-6]

DEFINITION

2-(Diethylamino)-*N*-(2,6-dimethylphenyl)acetamide.

Content: 99.0 per cent to 101.0 per cent (anhydrous substance).

CHARACTERS

Appearance: white or almost white, crystalline powder.

Solubility: practically insoluble in water, very soluble in ethanol (96 per cent) and in methylene chloride.

IDENTIFICATION

First identification: A.

Second identification: B, C.

A. Infrared absorption spectrophotometry (*2.2.24*).

Comparison: *lidocaine CRS.*

B. Melting point (*2.2.14*): 66 °C to 70 °C, determined without previous drying.

C. To about 5 mg add 0.5 ml of *fuming nitric acid R*. Evaporate to dryness on a water-bath, cool, and dissolve the residue in 5 ml of *acetone R*. Add 0.2 ml of *alcoholic potassium hydroxide solution R*. A green colour develops.

TESTS

Related substances. Liquid chromatography (*2.2.29*).

Test solution. Dissolve 50.0 mg of the substance to be examined in the mobile phase and dilute to 10.0 ml with the mobile phase.

Reference solution (a). Dissolve 50.0 mg of *2,6-dimethylaniline R* (impurity A) in the mobile phase and dilute to 100.0 ml with the mobile phase. Dilute 10.0 ml of this solution to 100.0 ml with the mobile phase.

Reference solution (b). Dissolve 5.0 mg of *2-chloro-N-(2,6-dimethylphenyl)acetamide R* (impurity H) in the mobile phase and dilute to 10.0 ml with the mobile phase.

Reference solution (c). Dilute 1.0 ml of the test solution to 10.0 ml with the mobile phase.

Reference solution (d). Mix 1.0 ml of reference solution (a), 1.0 ml of reference solution (b) and 1.0 ml of reference solution (c), then dilute to 100.0 ml with the mobile phase.

Column:

- *size*: l = 0.15 m, Ø = 3.9 mm;
- *stationary phase*: *end-capped polar-embedded octadecylsilyl amorphous organosilica polymer R* (5 µm);
- *temperature*: 30 °C.

Mobile phase: mix 30 volumes of *acetonitrile for chromatography R* and 70 volumes of a 4.85 g/l solution of *potassium dihydrogen phosphate R* previously adjusted to pH 8.0 with *strong sodium hydroxide solution R.*

Flow rate: 1.0 ml/min.

Detection: spectrophotometer at 230 nm.

Injection: 20 µl.

Run time: 3.5 times the retention time of lidocaine.

Relative retention with reference to lidocaine (retention time = about 17 min): impurity H = about 0.37; impurity A = about 0.40.

System suitability: reference solution (d):

- *resolution*: minimum 1.5 between the peaks due to impurities H and A.

Limits:

- *impurity A*: not more than the area of the corresponding peak in the chromatogram obtained with reference solution (d) (0.01 per cent);
- *unspecified impurities*: for each impurity, not more than the area of the peak due to lidocaine in the chromatogram obtained with reference solution (d) (0.10 per cent);
- *total*: not more than 5 times the area of the peak due to lidocaine in the chromatogram obtained with reference solution (d) (0.5 per cent);
- *disregard limit*: 0.5 times the area of the peak due to lidocaine in the chromatogram obtained with reference solution (d) (0.05 per cent).

Chlorides (*2.4.4*): maximum 35 ppm.

Dissolve 1.4 g in a mixture of 3 ml of *dilute nitric acid R* and 12 ml of *water R.*

Sulphates (*2.4.13*): maximum 0.1 per cent.

Dissolve 0.2 g in 5 ml of *ethanol (96 per cent) R* and dilute to 20 ml with *distilled water R.*

Water (*2.5.12*): maximum 1.0 per cent, determined on 1.00 g.

Sulphated ash (*2.4.14*): maximum 0.1 per cent, determined on 1.0 g.

ASSAY

To 0.200 g add 50 ml of *anhydrous acetic acid R* and stir until dissolution is complete. Titrate with *0.1 M perchloric acid,* determining the end-point potentiometrically (*2.2.20*).

1 ml of *0.1 M perchloric acid* is equivalent to 23.43 mg of $C_{14}H_{22}N_2O$.

IMPURITIES

Specified impurities: *A.*

Other detectable impurities (the following substances would, if present at a sufficient level, be detected by one or other of the tests in the monograph. They are limited by the general acceptance criterion for other/unspecified impurities and/or by the general monograph *Substances for pharmaceutical use (2034).* It is therefore not necessary to identify these impurities for demonstration of compliance. See also *5.10. Control of impurities in substances for pharmaceutical use*): *B, C, D, E, F, G, H, I, J.*

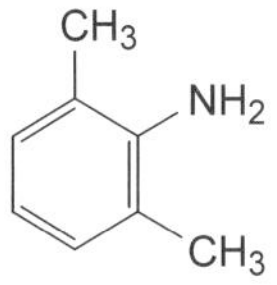

A. 2,6-dimethylaniline,

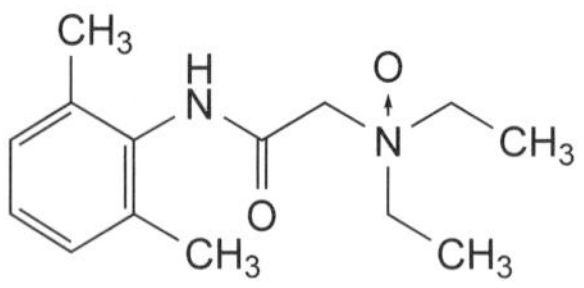

B. 2-(diethylazinoyl)-*N*-(2,6-dimethylphenyl)acetamide (lidocaine *N*-oxide),

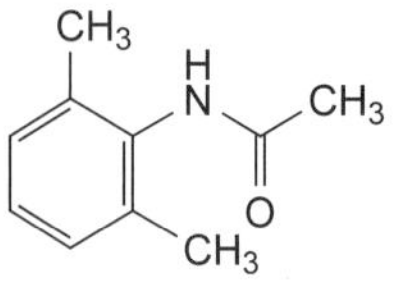

C. *N*-(2,6-dimethylphenyl)acetamide,

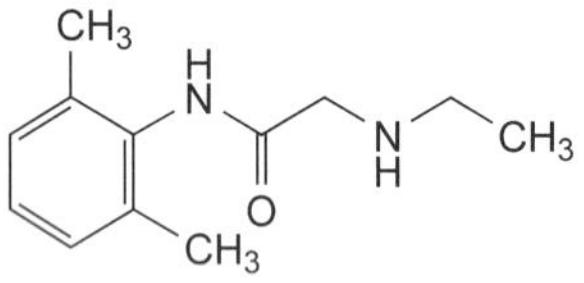

D. *N*-(2,6-dimethylphenyl)-2-(ethylamino)acetamide,

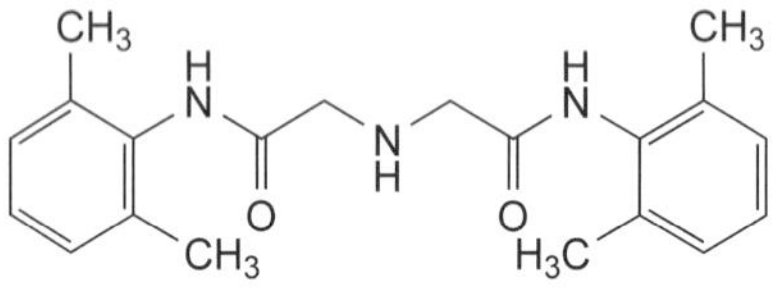

E. 2,2′-iminobis(*N*-(2,6-dimethylphenyl)acetamide),

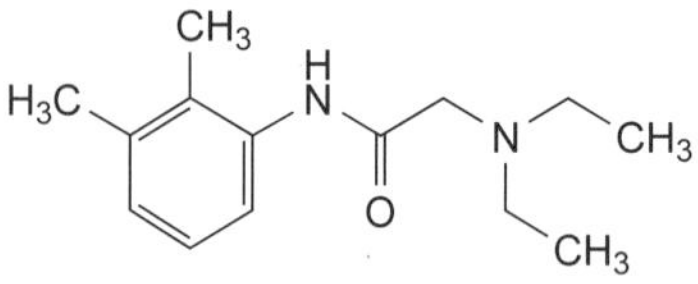

F. 2-(diethylamino)-*N*-(2,3-dimethylphenyl)acetamide,

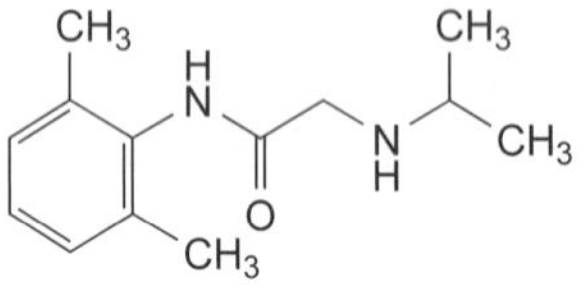

G. *N*-(2,6-dimethylphenyl)-2-((1-methylethyl)amino) acetamide,

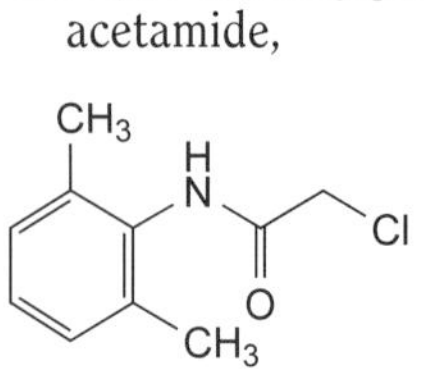

H. 2-chloro-*N*-(2,6-dimethylphenyl)acetamide,

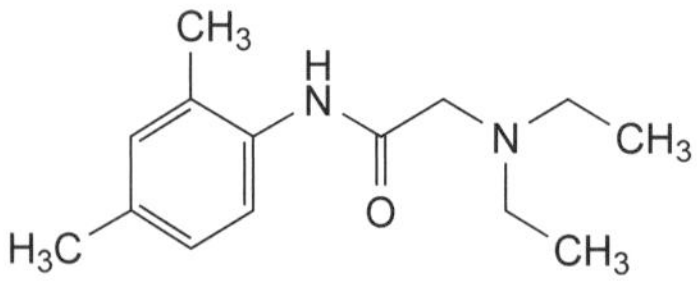

I. 2-(diethylamino)-*N*-(2,4-dimethylphenyl)acetamide,

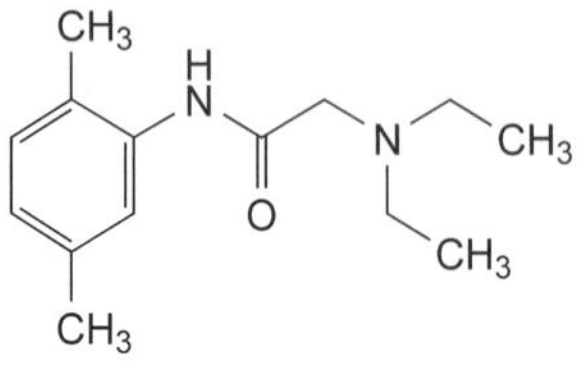

J. 2-(diethylamino)-*N*-(2,5-dimethylphenyl)acetamide.

04/2008:0728

LIOTHYRONINE SODIUM

Liothyroninum natricum

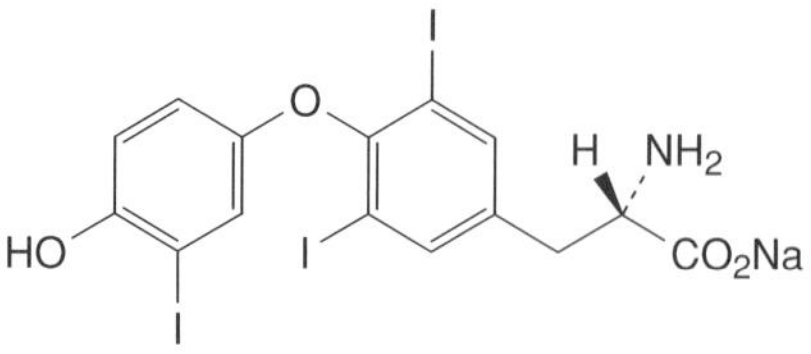

$C_{15}H_{11}I_3NNaO_4$ M_r 673

[55-06-1]

DEFINITION

Sodium (2*S*)-2-amino-3-[4-(4-hydroxy-3-iodophenoxy)-3,5-diiodophenyl]propanoate.

Content: 95.0 per cent to 102.0 per cent (dried substance).

CHARACTERS

Appearance: white or slightly coloured powder.

Solubility: practically insoluble in water, slightly soluble in ethanol (96 per cent). It dissolves in dilute solutions of alkali hydroxides.

IDENTIFICATION

First identification: A, C, E.

Second identification: A, B, D, E.

A. Specific optical rotation (see Tests).

B. Ultraviolet and visible absorption spectrophotometry (*2.2.25*).

Test solution. Dissolve 10.0 mg in *0.1 M sodium hydroxide* and dilute to 100.0 ml with the same solvent.

Spectral range: 230-350 nm.

Absorption maximum: at 319 nm.

Specific absorbance at the absorption maximum: 63 to 69 (dried substance).

C. Infrared absorption spectrophotometry (*2.2.24*).

Comparison: *liothyronine sodium CRS*.

D. To about 50 mg in a porcelain dish add a few drops of *sulphuric acid R* and heat. Violet vapour is evolved.

E. To 200 mg add 2 ml of *dilute sulphuric acid R*. Heat on a water-bath and then carefully over a naked flame, increasing the temperature gradually up to about 600 °C. Continue the ignition until most of the particles have disappeared. Dissolve the residue in 2 ml of *water R*. The solution gives reaction (a) of sodium (*2.3.1*).

TESTS

Specific optical rotation (*2.2.7*): + 18.0 to + 22.0 (dried substance).

Dissolve 0.200 g in a mixture of 1 volume of *1 M hydrochloric acid* and 4 volumes of *ethanol (96 per cent) R* and dilute to 20.0 ml with the same mixture of solvents.

Related substances. Liquid chromatography (*2.2.29*). *Protect the solutions from light throughout the test.*

Solution A. Mix 10 volumes of mobile phase A with 90 volumes of *methanol R*.

Solution B. Mix 30 volumes of mobile phase B and 70 volumes of mobile phase A. Mix equal volumes of this solution with solution A.

Test solution. Dissolve 20.0 mg of the substance to be examined in 20 ml of solution A. Dilute 4.0 ml of this solution to 20.0 ml with solution B.

Reference solution (a). Dissolve 2.5 mg of *levothyroxine sodium CRS* (impurity A) and 2.5 mg of *liothyronine sodium CRS* in solution A and dilute to 25 ml with the same solution. Dilute 1.0 ml of this solution to 50.0 ml with solution B.

Reference solution (b). Dilute 1.0 ml of reference solution (a) to 10.0 ml with solution B.

Reference solution (c). Dissolve the contents of a vial of *liothyronine for peak identification CRS* (containing impurities A, B, C, D and E) in solution B and dilute to 1.0 ml with the same solution.

Reference solution (d). Dissolve 20.0 mg of *liothyronine sodium CRS* in 20 ml of solution A. Dilute 4.0 ml of this solution to 20.0 ml with solution B.

Blank solution: solution B.

Column:

- *size*: *l* = 0.15 m, Ø = 4.0 mm;
- *stationary phase*: *end-capped octadecylsilyl silica gel for chromatography R* (3 μm).

Mobile phase:

- *mobile phase A*: dissolve 9.7 g of *sulphamic acid R* in *water R* and dilute to 2000 ml with the same solvent; add 1.5 g of *sodium hydroxide R* and adjust to pH 2.0 with *2 M sodium hydroxide*;
- *mobile phase B*: *acetonitrile R1*;

Time (min)	Mobile phase A (per cent *V/V*)	Mobile phase B (per cent *V/V*)
0 - 3	75	25
3 - 4	75 → 70	25 → 30
4 - 14	70	30
14 - 44	70 → 20	30 → 80
44 - 54	20	80

Flow rate: 1 ml/min.

Detection: spectrophotometer at 225 nm.

Injection: 25 μl of the test solution and reference solutions (a), (b) and (c).

Identification of impurities: use the chromatogram obtained with reference solution (c) to identify the peaks due to impurities A, B, C, D and E.

- *relative retention* with reference to liothyronine (retention time = about 14 min): impurity B = about 0.2; impurity E = about 0.5; impurity A = about 1.4; impurity C = about 2; impurity D = about 2.4.

System suitability:

- *resolution*: minimum 5.0 between the peaks due to impurity A and liothyronine in the chromatogram obtained with reference solution (a).

Limits:

- *impurity A*: not more than the area of the corresponding peak in the chromatogram obtained with reference solution (a) (1.0 per cent);
- *impurity E*: not more than 5 times the area of the peak due to liothyronine in the chromatogram obtained with reference solution (b) (0.5 per cent);
- *impurities B, C*: for each impurity, not more than 3 times the area of the peak due to liothyronine in the chromatogram obtained with reference solution (b) (0.3 per cent);
- *impurity D*: not more than twice the area of the peak due to liothyronine in the chromatogram obtained with reference solution (b) (0.2 per cent);
- *unspecified impurities*: for each impurity, not more than the area of the peak due to liothyronine in the chromatogram obtained with reference solution (b) (0.10 per cent);
- *total*: not more than twice the area of the peak due to liothyronine in the chromatogram obtained with reference solution (a) (2.0 per cent);
- *disregard limit*: 0.5 times the area of the peak due to liothyronine in the chromatogram obtained with reference solution (b) (0.05 per cent).

Chlorides: maximum 2.0 per cent, expressed as NaCl (dried substance).

Dissolve 0.500 g in a 2 g/l solution of *sodium hydroxide R* and dilute to 100 ml with the same solvent. Add 15 ml of *dilute nitric acid R* and titrate with *0.05 M silver nitrate*, determining the end-point potentiometrically (*2.2.20*).

1 ml of *0.05 M silver nitrate* is equivalent to 2.93 mg of NaCl.

Loss on drying (*2.2.32*): maximum 4.0 per cent, determined on 0.500 g by drying *in vacuo* at 60 °C for 4 h.

ASSAY

Liquid chromatography (*2.2.29*) as described in the test for related substances with the following modifications.

Injection: test solution and reference solution (d).

Calculate the percentage content of $C_{15}H_{11}I_3NNaO_4$ from the declared content of *liothyronine sodium CRS*.

STORAGE

In an airtight container, protected from light, at a temperature between 2 °C and 8 °C.

IMPURITIES

Specified impurities: A, B, C, D, E.

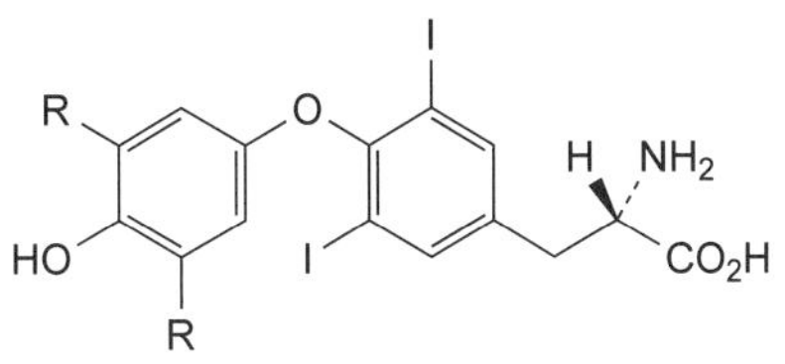

A. R = I: levothyroxine,

E. R = H: (2*S*)-2-amino-3-[4-(4-hydroxyphenoxy)-3,5-diiodophenyl]propanoic acid (diiodothyronine).

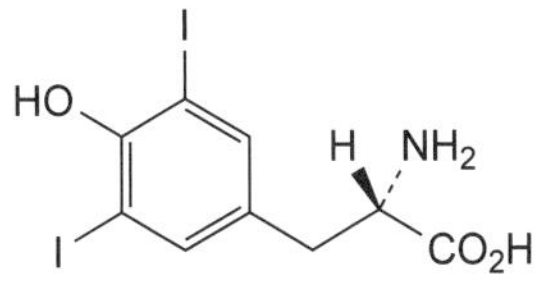

B. (2*S*)-2-amino-3-(4-hydroxy-3,5-diiodophenyl)propanoic acid (diiodotyrosine),

Monographs L-P

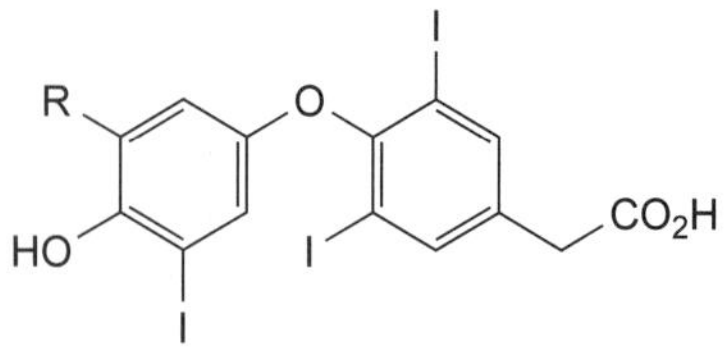

C. R = H: [4-(4-hydroxy-3-iodophenoxy)-3,5-diiodophenyl]acetic acid (triiodothyroacetic acid),

D. R = I: [4-(4-hydroxy-3,5-diiodophenoxy)-3,5-diiodophenyl]acetic acid (tetraiodothyroacetic acid),

04/2008:2378

LIQUORICE DRY EXTRACT FOR FLAVOURING PURPOSES

Liquiritiae extractum siccum ad saporandum

DEFINITION

Dry extract produced from *Liquorice root (0277).*

Content: 5.0 per cent to 7.0 per cent of 18β-glycyrrhizic acid ($C_{42}H_{62}O_{16}$; M_r 823) (dried extract).

PRODUCTION

The extract is produced from the cut herbal drug by a suitable procedure using water.

CHARACTERS

Appearance: yellowish-brown or brown powder.

Very sweet taste.

IDENTIFICATION

Thin-layer chromatography (*2.2.27*).

Solvent mixture: *ethyl acetate R, methanol R* (50:50 *V/V*).

Test solution. To 0.30 g of the extract to be examined add 30 ml of *hydrochloric acid R1* and boil on a water-bath under a reflux condenser for 60 min. After cooling, extract the mixture with 2 quantities, each of 20 ml, of *ethyl acetate R*. Combine the organic layers and filter through a filter covered with *anhydrous sodium sulphate R*. Evaporate the filtrate to dryness *in vacuo* and dissolve the residue in 2.0 ml of the solvent mixture.

Reference solution. Dissolve 5.0 mg of *glycyrrhetic acid R* and 5.0 mg of *thymol R* in 5.0 ml of the solvent mixture.

Plate: *TLC silica gel F_{254} plate R* (5-40 μm) [or *TLC silica gel F_{254} plate R* (2-10 μm)].

Mobile phase: *concentrated ammonia R, water R, ethanol (96 per cent) R, ethyl acetate R* (1:9:25:65 *V/V/V/V*).

Application: 20 μl [or 10 μl], as bands.

Development: over a path of 15 cm [or 7 cm].

Drying: in air for 5 min.

Detection: spray with *anisaldehyde solution R* and heat at 100-105 °C for 5-10 min; examine in daylight.

Results: see below the sequence of zones present in the chromatograms obtained with the reference solution and the test solution. Furthermore, other faint zones may be present in the chromatogram obtained with the test solution.

Top of the plate	
Thymol: a red zone	
	A yellow zone
———	———
———	———
Glycyrrhetic acid: a violet zone	A violet zone (glycyrrhetic acid)
Reference solution	**Test solution**

TESTS

Loss on drying (*2.8.17*): maximum 7.0 per cent.

ASSAY

Liquid chromatography (*2.2.29*).

Solvent mixture: *water R, methanol R* (20:80 *V/V*).

Test solution. Place 0.200 g of the extract to be examined in a 150 ml ground-glass conical flask. Add 100.0 ml of the solvent mixture and sonicate for 2 min. Filter through a membrane filter (nominal pore size 0.45 μm).

Reference solution. Dissolve 50.0 mg of *monoammonium glycyrrhizate CRS* in the solvent mixture and dilute to 50.0 ml with the solvent mixture. Dilute 1.0 ml of this solution to 10.0 ml with the solvent mixture.

Column:

– *size*: *l* = 0.10 m, Ø = 4.0 mm;

– *stationary phase*: *octadecylsilyl silica gel for chromatography R* (5 μm).

Mobile phase: *glacial acetic acid R, acetonitrile R, water R* (6:30:64 *V/V/V*).

Flow rate: 1.5 ml/min.

Detection: spectrophotometer at 254 nm.

Injection: 10 μl.

Run time: 3 times the retention time of 18β-glycyrrhizic acid.

Retention time: 18β-glycyrrhizic acid = about 9 min.

Identification of peaks: use the chromatogram supplied with *monoammonium glycyrrhizate CRS* and the chromatogram obtained with the reference solution to identify the peaks due to 18β-glycyrrhizic acid and 18α-glycyrrhizic acid.

System suitability: reference solution:

– the chromatogram obtained with the reference solution is similar to the chromatogram supplied with *monoammonium glycyrrhizate CRS*;

– *resolution*: minimum 2.0 between the peaks due to 18β-glycyrrhizic acid and 18α-glycyrrhizic acid.

Calculate the percentage content of 18β-glycyrrhizic acid, using the following expression:

$$\frac{A_1 \times m_2 \times p \times 0.979}{A_2 \times m_1 \times 5}$$

A_1 = area of the peak due to 18β-glycyrrhizic acid in the chromatogram obtained with the test solution;

A_2 = area of the peak due to 18β-glycyrrhizic acid in the chromatogram obtained with the reference solution;

m_1 = mass of the extract to be examined used to prepare the test solution, in grams;

m_2 = mass of *monoammonium glycyrrhizate CRS* used to prepare the reference solution, in grams;

p = percentage content of 18β-glycyrrhizic acid in *monoammonium glycyrrhizate CRS*;

0.979 = peak correlation factor between glycyrrhizic acid and monoammonium glycyrrhizate.

04/2008:1654

LYMECYCLINE

Lymecyclinum

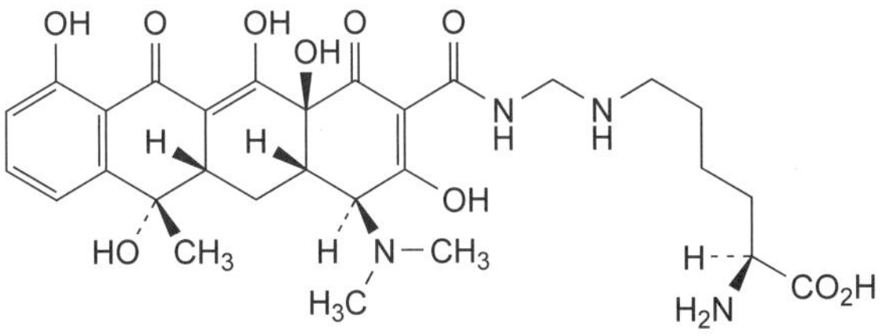

$C_{29}H_{38}N_4O_{10}$ M_r 603

[992-21-2]

DEFINITION

(2*S*)-2-Amino-6-[[[[(4*S*,4a*S*,5a*S*,6*S*,12a*S*)-4-(dimethylamino)-3,6,10,12,12a-pentahydroxy-6-methyl-1,11-dioxo-1,4,4a,5,5a,6,11,12a-octahydrotetracen-2-yl]carbonyl]amino]methyl]amino]hexanoic acid (reaction product of formaldehyde, lysine and tetracycline).

Semi-synthetic product derived from a fermentation product.

Content: 81.0 per cent to 102.0 per cent (equivalent to 60.0 per cent to 75.0 per cent of tetracycline) (anhydrous substance).

CHARACTERS

Appearance: yellow, hygroscopic powder.

Solubility: very soluble in water, slightly soluble in ethanol (96 per cent), practically insoluble in methylene chloride.

IDENTIFICATION

A. Thin-layer chromatography (*2.2.27*).

Test solution. Dissolve 5 mg of the substance to be examined in *methanol R* and dilute to 10 ml with the same solvent.

Reference solution (a). Dissolve 5 mg of *tetracycline hydrochloride CRS* in *methanol R* and dilute to 10 ml with the same solvent.

Reference solution (b). Dissolve 5 mg of *tetracycline hydrochloride CRS*, 5 mg of *demeclocycline hydrochloride R* and 5 mg of *oxytetracycline hydrochloride R* in *methanol R* and dilute to 10 ml with the same solvent.

Plate: *TLC octadecylsilyl silica gel F_{254} plate R* (2-10 μm).

Mobile phase: mix 20 volumes of *acetonitrile R*, 20 volumes of *methanol R* and 60 volumes of a 63 g/l solution of *oxalic acid R* previously adjusted to pH 2.0 with *concentrated ammonia R*.

Application: 2 μl.

Development: over half of the plate.

Drying: in air.

Detection: examine in ultraviolet light at 254 nm.

System suitability: reference solution (b):

– the chromatogram shows 3 clearly separated spots.

Results: the principal spot in the chromatogram obtained with the test solution is similar in position and size to the principal spot in the chromatogram obtained with reference solution (a).

B. Thin-layer chromatography (*2.2.27*).

Test solution. Dissolve 50 mg of the substance to be examined in 50 ml of *water R*.

Reference solution (a). Dissolve 10 mg of *lysine hydrochloride CRS* in *water R* and dilute to 50 ml with the same solvent.

Reference solution (b). Dissolve 10 mg of *arginine CRS* and 10 mg of *lysine hydrochloride CRS* in *water R* and dilute to 25 ml with the same solvent.

Plate: *TLC silica gel plate R*.

Mobile phase: *concentrated ammonia R*, *2-propanol R* (30:70 *V/V*).

Application: 5 μl.

Development: over 3/4 of the plate.

Drying: at 100-105 °C until the ammonia disappears completely.

Detection: spray with *ninhydrin solution R* and heat at 100-105 °C for 15 min.

System suitability: reference solution (b):

– the chromatogram shows 2 clearly separated principal spots.

Results: the principal spot in the chromatogram obtained with the test solution is similar in position, colour and size to the principal spot in the chromatogram obtained with reference solution (a).

C. Dissolve 0.2 g in 5 ml of *water R*, add 0.3 ml of *orthophosphoric acid R* and distil. To 1 ml of the distillate add 10 ml of *chromotropic acid-sulphuric acid solution R*. A violet colour is produced.

D. Specific optical rotation (see Tests).

TESTS

pH (*2.2.3*): 7.8 to 8.2.

Dissolve 0.1 g in 10 ml of *carbon dioxide-free water R*.

Specific optical rotation (*2.2.7*): – 180 to – 210 (anhydrous substance).

Dissolve 0.250 g in *water R* and dilute to 50.0 ml with the same solvent.

Free tetracycline (impurity H): maximum 2.5 per cent (anhydrous and methanol-free substance).

To 0.5 g add 50 ml of *butyl acetate R* and allow to stand at 25 °C for 1 h. Filter and extract the filtrate with 2 quantities, each of 25 ml, of *0.1 M hydrochloric acid*. Combine the extracts and dilute to 50.0 ml with *0.1 M hydrochloric acid*. Dilute 10.0 ml of this solution to 100.0 ml with *0.1 M hydrochloric acid*. The absorbance (*2.2.25*) measured at 355 nm is not greater than 0.64.

Monographs L-P

Light-absorbing impurities: the absorbance (*2.2.25*) is not greater than 0.50 at 430 nm (anhydrous and methanol-free substance).

Dissolve 25.0 mg in *0.01 M hydrochloric acid* and dilute to 10.0 ml with the same acid.

Related substances. Liquid chromatography (*2.2.29*). *Prepare the solutions immediately before use.*

Test solution. Dissolve 0.125 g of the substance to be examined in 5.0 ml of *water R*. Add 1.0 ml of a 40 g/l solution of *sodium metabisulphite R* and allow to stand in the dark at 20-25 °C for 16-24 h, without stirring. Add 50 ml of *0.05 M hydrochloric acid,* shake to dissolve the precipitate and dilute to 100.0 ml with *water R*.

Reference solution (a). Dissolve 25.0 mg of *tetracycline hydrochloride CRS* in *0.01 M hydrochloric acid* and dilute to 25.0 ml with the same acid.

Reference solution (b). Dissolve 12.5 mg of *4-epitetracycline hydrochloride CRS* (impurity A) in *0.01 M hydrochloric acid* and dilute to 50.0 ml with the same acid.

Reference solution (c). Dissolve 10.0 mg of *anhydrotetracycline hydrochloride CRS* (impurity C) in *0.01 M hydrochloric acid* and dilute to 100.0 ml with the same acid.

Reference solution (d). Dissolve 10.0 mg of *4-epianhydrotetracycline hydrochloride CRS* (impurity D) in *0.01 M hydrochloric acid* and dilute to 50.0 ml with the same acid.

Reference solution (e). Mix 1 ml of reference solution (a), 2 ml of reference solution (b) and 5 ml of reference solution (d) and dilute to 25 ml with *0.01 M hydrochloric acid.*

Reference solution (f). Mix 40.0 ml of reference solution (b), 20.0 ml of reference solution (c) and 5.0 ml of reference solution (d) and dilute to 200.0 ml with *0.01 M hydrochloric acid.*

Column:

- *size*: *l* = 0.25 m, Ø = 4.6 mm;
- *stationary phase*: *styrene-divinylbenzene copolymer R* (8 μm) with a pore size of 10 nm;
- *temperature*: 60 °C.

Mobile phase: weigh 80.0 g of *2-methyl-2-propanol R* and transfer to a 1000 ml volumetric flask with the aid of 200 ml of *water R*; add 100 ml of a 35 g/l solution of *dipotassium hydrogen phosphate R* adjusted to pH 8.0 with *dilute phosphoric acid R*, 200 ml of a 10 g/l solution of *tetrabutylammonium hydrogen sulphate R* adjusted to pH 8.0 with *dilute sodium hydroxide solution R*, and 10 ml of a 40 g/l solution of *sodium edetate R* adjusted to pH 8.0 with *dilute sodium hydroxide solution R*; dilute to 1000.0 ml with *water R*.

Flow rate: 1.0 ml/min.

Detection: spectrophotometer at 254 nm.

Injection: 20 μl of the test solution and reference solutions (e) and (f).

Run time: 5 times the retention time of the principal peak in the chromatogram obtained with the test solution.

Relative retention with reference to tetracycline (retention time = about 8 min): impurity E = about 0.50; impurity A = about 0.6; impurity F = about 0.68; impurity B (eluting on the tail of the principal peak) = about 1.2; impurity D = about 1.45; impurity G = about 1.45; impurity C = about 2.95.

System suitability: reference solution (e):

- *resolution*: minimum 3.0 between the 1st peak (impurity A) and the 2nd peak (tetracycline) and minimum 5.0 between the 2nd peak and the 3rd peak (impurity D); adjust the concentration of 2-methyl-2-propanol in the mobile phase if necessary;
- *symmetry factor*: maximum 1.25 for the peak due to tetracycline.

Limits:

- *impurity A*: not more than the area of the corresponding peak in the chromatogram obtained with reference solution (f) (5.0 per cent),
- *impurity C*: not more than the area of the corresponding peak in the chromatogram obtained with reference solution (f) (1.0 per cent),
- *impurities B, E, F*: for each impurity, not more than 0.1 times the area of the peak due to impurity A in the chromatogram obtained with reference solution (f) (0.5 per cent),
- *sum of impurities D and G*: not more than the area of the corresponding peak in the chromatogram obtained with reference solution (f) (0.5 per cent),
- *any other impurity*: for each impurity, not more than 0.04 times the area of the peak due to impurity A in the chromatogram obtained with reference solution (f) (0.2 per cent),
- *total*: not more than 1.6 times the area of the peak due to impurity A in the chromatogram obtained with reference solution (f) (8.0 per cent),
- *disregard limit*: 0.02 times the area of the peak due to impurity A in the chromatogram obtained with reference solution (f) (0.1 per cent).

Methanol (*2.4.24, System A*): maximum 1.5 per cent.

Water (*2.5.12*): maximum 5.0 per cent, determined on 0.20 g.

Sulphated ash (*2.4.14*): maximum 0.5 per cent, determined on 1.0 g.

ASSAY

Liquid chromatography (*2.2.29*) as described in the test for related substances with the following modifications.

Injection: test solution and reference solution (a).

System suitability:

- *repeatability*: maximum relative standard deviation of 1.0 per cent after 6 injections of reference solution (a).

Calculate the percentage content of tetracycline and multiply it by 1.356 to obtain the percentage content of lymecycline.

STORAGE

In an airtight container, protected from light.

IMPURITIES

Specified impurities: A, B, C, D, E, F, G, H.

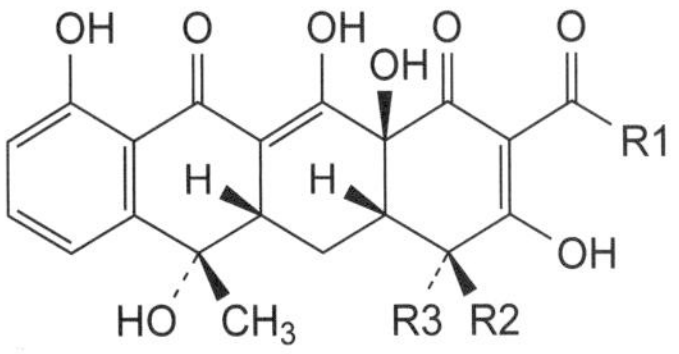

A. R1 = NH_2, R2 = H, R3 = $N(CH_3)_2$: (4*R*,4a*S*,5a*S*,6*S*,12a*S*)-4-(dimethylamino)-3,6,10,12,12a-pentahydroxy-6-methyl-1,11-dioxo-1,4,4a,5,5a,6,11,12a-octahydrotetracene-2-carboxamide (4-epitetracycline),

B. R1 = CH_3, R2 = $N(CH_3)_2$, R3 = H: (4*S*,4a*S*,5a*S*,6*S*,12a*S*)-2-acetyl-4-(dimethylamino)-3,6,10,12,12a-pentahydroxy-6-methyl-4a,5a,6,12a-tetrahydrotetracene-1,11(4*H*,5*H*)-dione (2-acetyl-2-decarbamoyltetracycline),

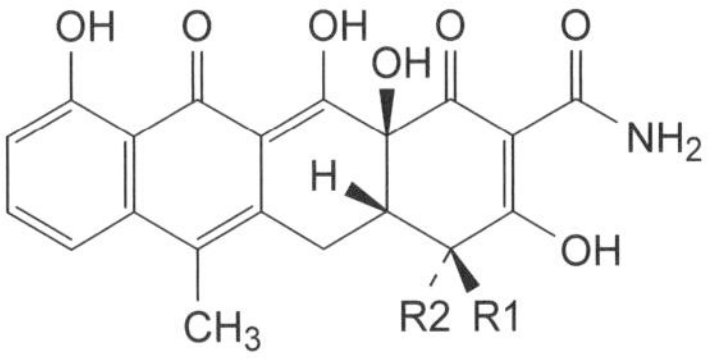

C. R1 = $N(CH_3)_2$, R2 = H: (4*S*,4a*S*,12a*S*)-4-(dimethylamino)-3,10,11,12a-tetrahydroxy-6-methyl-1,12-dioxo-1,4,4a,5,12,12a-hexahydrotetracene-2-carboxamide (anhydrotetracycline),

D. R1 = H, R2 = $N(CH_3)_2$: (4*R*,4a*S*,12a*S*)-4-(dimethylamino)-3,10,11,12a-tetrahydroxy-6-methyl-1,12-dioxo-1,4,4a,5,12,12a-hexahydrotetracene-2-carboxamide (4-epianhydrotetracycline),

E. unknown structure,

F. unknown structure,

G. chlortetracycline,

H. tetracycline.

Monographs L-P

M

04/2008:2161

MAGNESIUM GLUCONATE

Magnesii gluconas

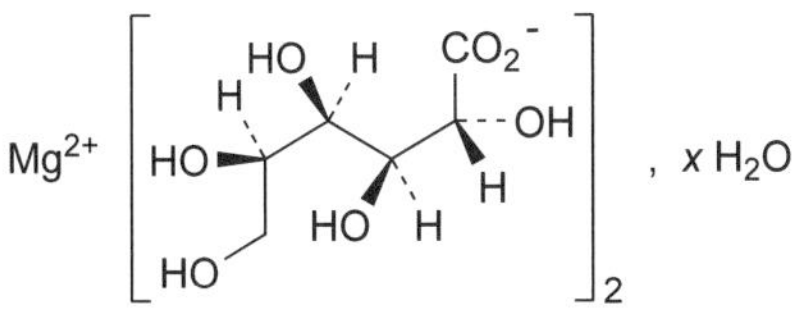

$C_{12}H_{22}MgO_{14},xH_2O$ M_r 414.6 (anhydrous substance)

DEFINITION

Anhydrous or hydrated magnesium D-gluconate.

Content: 98.0 per cent to 102.0 per cent (anhydrous substance).

CHARACTERS

Appearance: white or almost white, amorphous, hygroscopic, crystalline or granular powder.

Solubility: freely soluble in water, slightly soluble in ethanol (96 per cent), very slightly soluble in methylene chloride.

IDENTIFICATION

A. Thin-layer chromatography (*2.2.27*).

Test solution. Dissolve 20 mg of the substance to be examined in 1 ml of *water R*.

Reference solution. Dissolve 20 mg of *calcium gluconate CRS* in 1 ml of *water R*, heating if necessary in a water-bath at 60 °C.

Plate: *TLC silica gel plate R* (5-40 µm) [or *TLC silica gel plate R* (2-10 µm)].

Mobile phase: *concentrated ammonia R, ethyl acetate R, water R, ethanol (96 per cent) R* (10:10:30:50 *V/V/V/V*).

Application: 1 µl.

Development: over 3/4 of the plate.

Drying: at 100-105 °C for 20 min, then allow to cool to room temperature.

Detection: spray with a solution containing 25 g/l of *ammonium molybdate R* and 10 g/l of *cerium sulphate R* in *dilute sulphuric acid R*, then heat at 100-105 °C for about 10 min.

Results: the principal spot in the chromatogram obtained with the test solution is similar in position, colour and size to the principal spot in the chromatogram obtained with the reference solution.

B. To 10 ml of solution S (see Tests) add 3 ml of *ammonium chloride solution R*. A slight opalescence may be observed. Add 10 ml of *disodium hydrogen phosphate solution R*. A white precipitate is formed that does not dissolve upon the addition of 2 ml of *dilute ammonia R1*.

TESTS

Solution S. Dissolve 1.0 g in *water R* and dilute to 50 ml with the same solvent.

Appearance of solution. Solution S is clear (*2.2.1*) and not more intensely coloured than reference solution Y_7 (*2.2.2, Method II*).

Sucrose and reducing sugars. Dissolve 0.5 g in a mixture of 2 ml of *hydrochloric acid R1* and 10 ml of *water R*. Boil for 5 min, allow to cool, add 10 ml of *sodium carbonate solution R* and allow to stand for 10 min. Dilute to 25 ml with *water R* and filter. To 5 ml of the filtrate add 2 ml of *cupri-tartaric solution R* and boil for 1 min. Allow to stand for 2 min. No red precipitate is formed.

Chlorides (*2.4.4*): maximum 500 ppm.

Dilute 5 ml of solution S to 15 ml with *water R*.

Sulphates (*2.4.13*): maximum 500 ppm.

Dissolve 2.0 g in a mixture of 10 ml of *acetic acid R* and 90 ml of *distilled water R*.

Heavy metals (*2.4.8*): maximum 10 ppm.

Dissolve 2.0 g in 20 ml of *water R*. 12 ml of the solution complies with test A. Prepare the reference solution using *lead standard solution (1 ppm Pb) R*.

Water (*2.5.32*): maximum 12.0 per cent, determined on 80 mg.

Microbial contamination. Total viable aerobic count (*2.6.12*) not more than 10^3 micro-organisms per gram, determined by plate count.

ASSAY

Dissolve 0.350 g in 100 ml of *water R* and carry out the complexometric titration of magnesium (*2.5.11*).

1 ml of *0.1 M sodium edetate* is equivalent to 41.46 mg of $C_{12}H_{22}MgO_{14}$.

STORAGE

In an airtight container.

04/2008:2162

MANGANESE GLUCONATE

Mangani gluconas

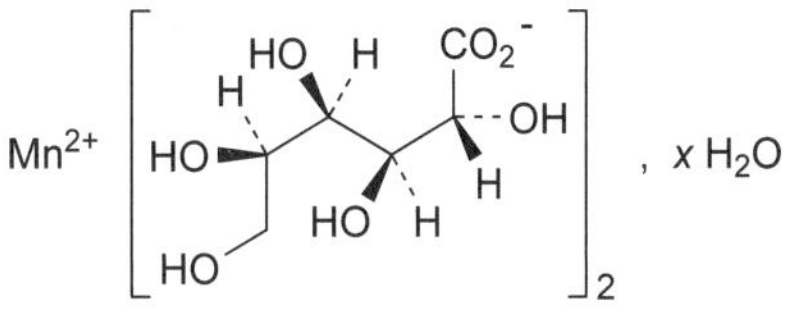

$C_{12}H_{22}MnO_{14},xH_2O$ M_r 445.2 (anhydrous substance)

DEFINITION

Anhydrous or hydrated manganese(II) D-gluconate.

Content: 98.0 per cent to 102.0 per cent (anhydrous substance).

CHARACTERS

Appearance: white or pale pink, slightly hygroscopic, crystalline powder.

Solubility: soluble in water, practically insoluble in anhydrous ethanol, insoluble in methylene chloride.

IDENTIFICATION

A. Thin-layer chromatography (*2.2.27*).

Test solution. Dissolve 20 mg of the substance to be examined in 1 ml of *water R*.

Reference solution. Dissolve 20 mg of *calcium gluconate CRS* in 1 ml of *water R*, heating if necessary in a water-bath at 60 °C.

Plate: *TLC silica gel plate R* (5-40 µm) [or *TLC silica gel plate R* (2-10 µm)].

Mobile phase: *concentrated ammonia R, ethyl acetate R, water R, ethanol (96 per cent) R* (10:10:30:50 *V/V/V/V*).

Application: 1 µl.

Monographs L-P

Development: over 3/4 of the plate.

Drying: at 100-105 °C for 20 min, then allow to cool to room temperature.

Detection: spray with a solution containing 25 g/l of *ammonium molybdate R* and 10 g/l of *cerium sulphate R* in *dilute sulphuric acid R*, and heat at 100-105 °C for about 10 min.

Results: the principal spot in the chromatogram obtained with the test solution is similar in position, colour and size to the principal spot in the chromatogram obtained with the reference solution.

B. Dissolve 50 mg in 5 ml of *water R*. Add 0.5 ml of *ammonium sulphide solution R*. A pale pink precipitate is formed that dissolves upon the addition of 1 ml of *glacial acetic acid R*.

TESTS

Solution S. Dissolve 1.0 g in *water R* and dilute to 50 ml with the same solvent.

Appearance of solution. Solution S is not more opalescent than reference suspension II (*2.2.1*) and not more intensely coloured than intensity 6 of the range of reference solutions of the most appropriate colour (*2.2.2, Method II*).

Sucrose and reducing sugars. Dissolve 0.5 g in a mixture of 2 ml of *hydrochloric acid R1* and 10 ml of *water R*. Boil for 5 min, allow to cool, add 10 ml of *sodium carbonate solution R* and allow to stand for 10 min. Dilute to 25 ml with *water R* and filter. To 5 ml of the filtrate add 2 ml of *cupri-tartaric solution R* and boil for 1 min. Allow to stand for 2 min. No red precipitate is formed.

Chlorides (*2.4.4*): maximum 500 ppm.

Dilute 5 ml of solution S to 15 ml with *water R*.

Sulphates (*2.4.13*): maximum 500 ppm.

Dissolve 2.0 g in a mixture of 10 ml of *acetic acid R* and 90 ml of *distilled water R*.

Zinc: maximum 50 ppm.

To 10 ml of solution S add 1 ml of *sulphuric acid R* and 0.1 ml of *potassium ferrocyanide solution R*. After 30 s, any opalescence in the solution is not more intense than that in a mixture of 1.0 ml of *zinc standard solution (10 ppm Zn) R*, 9 ml of *water R*, 1 ml of *sulphuric acid R* and 0.1 ml of *potassium ferrocyanide solution R*.

Heavy metals (*2.4.8*): maximum 10 ppm.

Dissolve 2.0 g in 20 ml of *water R*, heating in a water-bath at 60 °C. 12 ml of the solution complies with test A. Prepare the reference solution using *lead standard solution (1 ppm Pb) R*.

Water (*2.5.32*): maximum 9.0 per cent, determined on 80 mg.

Microbial contamination. Total viable aerobic count (*2.6.12*) not more than 10^3 micro-organisms per gram, determined by plate count.

ASSAY

Dissolve 0.400 g in 50 ml of *water R*. Add 10 mg of *ascorbic acid R*, 20 ml of *ammonium chloride buffer solution pH 10.0 R* and 0.2 ml of a 2 g/l solution of *mordant black 11 R* in *triethanolamine R*. Titrate with *0.1 M sodium edetate* until the colour changes from violet to pure blue.

1 ml of *0.1 M sodium edetate* is equivalent to 44.52 mg of $C_{12}H_{22}MnO_{14}$.

STORAGE

In a non-metallic, airtight container.

04/2008:2233

MARBOFLOXACIN FOR VETERINARY USE

Marbofloxacinum ad usum veterinarium

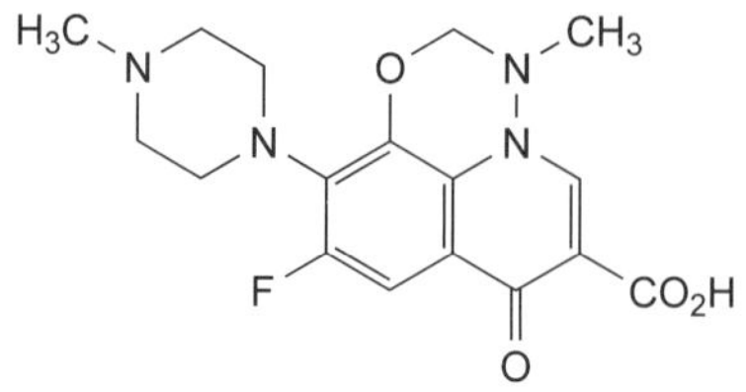

$C_{17}H_{19}FN_4O_4$ M_r 362.4

[115550-35-1]

DEFINITION

9-Fluoro-3-methyl-10-(4-methylpiperazin-1-yl)-7-oxo-2,3-dihydro-7*H*-pyrido[3,2,1-*ij*][4,1,2]benzoxadiazine-6-carboxylic acid.

Content: 99.0 per cent to 101.0 per cent (dried substance).

CHARACTERS

Appearance: light yellow, crystalline powder.

Solubility: slightly soluble in water, sparingly soluble or slightly soluble in methylene chloride, very slightly soluble in ethanol (96 per cent).

IDENTIFICATION

Infrared absorption spectrophotometry (*2.2.24*).

Comparison: *marbofloxacin CRS*.

TESTS

Absorbance (*2.2.25*): maximum 0.20, determined at 450 nm.

Dissolve 0.400 g in *borate buffer solution pH 10.4 R* and dilute to 10.0 ml with the same buffer solution.

Related substances. Liquid chromatography (*2.2.29*). *Carry out the test protected from light.*

Solvent mixture: *methanol R*, *water R* (23:77 *V/V*).

Test solution. To 0.100 g of the substance to be examined add 80 ml of the solvent mixture, sonicate until dissolution and dilute to 100.0 ml with the solvent mixture.

Reference solution (a). Dilute 5.0 ml of the test solution to 100.0 ml with the solvent mixture. Dilute 1.0 ml of this solution to 50.0 ml with the solvent mixture.

Reference solution (b). Dissolve 10 mg of *marbofloxacin for peak identification CRS* (containing impurities A, B, C, D and E) in the solvent mixture and dilute to 10 ml with the solvent mixture.

Column:

- *size*: *l* = 0.15 m, Ø = 4.6 mm;
- *stationary phase*: *end-capped polar-embedded octadecylsilyl amorphous organosilica polymer R* (3.5 μm);
- *temperature*: 40 °C.

Mobile phase: mix 230 volumes of *methanol R* and 5 volumes of *glacial acetic acid R* with 770 volumes of a 2.70 g/l solution of *sodium dihydrogen phosphate R* containing 3.50 g/l of *sodium octanesulphonate R* and previously adjusted to pH 2.5 with *phosphoric acid R*.

Flow rate: 1.2 ml/min.

Detection: spectrophotometer at 315 nm.

Injection: 10 μl.

Run time: 2.5 times the retention time of marbofloxacin.

Relative retention with reference to marbofloxacin (retention time = about 33 min): impurity B = about 0.5; impurity A = about 0.7; impurity C = about 0.9; impurity D = about 1.3; impurity E = about 1.5.

System suitability: reference solution (b):

- *resolution*: minimum 1.5 between the peaks due to impurity C and marbofloxacin, and minimum 4.0 between the peaks due to marbofloxacin and impurity D.

Limits:

- *correction factor*: for the calculation of content, multiply the peak area of impurity E by 1.5;
- *impurities C, D, E*: for each impurity, not more than twice the area of the principal peak in the chromatogram obtained with reference solution (a) (0.2 per cent);
- *impurities A, B*: for each impurity, not more than the area of the principal peak in the chromatogram obtained with reference solution (a) (0.1 per cent);
- *unspecified impurities*: for each impurity, not more than twice the area of the principal peak in the chromatogram obtained with reference solution (a) (0.2 per cent);
- *total*: not more than 5 times the area of the principal peak in the chromatogram obtained with reference solution (a) (0.5 per cent);
- *disregard limit*: the area of the principal peak in the chromatogram obtained with reference solution (a) (0.1 per cent).

Heavy metals (*2.4.8*): maximum 20 ppm.

Dissolve 0.5 g in *dilute acetic acid R* and dilute to 30 ml with the same solvent. Adding 2 ml of *water R* instead of 2 ml of *buffer solution pH 3.5 R*, the filtrate complies with test E. Prepare the reference solution using 5 ml of *lead standard solution (2 ppm Pb) R*.

Loss on drying (*2.2.32*): maximum 0.5 per cent, determined on 1.000 g by drying at 105 °C for 4 h.

Sulphated ash (*2.4.14*): maximum 0.1 per cent, determined on 1.0 g in a platinum crucible.

ASSAY

Dissolve 0.300 g in 80 ml of *glacial acetic acid R*. Titrate with *0.1 M perchloric acid*, determining the end-point potentiometrically (*2.2.20*).

1 ml of *0.1 M perchloric acid* is equivalent to 36.24 mg of $C_{17}H_{19}FN_4O_4$.

STORAGE

Protected from light.

IMPURITIES

Specified impurities: A, B, C, D, E.

Other detectable impurities (the following substances would, if present at a sufficient level, be detected by one or other of the tests in the monograph. They are limited by the general acceptance criterion for other/unspecified impurities and/or by the general monograph *Substances for pharmaceutical use (2034)*. It is therefore not necessary to identify these impurities for demonstration of compliance. See also *5.10. Control of impurities in substances for pharmaceutical use*): *F*.

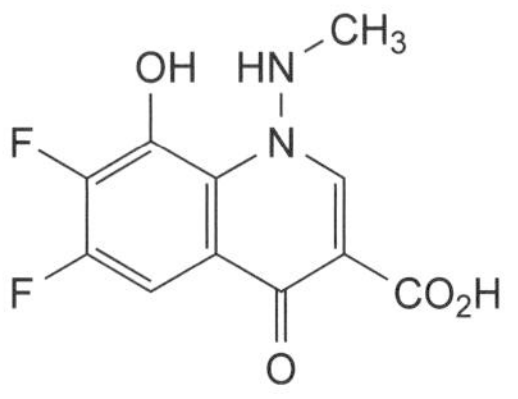

A. 6,7-difluoro-8-hydroxy-1-(methylamino)-4-oxo-1,4-dihydroquinoline-3-carboxylic acid,

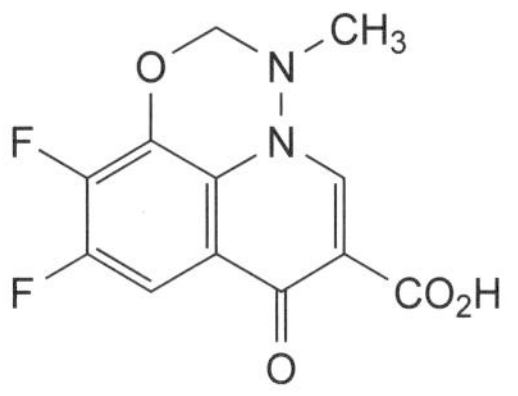

B. 9,10-difluoro-3-methyl-7-oxo-2,3-dihydro-7*H*-pyrido[3,2,1-*ij*][4,1,2]benzoxadiazine-6-carboxylic acid,

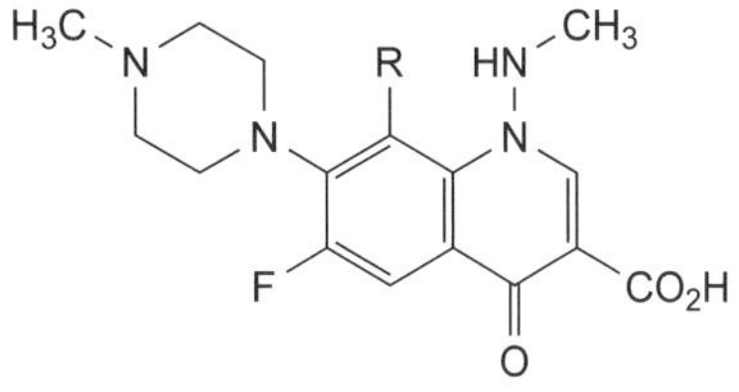

C. R = F: 6,8-difluoro-1-(methylamino)-7-(4-methylpiperazin-1-yl)-4-oxo-1,4-dihydroquinoline-3-carboxylic acid,

D. R = OH: 6-fluoro-8-hydroxy-1-(methylamino)-7-(4-methylpiperazin-1-yl)-4-oxo-1,4-dihydroquinoline-3-carboxylic acid,

E. R = O-C_2H_5: 8-ethoxy-6-fluoro-1-(methylamino)-7-(4-methylpiperazin-1-yl)-4-oxo-1,4-dihydroquinoline-3-carboxylic acid,

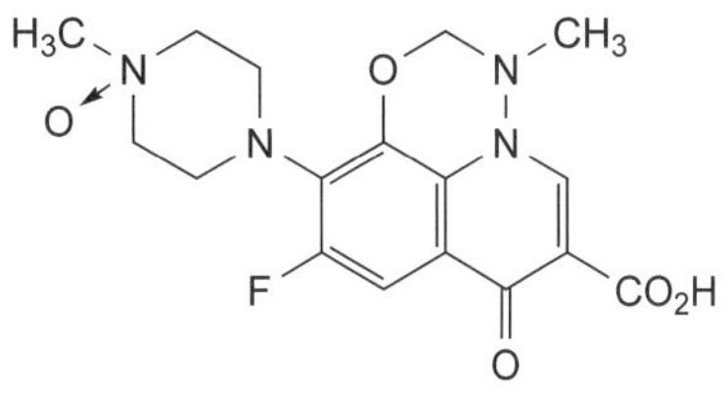

F. 4-[6-carboxy-9-fluoro-3-methyl-7-oxo-2,3-dihydro-7*H*-pyrido[3,2,1-*ij*][4,1,2]benzoxadiazin-10-yl]-1-methylpiperazine 1-oxide.

01/2008:0345
corrected 6.1

METHYLCELLULOSE

Methylcellulosum

[9004-67-5]

DEFINITION

Partly *O*-methylated cellulose.

CHARACTERS

Appearance: white, yellowish-white or greyish-white powder or granules, hygroscopic after drying.

Solubility: practically insoluble in hot water, in acetone, in anhydrous ethanol and in toluene. It dissolves in cold water giving a colloidal solution.

IDENTIFICATION

A. Evenly distribute 1.0 g onto the surface of 100 ml of *water R* in a beaker, tapping the top of the beaker gently if necessary to ensure a uniform layer on the surface. Allow to stand for 1-2 min: the powdered material aggregates on the surface.

B. Evenly distribute 1.0 g into 100 ml of boiling *water R*, and stir the mixture using a magnetic stirrer with a bar 25 mm long: a slurry is formed and the particles do not dissolve. Allow the slurry to cool to 5 °C and stir using a magnetic stirrer: a clear or slightly turbid solution occurs with its thickness dependent on the viscosity grade.

C. To 0.1 ml of the solution obtained in identification B add 9 ml of a 90 per cent *V/V* solution of *sulphuric acid R*, shake, heat on a water-bath for exactly 3 min, immediately cool in an ice-bath, carefully add 0.6 ml of a 20 g/l solution of *ninhydrin R*, shake and allow to stand at 25 °C: a red colour develops and does not change to purple within 100 min.

D. Place 2-3 ml of the solution obtained in identification B on a glass slide as a thin film and allow the water to evaporate: a coherent, clear film forms on the glass slide.

E. Add exactly 50 ml of the solution obtained in identification B to exactly 50 ml of *water R* in a beaker. Insert a thermometer into the solution. Stir the solution on a magnetic stirrer/hot plate and begin heating, increasing the temperature at a rate of 2-5 °C per minute. Determine the temperature at which a turbidity increase begins to occur and designate the temperature as the flocculation temperature: the flocculation temperature is higher than 50 °C.

TESTS

Solution S. While stirring, introduce a quantity of the substance to be examined equivalent to 1.0 g of the dried substance into 50 g of *carbon dioxide-free water R* heated to 90 °C. Allow to cool, adjust the mass of the solution to 100 g with *carbon dioxide-free water R* and stir until dissolution is complete. Allow to stand at 2-8 °C for 1 h before carrying out the test for appearance of solution.

Appearance of solution. Solution S is not more opalescent than reference suspension III (*2.2.1*) and not more intensely coloured than reference solution Y_6 (*2.2.2, Method II*).

pH (*2.2.3*): 5.0 to 8.0 for the solution prepared as described under Apparent viscosity.

Read the pH after the probe has been immersed for 5 ± 0.5 min.

Heavy metals (*2.4.8*): maximum 20 ppm.

1.0 g complies with test F. Prepare the reference solution using 2 ml of *lead standard solution (10 ppm Pb) R*.

Loss on drying (*2.2.32*): maximum 5.0 per cent, determined on 1.000 g by drying in an oven at 105 °C for 1 h.

Sulphated ash (*2.4.14*): maximum 1.5 per cent, determined on 1.0 g.

FUNCTIONALITY-RELATED CHARACTERISTICS

This section provides information on characteristics that are recognised as being relevant control parameters for one or more functions of the substance when used as an excipient. This section is a non-mandatory part of the monograph and it is not necessary to verify the characteristics to demonstrate compliance. Control of these characteristics can however contribute to the quality of a medicinal product by improving the consistency of the manufacturing process and the performance of the medicinal product during use. Where control methods are cited, they are recognised as being suitable for the purpose, but other methods can also be used. Wherever results for a particular characteristic are reported, the control method must be indicated.

The following characteristics may be relevant for methylcellulose used as binder, viscosity-enhancing agent or film former.

Apparent viscosity: minimum 80 per cent and maximum 120 per cent of the nominal value for samples with a viscosity of less than 600 mPa·s (Method 1); minimum 75 per cent and maximum 140 per cent of the nominal value for samples with a viscosity of 600 mPa·s or higher (Method 2).

Method 1, to be applied to samples with a viscosity of less than 600 mPa·s. Weigh accurately a quantity of the substance to be examined equivalent to 4.000 g of the dried substance. Transfer into a wide-mouthed bottle, and adjust the mass to 200.0 g with *water R*. Capping the bottle, stir by mechanical means at 400 ± 50 r/min for 10-20 min until the particles are thoroughly dispersed and wetted. Scrape down the insides of the bottle with a spatula if necessary, to ensure that there is no undissolved material on the sides of the bottle, and continue the stirring in a cooling water-bath maintained at a temperature below 5 °C for another 20-40 min. Adjust the solution mass if necessary to 200.0 g using cold *water R*. Centrifuge the solution if necessary to expel any entrapped air bubbles. Using a spatula remove any foam, if present. Determine the viscosity of this solution using the capillary viscometer method (*2.2.9*) to obtain the kinematic viscosity (ν). Separately, determine the density (ρ) (*2.2.5*) of the solution and calculate the dynamic viscosity (η), as $\eta = \rho\nu$.

Method 2, to be applied to samples with a viscosity of 600 mPa·s or higher. Weigh accurately a quantity of the substance to be examined equivalent to 10.00 g of the dried substance. Transfer into a wide-mouthed bottle, and adjust the mass to 500.0 g with *water R*. Capping the bottle, stir by mechanical means at 400 ± 50 r/min for 10-20 min until the particles are thoroughly dispersed and wetted. Scrape down the insides of the bottle with a spatula if necessary, to ensure that there is no undissolved material on the sides of the bottle, and continue the stirring in a cooling water-bath maintained at a temperature below 5 °C for another 20-40 min. Adjust the solution mass if necessary to 500.0 g using cold *water R*. Centrifuge the solution if necessary to expel any entrapped air bubbles. Using a spatula, remove any foam, if present. Determine the viscosity (*2.2.10*) of this solution at 20 ± 0.1 °C using a rotating viscometer.

Apparatus: single-cylinder type spindle viscometer.

Rotor number, revolution and calculation multiplier: apply the conditions specified in Table 0345.-1.

Table 0345.-1.

Nominal viscosity* (mPa·s)	Rotor number	Revolution (r/min)	Calculation multiplier
600 to less than 1400	3	60	20
1400 to less than 3500	3	12	100
3500 to less than 9500	4	60	100
9500 to less than 99 500	4	6	1000
99 500 or more	4	3	2000

*the nominal viscosity is based on the manufacturer's specifications.

Allow the spindle to rotate for 2 min before taking the measurement. Allow a rest period of 2 min between subsequent measurements. Repeat the measurement twice and determine the mean of the 3 readings.

Degree of substitution: 26.0 per cent to 33.0 per cent of methoxy groups (dried substance).

Gas chromatography (*2.2.28*).

Apparatus:

- *reaction vial*: a 5 ml pressure-tight vial, 50 mm in height, 20 mm in external diameter and 13 mm in internal diameter at the mouth, equipped with a pressure-tight butyl rubber membrane stopper coated with polytetrafluoroethylene and secured with an aluminium crimped cap or another sealing system providing a sufficient air-tightness;
- *heater*: a heating module with a square aluminium block having holes 20 mm in diameter and 32 mm in depth, so that the reaction vials fit; mixing of the contents of the vial is effected using a magnetic stirrer equipped in the heating module or using a reciprocal shaker that performs approximately 100 cycles/min.

Internal standard solution: 30 g/l solution of *octane R* in *xylene R*.

Test solution. Weigh 65.0 mg of the substance to be examined, place in a reaction vial, add 0.06-0.10 g of *adipic acid R*, 2.0 ml of the internal standard solution and 2.0 ml of a 570 g/l solution of *hydriodic acid R*, immediately cap and seal the vial, and weigh accurately. Using a magnetic stirrer, mix the contents of the vial continuously for 60 min while heating the block so that the temperature of the contents is maintained at 130 ± 2 °C. If a reciprocal shaker or magnetic stirrer cannot be used, shake the vial well by hand at 5-minute intervals during the initial 30 min of the heating time. Allow the vial to cool, and again weigh accurately. If the loss of mass is less than 0.50 per cent of the contents and there is no evidence of a leak, use the upper layer of the mixture as the test solution.

Reference solution. Place 0.06-0.10 g of *adipic acid R*, 2.0 ml of the internal standard solution and 2.0 ml of *hydroiodic acid R* in another reaction vial, cap and seal the vial, and weigh accurately. Add 45 μl of *methyl iodide R* through the septum with a syringe, and weigh accurately. Shake the reaction vial well, and use the upper layer as the reference solution.

Column:

- *size*: l = 1.8-3 m, Ø = 3-4 mm;
- *stationary phase*: *diatomaceous earth for gas chromatography R* impregnated with 10-20 per cent of *poly(dimethyl)(75)(diphenyl)(25)siloxane R* (film thickness 125-150 μm);
- *temperature*: 100 °C.

Carrier gas: *helium for chromatography R* (thermal conductivity); *helium for chromatography R* or *nitrogen for chromatography R* (flame ionisation).

Flow rate: adjusted so that the retention time of the internal standard is about 10 min.

Detection: flame ionisation or thermal conductivity.

Injection: 1-2 μl.

System suitability: reference solution:

- *resolution*: well-resolved peaks of methyl iodide (1st peak) and internal standard (2nd peak).

Calculation:

- *methoxy groups*: calculate the ratio (Q) of the area of the peak due to methyl iodide to the area of the peak due to the internal standard in the chromatogram obtained with the test solution, and the ratio (Q_1) of the area of the peak due to methyl iodide to the area of the peak due to the internal standard in the chromatogram obtained with the reference solution.

  Calculate the percentage content of methoxy groups using the following expression:

$$\frac{Q \times m_1}{Q_1 \times m} \times 21.864$$

m_1 = mass of methyl iodide in the reference solution, in milligrams;

m = mass of the sample (dried substance), in milligrams.

04/2008:1701

MOLSIDOMINE

Molsidominum

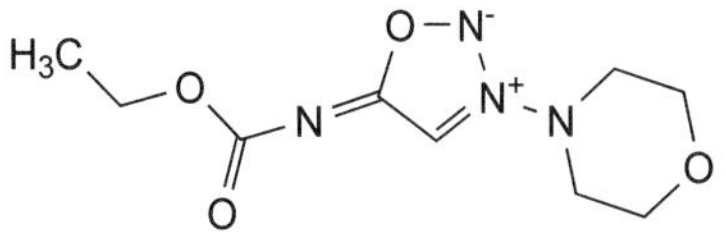

$C_9H_{14}N_4O_4$ M_r 242.2

[25717-80-0]

DEFINITION

N-(Ethoxycarbonyl)-3-(morpholin-4-yl)sydnonimine.

Content: 99.0 per cent to 101.0 per cent (dried substance).

CHARACTERS

Appearance: white or almost white, crystalline powder.

Solubility: sparingly soluble in water, soluble in anhydrous ethanol and in methylene chloride.

mp: about 142 °C.

IDENTIFICATION

Infrared absorption spectrophotometry (*2.2.24*).

Comparison: *molsidomine CRS*.

Monographs L-P

TESTS

Appearance of solution. The solution is clear (*2.2.1*) and not more intensely coloured than reference solution B_7 (*2.2.2, Method II*).

Dissolve 1.0 g in *anhydrous ethanol R* and dilute to 20.0 ml with the same solvent.

pH (*2.2.3*): 5.5 to 7.5.

Dissolve 0.50 g in *carbon dioxide-free water R* and dilute to 50.0 ml with the same solvent.

Impurity B. Liquid chromatography (*2.2.29*) as described in the test for related substances with the following modifications.

Detection: spectrophotometer at 240 nm.

Injection: 20 µl of test solution (a) and reference solution (b).

Relative retention with reference to molsidomine (retention time = about 9 min): impurity B = about 0.43.

System suitability: reference solution (b):

– *signal-to-noise ratio*: minimum 20 for the principal peak.

Limit:

– *impurity B*: not more than the area of the corresponding peak in the chromatogram obtained with reference solution (b) (3 ppm).

Impurity E. Liquid chromatography (*2.2.29*).

Test solution. Dissolve 0.200 g of the substance to be examined in the mobile phase and dilute to 100.0 ml with the mobile phase.

Reference solution (a). Dissolve 50.0 mg of *morpholine for chromatography R* in 500.0 ml of *water for chromatography R*. Dilute 20.0 ml of the solution to 500.0 ml with *water for chromatography R*. Dilute 5.0 ml of this solution to 100.0 ml with *water for chromatography R*.

Reference solution (b). Mix 10.0 ml of the test solution with 10.0 ml of reference solution (a).

Column:

– *size*: *l* = 0.25 m, Ø = 4.0 mm;

– *stationary phase*: *resin for reversed-phase ion chromatography R*;

– *temperature*: 25 °C.

Mobile phase: mix 3.0 ml of *methanesulphonic acid R* and 75 ml of *acetonitrile R* in *water for chromatography R* and dilute to 1000 ml with *water for chromatography R*.

Suppressor regenerant: *water for chromatography R*.

Flow rate: 1.0 ml/min.

Expected background conductivity: less than 0.5 µS.

Detection: conductivity detector at 10 µS.

Injection: 50 µl.

Run time: 20 min.

Relative retention with reference to molsidomine (retention time = about 3 min): impurity E = about 2.4.

System suitability: reference solution (b):

– *signal-to-noise ratio*: minimum 6 for the peak due to impurity E.

Limit:

– *impurity E*: not more than the area of the principal peak in the chromatogram obtained with reference solution (a) (0.01 per cent).

Related substances. Liquid chromatography (*2.2.29*). *Protect the solutions from light.*

Solvent mixture: *methanol R*, mobile phase A (10:90 *V/V*).

Test solution (a). Dissolve 0.200 g of the substance to be examined in 2.5 ml of *methanol R* and dilute to 5.0 ml with mobile phase A.

Test solution (b). Dilute 1.0 ml of test solution (a) to 20.0 ml with the solvent mixture.

Reference solution (a). Dilute 1.0 ml of test solution (b) to 100.0 ml with the solvent mixture. Dilute 1.0 ml of this solution to 10.0 ml with the solvent mixture.

Reference solution (b). Dissolve 2.4 mg of *molsidomine impurity B CRS* in 80 ml of *methanol R* and dilute to 100.0 ml with *methanol R*. Dilute 2.0 ml of the solution to 100.0 ml with the solvent mixture. Dilute 5.0 ml of this solution to 20.0 ml with the solvent mixture.

Reference solution (c). Dissolve 10 mg of *linsidomine hydrochloride R* (impurity A) and 5 mg of *molsidomine impurity D CRS* in 10 ml of *methanol R* and dilute to 50.0 ml with the solvent mixture. Dilute 5.0 ml of this solution to 50.0 ml with the solvent mixture.

Column:

– *size*: *l* = 0.15 m, Ø = 4.6 mm;

– *stationary phase*: *end-capped octadecylsilyl silica gel for chromatography R* (5 µm);

– *temperature*: 30 °C.

Mobile phase:

– *mobile phase A*: dissolve 4.0 g of *potassium dihydrogen phosphate R* in *water for chromatography R* and dilute to 1000 ml with the same solvent;

– *mobile phase B*: *methanol R1*;

Time (min)	Mobile phase A (per cent *V/V*)	Mobile phase B (per cent *V/V*)
0 - 3	90	10
3 - 10	90 → 20	10 → 80
10 - 13	20	80

Flow rate: 1.3 ml/min.

Detection: spectrophotometer at 210 nm.

Injection: 20 µl of test solution (b) and reference solutions (a) and (c).

Relative retention with reference to molsidomine (retention time = about 9 min): impurity A = about 0.2; impurity D = about 0.3.

System suitability: reference solution (c):

– *resolution*: minimum 3.5 between the peaks due to impurities A and D.

Limits:

– *unspecified impurities*: for each impurity, not more than the area of the peak due to molsidomine in the chromatogram obtained with reference solution (a) (0.10 per cent);

– *total*: not more than 3 times the area of the peak due to molsidomine in the chromatogram obtained with reference solution (a) (0.3 per cent);

– *disregard limit*: 0.5 times the area of the peak due to molsidomine in the chromatogram obtained with reference solution (a) (0.05 per cent).

Heavy metals: maximum 20 ppm.

Prescribed solution. Dissolve 0.5 g in 20 ml of *ethanol (96 per cent) R*.

Test solution. 12 ml of the prescribed solution.

Reference solution. Mix 6 ml of lead standard solution (1 ppm Pb) (obtained by diluting *lead standard solution (100 ppm Pb) R* with *ethanol (96 per cent) R*) with 2 ml of the prescribed solution and 4 ml of *water R*.

Blank solution. Mix 10 ml of *ethanol (96 per cent) R* and 2 ml of the prescribed solution.

To each solution, add 2 ml of *buffer solution pH 3.5 R.* Mix and add to 1.2 ml of *thioacetamide reagent R.* Mix immediately. Filter the solutions through a membrane filter (pore size 0.45 µm) (*2.4.8*). Carry out the filtration slowly and uniformly, applying moderate and constant pressure to the piston. Compare the spots on the filters obtained with the different solutions. The test is invalid if the reference solution does not show a slight brown colour compared to the blank solution. The substance to be examined complies with the test if the brown colour of the spot resulting from the test solution is not more intense than that of the spot resulting from the reference solution.

Loss on drying (*2.2.32*): maximum 0.5 per cent, determined on 1.000 g by drying in an oven at 105 °C.

Sulphated ash (*2.4.14*): maximum 0.1 per cent, determined on 1.0 g.

ASSAY

Dissolve 0.200 g in a mixture of 5 ml of *acetic anhydride R* and 50 ml of *anhydrous acetic acid R.* Titrate with *0.1 M perchloric acid,* determining the end-point potentiometrically (*2.2.20*).

1 ml of *0.1 M perchloric acid* is equivalent to 24.22 mg of $C_9H_{14}N_4O_4$.

STORAGE

Protected from light.

IMPURITIES

Specified impurities: B, E.

Other detectable impurities (the following substances would, if present at a sufficient level, be detected by one or other of the tests in the monograph. They are limited by the general acceptance criterion for other/unspecified impurities and/or by the general monograph *Substances for pharmaceutical use (2034).* It is therefore not necessary to identify these impurities for demonstration of compliance. See also *5.10. Control of impurities in substances for pharmaceutical use*)*: A, C, D.*

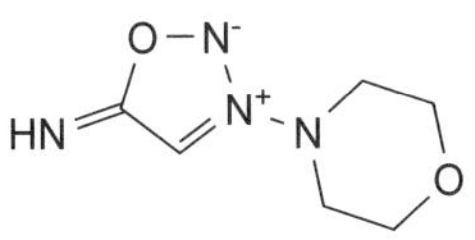

A. 3-(morpholin-4-yl)sydnonimine (linsidomine),

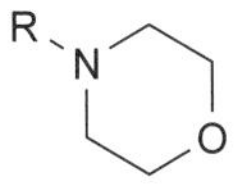

B. R = NO: 4-nitrosomorpholine,

D. R = CHO: morpholine-4-carbaldehyde,

E. R = H: morpholine,

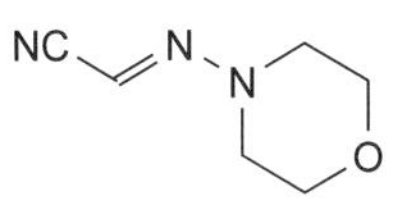

C. (2*E*)-(morpholin-4-ylimino)acetonitrile.

04/2008:0097

MORPHINE HYDROCHLORIDE

Morphini hydrochloridum

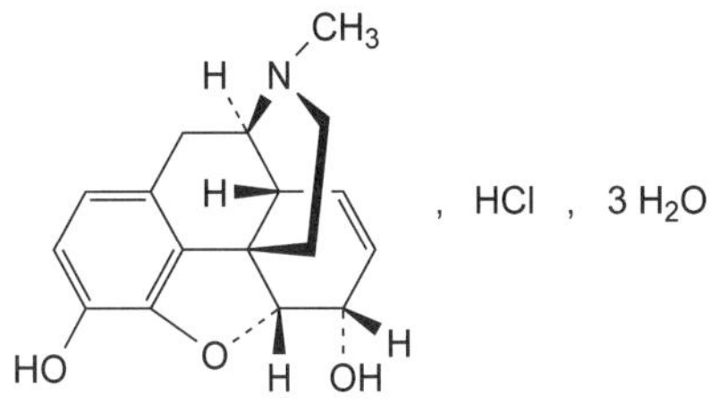

$C_{17}H_{20}ClNO_3,3H_2O$ M_r 375.8

[6055-06-7]

DEFINITION

7,8-Didehydro-4,5α-epoxy-17-methylmorphinan-3,6α-diol hydrochloride trihydrate.

Content: 98.0 per cent to 102.0 per cent (anhydrous substance).

CHARACTERS

Appearance: white or almost white, crystalline powder or colourless, silky needles or cubical masses, efflorescent in a dry atmosphere.

Solubility: soluble in water, slightly soluble in ethanol (96 per cent), practically insoluble in toluene.

IDENTIFICATION

First identification: A, E.

Second identification: B, C, D, E.

A. Infrared absorption spectrophotometry (*2.2.24*).

Comparison: *morphine hydrochloride CRS.*

B. Ultraviolet and visible absorption spectrophotometry (*2.2.25*).

Solution A. Dissolve 25.0 mg in *water R* and dilute to 25.0 ml with the same solvent.

Test solution (a). Dilute 10.0 ml of solution A to 100.0 ml with *water R.*

Test solution (b). Dilute 10.0 ml of solution A to 100.0 ml with *0.1 M sodium hydroxide.*

Spectral range: 250-350 nm for test solutions (a) and (b).

Absorption maximum: at 285 nm for test solution (a); at 298 nm for test solution (b).

Specific absorbance at the absorption maximum: 37 to 43 for test solution (a); 64 to 72 for test solution (b).

C. To about 1 mg of powdered substance in a porcelain dish add 0.5 ml of *sulphuric acid-formaldehyde reagent R.* A purple colour develops and becomes violet.

D. It gives the reaction of alkaloids (*2.3.1*).

E. It gives reaction (a) of chlorides (*2.3.1*).

TESTS

Solution S. Dissolve 0.500 g in *carbon dioxide-free water R* and dilute to 25.0 ml with the same solvent.

Appearance of solution. Solution S is clear (*2.2.1*) and not more intensely coloured than reference solution Y_6 or BY_6 (*2.2.2, Method II*).

Acidity or alkalinity. To 10 ml of solution S add 0.05 ml of *methyl red solution R*. Not more than 0.2 ml of *0.02 M sodium hydroxide* or *0.02 M hydrochloric acid* is required to change the colour of the indicator.

Specific optical rotation (*2.2.7*): – 110 to – 115 (anhydrous substance), determined on solution S.

Related substances. Liquid chromatography (*2.2.29*).

Test solution. Dissolve 0.125 g of the substance to be examined in a 1 per cent *V/V* solution of *acetic acid R* and dilute to 50 ml with the same solution.

Reference solution (a). Dilute 1.0 ml of the test solution to 100.0 ml with a 1 per cent *V/V* solution of *acetic acid R*. Dilute 2.0 ml of this solution to 10.0 ml with a 1 per cent *V/V* solution of *acetic acid R*.

Reference solution (b). Dissolve 5 mg of *morphine for system suitability CRS* (containing impurities B, C, E and F) in a 1 per cent *V/V* solution of *acetic acid R* and dilute to 2 ml with the same solution.

Column:
- *size*: l = 0.15 m, Ø = 4.6 mm;
- *stationary phase*: *end-capped octadecylsilyl silica gel for chromatography R* (5 μm);
- *temperature*: 35 °C.

Mobile phase:
- *mobile phase A*: 1.01 g/l solution of *sodium heptanesulphonate R* adjusted to pH 2.6 with a 50 per cent *V/V* solution of *phosphoric acid R*;
- *mobile phase B*: *methanol R*;

Time (min)	Mobile phase A (per cent *V/V*)	Mobile phase B (per cent *V/V*)
0 - 2	85	15
2 - 35	85 → 50	15 → 50
35 - 40	50	50

Flow rate: 1.5 ml/min.

Detection: spectrophotometer at 230 nm.

Injection: 10 μl.

Identification of impurities: use the chromatogram supplied with *morphine for system suitability CRS* and the chromatogram obtained with reference solution (b) to identify the peaks due to impurities B, C, E and F.

Relative retention with reference to morphine (retention time = about 12.5 min): impurity F = about 0.95; impurity E = about 1.1; impurity C = about 1.6; impurity B = about 1.9.

System suitability: reference solution (b):
- *peak-to-valley ratio*: minimum 2, where H_p = height above the baseline of the peak due to impurity F and H_v = height above the baseline of the lowest point of the curve separating this peak from the peak due to morphine.

Limits:
- *correction factors*: for the calculation of content, multiply the peak areas of the following impurities by the corresponding correction factor: impurity B = 0.25; impurity C = 0.4; impurity E = 0.5;
- *impurity B*: not more than twice the area of the principal peak in the chromatogram obtained with reference solution (a) (0.4 per cent);
- *impurities C, E*: for each impurity, not more than the area of the principal peak in the chromatogram obtained with reference solution (a) (0.2 per cent);
- *any other impurity*: for each impurity, not more than the area of the principal peak in the chromatogram obtained with reference solution (a) (0.2 per cent);
- *total*: not more than 5 times the area of the principal peak in the chromatogram obtained with reference solution (a) (1.0 per cent);
- *disregard limit*: 0.25 times the area of the principal peak in the chromatogram obtained with reference solution (a) (0.05 per cent).

The thresholds indicated under Related substances (Table 2034.-1) in the general monograph *Substances for pharmaceutical use (2034)* do not apply.

Water (*2.5.12*): 12.5 per cent to 15.5 per cent, determined on 0.10 g.

Sulphated ash (*2.4.14*): maximum 0.1 per cent, determined on 1.0 g.

ASSAY

Dissolve 0.300 g in a mixture of 5 ml of *0.01 M hydrochloric acid* and 30 ml of *ethanol (96 per cent) R*. Carry out a potentiometric titration (*2.2.20*), using *0.1 M sodium hydroxide*. Read the volume added between the 2 points of inflexion.

1 ml of *0.1 M sodium hydroxide* is equivalent to 32.18 mg of $C_{17}H_{20}ClNO_3$.

STORAGE

Protected from light.

IMPURITIES

Specified impurities: B, C, E.

Other detectable impurities (the following substances would, if present at a sufficient level, be detected by one or other of the tests in the monograph. They are limited by the general acceptance criterion for other/unspecified impurities and/or by the general monograph *Substances for pharmaceutical use (2034)*. It is therefore not necessary to identify these impurities for demonstration of compliance. See also *5.10. Control of impurities in substances for pharmaceutical use*): *A, D, F.*

A. codeine,

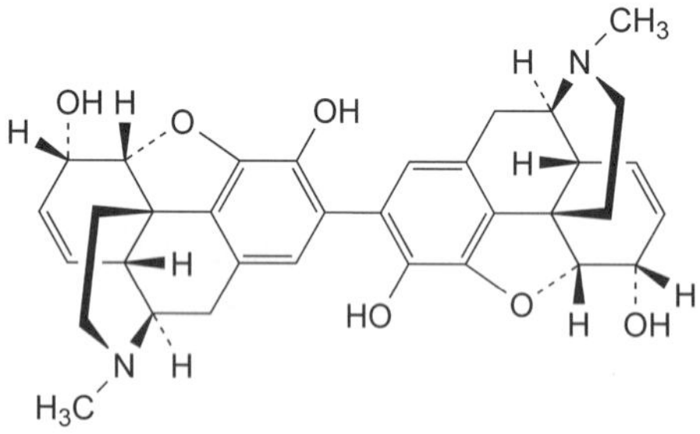

B. 7,7′,8,8′-tetradehydro-4,5α:4′,5′α-diepoxy-17,17′-dimethyl-2,2′-bimorphinanyl-3,3′,6α,6′α-tetrol (2,2′-bimorphine),

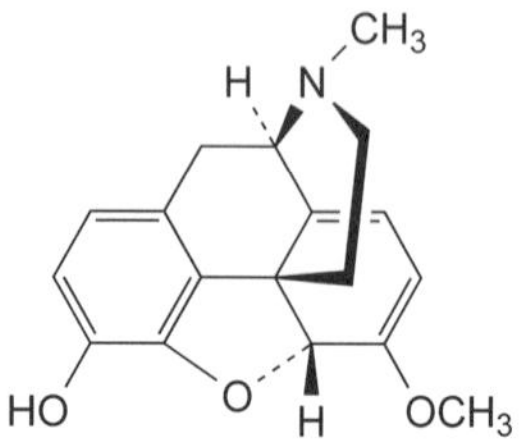

C. 6,7,8,14-tetradehydro-4,5α-epoxy-6-methoxy-17-methylmorphinan-3-ol (oripavine),

Monographs L-P

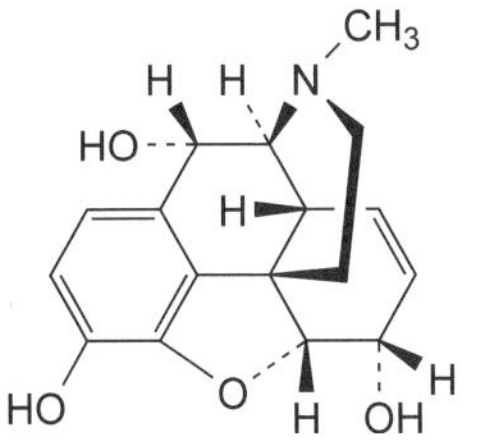

D. 7,8-didehydro-4,5α-epoxy-17-methylmorphinan-3,6α,10α-triol (10*S*-hydroxymorphine),

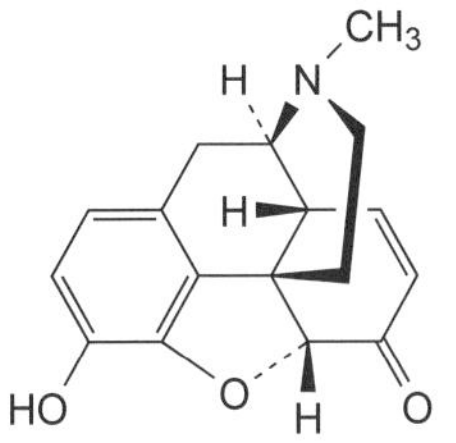

E. 7,8-didehydro-4,5α-epoxy-3-hydroxy-17-methylmorphinan-6-one (morphinone),

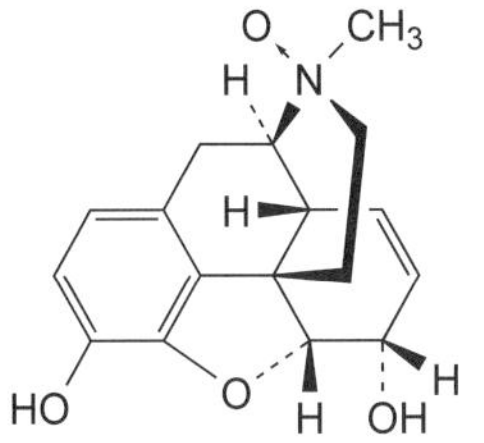

F. (17*S*)-7,8-didehydro-4,5α-epoxy-17-methylmorphinan-3,6α-diol 17-oxide (morphine *N*-oxide).

04/2008:1244

MORPHINE SULPHATE

Morphini sulfas

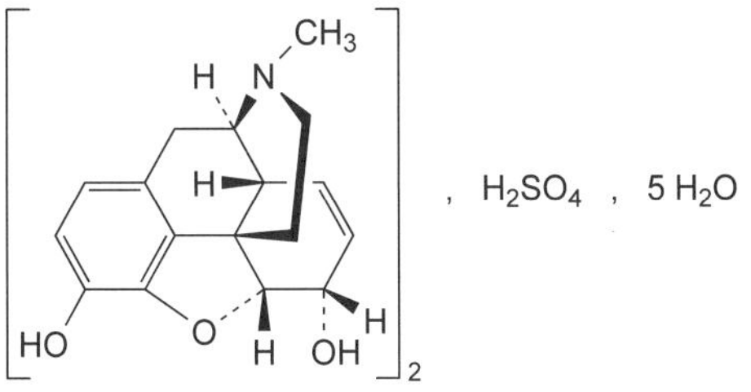

$C_{34}H_{40}N_2O_{10}S,5H_2O$ M_r 759
[6211-15-0]

DEFINITION

Di(7,8-didehydro-4,5α-epoxy-17-methylmorphinan-3,6α-diol) sulphate pentahydrate.

Content: 98.0 per cent to 102.0 per cent (anhydrous substance).

CHARACTERS

Appearance: white or almost white, crystalline powder.

Solubility: soluble in water, very slightly soluble in ethanol (96 per cent), practically insoluble in toluene.

IDENTIFICATION

First identification: A, E.

Second identification: B, C, D, E.

A. Infrared absorption spectrophotometry (*2.2.24*).

Preparation: dissolve 20 mg in 1 ml of *water R*, add 0.05 ml of *1 M sodium hydroxide* and shake. A precipitate is formed. Filter, wash with 2 quantities, each of 0.5 ml, of *water R* and dry the precipitate at 145 °C for 1 h. Prepare discs using the dried precipitate.

Comparison: repeat the operations using 20 mg of *morphine sulphate CRS*.

B. Ultraviolet and visible absorption spectrophotometry (*2.2.25*).

Solution A. Dissolve 25.0 mg in *water R* and dilute to 25.0 ml with the same solvent.

Test solution (a). Dilute 10.0 ml of solution A to 100.0 ml with *water R*.

Test solution (b). Dilute 10.0 ml of solution A to 100.0 ml with *0.1 M sodium hydroxide*.

Spectral range: 250-350 nm for test solutions (a) and (b).

Absorption maximum: at 285 nm for test solution (a); at 298 nm for test solution (b).

Specific absorbance at the absorption maximum: 37 to 43 for test solution (a); 64 to 72 for test solution (b).

C. To about 1 mg of powdered substance in a porcelain dish add 0.5 ml of *sulphuric acid-formaldehyde reagent R*. A purple colour develops and becomes violet.

D. It gives the reaction of alkaloids (*2.3.1*).

E. It gives the reactions of sulphates (*2.3.1*).

TESTS

Solution S. Dissolve 0.500 g in *carbon dioxide-free water R* and dilute to 25.0 ml with the same solvent.

Appearance of solution. Solution S is clear (*2.2.1*) and not more intensely coloured than reference solution Y_6 or BY_6 (*2.2.2, Method II*).

Acidity or alkalinity. To 10 ml of solution S add 0.05 ml of *methyl red solution R*. Not more than 0.2 ml of *0.02 M sodium hydroxide* or *0.02 M hydrochloric acid* is required to change the colour of the indicator.

Specific optical rotation (*2.2.7*): – 107 to – 110 (anhydrous substance), determined on solution S.

Related substances. Liquid chromatography (*2.2.29*).

Test solution. Dissolve 0.125 g of the substance to be examined in a 1 per cent *V/V* solution of *acetic acid R* and dilute to 50 ml with the same solution.

Reference solution (a). Dilute 1.0 ml of the test solution to 100.0 ml with a 1 per cent *V/V* solution of *acetic acid R*. Dilute 2.0 ml of this solution to 10.0 ml with a 1 per cent *V/V* solution of *acetic acid R*.

Reference solution (b). Dissolve 5 mg of *morphine for system suitability CRS* (containing impurities B, C, E and F) in a 1 per cent *V/V* solution of *acetic acid R* and dilute to 2 ml with the same solution.

Column:

- *size*: *l* = 0.15 m, Ø = 4.6 mm;
- *stationary phase*: *end-capped octadecylsilyl silica gel for chromatography R* (5 μm);
- *temperature*: 35 °C.

Mobile phase:

- *mobile phase A*: 1.01 g/l solution of *sodium heptanesulphonate R* adjusted to pH 2.6 with a 50 per cent *V/V* solution of *phosphoric acid R*;
- *mobile phase B*: *methanol R*;

Monographs L-P

Time (min)	Mobile phase A (per cent *V/V*)	Mobile phase B (per cent *V/V*)
0 - 2	85	15
2 - 35	85 → 50	15 → 50
35 - 40	50	50

Flow rate: 1.5 ml/min.

Detection: spectrophotometer at 230 nm.

Injection: 10 μl.

Identification of impurities: use the chromatogram supplied with *morphine for system suitability CRS* and the chromatogram obtained with reference solution (b) to identify the peaks due to impurities B, C, E and F.

Relative retention with reference to morphine (retention time = about 12.5 min): impurity F = about 0.95; impurity E = about 1.1; impurity C = about 1.6; impurity B = about 1.9.

System suitability: reference solution (b):

- *peak-to-valley ratio*: minimum 2, where H_p = height above the baseline of the peak due to impurity F and H_v = height above the baseline of the lowest point of the curve separating this peak from the peak due to morphine.

Limits:

- *correction factors*: for the calculation of content, multiply the peak areas of the following impurities by the corresponding correction factor: impurity B = 0.25; impurity C = 0.4; impurity E = 0.5;
- *impurity B*: not more than twice the area of the principal peak in the chromatogram obtained with reference solution (a) (0.4 per cent);
- *impurities C, E*: for each impurity, not more than the area of the principal peak in the chromatogram obtained with reference solution (a) (0.2 per cent);
- *any other impurity*: for each impurity, not more than the area of the principal peak in the chromatogram obtained with reference solution (a) (0.2 per cent);
- *total*: not more than 5 times the area of the principal peak in the chromatogram obtained with reference solution (a) (1.0 per cent);
- *disregard limit*: 0.25 times the area of the principal peak in the chromatogram obtained with reference solution (a) (0.05 per cent).

The thresholds indicated under Related substances (Table 2034.-1) in the general monograph *Substances for pharmaceutical use (2034)* do not apply.

Iron (*2.4.9*): maximum 5 ppm.

Dissolve the residue from the test for sulphated ash in *water R* and dilute to 10.0 ml with the same solvent.

Water (*2.5.12*): 10.4 per cent to 13.4 per cent, determined on 0.10 g.

Sulphated ash (*2.4.14*): maximum 0.1 per cent, determined on 1.0 g.

ASSAY

Dissolve 0.500 g in 120 ml of *anhydrous acetic acid R*. Titrate with *0.1 M perchloric acid*, determining the end-point potentiometrically (*2.2.20*).

1 ml of *0.1 M perchloric acid* is equivalent to 66.88 mg of $C_{34}H_{40}N_2O_{10}S$.

STORAGE

Protected from light.

IMPURITIES

Specified impurities: B, C, E.

Other detectable impurities (the following substances would, if present at a sufficient level, be detected by one or other of the tests in the monograph. They are limited by the general acceptance criterion for other/unspecified impurities and/or by the general monograph *Substances for pharmaceutical use (2034)*. It is therefore not necessary to identify these impurities for demonstration of compliance. See also *5.10. Control of impurities in substances for pharmaceutical use*): *A, D, F.*

A. codeine,

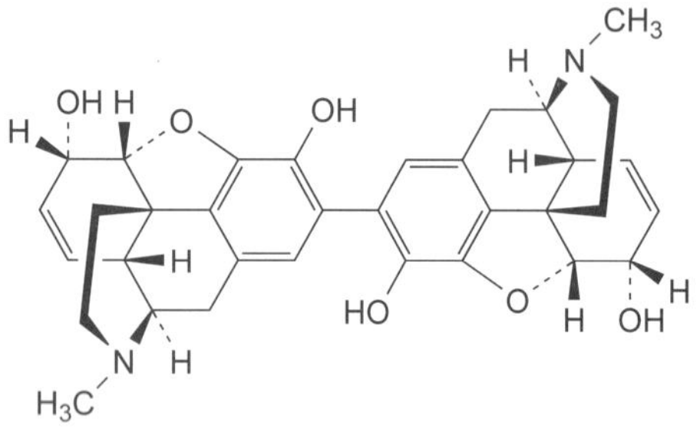

B. 7,7′,8,8′-tetradehydro-4,5α:4′,5′α-diepoxy-17,17′-dimethyl-2,2′-bimorphinanyl-3,3′,6α,6′α-tetrol (2,2′-bimorphine),

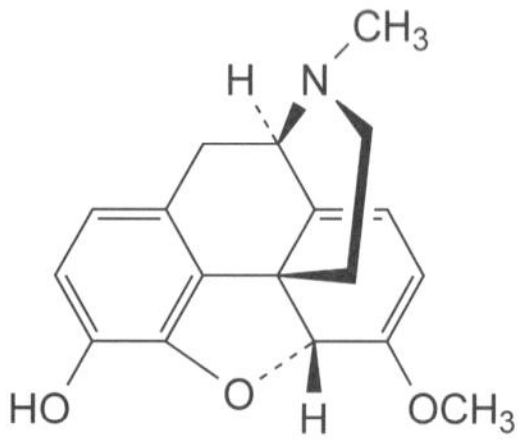

C. 6,7,8,14-tetradehydro-4,5α-epoxy-6-methoxy-17-methylmorphinan-3-ol (oripavine),

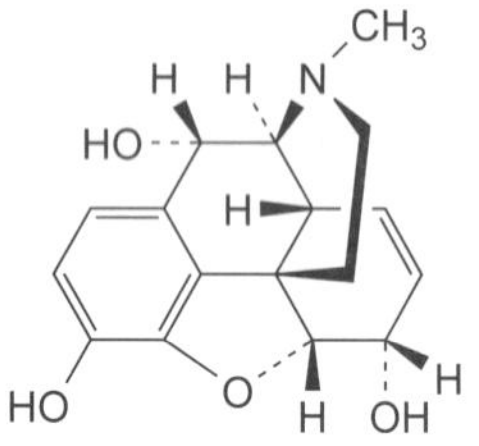

D. 7,8-didehydro-4,5α-epoxy-17-methylmorphinan-3,6α,10α-triol (10*S*-hydroxymorphine),

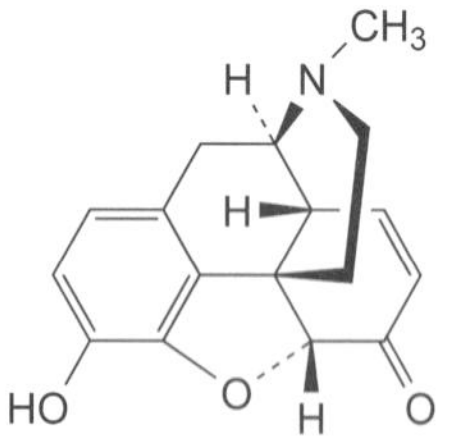

E. 7,8-didehydro-4,5α-epoxy-3-hydroxy-17-methylmorphinan-6-one (morphinone),

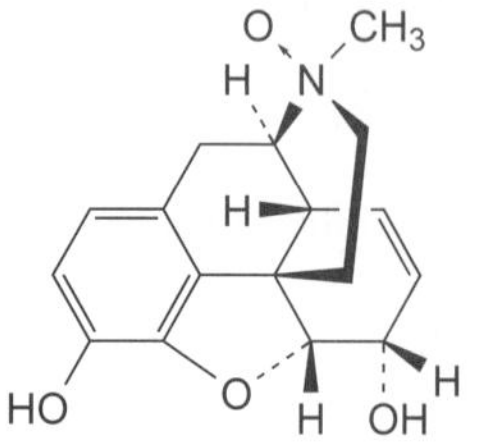

F. (17*S*)-7,8-didehydro-4,5α-epoxy-17-methylmorphinan-3,6α-diol 17-oxide (morphine *N*-oxide).

N

01/2008:1702
corrected 6.1

NAPROXEN SODIUM

Naproxenum natricum

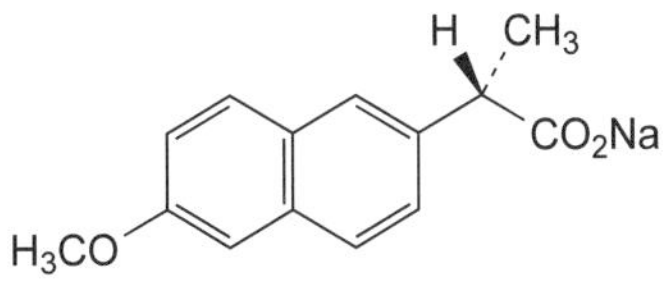

$C_{14}H_{13}O_3Na$ M_r 252.2

DEFINITION

Sodium (2*S*)-2-(6-methoxynaphthalen-2-yl)propanoate.

Content: 98.0 per cent to 101.0 per cent (dried substance).

CHARACTERS

Appearance: white or almost white, hygroscopic, crystalline powder.

Solubility: freely soluble in water, freely soluble or soluble in methanol, sparingly soluble in ethanol (96 per cent).

IDENTIFICATION

First identification: A, C, D.

Second identification: A, B, D.

A. Specific optical rotation (*2.2.7*): – 14.7 to – 17.0 (dried substance).

Dissolve 0.50 g in a 4.2 g/l solution of *sodium hydroxide R* and dilute to 25.0 ml with the same solution.

B. Ultraviolet and visible absorption spectrophotometry (*2.2.25*).

Test solution. Dissolve 40.0 mg in *methanol R* and dilute to 100.0 ml with the same solvent. Dilute 10.0 ml of this solution to 100.0 ml with *methanol R*.

Spectral range: 230-350 nm.

Absorption maxima: at 262 nm, 271 nm, 316 nm and 331 nm.

Specific absorbance at the absorption maxima:

- at 262 nm: 207 to 227;
- at 271 nm: 200 to 220;
- at 316 nm: 56 to 68;
- at 331 nm: 72 to 84.

C. Infrared absorption spectrophotometry (*2.2.24*).

Preparation. Dissolve 50 mg in 5 ml of *water R*. Add 1 ml of *dilute sulphuric acid R* and 5 ml of *ethyl acetate R*. Shake vigorously. Allow the 2 layers to separate. Evaporate the upper layer to dryness and subsequently dry at 60 °C for 15 min. Record the spectrum using the residue.

Comparison: *naproxen CRS*.

D. It gives reaction (a) of sodium (*2.3.1*).

TESTS

Appearance of solution. The solution is clear (*2.2.1*) and not more intensely coloured than reference solution BY_7 (*2.2.2, Method II*).

Dissolve 1.25 g in *water R* and dilute to 25 ml with the same solvent.

pH (*2.2.3*): 7.0 to 9.8.

Dissolve 0.5 g in *carbon dioxide-free water R* and dilute to 25 ml with the same solvent.

Enantiomeric purity. Liquid chromatography (*2.2.29*). *Protect the solutions from light.*

Test solution. Dissolve 25.0 mg of the substance to be examined in 15 ml of *water R* and add 1 ml of *hydrochloric acid R*. Shake with 2 quantities, each of 10 ml, of *ethyl acetate R*, combine the upper layers and evaporate to dryness under reduced pressure. Dissolve the residue in 50.0 ml of *tetrahydrofuran R*. Dilute 2.0 ml of this solution to 20.0 ml with the mobile phase.

Reference solution (a). Dilute 2.5 ml of the test solution to 100.0 ml with the mobile phase.

Reference solution (b). Dissolve 5 mg of *racemic naproxen CRS* in 10 ml of *tetrahydrofuran R* and dilute to 100 ml with the mobile phase.

Column:

- *size*: *l* = 0.25 m, Ø = 4.6 mm;
- *stationary phase*: *silica gel π-acceptor/π-donor for chiral separations R* (5 µm) (*S,S*);
- *temperature*: 25 °C.

Mobile phase: *glacial acetic acid R, acetonitrile R, 2-propanol R, hexane R* (5:50:100:845 *V/V/V/V*).

Flow rate: 2 ml/min.

Detection: spectrophotometer at 263 nm.

Injection: 20 µl.

Run time: 1.5 times the retention time of naproxen (retention time = about 5 min).

System suitability: reference solution (b):

- *resolution*: minimum 3 between the peaks due to impurity G and naproxen.

Limit:

- *impurity G*: not more than the area of the principal peak in the chromatogram obtained with reference solution (a) (2.5 per cent).

Related substances. Liquid chromatography (*2.2.29*). *Protect the solutions from light.*

Test solution. Dissolve 12 mg of the substance to be examined in the mobile phase and dilute to 20 ml with the mobile phase.

Reference solution (a). Dilute 1.0 ml of the test solution to 50.0 ml with the mobile phase. Dilute 1.0 ml of this solution to 20.0 ml with the mobile phase.

Reference solution (b). Dissolve 6 mg of *bromomethoxynaphthalene R* (impurity N), 6.0 mg of *naproxen impurity L CRS* and 6 mg of *(1RS)-1-(6-methoxynaphthalen-2-yl)ethanol R* (impurity K) in *acetonitrile R* and dilute to 10 ml with the same solvent. To 1 ml of the solution add 1 ml of the test solution and dilute to 50 ml with the mobile phase. Dilute 1 ml of this solution to 20 ml with the mobile phase.

Column:

- *size*: *l* = 0.10 m, Ø = 4.0 mm;
- *stationary phase*: *octadecylsilyl silica gel for chromatography R* (3 µm);
- *temperature*: 50 °C.

Mobile phase: mix 42 volumes of *acetonitrile R* and 58 volumes of a 1.36 g/l solution of *potassium dihydrogen phosphate R* previously adjusted to pH 2.0 with *phosphoric acid R*.

Flow rate: 1.5 ml/min.

Detection: spectrophotometer at 230 nm.

Injection: 20 µl.

Run time: 1.5 times the retention time of impurity N.

Monographs L-P

Relative retention with reference to naproxen (retention time = about 2.5 min): impurity K = about 0.9; impurity L = about 1.4; impurity N = about 5.3.

System suitability: reference solution (b):

– *resolution*: minimum 2.2 between the peaks due to impurity K and naproxen.

Limits:

– *impurity L*: not more than the area of the corresponding peak in the chromatogram obtained with reference solution (b) (0.1 per cent);
– *unspecified impurities*: for each impurity, not more than the area of the principal peak in the chromatogram obtained with reference solution (a) (0.10 per cent);
– *total*: not more than 3 times the area of the principal peak in the chromatogram obtained with reference solution (a) (0.3 per cent);
– *disregard limit*: 0.5 times the area of the principal peak in the chromatogram obtained with reference solution (a) (0.05 per cent).

Heavy metals (*2.4.8*): maximum 20 ppm.

Dissolve 2.0 g in 20.0 ml of *water R*. 12 ml of the solution complies with test A. Prepare the reference solution using 2 ml of *lead standard solution (10 ppm Pb) R*.

After the addition of *buffer solution pH 3.5 R*, the substance precipitates. Dilute each solution to 40 ml with *anhydrous ethanol R*: the substance dissolves completely. Proceed as described in the test, filtering the solutions to evaluate the result.

Loss on drying (*2.2.32*): maximum 1.0 per cent, determined on 1.000 g by drying in an oven at 105 °C for 3 h.

ASSAY

Dissolve 0.200 g in 50 ml of *anhydrous acetic acid R*. Titrate with *0.1 M perchloric acid*, determining the end-point potentiometrically (*2.2.20*).

1 ml of *0.1 M perchloric acid* is equivalent to 25.22 mg of $C_{14}H_{13}O_3Na$.

STORAGE

In an airtight container, protected from light.

IMPURITIES

Specified impurities: G, L.

Other detectable impurities (the following substances would, if present at a sufficient level, be detected by one or other of the tests in the monograph. They are limited by the general acceptance criterion for other/unspecified impurities and/or by the general monograph *Substances for pharmaceutical use (2034)*. It is therefore not necessary to identify these impurities for demonstration of compliance. See also *5.10. Control of impurities in substances for pharmaceutical use*): *A, B, C, D, E, F, H, I, J, K, M, N.*

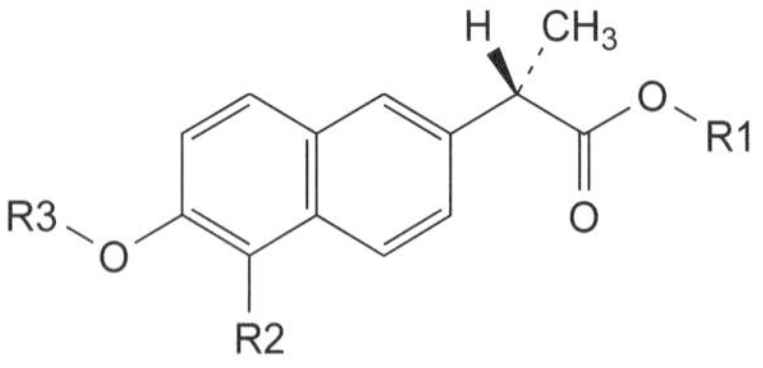

A. R1 = R2 = R3 = H: (2*S*)-2-(6-hydroxynaphthalen-2-yl)propanoic acid,

B. R1 = H, R2 = Cl, R3 = CH_3: (2*S*)-2-(5-chloro-6-methoxynaphthalen-2-yl)propanoic acid,

C. R1 = H, R2 = Br, R3 = CH_3: (2*S*)-2-(5-bromo-6-methoxynaphthalen-2-yl)propanoic acid,

D. R1 = H, R2 = I, R3 = CH_3: (2*S*)-2-(5-iodo-6-methoxynaphthalen-2-yl)propanoic acid,

E. R1 = R3 = CH_3, R2 = H: methyl (2*S*)-2-(6-methoxynaphthalen-2-yl)propanoate,

F. R1 = C_2H_5, R2 = H, R3 = CH_3: ethyl (2*S*)-2-(6-methoxynaphthalen-2-yl)propanoate,

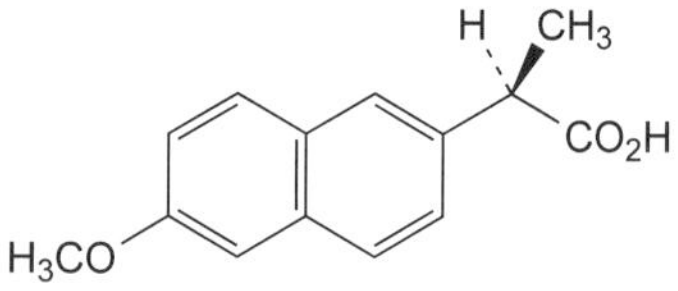

G. (2*R*)-2-(6-methoxynaphthalen-2-yl)propanoic acid,

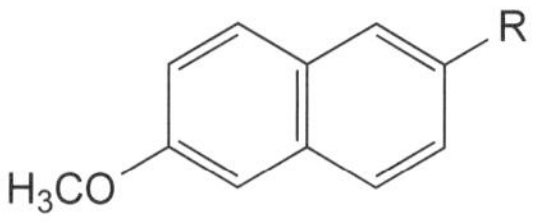

H. R = OH: 6-methoxynaphthalen-2-ol,

I. R = CH_2-CO_2H: (6-methoxynaphthalen-2-yl)acetic acid,

J. R = C_2H_5: 2-ethyl-6-methoxynaphthalene,

K. R = CHOH-CH_3: (1*RS*)-1-(6-methoxynaphthalen-2-yl)ethanol,

L. R = CO-CH_3: 1-(6-methoxynaphthalen-2-yl)ethanone,

M. R = H: 2-methoxynaphthalene (nerolin),

N. R = Br: 2-bromo-6-methoxynaphthalene.

04/2008:2115

NIFLUMIC ACID

Acidum niflumicum

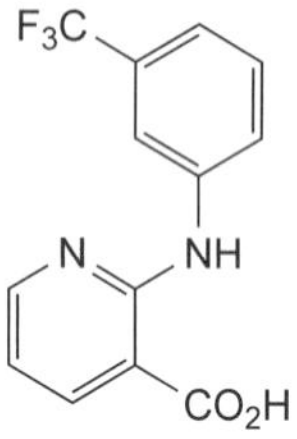

$C_{13}H_9F_3N_2O_2$ M_r 282.2
[4394-00-7]

DEFINITION

2-[[3-(Trifluoromethyl)phenyl]amino]pyridine-3-carboxylic acid.

Content: 98.5 per cent to 101.5 per cent (dried substance).

CHARACTERS

Appearance: pale yellow, crystalline powder.

Solubility: practically insoluble in water, freely soluble in acetone, soluble in ethanol (96 per cent) and in methanol.

mp: about 204 °C.

IDENTIFICATION

Infrared absorption spectrophotometry (*2.2.24*).

Comparison: *niflumic acid CRS*.

TESTS

Impurity C. Thin-layer chromatography (*2.2.27*).

Test solution. Dissolve 0.50 g of the substance to be examined in 5 ml of *methanol R* and dilute to 10.0 ml with the same solvent.

Reference solution. Dissolve 25 mg of *3-trifluoromethyl-aniline R* (impurity C) in 20 ml of *methanol R* and dilute to 100 ml with the same solvent. Dilute 1.0 ml of this solution to 100 ml with *methanol R.*

Plate: *TLC silica gel F_{254} plate R.*

Mobile phase: *acetic acid R, ethyl acetate R, toluene R* (5:25:90 *V/V/V*).

Application: 10 µl.

Development: over 3/4 of the plate.

Drying: in air, until the solvents have evaporated.

Detection: spray with *4-dimethylaminocinnamaldehyde solution R* and heat at 60 °C for 10 min.

Limit:

– *impurity C*: any spot due to impurity C is not more intense than the principal spot in the chromatogram obtained with the reference solution (50 ppm).

Related substances. Liquid chromatography (*2.2.29*).

Test solution. Dissolve 20.0 mg of the substance to be examined in 10 ml of *acetonitrile R* and dilute to 20.0 ml with *water R.*

Reference solution. Dissolve 5.0 mg of *niflumic acid impurity A CRS,* 5.0 mg of *niflumic acid impurity B CRS* and 6.0 mg of *niflumic acid impurity E CRS* in 20 ml of *acetonitrile R,* add 5.0 ml of the test solution and dilute to 50.0 ml with *water R.* Dilute 1.0 ml of this solution to 100.0 ml with a mixture of equal volumes of *acetonitrile R* and *water R.*

Column:

– *size*: *l* = 0.125 m, Ø = 4.0 mm;

– *stationary phase*: *octylsilyl silica gel for chromatography R* (5 µm);

– *temperature*: 25 °C.

Mobile phase: *phosphoric acid R, acetonitrile R, water R* (2.5:500:500 *V/V/V*).

Flow rate: 1.0 ml/min.

Detection: spectrophotometer at 267 nm.

Injection: 10 µl.

Run time: 4 times the retention time of niflumic acid.

Relative retention with reference to niflumic acid (retention time = about 5.5 min): impurity A = about 0.25; impurity B = about 0.57; impurity E = about 0.64.

System suitability: reference solution:

– *resolution*: minimum 1.5 between the peaks due to impurities B and E.

Limits:

– *impurity B*: not more than 4 times the area of the corresponding peak in the chromatogram obtained with the reference solution (0.4 per cent);

– *impurity A*: not more than the area of the corresponding peak in the chromatogram obtained with the reference solution (0.1 per cent);

– *unspecified impurities*: for each impurity, not more than the area of the peak due to niflumic acid in the chromatogram obtained with the reference solution (0.10 per cent);

– *sum of impurities other than B*: not more than twice the area of the peak due to niflumic acid in the chromatogram obtained with the reference solution (0.2 per cent);

– *disregard limit*: 0.5 times the area of the peak due to niflumic acid in the chromatogram obtained with the reference solution (0.05 per cent).

Chlorides (*2.4.4*): maximum 200 ppm.

Dissolve 0.5 g in a mixture of 1 ml of *nitric acid R* and 10 ml of *methanol R,* and dilute to 20 ml with *water R.* To 10 ml of this solution add 5 ml of *water R.*

Phosphates (*2.4.11*): maximum 100 ppm.

Dilute 1.0 ml of the solution prepared in the test for heavy metals to 100 ml with *water R.*

Heavy metals (*2.4.8*): maximum 10 ppm.

2.0 g complies with test C. Prepare the reference solution using 2 ml of *lead standard solution (10 ppm Pb) R.*

Loss on drying (*2.2.32*): maximum 0.3 per cent, determined on 2.000 g by drying in an oven at 105 °C.

Sulphated ash (*2.4.14*): maximum 0.1 per cent, determined on 1.0 g in a platinum crucible.

ASSAY

Dissolve 0.200 g in a mixture of 10 ml of *water R* and 40 ml of *ethanol (96 per cent) R.* Titrate with *0.1 M sodium hydroxide,* determining the end-point potentiometrically (*2.2.20*).

1 ml of *0.1 M sodium hydroxide* is equivalent to 28.22 mg of $C_{13}H_9F_3N_2O_2$.

IMPURITIES

Specified impurities: A, B, C.

Other detectable impurities (the following substances would, if present at a sufficient level, be detected by one or other of the tests in the monograph. They are limited by the general acceptance criterion for other/unspecified impurities and/or by the general monograph *Substances for pharmaceutical use (2034).* It is therefore not necessary to identify these impurities for demonstration of compliance. See also *5.10. Control of impurities in substances for pharmaceutical use*): *E, F.*

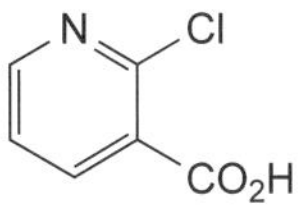

A. 2-chloropyridine-3-carboxylic acid,

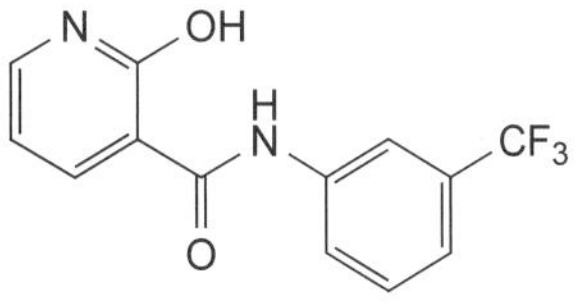

B. 2-hydroxy-*N*-[3-(trifluoromethyl)phenyl]pyridine-3-carboxamide,

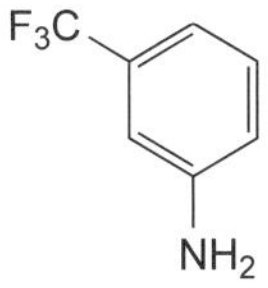

C. 3-(trifluoromethyl)aniline,

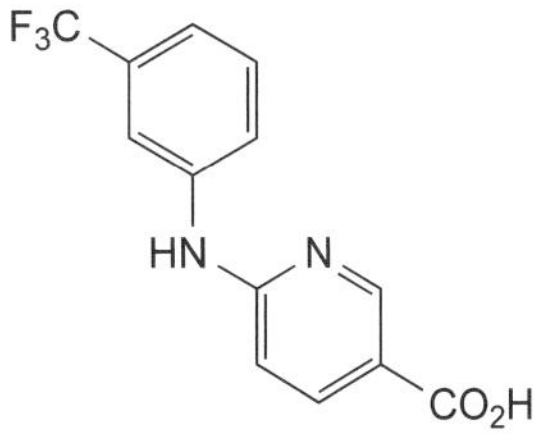

E. 6-[[3-(trifluoromethyl)phenyl]amino]pyridine-3-carboxylic acid,

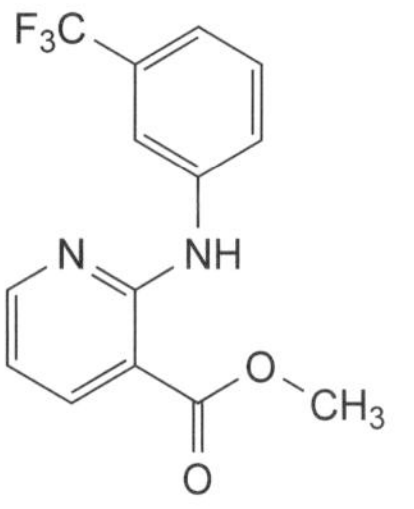

F. methyl 2-[[3-(trifluoromethyl)phenyl]amino]pyridine-3-carboxylate.

04/2008:1999

NIFUROXAZIDE

Nifuroxazidum

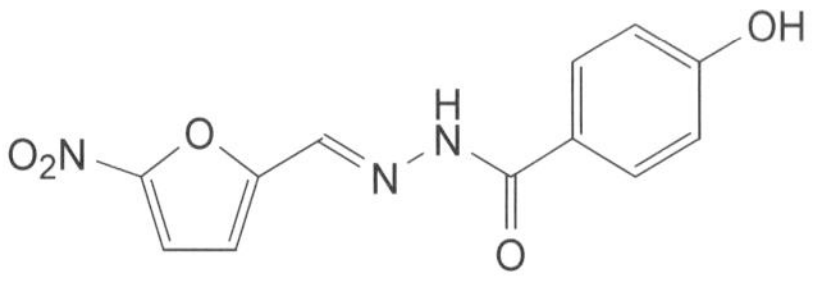

$C_{12}H_9N_3O_5$ M_r 275.2
[965-52-6]

DEFINITION

(*E*)-4-Hydroxy-*N*′-[(5-nitrofuran-2-yl)methylidene]-benzohydrazide.

Content: 98.5 per cent to 101.5 per cent (dried substance).

CHARACTERS

Appearance: bright yellow, crystalline powder.

Solubility: practically insoluble in water, slightly soluble in ethanol (96 per cent), practically insoluble in methylene chloride.

IDENTIFICATION

Infrared absorption spectrophotometry (*2.2.24*).

Comparison: *nifuroxazide CRS.*

TESTS

Specific absorbance (*2.2.25*): 940 to 1000 at the absorption maximum at 367 nm.

Protected from light, dissolve 10.0 mg in 10 ml of *ethylene glycol monomethyl ether R* and dilute to 100.0 ml with *methanol R*. Dilute 5.0 ml of this solution to 100.0 ml with *methanol R*.

Impurity A: maximum 0.05 per cent.

Test solution (a). Dissolve 1.0 g of the substance to be examined in *dimethyl sulphoxide R* and dilute to 10.0 ml with the same solvent.

Test solution (b). To 5.5 ml of test solution (a) add 50.0 ml of *water R* while stirring. Allow to stand for 15 min and filter.

Reference solution. To 0.5 ml of test solution (a) add 5.0 ml of a 50 mg/l solution of *4-hydroxybenzohydrazide R* (impurity A) in *dimethyl sulphoxide R*. Add 50.0 ml of *water R* while stirring. Allow to stand for 15 min and filter.

Add 0.5 ml of *phosphomolybdotungstic reagent R* and 10.0 ml of *sodium carbonate solution R* separately to 10.0 ml of test solution (b) and to 10.0 ml of the reference solution. Allow to stand for 1 h. Examine the 2 solutions at 750 nm. The absorbance (*2.2.25*) of the solution obtained with test solution (b) is not greater than that obtained with the reference solution.

Related substances. Liquid chromatography (*2.2.29*). *Use amber volumetric flasks, unless otherwise specified.*

Solvent mixture: *acetonitrile R, water R* (40:60 *V/V*).

Test solution. Dissolve 10.0 mg of the substance to be examined in the solvent mixture, using sonication for not more than 5 min, and dilute to 100.0 ml with the solvent mixture.

Reference solution (a). Dilute 1.0 ml of the test solution to 100.0 ml with the solvent mixture. Dilute 1.0 ml of this solution to 10.0 ml with the solvent mixture.

Reference solution (b). In order to prepare impurity E *in situ*, dissolve 5 mg of the substance to be examined in the solvent mixture in a colourless volumetric flask, using sonication for 5 min, and dilute to 50 ml with the solvent mixture. Allow to stand in ambient light for 1 h.

Reference solution (c). Dissolve 5.0 mg of *methyl parahydroxybenzoate CRS* (impurity B) in the solvent mixture and dilute to 100.0 ml with the solvent mixture. Dilute 1.0 ml of this solution to 100.0 ml with the solvent mixture.

Column:

- *size*: *l* = 0.25 m, Ø = 4.6 mm;
- *stationary phase*: spherical *octadecylsilyl silica gel for chromatography R* (5 µm);
- *temperature*: 10 °C.

Mobile phase:

- *mobile phase A*: *tetrahydrofuran R, water R* (5:95 *V/V*);
- *mobile phase B*: *acetonitrile R*;

Time (min)	Mobile phase A (per cent *V/V*)	Mobile phase B (per cent *V/V*)
0 - 10	67	33
10 - 30	67 → 43	33 → 57

Flow rate: 1.0 ml/min.

Detection: spectrophotometer at 280 nm.

Injection: 50 µl.

Relative retention with reference to nifuroxazide (retention time = about 8 min): impurity A (keto-enol tautomers) = about 0.36 and 0.39; impurity E = about 0.9; impurity B = about 1.2; impurity C = about 2.6; impurity D = about 3.4.

System suitability: reference solution (b):

- *resolution*: minimum 2.0 between the peaks due to impurity E and nifuroxazide.

Limits:

- *impurity E*: not more than 3 times the area of the principal peak in the chromatogram obtained with reference solution (a) (0.3 per cent);
- *impurities B, C, D*: for each impurity, not more than 0.6 times the area of the principal peak in the chromatogram obtained with reference solution (c) (0.3 per cent), and not more than 1 such peak has an area greater than 0.2 times the area of the principal peak in the chromatogram obtained with reference solution (c) (0.1 per cent);
- *unspecified impurities*: for each impurity, not more than the area of the principal peak in the chromatogram obtained with reference solution (a) (0.10 per cent);

- *sum of impurities other than E*: not more than the area of the principal peak in the chromatogram obtained with reference solution (c) (0.5 per cent);
- *disregard limit*: 0.1 times the area of the principal peak in the chromatogram obtained with reference solution (c) (0.05 per cent); disregard the peaks due to impurity A.

Heavy metals (*2.4.8*): maximum 20 ppm.

1.0 g complies with test D. Prepare the reference solution using 2 ml of *lead standard solution (10 ppm Pb) R*.

Loss on drying (*2.2.32*): maximum 0.5 per cent, determined on 1.000 g by drying in an oven at 105 °C for 3 h.

Sulphated ash (*2.4.14*): maximum 0.1 per cent, determined on 1.0 g.

ASSAY

Dissolve 0.200 g, with heating if necessary, in 30 ml of *dimethylformamide R* and add 20 ml of *water R*. Titrate with *0.1 M sodium hydroxide*, determining the end-point potentiometrically (*2.2.20*).

1 ml of *0.1 M sodium hydroxide* is equivalent to 27.52 mg of $C_{12}H_9N_3O_5$.

STORAGE

Protected from light.

IMPURITIES

Specified impurities: A, B, C, D, E.

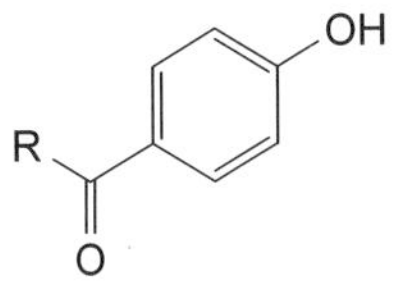

A. R = $NH\text{-}NH_2$: 4-hydroxybenzohydrazide (*p*-hydroxybenzohydrazide),

B. R = OCH_3: methyl 4-hydroxybenzoate (methyl parahydroxybenzoate),

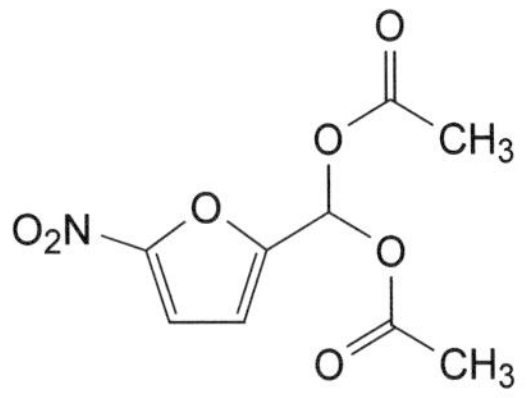

C. (5-nitrofuran-2-yl)methylidene diacetate,

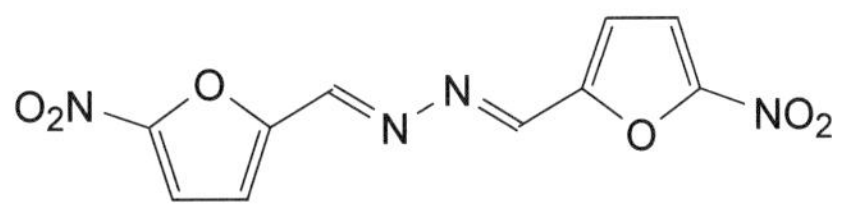

D. (*E,E*)-*N,N'*-bis[(5-nitrofuran-2-yl)methylidene]hydrazine (5-nitrofurfural azine),

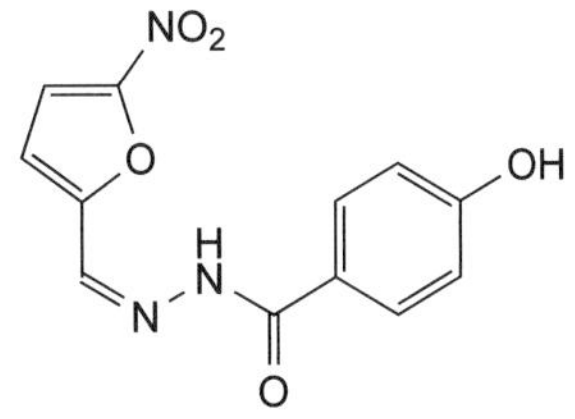

E. (*Z*)-4-hydroxy-*N'*-[(5-nitrofuran-2-yl)methylidene]-benzohydrazide.

Monographs L-P

P

01/2008:1794
corrected 6.1

PACLITAXEL

Paclitaxelum

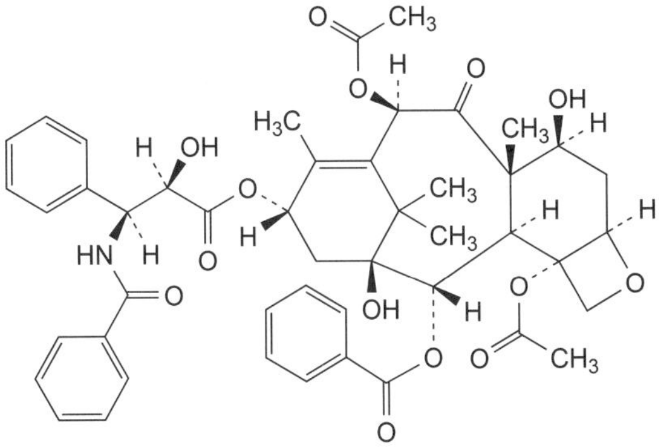

$C_{47}H_{51}NO_{14}$ M_r 854

DEFINITION

5β,20-Epoxy-1,7β-dihydroxy-9-oxotax-11-ene-2α,4,10β,13α-tetrayl 4,10-diacetate 2-benzoate 13-[(2*R*,3*S*)-3-(benzoylamino)-2-hydroxy-3-phenylpropanoate].

It is isolated from natural sources or produced by fermentation or by a semi-synthetic process.

Content: 97.0 per cent to 102.0 per cent (anhydrous substance).

CHARACTERS

Appearance: white or almost white, crystalline powder.

Solubility: practically insoluble in water, soluble in methanol and freely soluble in methylene chloride.

IDENTIFICATION

A. Specific optical rotation (see Tests).

B. Infrared absorption spectrophotometry (*2.2.24*).

Comparison: *paclitaxel CRS.*

If the spectra obtained in the solid state show differences, dissolve 10 mg of the substance to be examined and the reference substance separately in 0.4 ml of *methylene chloride R*, evaporate to dryness and record new spectra using the residues.

TESTS

Appearance of the solution. The solution is clear (*2.2.1*) and colourless (*2.2.2, Method II*).

Dissolve 0.1 g in 10 ml of *methanol R.*

Specific optical rotation (*2.2.7*): – 49.0 to – 55.0 (anhydrous substance).

Dissolve 0.250 g in *methanol R* and dilute to 25.0 ml with the same solvent.

Related substances. Liquid chromatography (*2.2.29*).

A. Paclitaxel isolated from natural sources or produced by fermentation.

Test solution (a). Dissolve 20.0 mg of the substance to be examined in *acetonitrile R* and dilute to 10.0 ml with the same solvent.

Test solution (b). Dilute 1.0 ml of test solution (a) to 20.0 ml with *acetonitrile R.*

Reference solution (a). Dilute 1.0 ml of test solution (a) to 10.0 ml with *acetonitrile R*. Dilute 1.0 ml of this solution to 100.0 ml with *acetonitrile R.*

Reference solution (b). Dissolve 5.0 mg of *paclitaxel CRS* in *acetonitrile R* and dilute to 5.0 ml with the same solvent. Dilute 2.0 ml of this solution to 20.0 ml with *acetonitrile R.*

Reference solution (c). Dissolve 2.0 mg of *paclitaxel impurity C CRS* in *acetonitrile R* and dilute to 20.0 ml with the same solvent.

Reference solution (d). Dilute 1.0 ml of reference solution (c) to 50.0 ml with *acetonitrile R.*

Reference solution (e). To 1 ml of reference solution (b) add 1 ml of reference solution (c).

Reference solution (f). Dissolve 5 mg of *paclitaxel natural for peak identification CRS* (containing impurities A, B, C, D, E, F, H, O, P, Q and R) in *acetonitrile R* and dilute to 5 ml with the same solvent.

Column:

- *size*: *l* = 0.25 m, Ø = 4.6 mm;
- *stationary phase*: *diisopropylcyanopropylsilyl silica gel for chromatography R* (5 μm) with a specific surface area of 180 m²/g and a pore size of 80 Å;
- *temperature*: 20 ± 1 °C.

Mobile phase:

- *mobile phase A*: *methanol R, water R* (200:800 *V/V*);
- *mobile phase B*: *methanol R, acetonitrile for chromatography R* (200:800 *V/V*);

Time (min)	Mobile phase A (per cent *V/V*)	Mobile phase B (per cent *V/V*)
0 - 60	85 → 56	15 → 44
60 - 61	56 → 85	44 → 15
61 - 75	85	15

Flow rate: 1.0 ml/min.

Detection: spectrophotometer at 227 nm.

Injection: 10 μl of test solution (a) and reference solutions (a), (d), (e) and (f).

Identification of impurities: use the chromatogram supplied with *paclitaxel natural for peak identification CRS* and the chromatogram obtained with reference solution (f) to identify the peaks due to impurities A, B, C, D, E, F, H, O, P, Q and R.

Relative retention with reference to paclitaxel (retention time = about 50 min): impurities A and B = about 0.90; impurity R = about 0.93; impurity H = about 0.96; impurities Q and P = about 1.02; impurity C = about 1.05; impurity D = about 1.07; impurities O and E = about 1.15; impurity F = about 1.20.

System suitability: reference solution (e):

- *resolution*: minimum 3.5 between the peaks due to paclitaxel and impurity C.

Monographs L-P

Limits:

- *sum of impurities A and B*: not more than 4 times the area of the principal peak in the chromatogram obtained with reference solution (a) (0.4 per cent);
- *impurity C*: not more than 3 times the area of the corresponding peak in the chromatogram obtained with reference solution (d) (0.3 per cent);
- *impurity D*: not more than twice the area of the principal peak in the chromatogram obtained with reference solution (a) (0.2 per cent);
- *sum of impurities E and O*: not more than 5 times the area of the principal peak in the chromatogram obtained with reference solution (a) (0.5 per cent);
- *impurity F*: not more than the area of the principal peak in the chromatogram obtained with reference solution (d) (0.1 per cent);
- *sum of impurities P and Q*: not more than twice the area of the principal peak in the chromatogram obtained with reference solution (a) (0.2 per cent);
- *impurity R*: not more than 5 times the area of the principal peak in the chromatogram obtained with reference solution (a) (0.5 per cent);
- *unspecified impurities*: for each impurity, not more than the area of the principal peak in the chromatogram obtained with reference solution (a) (0.10 per cent);
- *total*: not more than 15 times the area of the principal peak in the chromatogram obtained with reference solution (a) (1.5 per cent);
- *disregard limit*: 0.5 times the area of the principal peak in the chromatogram obtained with reference solution (a) (0.05 per cent).

B. Paclitaxel produced by a semi-synthetic process.

Test solution. Dissolve 10.0 mg of the substance to be examined in *acetonitrile R* and dilute to 10.0 ml with the same solvent.

Reference solution (a). Dilute 1.0 ml of the test solution to 10.0 ml with *acetonitrile R*. Dilute 1.0 ml of this solution to 100.0 ml with *acetonitrile R*.

Reference solution (b). Dissolve 5.0 mg of *paclitaxel CRS* in *acetonitrile R* and dilute to 5.0 ml with the same solvent.

Reference solution (c). Dissolve 5 mg of *paclitaxel semi-synthetic for peak identification CRS* (containing impurities A, G, I and L) in *acetonitrile R* and dilute to 5 ml with the same solvent.

Reference solution (d). Dissolve 5.0 mg of *paclitaxel semi-synthetic for system suitability CRS* (containing impurities E, H and N) in *acetonitrile R* and dilute to 5.0 ml with the same solvent.

Column:

- *size*: *l* = 0.15 m, Ø = 4.6 mm;
- *stationary phase*: *end-capped octadecylsilyl silica gel for chromatography R* (3 μm) with a specific surface area of 300 m²/g and a pore size of 120 Å;
- temperature: 35 °C.

Mobile phase:

- *mobile phase A*: *acetonitrile for chromatography R*, *water R* (400:600 *V/V*);
- *mobile phase B*: *acetonitrile for chromatography R*;

Time (min)	Mobile phase A (per cent *V/V*)	Mobile phase B (per cent *V/V*)
0 - 20	100	0
20 - 60	100 → 10	0 → 90
60 - 62	10 → 100	90 → 0
62 - 70	100	0

Flow rate: 1.2 ml/min.

Detection: spectrophotometer at 227 nm.

Injection: 15 μl of the test solution and reference solutions (a), (c) and (d).

Identification of impurities: use the chromatogram supplied with *paclitaxel semi-synthetic for peak identification CRS* and the chromatogram obtained with reference solution (c) to identify the peaks due to impurities A, G, I and L; use the chromatogram supplied with *paclitaxel semi-synthetic for system suitability CRS* and the chromatogram obtained with reference solution (d) to identify the peaks due to impurities E, H and N.

Relative retention with reference to paclitaxel (retention time = about 23 min): impurity N = about 0.2; impurity G = about 0.5; impurity A = about 0.8; impurities M, J and H = about 0.9; impurity E = about 1.3; impurity I = about 1.4; impurity L = about 1.5; impurity K = about 2.2.

System suitability: reference solution (d):

- *resolution*: minimum 1.5 between the peaks due to impurity H and paclitaxel.

Limits:

- *correction factor*: for the calculation of content, multiply the peak area of impurity N by 1.29;
- *impurity A*: not more than 7 times the area of the principal peak in the chromatogram obtained with reference solution (a) (0.7 per cent);
- *impurities E, I*: for each impurity, not more than 4 times the area of the principal peak in the chromatogram obtained with reference solution (a) (0.4 per cent);
- *impurities G, K, N*: for each impurity, not more than twice the area of the principal peak in the chromatogram obtained with reference solution (a) (0.2 per cent);
- *sum of impurities H, J and M*: not more than 4 times the area of the principal peak in the chromatogram obtained with reference solution (a) (0.4 per cent);
- *impurity L*: not more than 5 times the area of the principal peak in the chromatogram obtained with reference solution (a) (0.5 per cent);
- *unspecified impurities*: for each impurity, not more than the area of the principal peak in the chromatogram obtained with reference solution (a) (0.10 per cent);
- *total*: not more than 12 times the area of the principal peak in the chromatogram obtained with reference solution (a) (1.2 per cent);
- *disregard limit*: 0.5 times the area of the principal peak in the chromatogram obtained with reference solution (a) (0.05 per cent).

Heavy metals (*2.4.8*): maximum 20 ppm.

Dissolve 1.0 g in *methanol R* and dilute to 20 ml with the same solvent. 12 ml of the solution complies with test B. Prepare the reference solution using 10 ml of lead standard solution (1 ppm Pb), obtained by diluting *lead standard*

Monographs L-P

solution (100 ppm Pb) R with *methanol R* and 2 ml of the test solution. To 12 ml of each solution, add 2 ml of *buffer solution pH 3.5 R*. Mix. Add 1.2 ml of *thioacetamide reagent R*. The substance will precipitate. Dilute to 40 ml with *methanol R*; the substance re-dissolves completely. Filter the solution through a membrane filter (pore size: 0.45 μm). Compare the spots on the filters obtained with the different solutions. The substance to be examined complies with the test if any brownish-black colour in the spot of the test solution is not more intense than that in the reference solution.

Water (*2.5.32*): maximum 3.0 per cent, determined on 0.050 g.

Microbial contamination. Total viable aerobic count (*2.6.12*) not more than 10^2 bacteria and not more than 10^1 fungi per gram determined by plate count. It complies with the tests for *Escherichia coli, Salmonella, Pseudomonas aeruginosa* and *Staphylococcus aureus* (*2.6.13*).

Bacterial endotoxins (*2.6.14*): less than 0.4 IU/mg.

ASSAY

A. Paclitaxel isolated from natural sources or produced by fermentation.

Liquid chromatography (*2.2.29*) as described in test A for related substances with the following modification.

Injection: test solution (b) and reference solution (b).

Calculate the percentage content of $C_{47}H_{51}NO_{14}$ from the declared content of *paclitaxel CRS*.

B. Paclitaxel produced by a semi-synthetic process.

Liquid chromatography (*2.2.29*) as described in test B for related substances with the following modification.

Injection: 10 μl of the test solution and reference solution (b).

Calculate the percentage content of $C_{47}H_{51}NO_{14}$ from the declared content of *paclitaxel CRS*.

STORAGE

In an airtight container, protected from light.

LABELLING

The label states the origin of the substance:

- isolated from natural sources;
- produced by fermentation;
- produced by a semi-synthetic process.

IMPURITIES

Test A

Specified impurities: *A, B, C, D, E, F, O, P, Q, R.*

Other detectable impurities (the following substances would, if present at a sufficient level, be detected by one or other of the tests in the monograph. They are limited by the general acceptance criterion for other/unspecified impurities and/or by the general monograph *Substances for pharmaceutical use (2034)*. It is therefore not necessary to identify these impurities for demonstration of compliance. See also *5.10. Control of impurities in substances for pharmaceutical use*): *H.*

Test B

Specified impurities: A, E, G, H, I, J, K ,L, M, N.

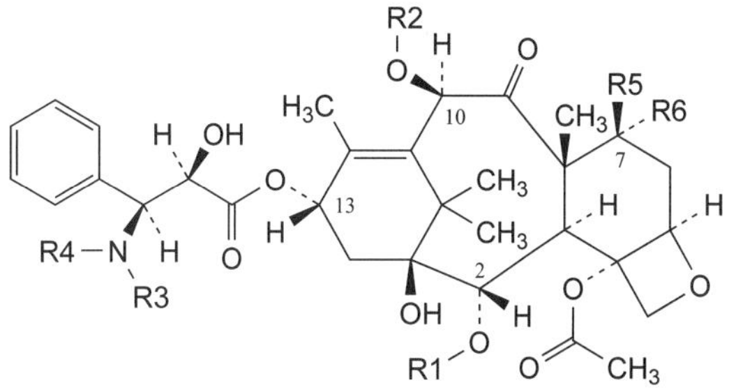

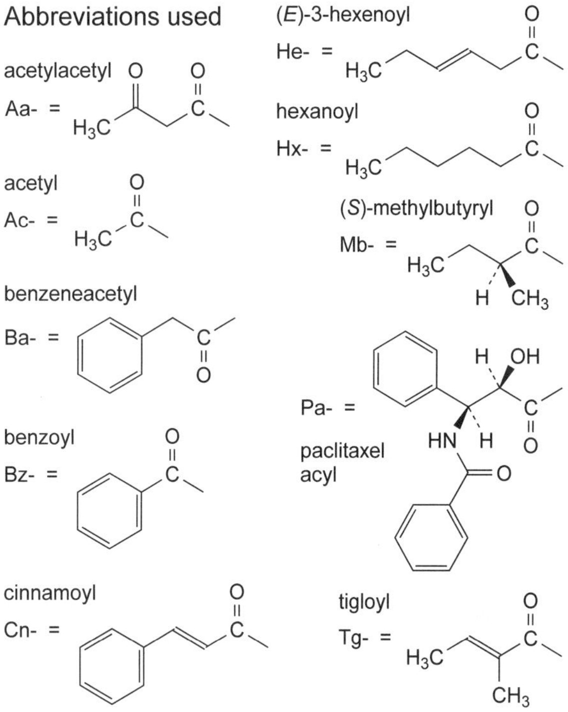

A. R1 = Tg, R2 = Ac, R3 = Bz, R4 = R6 = H, R5 = OH: 2-*O*-debenzoyl-2-*O*-tigloylpaclitaxel,

B. R1 = Bz, R2 = Ac, R3 = Tg, R4 = R6 = H, R5 = OH: *N*-debenzoyl-*N*-tigloylpaclitaxel (cephalomannine),

C. R1 = Bz, R2 = Ac, R3 = Hx, R4 = R6 = H, R5 = OH: *N*-debenzoyl-*N*-hexanoylpaclitaxel (paclitaxel C),

D. R1 = Bz, R2 = Ac, R3 = Tg, R4 = R5 = H, R6 = OH: *N*-debenzoyl-*N*-tigloyl-7-*epi*-paclitaxel (7-*epi*-cephalomannine),

E. R1 = R3 = Bz, R2 = Ac, R4 = R5 = H, R6 = OH: 7-*epi*-paclitaxel,

F. R1 = Bz, R2 = Ac, R3 = Hx, R4 = CH_3, R5 = OH, R6 = H: *N*-debenzoyl-*N*-hexanoyl-*N*-methylpaclitaxel (*N*-methylpaclitaxel C),

G. R1 = R3 = Bz, R2 = R4 = R6 = H, R5 = OH: 10-*O*-deacetylpaclitaxel,

H. R1 = R3 = Bz, R2 = R4 = R5 = H, R6 = OH: 10-*O*-deacetyl-7-*epi*-paclitaxel,

I. R1 = R3 = Bz, R2 = Pa, R4 = R6 = H, R5 = OH: 10-*O*-[(2*R*,3*S*)-3-(benzoylamino)-2-hydroxy-3-phenylpropanoyl]-10-*O*-deacetylpaclitaxel,

J. R1 = R3 = Bz, R2 = Aa, R4 = R6 = H, R5 = OH: 10-*O*-deacetyl-10-*O*-(3-oxobutanoyl)paclitaxel,

K. R1 = R3 = Bz, R2 = Ac, R4 = R6 = H, R5 = O-Si(C_2H_5)$_3$: 7-*O*-(triethylsilanyl)paclitaxel,

L. R1 = R3 = Bz, R2 = Ac, R4 = R6 = H, R5 = O-CO-CH_3: 7-*O*-acetylpaclitaxel,

O. R1 = Bz, R2 = Ac, R3 = Cn, R4 = R6 = H, R5 = OH: *N*-cinnamoyl-*N*-debenzoylpaclitaxel,

P. R1 = Bz, R2 = Ac, R3 = Ba, R4 = R6 = H, R5 = OH: *N*-debenzoyl-*N*-(phenylacetyl)paclitaxel,

Q. R1 = Bz, R2 = Ac, R3 = He, R4 = R6 = H, R5 = OH: *N*-debenzoyl-*N*-[(3*E*)-hex-3-enoyl]paclitaxel,

R. R1 = Bz, R2 = Ac, R3 = Mb, R4 = R6 = H, R5 = OH: *N*-debenzoyl-*N*-[(2*S*)-2-methylbutanoyl]paclitaxel,

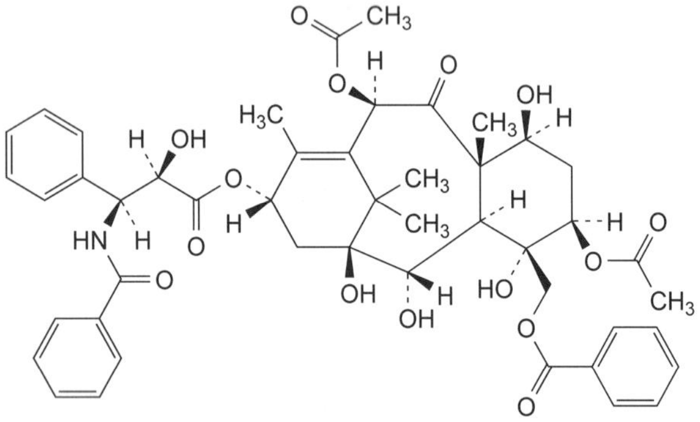

M. 1,2α,4,7β-dihydroxy-9-oxotax-11-ene-5β,10β,13α,20-tetrayl 5,10-diacetate 20-benzoate 13-[(2*R*,3*S*)-3-(benzoylamino)-2-hydroxy-3-phenylpropanoate],

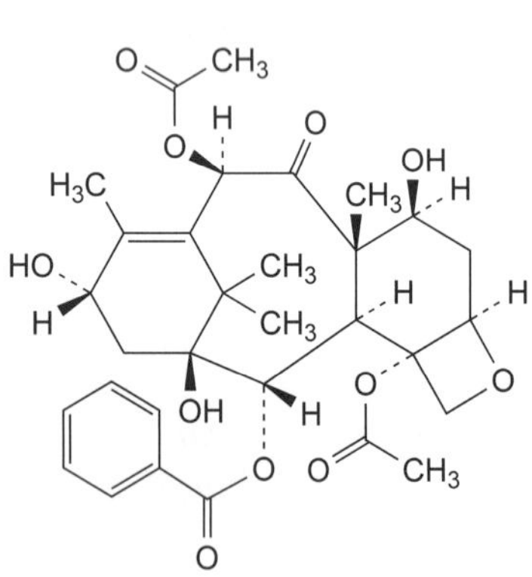

N. 13-*O*-de[(2*R*,3*S*)-3-(benzoylamino)-2-hydroxy-3-phenylpropanoyl]paclitaxel (baccatin III).

04/2008:2296

PANTOPRAZOLE SODIUM SESQUIHYDRATE

Pantoprazolum natricum sesquihydricum

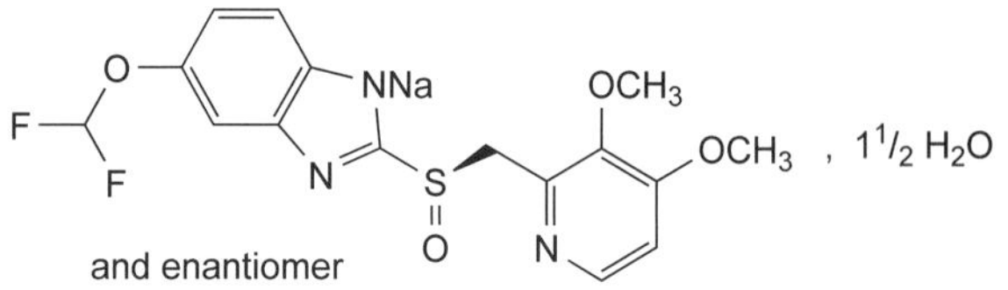

$C_{16}H_{14}F_2N_3NaO_4S,1^1/_2H_2O$ — M_r 432.4

[164579-32-2]

DEFINITION

Sodium 5-(difluoromethoxy)-2-[(*RS*)-[(3,4-dimethoxypyridin-2-yl)methyl]sulphinyl]benzimidazol-1-ide sesquihydrate.

Content: 99.0 per cent to 101.0 per cent (anhydrous substance).

PRODUCTION

It is produced by methods of manufacture designed to guarantee the proper hydrate form and it complies, if tested, with a suitable test that demonstrates its sesquihydrate nature (for example near-infrared spectrophotometry (*2.2.40*) or X-ray powder diffraction (*2.9.33*)).

CHARACTERS

Appearance: white or almost white powder.

Solubility: freely soluble in water and in ethanol (96 per cent), practically insoluble in hexane.

IDENTIFICATION

A. Infrared absorption spectrophotometry (*2.2.24*).

Comparison: *pantoprazole sodium sesquihydrate CRS.*

B. It gives reaction (a) of sodium (*2.3.1*).

TESTS

Appearance of solution. The solution is clear (*2.2.1*) and not more intensely coloured than reference solution B_6 (*2.2.2, Method II*).

Dissolve 0.20 g in *water R* and dilute to 20.0 ml with the same solvent.

Optical rotation (*2.2.7*): − 0.4° to + 0.4°.

Dissolve 0.2 g in 10 ml of *water R*. Adjust to pH 11.5-12.0 with an 8 g/l solution of *sodium hydroxide R*. Dilute to 20.0 ml with *water R*.

Related substances. Liquid chromatography (*2.2.29*).

Solvent mixture: *acetonitrile for chromatography R*, 40 mg/l solution of *sodium hydroxide R* (50:50 *V/V*).

Test solution. Dissolve 23 mg of the substance to be examined in the solvent mixture and dilute to 50.0 ml with the solvent mixture.

Reference solution (a). Dilute 1.0 ml of the test solution to 100.0 ml with the solvent mixture. Dilute 1.0 ml of this solution to 10.0 ml with the solvent mixture.

Reference solution (b). Dissolve the contents of a vial of *pantoprazole for system suitability CRS* (containing impurities A, B, C, D and E) in 1.0 ml of the solvent mixture.

Column:

– *size*: *l* = 0.125 m, Ø = 4 mm;

– *stationary phase*: *octadecylsilyl silica gel for chromatography R* (5 µm);

– *temperature*: 40 °C.

Mobile phase:

– *mobile phase A*: 1.74 g/l solution of *dipotassium hydrogen phosphate R* adjusted to pH 7.00 ± 0.05 with a 330 g/l solution of *phosphoric acid R*;

– *mobile phase B*: *acetonitrile for chromatography R*;

Time (min)	Mobile phase A (per cent *V/V*)	Mobile phase B (per cent *V/V*)
0 - 40	80 → 20	20 → 80
40 - 45	20 → 80	80 → 20

Flow rate: 1.0 ml/min.

Detection: spectrophotometer at 290 nm and, for impurity C, at 305 nm.

Injection: 20 μl.

Identification of impurities: use the chromatogram supplied with *pantoprazole for system suitability CRS* and the chromatogram obtained with reference solution (b) to identify the peaks due to impurities A, B, C, D + F and E.

Relative retention with reference to pantoprazole (retention time = about 11 min): impurity C = about 0.6; impurity A = about 0.9; impurities D and F = about 1.2; impurity E = about 1.3; impurity B = about 1.5.

System suitability: reference solution (b):

– *resolution*: minimum 1.5 between the peaks due to impurities E and D + F;

– the chromatogram obtained is similar to the chromatogram supplied with *pantoprazole for system suitability CRS*.

Limits:

– *correction factor*: for the calculation of content, multiply the peak area of impurity C by 0.3;

– *impurity A*: not more than twice the area of the principal peak in the chromatogram obtained with reference solution (a) (0.2 per cent);

– *sum of impurities D and F*: not more than twice the area of the principal peak in the chromatogram obtained with reference solution (a) (0.2 per cent);

– *impurities B, C, E*: for each impurity, not more than the area of the principal peak in the chromatogram obtained with reference solution (a) (0.1 per cent);

– *unspecified impurities*: for each impurity, not more than the area of the principal peak in the chromatogram obtained with reference solution (a) (0.10 per cent);

– *total*: not more than 5 times the area of the principal peak in the chromatogram obtained with reference solution (a) (0.5 per cent);

– *disregard limit*: 0.5 times the area of the principal peak in the chromatogram obtained with reference solution (a) (0.05 per cent).

Heavy metals (*2.4.8*): maximum 20 ppm.

1.0 g complies with test C. Prepare the reference solution using 2 ml of *lead standard solution (10 ppm Pb) R*.

Water (*2.5.12*): 5.9 per cent to 6.9 per cent, determined on 0.150 g.

ASSAY

Dissolve 0.200 g in 80 ml of *anhydrous acetic acid R*, add 5 ml of *acetic anhydride R* and mix for at least 10 min. Titrate with *0.1 M perchloric acid*, determining the end-point potentiometrically (*2.2.20*).

1 ml of *0.1 M perchloric acid* is equivalent to 20.27 mg of $C_{16}H_{14}F_2N_3NaO_4S$.

STORAGE

Protected from light.

IMPURITIES

Specified impurities: A, B, C, D, E, F.

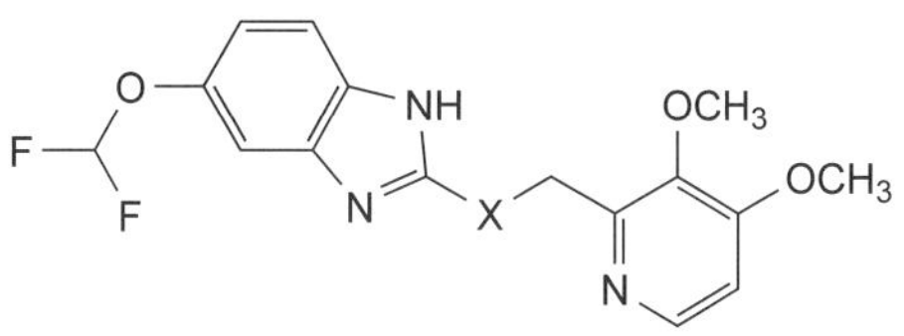

A. X = SO_2: 5-(difluoromethoxy)-2-[[(3,4-dimethoxypyridin-2-yl)methyl]sulphonyl]-1*H*-benzimidazole,

B. X = S: 5-(difluoromethoxy)-2-[[(3,4-dimethoxypyridin-2-yl)methyl]sulphanyl]-1*H*-benzimidazole,

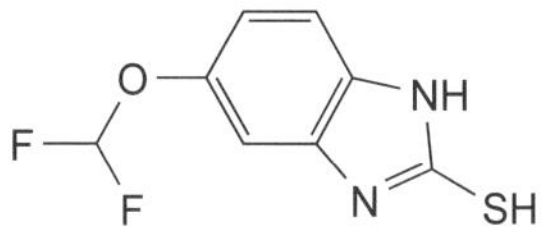

C. 5-(difluoromethoxy)-1*H*-benzimidazole-2-thiol,

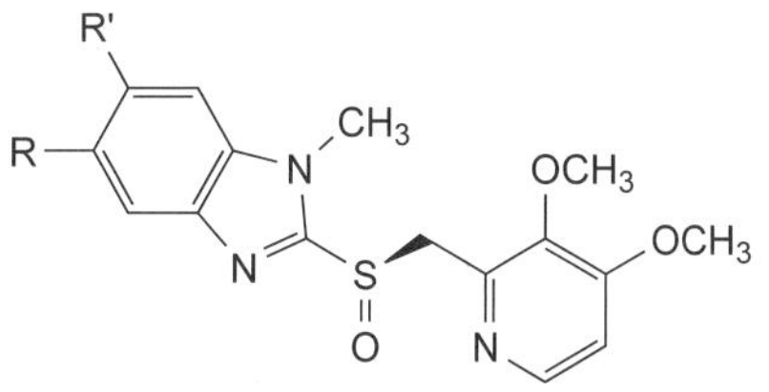

and enantiomer

D. R = $OCHF_2$, R′ = H: 5-(difluoromethoxy)-2-[(*RS*)-[(3,4-dimethoxypyridin-2-yl)methyl]sulphinyl]-1-methyl-1*H*-benzimidazole,

F. R = H, R′ = $OCHF_2$: 6-(difluoromethoxy)-2-[(*RS*)-[(3,4-dimethoxypyridin-2-yl)methyl]sulphinyl]-1-methyl-1*H*-benzimidazole,

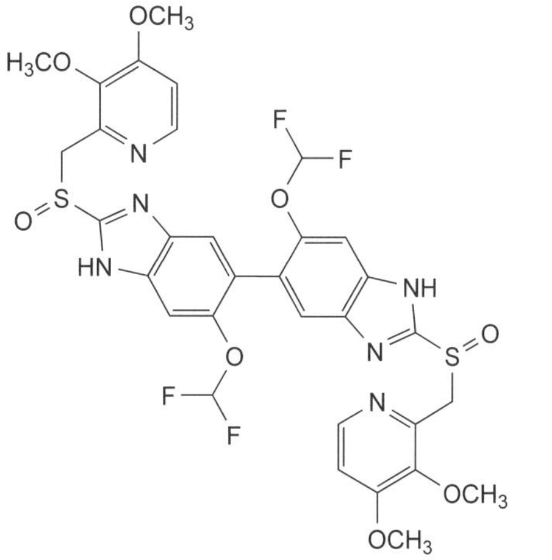

E. mixture of the stereoisomers of 6,6′-bis(difluoromethoxy)-2,2′-bis[[(3,4-dimethoxypyridin-2-yl)methyl]sulphinyl]-1*H*,1′*H*-5,5′-bibenzimidazolyl.

01/2008:0148
corrected 6.1

PHENOXYMETHYLPENICILLIN

Phenoxymethylpenicillinum

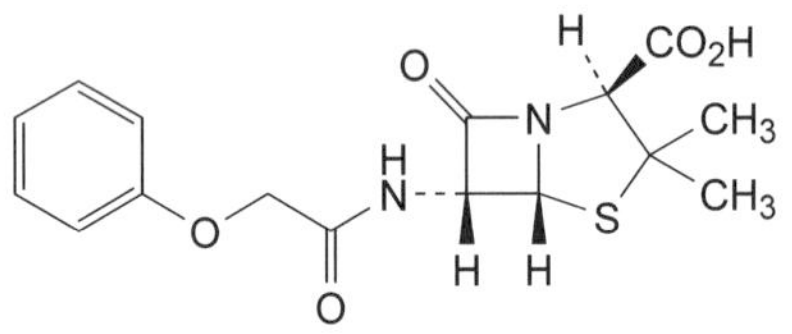

$C_{16}H_{18}N_2O_5S$ M_r 350.4
[87-08-1]

DEFINITION

(2*S*,5*R*,6*R*)-3,3-Dimethyl-7-oxo-6-[(phenoxyacetyl)amino]-4-thia-1-azabicyclo[3.2.0]heptane-2-carboxylic acid.

Substance produced by the growth of certain strains of *Penicillium notatum* or related organisms on a culture medium containing an appropriate precursor, or obtained by any other means.

Content: 95.0 per cent to 102.0 per cent for the sum of the percentage contents of phenoxymethylpenicillin and 4-hydroxyphenoxymethylpenicillin (anhydrous substance).

CHARACTERS

Appearance: white or almost white, slightly hygroscopic, crystalline powder.

Solubility: very slightly soluble in water, soluble in ethanol (96 per cent).

IDENTIFICATION

First identification: B.

Second identification: A, C, D.

A. pH (see Tests).

B. Infrared absorption spectrophotometry (*2.2.24*).

Comparison: *phenoxymethylpenicillin CRS.*

C. Thin-layer chromatography (*2.2.27*).

Test solution. Dissolve 25 mg of the substance to be examined in 5 ml of *acetone R*.

Reference solution (a). Dissolve 25 mg of *phenoxymethylpenicillin CRS* in 5 ml of *acetone R*.

Reference solution (b). Dissolve 25 mg of *benzylpenicillin potassium CRS* and 25 mg of *phenoxymethylpenicillin potassium CRS* in 5 ml of *water R*.

Plate: *TLC silanised silica gel plate R.*

Mobile phase: mix 30 volumes of *acetone R* and 70 volumes of a 154 g/l solution of *ammonium acetate R* adjusted to pH 5.0 with *glacial acetic acid R*.

Application: 1 μl.

Development: over a path of 15 cm.

Drying: in air.

Detection: expose to iodine vapour until the spots appear and examine in daylight.

System suitability: reference solution (b):

– the chromatogram shows 2 clearly separated spots.

Results: the principal spot in the chromatogram obtained with the test solution is similar in position, colour and size to the principal spot in the chromatogram obtained with reference solution (a).

D. Place about 2 mg in a test-tube about 150 mm long and 15 mm in diameter. Moisten with 0.05 ml of *water R* and add 2 ml of *sulphuric acid-formaldehyde reagent R*. Mix the contents of the tube by swirling; the solution is reddish-brown. Place the test-tube on a water-bath for 1 min; a dark reddish-brown colour develops.

TESTS

pH (*2.2.3*): 2.4 to 4.0.

Suspend 50 mg in 10 ml of *carbon dioxide-free water R*.

Specific optical rotation (*2.2.7*): + 186 to + 200 (anhydrous substance).

Dissolve 0.250 g in *butanol R* and dilute to 25.0 ml with the same solvent.

Related substances. Liquid chromatography (*2.2.29*).

Dissolution mixture. To 250 ml of *0.2 M potassium dihydrogen phosphate R* add 500 ml of *water R*, adjust to pH 6.5 with an 8.4 g/l solution of *sodium hydroxide R* and dilute to 1000 ml with *water R*.

Test solution (a). Dissolve 50.0 mg of the substance to be examined in the dissolution mixture and dilute to 50.0 ml with the dissolution mixture.

Test solution (b). Prepare immediately before use. Dissolve 80.0 mg of the substance to be examined in the dissolution mixture and dilute to 20.0 ml with the dissolution mixture.

Reference solution (a). Dissolve 55.0 mg of *phenoxymethylpenicillin potassium CRS* in the dissolution mixture and dilute to 50.0 ml with the dissolution mixture.

Reference solution (b). Dissolve 4.0 mg of *4-hydroxyphenoxymethylpenicillin potassium CRS* in the dissolution mixture and dilute to 10.0 ml with the dissolution mixture. Dilute 5.0 ml of this solution to 100.0 ml with the dissolution mixture.

Reference solution (c). Dissolve 10 mg of *phenoxymethylpenicillin potassium CRS* and 10 mg of *benzylpenicillin sodium CRS* (impurity A) in the dissolution mixture and dilute to 50 ml with the dissolution mixture.

Reference solution (d). Dilute 1.0 ml of reference solution (a) to 20 ml with the dissolution mixture. Dilute 1.0 ml of this solution to 50 ml with the dissolution mixture.

Reference solution (e). Dilute 1.0 ml of reference solution (a) to 25.0 ml with the dissolution mixture.

Column:

– *size*: *l* = 0.25 m, Ø = 4.6 mm;

– *stationary phase*: *octadecylsilyl silica gel for chromatography R* (5 μm).

Mobile phase:

– *mobile phase A*: *phosphate buffer solution pH 3.5 R, methanol R, water R* (10:30:60 *V/V/V*);

– *mobile phase B*: *phosphate buffer solution pH 3.5 R, water R, methanol R* (10:35:55 *V/V/V*);

Time (min)	Mobile phase A (per cent *V/V*)	Mobile phase B (per cent *V/V*)
0 - t_R	60	40
t_R - (t_R + 20)	60 → 0	40 → 100
(t_R + 20) - (t_R + 35)	0	100
(t_R + 35) - (t_R + 50)	0 → 60	100 → 40

t_R = retention time of phenoxymethylpenicillin determined with reference solution (d)

Monographs L-P

If the mobile phase composition has been adjusted to achieve the required resolution, the adjusted composition will apply at time zero in the gradient and in the assay.

Flow rate: 1.0 ml/min.

Detection: spectrophotometer at 254 nm.

Injection: 20 µl of reference solutions (c), (d) and (e) with isocratic elution at the initial mobile phase composition and 20 µl of test solution (b) according to the elution gradient described under Mobile phase; inject the dissolution mixture as a blank according to the elution gradient described under Mobile phase.

System suitability:

- *resolution*: minimum 6.0 between the peaks due to impurity A and phenoxymethylpenicillin in the chromatogram obtained with reference solution (c); if necessary, adjust the ratio A:B of the mobile phase;
- *signal-to-noise ratio*: minimum 3 for the principal peak in the chromatogram obtained with reference solution (d);
- *mass distribution ratio*: 5.0 to 7.0 for the peak due to phenoxymethylpenicillin (2nd peak) in the chromatogram obtained with reference solution (c).

Limits:

- *any impurity*: for each impurity, not more than the area of the principal peak in the chromatogram obtained with reference solution (e) (1 per cent);
- *disregard limit*: disregard the peak due to 4-hydroxyphenoxymethylpenicillin.

4-Hydroxyphenoxymethylpenicillin. Liquid chromatography (*2.2.29*) as described in the test for related substances with the following modifications.

Mobile phase: initial composition of the mixture of mobile phases A and B, adjusted where applicable.

Injection: test solution (a) and reference solution (b).

Limit:

- *4-hydroxyphenoxymethylpenicillin*: maximum 4.0 per cent (anhydrous substance).

Calculate the percentage content by multiplying, if necessary, by the correction factor supplied with the CRS.

Water (*2.5.12*): maximum 0.5 per cent, determined on 1.000 g.

ASSAY

Liquid chromatography (*2.2.29*) as described in the test for related substances with the following modifications.

Mobile phase: initial composition of the mixture of mobile phases A and B, adjusted where applicable.

Injection: test solution (a) and reference solutions (a) and (b).

System suitability: reference solution (a):

- *repeatability*: maximum relative standard deviation of 1.0 per cent after 6 injections.

Calculate the percentage content of phenoxymethylpenicillin by multiplying the percentage content of phenoxymethylpenicillin potassium by 0.902. Calculate the percentage content of 4-hydroxyphenoxymethylpenicillin by multiplying, if necessary, by the correction factor supplied with the CRS.

STORAGE

In an airtight container.

IMPURITIES

A. benzylpenicillin,

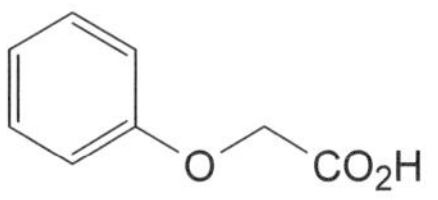

B. phenoxyacetic acid,

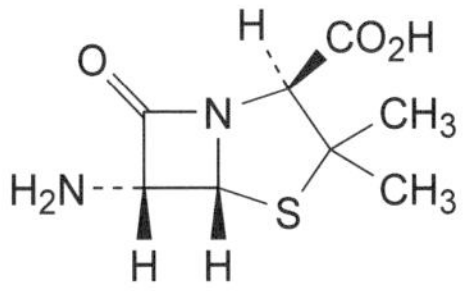

C. (2*S*,5*R*,6*R*)-6-amino-3,3-dimethyl-7-oxo-4-thia-1-azabicyclo[3.2.0]heptane-2-carboxylic acid (6-aminopenicillanic acid),

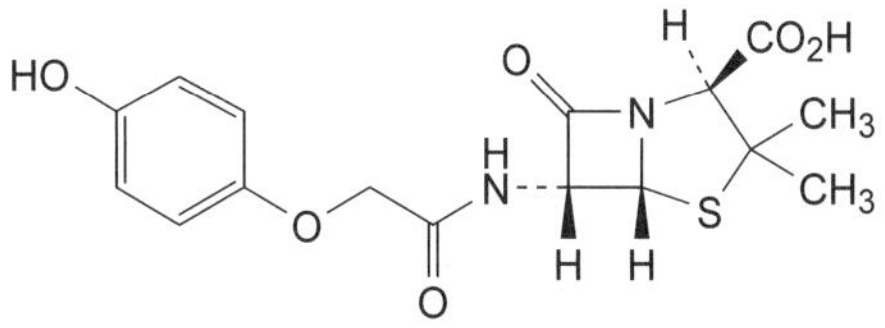

D. (2*S*,5*R*,6*R*)-3,3-dimethyl-7-oxo-6-[[2-(4-hydroxyphenoxy)acetyl]amino]-4-thia-1-azabicyclo[3.2.0]heptane-2-carboxylic acid (4-hydroxyphenoxymethylpenicillin),

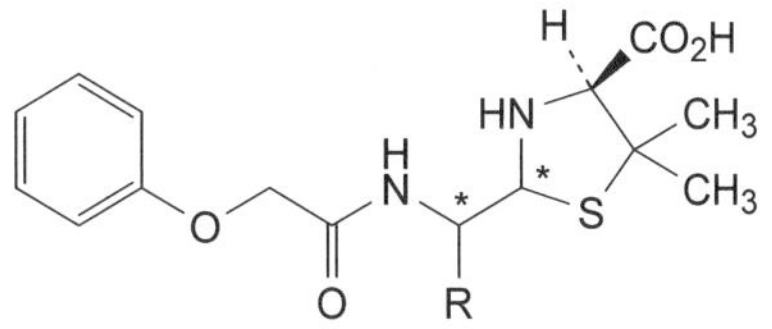

E. R = CO_2H: (4*S*)-2-[carboxy[(phenoxyacetyl)amino]methyl]-5,5-dimethylthiazolidine-4-carboxylic acid (penicilloic acids of phenoxymethylpenicillin),

F. R = H: (2*RS*,4*S*)-5,5-dimethyl-2-[[(phenoxyacetyl)amino]-methyl]thiazolidine-4-carboxylic acid (penilloic acids of phenoxymethylpenicillin).

01/2008:0149
corrected 6.1

PHENOXYMETHYLPENICILLIN POTASSIUM

Phenoxymethylpenicillinum kalicum

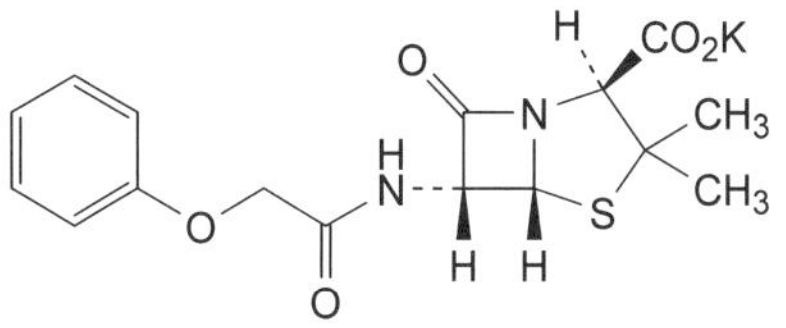

$C_{16}H_{17}KN_2O_5S$ M_r 388.5
[132-98-9]

DEFINITION

Potassium salt of (2*S*,5*R*,6*R*)-3,3-dimethyl-7-oxo-6-[(phenoxyacetyl)amino]-4-thia-1-azabicyclo[3.2.0]heptane-2-carboxylic acid.

Substance produced by the growth of certain strains of *Penicillium notatum* or related organisms on a culture medium containing an appropriate precursor, or obtained by any other means.

Content: 95.0 per cent to 102.0 per cent for the sum of the percentage contents of phenoxymethylpenicillin potassium and 4-hydroxyphenoxymethylpenicillin potassium (anhydrous substance).

CHARACTERS

Appearance: white or almost white, crystalline powder.

Solubility: freely soluble in water, practically insoluble in ethanol (96 per cent).

IDENTIFICATION

First identification: A, D.

Second identification: B, C, D.

A. Infrared absorption spectrophotometry (*2.2.24*).

Comparison: *phenoxymethylpenicillin potassium CRS.*

B. Thin-layer chromatography (*2.2.27*).

Test solution. Dissolve 25 mg of the substance to be examined in 5 ml of *water R.*

Reference solution (a). Dissolve 25 mg of *phenoxymethylpenicillin potassium CRS* in 5 ml of *water R.*

Reference solution (b). Dissolve 25 mg of *benzylpenicillin potassium CRS* and 25 mg of *phenoxymethylpenicillin potassium CRS* in 5 ml of *water R.*

Plate: *TLC silanised silica gel plate R.*

Mobile phase: mix 30 volumes of *acetone R* and 70 volumes of a 154 g/l solution of *ammonium acetate R* adjusted to pH 5.0 with *glacial acetic acid R.*

Application: 1 μl.

Development: over a path of 15 cm.

Drying: in air.

Detection: expose to iodine vapour until the spots appear and examine in daylight.

System suitability: reference solution (b):

– the chromatogram shows 2 clearly separated spots.

Results: the principal spot in the chromatogram obtained with the test solution is similar in position, colour and size to the principal spot in the chromatogram obtained with reference solution (a).

C. Place about 2 mg in a test-tube about 150 mm long and 15 mm in diameter. Moisten with 0.05 ml of *water R* and add 2 ml of *sulphuric acid-formaldehyde reagent R.* Mix the contents of the tube by swirling; the solution is reddish-brown. Place the test-tube in a water-bath for 1 min; a dark reddish-brown colour develops.

D. It gives reaction (a) of potassium (*2.3.1*).

TESTS

pH (*2.2.3*): 5.5 to 7.5.

Dissolve 50 mg in *carbon dioxide-free water R* and dilute to 10 ml with the same solvent.

Specific optical rotation (*2.2.7*): + 215 to + 230 (anhydrous substance).

Dissolve 0.250 g in *carbon dioxide-free water R* and dilute to 25.0 ml with the same solvent.

Related substances. Liquid chromatography (*2.2.29*).

Dissolution mixture. To 250 ml of *0.2 M potassium dihydrogen phosphate R* add 500 ml of *water R* and adjust to pH 6.5 with an 8.4 g/l solution of *sodium hydroxide R.* Dilute to 1000 ml with *water R.*

Test solution (a). Dissolve 50.0 mg of the substance to be examined in the dissolution mixture and dilute to 50.0 ml with the dissolution mixture.

Test solution (b). Prepare immediately before use. Dissolve 80.0 mg of the substance to be examined in the dissolution mixture and dilute to 20.0 ml with the dissolution mixture.

Reference solution (a). Dissolve 50.0 mg of *phenoxymethylpenicillin potassium CRS* in the dissolution mixture and dilute to 50.0 ml with the dissolution mixture.

Reference solution (b). Dissolve 4.0 mg of *4-hydroxyphenoxymethylpenicillin potassium CRS* in the dissolution mixture and dilute to 10.0 ml with the dissolution mixture. Dilute 5.0 ml of this solution to 100.0 ml with the dissolution mixture.

Reference solution (c). Dissolve 10 mg of *phenoxymethylpenicillin potassium CRS* and 10 mg of *benzylpenicillin sodium CRS* (impurity A) in the dissolution mixture and dilute to 50 ml with the dissolution mixture.

Reference solution (d). Dilute 1.0 ml of reference solution (a) to 20 ml with the dissolution mixture. Dilute 1.0 ml of this solution to 50 ml with the dissolution mixture.

Reference solution (e). Dilute 1.0 ml of reference solution (a) to 25.0 ml with the dissolution mixture.

Column:

– *size*: *l* = 0.25 m, Ø = 4.6 mm;

– *stationary phase*: *octadecylsilyl silica gel for chromatography R* (5 μm).

Mobile phase:

– *mobile phase A*: *phosphate buffer solution pH 3.5 R, methanol R, water R* (10:30:60 *V/V/V*);

– *mobile phase B*: *phosphate buffer solution pH 3.5 R, water R, methanol R* (10:35:55 *V/V/V*);

Time (min)	Mobile phase A (per cent *V/V*)	Mobile phase B (per cent *V/V*)
0 - t_R	60	40
t_R - (t_R + 20)	60 → 0	40 → 100
(t_R + 20) - (t_R+ 35)	0	100
(t_R + 35) - (t_R + 50)	0 → 60	100 → 40

t_R = retention time of phenoxymethylpenicillin determined with reference solution (d)

If the mobile phase composition has been adjusted to achieve the required resolution, the adjusted composition will apply at time zero in the gradient and in the assay.

Flow rate: 1.0 ml/min.

Detection: spectrophotometer at 254 nm.

Injection: 20 μl of reference solutions (c), (d) and (e) with isocratic elution at the initial mobile phase composition and 20 μl of test solution (b) according to the elution gradient described under Mobile phase; inject the dissolution mixture as a blank according to the elution gradient described under Mobile phase.

System suitability:

– *resolution*: minimum 6.0 between the peaks due to impurity A and phenoxymethylpenicillin in the chromatogram obtained with reference solution (c); if necessary, adjust the ratio A:B of the mobile phase;

– *signal-to-noise ratio*: minimum 3 for the principal peak in the chromatogram obtained with reference solution (d);

– *mass distribution ratio*: 5.0 to 7.0 for the peak due to phenoxymethylpenicillin (2nd peak) in the chromatogram obtained with reference solution (c).

Limits:

– *any impurity*: for each impurity, not more than the area of the principal peak in the chromatogram obtained with reference solution (e) (1 per cent);
– *disregard limit*: disregard the peak due to 4-hydroxyphenoxymethylpenicillin.

4-Hydroxyphenoxymethylpenicillin potassium. Liquid chromatography (*2.2.29*) as described in the test for related substances with the following modifications.

Mobile phase: initial composition of the mixture of mobile phases A and B, adjusted where applicable.

Injection: test solution (a) and reference solution (b).

Limit:

– *4-hydroxyphenoxymethylpenicillin potassium*: maximum 4.0 per cent (anhydrous substance).

Calculate the percentage content by multiplying, if necessary, by the correction factor supplied with the CRS.

Water (*2.5.12*): maximum 1.0 per cent, determined on 1.000 g.

ASSAY

Liquid chromatography (*2.2.29*) as described in the test for related substances with the following modifications.

Mobile phase: initial composition of the mixture of mobile phases A and B, adjusted where applicable.

Injection: test solution (a) and reference solutions (a) and (b).

System suitability: reference solution (a):

– *repeatability*: maximum relative standard deviation of 1.0 per cent after 6 injections.

Calculate the percentage content of phenoxymethylpenicillin potassium and of 4-hydroxyphenoxymethylpenicillin potassium.

IMPURITIES

A. benzylpenicillin,

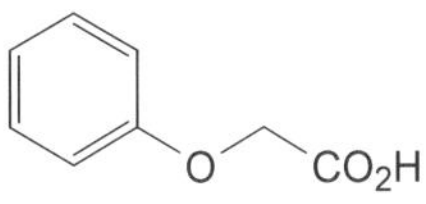

B. phenoxyacetic acid,

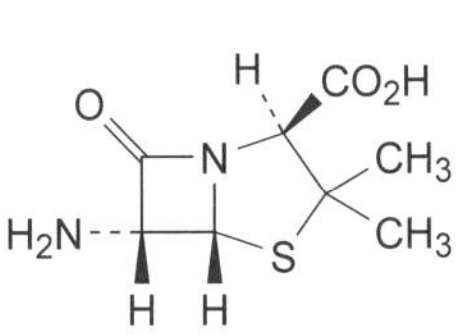

C. (2*S*,5*R*,6*R*)-6-amino-3,3-dimethyl-7-oxo-4-thia-1-azabicyclo[3.2.0]heptane-2-carboxylic acid (6-aminopenicillanic acid),

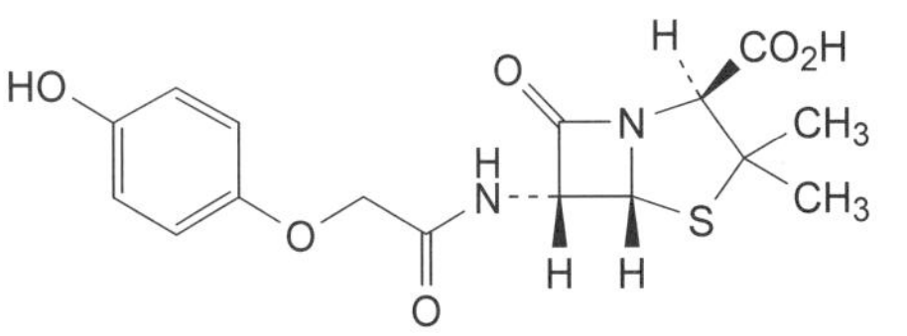

D. (2*S*,5*R*,6*R*)-3,3-dimethyl-7-oxo-6-[[2-(4-hydroxyphenoxy)acetyl]amino]-4-thia- 1-azabicyclo[3.2.0]heptane-2-carboxylic acid (4-hydroxyphenoxymethylpenicillin),

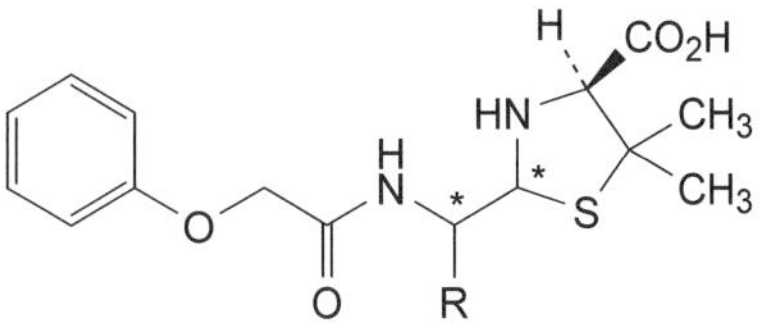

E. R = CO_2H: (4*S*)-2-[carboxy[(phenoxyacetyl)amino]methyl]-5,5dimethylthiazolidine-4-carboxylic acid (penicilloic acids of phenoxymethylpenicillin),

F. R = H: (2*RS*,4*S*)-5,5-dimethyl-2-[[(phenoxyacetyl)amino]-methyl]thiazolidine-4-carboxylic acid (penilloic acids of phenoxymethylpenicillin).

04/2008:0685

POVIDONE

Povidonum

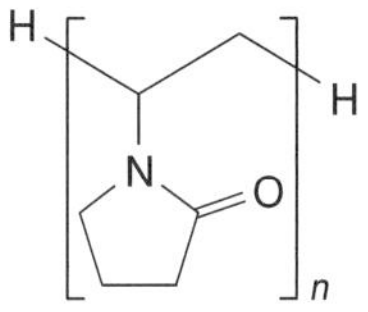

$C_{6n}H_{9n+2}N_nO_n$
[9003-39-8]

DEFINITION

α-Hydro-ω-hydropoly[1-(2-oxopyrrolidin-1-yl)ethylene]. It consists of linear polymers of 1-ethenylpyrrolidin-2-one.

Content: 11.5 per cent to 12.8 per cent of nitrogen (N; A_r 14.01) (anhydrous substance).

The different types of povidone are characterised by their viscosity in solution expressed as a K-value.

CHARACTERS

Appearance: white or yellowish-white, hygroscopic powder or flakes.

Solubility: freely soluble in water, in ethanol (96 per cent) and in methanol, very slightly soluble in acetone.

IDENTIFICATION

First identification: A, E.

Second identification: B, C, D, E.

A. Infrared absorption spectrophotometry (*2.2.24*).

Preparation: dry the substances beforehand at 105 °C for 6 h. Record the spectra using 4 mg of substance.

Comparison: *povidone CRS*.

B. To 0.4 ml of solution S1 (see Tests) add 10 ml of *water R*, 5 ml of *dilute hydrochloric acid R* and 2 ml of *potassium dichromate solution R*. An orange-yellow precipitate is formed.

C. To 1 ml of solution S1 add 0.2 ml of *dimethylaminobenzaldehyde solution R1* and 0.1 ml of *sulphuric acid R*. A pink colour is produced.

D. To 0.1 ml of solution S1 add 5 ml of *water R* and 0.2 ml of *0.05 M iodine*. A red colour is produced.

E. To 0.5 g add 10 ml of *water R* and shake. The substance dissolves.

TESTS

Solution S. Dissolve 1.0 g in *carbon dioxide-free water R* and dilute to 20 ml with the same solvent. Add the substance to be examined to the water in small portions, stirring using a magnetic stirrer.

Solution S1. Dissolve 2.5 g in *carbon dioxide-free water R* and dilute to 25 ml with the same solvent. Add the substance to be examined to the water in small portions, stirring using a magnetic stirrer.

Appearance of solution. Solution S is clear (*2.2.1*) and not more intensely coloured than reference solution B_6, BY_6 or R_6 (*2.2.2, Method II*).

pH (*2.2.3*): 3.0 to 5.0 for solution S, for povidone having a stated *K*-value of not more than 30; 4.0 to 7.0 for solution S, for povidone having a stated *K*-value of more than 30.

Viscosity, expressed as *K*-value. For povidone having a stated value of 18 or less, use a 50 g/l solution. For povidone having a stated value of more than 18 and not more than 95, use a 10 g/l solution. For povidone having a stated value of more than 95, use a 1.0 g/l solution. Allow to stand for 1 h and determine the viscosity (*2.2.9*) of the solution at 25 °C, using viscometer No.1 with a minimum flow time of 100 s. Calculate the *K*-value using the following expression:

$$\frac{1.5\log\eta - 1}{0.15 + 0.003c} + \frac{\sqrt{300c\log\eta + (c + 1.5c\log\eta)^2}}{0.15c + 0.003c^2}$$

c = concentration of the substance to be examined, calculated with reference to the anhydrous substance, in grams per 100 ml;

η = kinematic viscosity of the solution relative to that of *water R*.

The *K*-value of povidone having a stated *K*-value of 15 or less is 85.0 per cent to 115.0 per cent of the stated value.

The *K*-value of povidone having a stated *K*-value or a stated *K*-value range with an average of more than 15 is 90.0 per cent to 108.0 per cent of the stated value or of the average of the stated range.

Aldehydes: maximum 5.0×10^2 ppm, expressed as acetaldehyde.

Test solution. Dissolve 1.0 g of the substance to be examined in *phosphate buffer solution pH 9.0 R* and dilute to 100.0 ml with the same solvent. Stopper the flask tightly and heat at 60 °C for 1 h. Allow to cool to room temperature.

Reference solution. Dissolve 0.140 g of *acetaldehyde ammonia trimer trihydrate R* in *water R* and dilute to 200.0 ml with the same solvent. Dilute 1.0 ml of this solution to 100.0 ml with *phosphate buffer solution pH 9.0 R*.

Into 3 identical spectrophotometric cells with a path length of 1 cm, introduce separately 0.5 ml of the test solution, 0.5 ml of the reference solution and 0.5 ml of *water R* (blank). To each cell, add 2.5 ml of *phosphate buffer solution pH 9.0 R* and 0.2 ml of *nicotinamide-adenine dinucleotide solution R*. Mix and stopper tightly. Allow to stand at 22 ± 2 °C for 2-3 min and measure the absorbance (*2.2.25*) of each solution at 340 nm, using *water R* as the compensation liquid. To each cell, add 0.05 ml of *aldehyde dehydrogenase solution R*, mix and stopper tightly. Allow to stand at 22 ± 2 °C for 5 min. Measure the absorbance of each solution at 340 nm using *water R* as the compensation liquid.

Calculate the content of aldehydes using the following expression:

$$\frac{(A_{t2} - A_{t1}) - (A_{b2} - A_{b1})}{(A_{s2} - A_{s1}) - (A_{b2} - A_{b1})} \times \frac{100\,000 \times C}{m}$$

A_{t1} = absorbance of the test solution before the addition of aldehyde dehydrogenase;

A_{t2} = absorbance of the test solution after the addition of aldehyde dehydrogenase;

A_{S1} = absorbance of the reference solution before the addition of aldehyde dehydrogenase;

A_{S2} = absorbance of the reference solution after the addition of aldehyde dehydrogenase;

A_{b1} = absorbance of the blank before the addition of aldehyde dehydrogenase;

A_{b2} = absorbance of the blank after the addition of aldehyde dehydrogenase;

m = mass of povidone calculated with reference to the anhydrous substance, in grams;

C = concentration of acetaldehyde in the reference solution, calculated from the weight of the acetaldehyde ammonia trimer trihydrate with the factor 0.72, in milligrams per millilitre.

Peroxides: maximum 400 ppm, expressed as H_2O_2.

Dissolve a quantity of the substance to be examined equivalent to 4.0 g of the anhydrous substance in 100 ml of *water R*. To 25 ml of this solution, add 2 ml of *titanium trichloride-sulphuric acid reagent R*. Allow to stand for 30 min. The absorbance (*2.2.25*) of the solution, measured at 405 nm using a mixture of 25 ml of a 40 g/l solution of the substance to be examined and 2 ml of a 13 per cent *V/V* solution of *sulphuric acid R* as the compensation liquid, is not greater than 0.35.

Formic acid. Liquid chromatography (*2.2.29*).

Test solution. Dissolve a quantity of the substance to be examined equivalent to 2.0 g of the anhydrous substance in *water R* and dilute to 100.0 ml with the same solvent (test stock solution). Transfer a suspension of *strongly acidic ion exchange resin R* for column chromatography in *water R* to a glass tube 0.8 cm in internal diameter and about 20 mm long and keep the strongly acidic ion exchange resin layer constantly immersed in *water R*. Pour 5 ml of *water R* and adjust the flow rate so that the water drops at a rate of about 20 drops per min. When the level of the water comes down to near the top of the strongly acidic ion exchange resin layer, put the test stock solution into the column.

After dropping 2 ml of the solution, collect 1.5 ml of the solution and use this solution as the test solution.

Reference solution. Dissolve 100 mg of *formic acid R* and dilute to 100.0 ml with *water R*. Dilute 1.0 ml of this solution to 100.0 ml with *water R*.

Column:

- *material*: stainless steel,
- *size*: *l* = 0.25-0.30 m, Ø = 4-8 mm,
- *stationary phase*: *strongly acidic ion exchange resin for chromatography R* (5-10 µm),
- *temperature*: 30 °C.

Mobile phase: dilute 5 ml of *perchloric acid R* to 1000 ml with *water R*.

Flow rate: adjusted so that the retention time of formic acid is about 11 min.

Detection: spectrophotometer at 210 nm.

Injection: 50 µl each of the test and reference solutions.

System suitability:

- *repeatability*: maximum relative standard deviation of 2.0 per cent after 6 injections of the reference solution.

Limits:

- *formic acid*: not more than 10 times the area of the principal peak in the chromatogram obtained with the reference solution (0.5 per cent).

Hydrazine. Thin-layer chromatography (*2.2.27*). *Use freshly prepared solutions.*

Test solution. Dissolve a quantity of the substance to be examined equivalent to 2.5 g of the anhydrous substance in 25 ml of *water R*. Add 0.5 ml of a 50 g/l solution of *salicylaldehyde R* in *methanol R*, mix and heat in a water-bath at 60 °C for 15 min. Allow to cool, add 2.0 ml of *toluene R*, shake for 2 min and centrifuge. Use the upper layer of the mixture.

Reference solution. Dissolve 90 mg of *salicylaldehyde azine R* in *toluene R* and dilute to 100 ml with the same solvent. Dilute 1 ml of this solution to 100 ml with *toluene R*.

Plate: *TLC silanised silica gel plate F_{254} R.*

Mobile phase: *water R, methanol R* (1:2 *V/V*).

Application: 10 µl.

Development: over 2/3 of the plate.

Drying: in air.

Detection: examine in ultraviolet light at 365 nm.

Retardation factor: salicylaldehyde azine = about 0.3.

Limit:

- *hydrazine*: any spot corresponding to salicylaldehyde azine in the chromatogram obtained with the test solution is not more intense than the spot in the chromatogram obtained with the reference solution (1 ppm).

Impurity A. Liquid chromatography (*2.2.29*).

Test solution. Dissolve a quantity of the substance to be examined equivalent to 0.250 g of the anhydrous substance in the mobile phase and dilute to 10.0 ml with the mobile phase.

Reference solution (a). Dissolve 50 mg of *1-vinylpyrrolidin-2-one R* in *methanol R* and dilute to 100.0 ml with the same solvent. Dilute 1.0 ml of the solution to 100.0 ml with *methanol R*. Dilute 5.0 ml of this solution to 100.0 ml with the mobile phase.

Reference solution (b). Dissolve 10 mg of *1-vinylpyrrolidin-2-one R* and 0.5 g of *vinyl acetate R* in *methanol R* and dilute to 100.0 ml with the same solvent. Dilute 1.0 ml of the solution to 100.0 ml with the mobile phase.

Precolumn:

- *size*: l = 0.025 m, Ø = 4 mm;
- *stationary phase*: *octadecylsilyl silica gel for chromatography R* (5 µm).

Column:

- *size*: l = 0.25 m, Ø = 4 mm;
- *stationary phase*: *octadecylsilyl silica gel for chromatography R* (5 µm);
- *temperature*: 40 °C.

Mobile phase: *acetonitrile R, water R* (10:90 *V/V*).

Flow rate: adjusted so that the retention time of the peak corresponding to impurity A is about 10 min.

Detection: spectrophotometer at 235 nm.

Injection: 50 µl. After injection of the test solution, wait for about 2 min and wash the precolumn by passing the mobile phase backwards, at the same flow rate applied in the test, for 30 min.

System suitability:

- *resolution*: minimum 2.0 between the peaks due to impurity A and to vinyl acetate in the chromatogram obtained with reference solution (b);
- *repeatability*: maximum relative standard deviation of 2.0 per cent after 6 injections of reference solution (a).

Limit:

- *impurity A*: not more than the area of the principal peak in the chromatogram obtained with reference solution (a) (10 ppm).

Impurity B. Liquid chromatography (*2.2.29*).

Test solution. Dissolve a quantity of the substance to be examined equivalent to 100 mg of the anhydrous substance in *water R* and dilute to 50.0 ml with the same solvent.

Reference solution. Dissolve 100 mg of *2-pyrrolidone R* in *water R* and dilute to 100.0 ml with the same solvent. Dilute 3.0 ml of this solution to 50.0 ml with *water R*.

Precolumn:

- *size*: l = 0.025 m, Ø = 3 mm;
- *stationary phase*: *end-capped octadecylsilyl silica gel for chromatography R* (5 µm).

Column:

- *size*: l = 0.25 m, Ø = 3 mm;
- *stationary phase*: *end-capped octadecylsilyl silica gel for chromatography R* (5 µm);
- *temperature*: 30 °C.

Mobile phase: *water R*, adjusted to pH 2.4 with *phosphoric acid R*.

Flow rate: adjusted so that the retention time of impurity B is about 11 min.

Detection: spectrophotometer at 205 nm.

Injection: 50 µl. After each injection of the test solution, wash away the polymeric material of povidone from the guard column by passing the mobile phase through the column backwards for about 30 min at the same flow rate as applied in the test.

System suitability:

- *repeatability*: maximum relative standard deviation of 2.0 per cent after 6 injections of the reference solution.

Limit:

- *impurity B*: not more than the area of the principal peak in the chromatogram obtained with the reference solution (3.0 per cent).

Heavy metals (*2.4.8*): maximum 10 ppm.

2.0 g complies with test D. Prepare the reference solution using 2.0 ml of *lead standard solution (10 ppm Pb) R*.

Water (*2.5.12*): maximum 5.0 per cent, determined on 0.500 g.

Sulphated ash (*2.4.14*): maximum 0.1 per cent, determined on 1.0 g.

ASSAY

Place 100.0 mg of the substance to be examined (*m* mg) in a combustion flask, add 5 g of a mixture of 1 g of *copper sulphate R*, 1 g of *titanium dioxide R* and 33 g of *dipotassium sulphate R*, and 3 glass beads. Wash any adhering particles from the neck into the flask with a small quantity of *water R*. Add 7 ml of *sulphuric acid R*, allowing it to run down the insides of the flask. Heat the flask gradually until the solution has a clear, yellowish-green colour, and the inside wall of the flask is free from a carbonised material, and then heat for a further 45 min. After cooling, add cautiously 20 ml of *water R*, and connect the flask to the distillation

Monographs L-P

apparatus previously washed by passing steam through it. To the absorption flask add 30 ml of a 40 g/l solution of *boric acid R,* 3 drops of *bromocresol green-methyl red solution R* and sufficient water to immerse the lower end of the condenser tube. Add 30 ml of a solution of *strong sodium hydroxide solution R* through the funnel, rinse the funnel cautiously with 10 ml of *water R,* immediately close the clamp on the rubber tube, then start distillation with steam to obtain 80-100 ml of distillate. Remove the absorption flask from the lower end of the condenser tube, rinsing the end part with a small quantity of *water R,* and titrate the distillate with *0.025 M sulphuric acid* until the colour of the solution changes from green through pale greyish blue to pale greyish reddish-purple. Carry out a blank determination.

1 ml of *0.025 M sulphuric acid* is equivalent to 0.7004 mg of N.

STORAGE

In an airtight container.

LABELLING

The label indicates the nominal *K*-value.

IMPURITIES

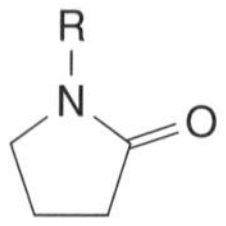

A. R = CH=CH_2: 1-ethenylpyrrolidin-2-one (1-vinylpyrrolidin-2-one),

B. R = H: pyrrolidin-2-one (2-pyrrolidone).

Monographs L-P

R

04/2008:1623

ROSELLE

Hibisci sabdariffae flos

DEFINITION

Whole or cut dried calyces and epicalyces of *Hibiscus sabdariffa* L. collected during fruiting.

Content: minimum 13.5 per cent of acids, expressed as citric acid ($C_6H_8O_7$; M_r 192.1) (dried drug).

CHARACTERS

Acidic taste.

IDENTIFICATION

A. The calyx is joined in the lower half to form an urceolate structure, the upper half dividing to form 5 long acuminate recurved tips. The tips have a prominent, slightly protruding midrib and a large, thick nectary gland about 1 mm in diameter. The epicalyx consists of 8-12 small, obovate leaflets, which are adnate to the base of the calyx. The calyx and epicalyx are fleshy, dry, easily fragmented and bright red or deep purple, somewhat lighter at the base of the inner side.

B. Reduce to a powder (355) (*2.9.12*). The powder is red or purplish-red. Examine under a microscope using *chloral hydrate solution R*. The powder shows the following diagnostic characters: predominantly red fragments of the parenchyma containing numerous crystal clusters of calcium oxalate and, sporadically, mucilage-filled cavities, sometimes associated with polygonal epidermal cells and anisocytic stomata (*2.8.3*); numerous fragments of vascular bundles with spiral and reticulate vessels; sclerenchymatous fibres with a wide lumen; rarely, rectangular, pitted parenchymatous cells; fragments of unicellular, smooth, bent covering trichomes and occasional glandular trichomes; rounded pollen grains with a spiny exine.

C. Thin-layer chromatography (*2.2.27*).

Test solution. To 1.0 g of the powdered drug (355) (*2.9.12*) add 10 ml of *ethanol (60 per cent V/V) R*. Shake for 15 min and filter.

Reference solution. Dissolve 2.5 mg of *quinaldine red R* and 2.5 mg of *sulphan blue R* in 10 ml of *methanol R*.

Plate: *TLC silica gel plate R* (5-40 μm) [or *TLC silica gel plate R* (2-10 μm)].

Mobile phase: *anhydrous formic acid R, water R, butanol R* (10:12:40 *V/V/V*).

Application: 5 μl as bands of 10 mm [or 2 μl as bands of 8 mm].

Development: over a path of 10 cm [or 6 cm].

Drying: in air.

Detection: examine immediately in daylight.

Results: see below the sequence of zones present in the chromatograms obtained with the reference solution and the test solution. Furthermore, other faint zones may be present in the chromatogram obtained with the test solution.

Top of the plate	
_______	_______
Quinaldine red: an orange-red zone	
	An intense violet zone
Sulphan blue: a blue zone	
	An intense violet-blue zone
_______	_______
Reference solution	**Test solution**

TESTS

Foreign matter (*2.8.2*): maximum 2 per cent of fragments of fruits (red funicles and parts of the 5-caverned capsule with yellowish-grey pericarp, whose thin walls consist of several layers of differently directed fibres; flattened, reniform seeds with a dotted surface).

Loss on drying (*2.2.32*): maximum 11.0 per cent, determined on 1.000 g of the powdered drug (355) (*2.9.12*) by drying in an oven at 105 °C for 2 h.

Total ash (*2.4.16*): maximum 10.0 per cent.

Colouring intensity. Reduce 100 g to a coarse powder (1400) (*2.9.12*) and homogenise. Reduce about 10 g of this mixture to a powder (355) (*2.9.12*). To 1.0 g of the powdered drug (355) (*2.9.12*) add 25 ml of boiling *water R* in a 100 ml flask and heat for 15 min on a water-bath with frequent shaking. Filter the hot mixture into a 50 ml graduated flask; rinse successively the 100 ml flask and the filter with 3 quantities, each of 5 ml, of warm *water R*. After cooling, dilute to 50 ml with *water R*. Dilute 5 ml of this solution to 50 ml with *water R*. Measure the absorbance (*2.2.25*) at 520 nm using *water R* as the compensation liquid. The absorbance is not less than 0.350 for the whole drug and not less than 0.250 for the cut drug.

ASSAY

Shake 1.000 g of the powdered drug (355) (*2.9.12*) with 100 ml of *carbon dioxide-free water R* for 15 min. Filter. To 50.0 ml of the filtrate add 100 ml of *carbon dioxide-free water R*. Titrate with *0.1 M sodium hydroxide* to pH 7.0, determining the end-point potentiometrically (*2.2.20*).

1 ml of *0.1 M sodium hydroxide* is equivalent to 6.4 mg of citric acid.

Monographs
Q-Z

S

04/2008:2385

SANGUISORBA ROOT

Sanguisorbae radix

DEFINITION

Whole or fragmented, dried underground parts of *Sanguisorba officinalis* L. without rootlets.

Content: minimum 5.0 per cent of tannins, expressed as pyrogallol ($C_6H_6O_3$; M_r 126.1) (dried drug).

CHARACTERS

The adventitious roots are about 5-25 cm long and up to 2 cm in diameter.

IDENTIFICATION

A. The whole drug consists of the rhizome, often ramified, thick, short, fusiform or cylindrical and the adventitious roots whose surface is reddish-brown or blackish-brown, with longitudinal striations, sometimes with transverse fissures, and showing rootlet scars.

It may also be found as more or less cylindrical fragments up to 2 cm long or elliptical or irregular discs. The fracture is light-coloured and very fibrous.

B. Reduce to a powder (355) (*2.9.12*). The powder is light yellowish-brown. Examine under a microscope using *chloral hydrate solution R*. The powder shows the following diagnostic characters: numerous, whole or fragmented phloem fibres, usually isolated, narrow, sometimes more than 500 µm long and often rough-walled; calcium oxalate cluster crystals, free or inside parenchyma cells; a few reticulate lignified vessels; rare cork fragments. Examine under a microscope using a 50 per cent *V/V* solution of *glycerol R*. The powder shows rounded or ovoid starch granules, single or in groups of 2-4; the diameter of a component granule may reach 30 µm. Some starch granules are found in the parenchyma cells or in cells of the medullary rays.

C. Thin-layer chromatography (*2.2.27*).

Test solution. To 2.0 g of the powdered drug (355) (*2.9.12*) add 50 ml of *water R* and boil under a reflux condenser for 30 min. Cool the solution and centrifuge for 10 min. Shake the supernatant with 2 quantities, each of 15 ml, of *di-isopropyl ether R* saturated with *hydrochloric acid R*. Combine the ether layers. Evaporate to dryness and dissolve the residue in 1.0 ml of *methanol R*. Filter through a polypropylene syringe filter (nominal pore size 0.45 µm).

Reference solution. Dissolve 5 mg of *gallic acid R* and 20 mg of *resorcinol R* in 20 ml of *methanol R*.

Plate: *TLC silica gel F_{254} plate R* (5-40 µm) [or *TLC silica gel F_{254} plate R* (2-10 µm)].

Mobile phase: *anhydrous formic acid R, ethyl acetate R, toluene R* (10:30:60 *V/V/V*).

Application: 10 µl [or 4 µl] as bands.

Development: over a path of 10 cm [or 6 cm].

Drying: in air.

Detection A: examine in ultraviolet light at 254 nm.

Results A: see below the sequence of quenching zones present in the chromatograms obtained with the reference solution and the test solution. Furthermore, other faint quenching zones may be present in the chromatogram obtained with the test solution.

Top of the plate	
	A quenching zone
_______	_______
Resorcinol: a quenching zone	
	A quenching zone
_______	_______
Gallic acid: a quenching zone	A quenching zone (gallic acid)
	A quenching zone
	A quenching zone
Reference solution	**Test solution**

Detection B: spray with a 10 g/l solution of *ferric chloride R* in *anhydrous ethanol R* and heat at 100-105 °C for 15 min; examine in daylight.

Results B: see below the sequence of the zones present in the chromatograms obtained with the reference solution and the test solution. Furthermore, other faint zones may be present in the chromatogram obtained with the test solution.

Top of the plate	
_______	_______
Resorcinol: a brown zone	
	A blackish-blue zone
_______	_______
Gallic acid: a blackish-blue zone	A blackish-blue zone (gallic acid)
	A blackish-blue zone
Reference solution	**Test solution**

TESTS

Loss on drying (*2.2.32*): maximum 12.0 per cent, determined on 1.000 g of the powdered drug (355) (*2.9.12*) by drying in an oven at 105 °C.

Total ash (*2.4.16*): maximum 10.0 per cent.

Ash insoluble in hydrochloric acid (*2.8.1*): maximum 2.0 per cent.

ASSAY

Carry out the determination of tannins in herbal drugs (*2.8.14*). Use 0.500 g of the powdered drug (180) (*2.9.12*).

Monographs Q-Z

04/2008:2268

SELAMECTIN FOR VETERINARY USE

Selamectinum ad usum veterinarium

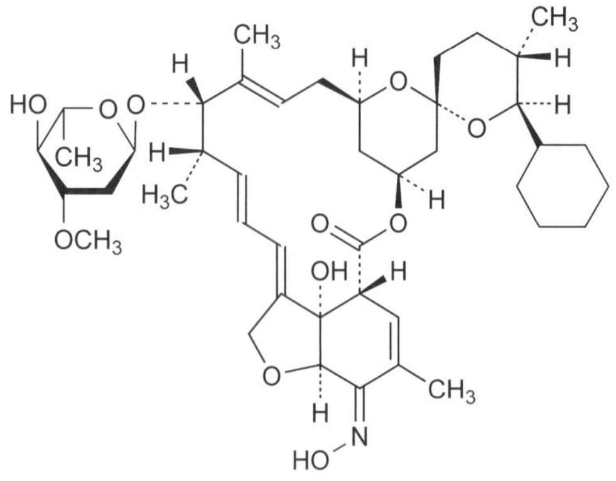

$C_{43}H_{63}NO_{11}$ M_r 770

[165108-07-6]

DEFINITION

(2a*E*,2′*R*,4*E*,5′*S*,6*S*,6′*S*,7*S*,8*E*,11*R*,15*S*,17a*R*,20*Z*,20a*R*,20b*S*)-6′-cyclohexyl-7-[(2,6-dideoxy-3-*O*-methyl-α-L-*arabino*-hexopyranosyl)oxy]-20b-hydroxy-20-(hydroxyimino)-5′,6,8,19-tetramethyl-3′,4′,5′,6,6′,7,10,11,14,15,17a,20,20a,20b-tetradecahydrospiro[2*H*,17*H*-11,15-methanofuro[4,3,2-*pq*][2,6]benzodioxacyclooctadecine-13,2′-pyran]-17-one ((5*Z*,25*S*)-25-cyclohexyl-4′-*O*-de(2,6-dideoxy-3-*O*-methyl-α-L-*arabino*-hexopyranosyl)-5-demethoxy-25-de(1-methylpropyl)-22,23-dihydro-5-(hydroxyimino)avermectin A_{1a}).

Semi-synthetic product derived from a fermentation product.

Content: 96.0 per cent to 102.0 per cent (anhydrous substance).

CHARACTERS

Appearance: white or almost white, hygroscopic powder.

Solubility: practically insoluble in water, freely soluble in isopropyl alcohol, soluble in acetone and in methylene chloride, sparingly soluble in methanol.

IDENTIFICATION

Infrared absorption spectrophotometry (*2.2.24*).

Comparison: *selamectin CRS*.

TESTS

Related substances. Liquid chromatography (*2.2.29*).

Solvent mixture: *water R, acetonitrile R* (40:60 *V/V*).

Test solution. Dissolve 25 mg of the substance to be examined in the solvent mixture and dilute to 50 ml with the solvent mixture.

Reference solution (a). Dilute 1.0 ml of the test solution to 100.0 ml with the solvent mixture.

Reference solution (b). Dissolve 2.5 mg of *selamectin for system suitability CRS* (containing impurities A, B, C and D) in the solvent mixture and dilute to 5 ml with the solvent mixture.

Column:
- *size*: *l* = 0.15 m, Ø = 3.9 mm;
- *stationary phase*: *end-capped octadecylsilyl silica gel for chromatography R* (4 µm);
- *temperature*: 30 °C.

Mobile phase:
- *mobile phase A*: *water R*;
- *mobile phase B*: *acetonitrile R*;

Time (min)	Mobile phase A (per cent *V/V*)	Mobile phase B (per cent *V/V*)
0 - 28	40	60
28 - 45	40 → 20	60 → 80

Flow rate: 2.0 ml/min.

Detection: spectrophotometer at 243 nm.

Injection: 20 µl.

Identification of impurities: use the chromatogram supplied with *selamectin for system suitability CRS* and the chromatogram obtained with reference solution (b) to identify the peaks due to impurities A, B, C and D.

Relative retention with reference to selamectin (retention time = about 22 min): impurity A = about 0.2; impurity B = about 0.4; impurity C = about 0.5; impurity D = about 1.7.

System suitability: reference solution (b):
- *resolution*: minimum 4.0 between the peaks due to impurities B and C.

Limits:
- *correction factor*: for the calculation of content, multiply the peak area of impurity D by 1.5;
- *impurities A, B*: for each impurity, not more than twice the area of the principal peak in the chromatogram obtained with reference solution (a) (2.0 per cent);
- *impurities C, D*: for each impurity, not more than 1.5 times the area of the principal peak in the chromatogram obtained with reference solution (a) (1.5 per cent);
- *any other impurity*: for each impurity, not more than the area of the principal peak in the chromatogram obtained with reference solution (a) (1.0 per cent);
- *total*: not more than 4 times the area of the principal peak in the chromatogram obtained with reference solution (a) (4.0 per cent);
- *disregard limit*: 0.2 times the area of the principal peak in the chromatogram obtained with reference solution (a) (0.2 per cent).

Heavy metals (*2.4.8*): maximum 20 ppm.

Dissolve 2.0 g in *ethanol (96 per cent) R* and dilute to 20.0 ml with the same solvent. 12 ml of the solution complies with test B. Prepare the reference solution using lead standard solution (2 ppm Pb) obtained by diluting *lead standard solution (100 ppm Pb) R* with *ethanol (96 per cent) R*. Filter the solution through a membrane filter (pore size: 0.45 µm). Compare the spots on the filters obtained with the different solutions. Any brownish-black colour in the spot from the test solution is not more intense than that in the spot from the reference solution.

Water (*2.5.12, Method A*): maximum 4.0 per cent, determined on 0.20 g.

Sulphated ash (*2.4.14*): maximum 0.1 per cent, determined on 1.0 g.

ASSAY

Liquid chromatography (*2.2.29*).

Test solution. Dissolve 50.0 mg of the substance to be examined in the mobile phase and dilute to 250.0 ml with the mobile phase.

Reference solution. Dissolve 50.0 mg of *selamectin CRS* in the mobile phase and dilute to 250.0 ml with the mobile phase.

Column:
- *size*: *l* = 0.15 m, Ø = 3.9 mm;

– *stationary phase*: *end-capped octadecylsilyl silica gel for chromatography R* (4 μm);
– *temperature*: 30 °C.

Mobile phase: *water R, acetonitrile R* (20:80 *V/V*).

Flow rate: 1.0 ml/min.

Detection: spectrophotometer at 243 nm.

Injection: 20 μl.

Run time: twice the retention time of selamectin.

Retention time: selamectin = about 9 min.

Calculate the percentage content of $C_{43}H_{63}NO_{11}$ from the declared content of *selamectin CRS*.

STORAGE

In an airtight container.

IMPURITIES

Specified impurities: A, B, C, D.

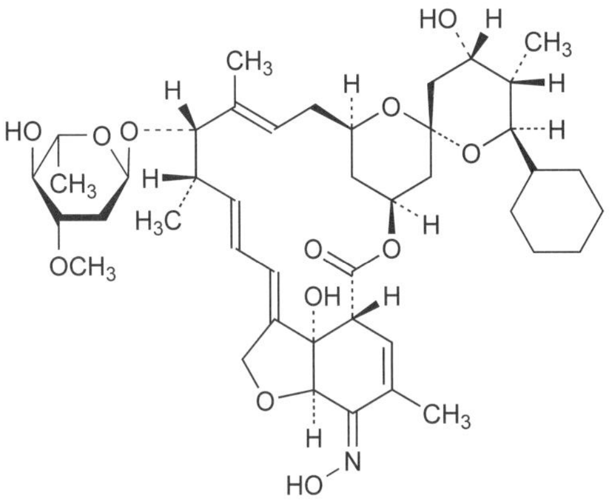

A. (2a*E*,2′*R*,4*E*,4′*S*,5′*S*,6*S*,6′*R*,7*S*,8*E*,11*R*,15*S*,17a*R*,20*Z*,20a*R*,20b*S*)-6′-cyclohexyl-7-[(2,6-dideoxy-3-*O*-methyl-α-L-*arabino*-hexopyranosyl)oxy]-4′,20b-dihydroxy-20-(hydroxyimino)-5′,6,8,19-tetramethyl-3′,4′,5′,6,6′,7,10,11,14,15,17a,20,20a,20b-tetradecahydrospiro[2*H*,17*H*-11,15-methanofuro[4,3,2-*pq*][2,6]benzodioxacyclooctadecine-13,2′-pyran]-17-one ((5*Z*,21*R*,23*S*,25*R*)-25-cyclohexyl-4′-*O*-de(2,6-dideoxy-3-*O*-methyl-α-L-*arabino*-hexopyranosyl)-5-demethoxy-25-de(1-methylpropyl)-22,23-dihydro-23-hydroxy-5-(hydroxyimino)avermectin A_{1a}),

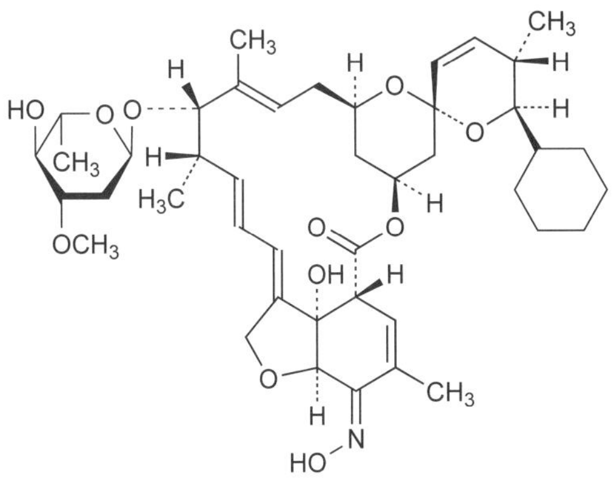

B. (2a*E*,2′*S*,4*E*,5′*S*,6*S*,6′*R*,7*S*,8*E*,11*R*,15*S*,17a*R*,20*Z*,20a*R*,20b*S*)-6′-cyclohexyl-7-[(2,6-dideoxy-3-*O*-methyl-α-L-*arabino*-hexopyranosyl)oxy]-20b-hydroxy-20-(hydroxyimino)-5′,6,8,19-tetramethyl-5′,6,6′,7,10,11,14,15,17a,20,20a,20b-dodecahydrospiro[2*H*,17*H*-11,15-methanofuro[4,3,2-*pq*][2,6]benzodioxacyclooctadecine-13,2′-pyran]-17-one ((5*Z*,25*R*)-25-cyclohexyl-4′-*O*-de(2,6-dideoxy-3-*O*-methyl-α-L-*arabino*-hexopyranosyl)-5-demethoxy-25-de(1-methylpropyl)-5-(hydroxyimino)avermectin A_{1a}),

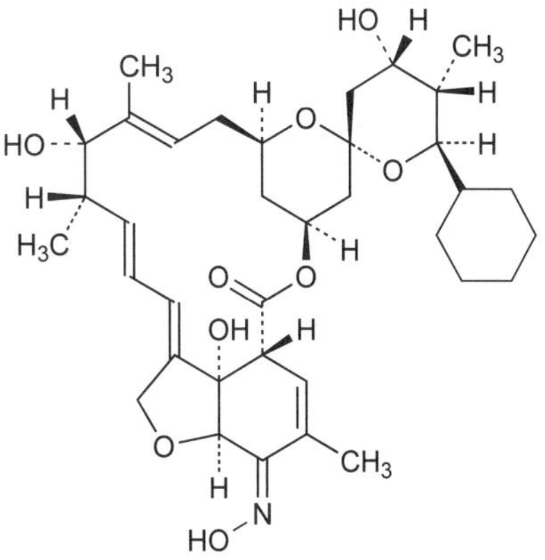

C. (2a*E*,2′*R*,4*E*,4′*S*,5′*S*,6*S*,6′*R*,7*S*,8*E*,11*R*,15*S*,17a*R*,20*Z*,20a*R*,20b*S*)-6′-cyclohexyl-4′,7,20b-trihydroxy-20-(hydroxyimino)-5′,6,8,19-tetramethyl-3′,4′,5′,6,6′,7,10,11,14,15,17a,20,20a,20b-tetradecahydrospiro[2*H*,17*H*-11,15-methanofuro[4,3,2-*pq*][2,6]benzodioxacyclooctadecine-13,2′-pyran]-17-one ((5*Z*,13*S*,25*R*)-25-cyclohexyl-25-demethyl-5-deoxy-13-hydroxy-5-(hydroxyimino)milbemycin α_1),

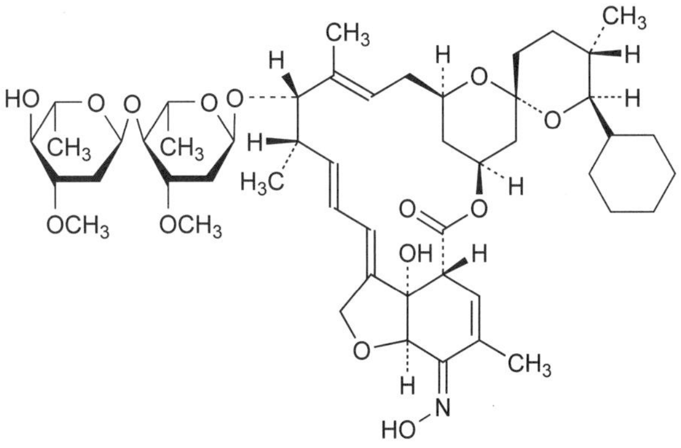

D. (2a*E*,2′*R*,4*E*,5′*S*,6*S*,6′*S*,7*S*,8*E*,11*R*,15*S*,17a*R*,20*Z*,20a*R*,20b*S*)-6′-cyclohexyl-7-[(2,6-dideoxy-3-*O*-methyl-α-L-*arabino*-hexopyranosyl-(1→4)-2,6-dideoxy-3-*O*-methyl-α-L-*arabino*-hexopyranosyl)oxy]-20b-hydroxy-20-(hydroxyimino)-5′,6,8,19-tetramethyl-3′,4′,5′,6,6′,7,10,11,14,15,17a,20,20a,20b-tetradecahydrospiro[2*H*,17*H*-11,15-methanofuro[4,3,2-*pq*][2,6]benzodioxacyclooctadecine-13,2′-pyran]-17-one ((5*Z*,21*R*,25*S*)-25-cyclohexyl-5-demethoxy-25-de(1-methylpropyl)-22,23-dihydro-5-(hydroxyimino)avermectin A_{1a}).

01/2008:1148
corrected 6.1

SERTACONAZOLE NITRATE

Sertaconazoli nitras

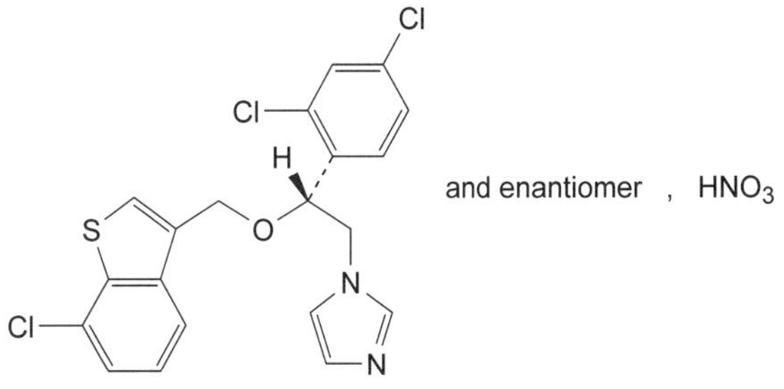

$C_{20}H_{16}Cl_3N_3O_4S$ M_r 500.8
[99592-39-9]

DEFINITION

(*RS*)-1-[2-[(7-Chloro-1-benzothiophen-3-yl)methoxy]-2-(2,4-dichlorophenyl)ethyl]-1*H*-imidazole nitrate.

Content: 98.5 per cent to 101.0 per cent (anhydrous substance).

CHARACTERS

Appearance: white or almost white powder.

Solubility: practically insoluble in water, soluble in methanol, sparingly soluble in ethanol (96 per cent) and in methylene chloride.

IDENTIFICATION

First identification: A, C.

Second identification: A, B, D, E.

A. Melting point (*2.2.14*): 156 °C to 161 °C.

B. Ultraviolet and visible absorption spectrophotometry (*2.2.25*).

Test solution. Dissolve 0.1 g in *methanol R* and dilute to 100 ml with the same solvent. Dilute 10 ml of this solution to 100 ml with *methanol R*.

Spectral range: 240-320 nm.

Absorption maxima: at 260 nm, 293 nm and 302 nm.

Absorbance ratio: A_{302}/A_{293} = 1.16 to 1.28.

C. Infrared absorption spectrophotometry (*2.2.24*).

Preparation: dry the substances at 100-105 °C for 2 h and examine as discs of *potassium bromide R*.

Comparison: *sertaconazole nitrate CRS*.

D. Thin-layer chromatography (*2.2.27*).

Solvent mixture: *concentrated ammonia R, methanol R* (10:90 *V/V*).

Test solution. Dissolve 40 mg of the substance to be examined in the solvent mixture and dilute to 10 ml with the solvent mixture.

Reference solution (a). Dissolve 40 mg of *sertaconazole nitrate CRS* in the solvent mixture and dilute to 10 ml with the solvent mixture.

Reference solution (b). Dissolve 20 mg of *miconazole nitrate CRS* in reference solution (a) and dilute to 5 ml with reference solution (a).

Plate: *TLC silica gel G plate R*.

Mobile phase: *concentrated ammonia R, toluene R, dioxan R* (1:40:60 *V/V/V*).

Application: 5 µl.

Development: over a path of 15 cm.

Drying: in a current of air for 15 min.

Detection: expose to iodine vapour for 30 min.

System suitability: reference solution (b):

– the chromatogram shows 2 clearly separated spots.

Results: the principal spot in the chromatogram obtained with the test solution is similar in position, colour and size to the principal spot in the chromatogram obtained with reference solution (a).

E. About 1 mg gives the reaction of nitrates (*2.3.1*).

TESTS

Appearance of solution. The solution is clear (*2.2.1*) and not more intensely coloured than reference solution Y_5 (*2.2.2, Method II*).

Dissolve 0.1 g in *ethanol (96 per cent) R* and dilute to 10 ml with the same solvent.

Related substances. Liquid chromatography (*2.2.29*).

Test solution. Dissolve 10.0 mg of the substance to be examined in the mobile phase and dilute to 10.0 ml with the mobile phase.

Reference solution (a). Dilute 5.0 ml of the test solution to 100.0 ml with the mobile phase. Dilute 1.0 ml of this solution to 20.0 ml with the mobile phase.

Reference solution (b). Dissolve 5.0 mg of *sertaconazole nitrate CRS* and 5.0 mg of *miconazole nitrate CRS* in the mobile phase and dilute to 20.0 ml with the mobile phase. Dilute 1.0 ml of this solution to 50.0 ml with the mobile phase.

Column:

– *size*: *l* = 0.25 m, Ø = 4.0 mm;

– *stationary phase*: *nitrile silica gel for chromatography R1* (10 µm).

Mobile phase: *acetonitrile R1*, 1.5 g/l solution of *sodium dihydrogen phosphate R* (37:63 *V/V*).

Flow rate: 1.6 ml/min.

Detection: spectrophotometer at 220 nm.

Injection: 20 µl.

Run time: 1.3 times the retention time of sertaconazole.

Retention time: nitrate ion = about 1 min; miconazole = about 17 min; sertaconazole = about 19 min.

System suitability: reference solution (b):

– *resolution*: minimum 2.0 between the peaks due to miconazole and sertaconazole.

Limits:

– *impurities A, B, C*: for each impurity, not more than the area of the principal peak in the chromatogram obtained with reference solution (a) (0.25 per cent);

– *total*: not more than twice the area of the principal peak in the chromatogram obtained with reference solution (a) (0.5 per cent);

– *disregard limit*: 0.2 times the area of the principal peak in the chromatogram obtained with reference solution (a) (0.05 per cent); disregard the peak due to the nitrate ion.

Water (*2.5.12*): maximum 1.0 per cent, determined on 0.50 g.

Sulphated ash (*2.4.14*): maximum 0.1 per cent, determined on 1.0 g.

ASSAY

Dissolve 0.400 g in 50 ml of a mixture of equal volumes of *anhydrous acetic acid R* and *methyl ethyl ketone R*. Titrate with *0.1 M perchloric acid*, determining the end-point potentiometrically (*2.2.20*). Carry out a blank titration.

1 ml of *0.1 M perchloric acid* is equivalent to 50.08 mg of $C_{20}H_{16}Cl_3N_3O_4S$.

STORAGE

Protected from light.

IMPURITIES

Specified impurities: *A, B, C.*

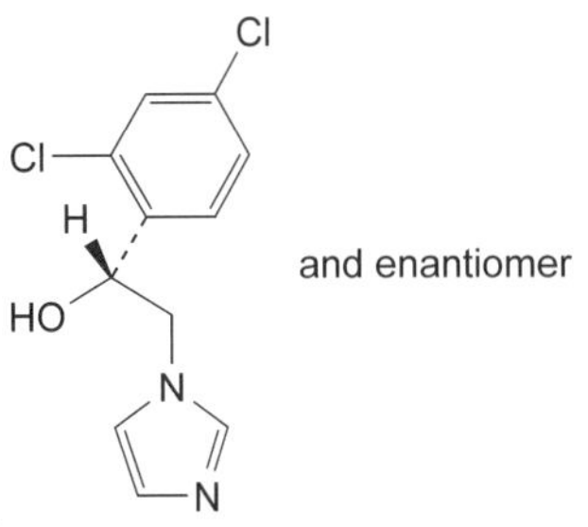

A. (1*RS*)-1-(2,4-dichlorophenyl)-2-(1*H*-imidazol-1-yl)ethanol,

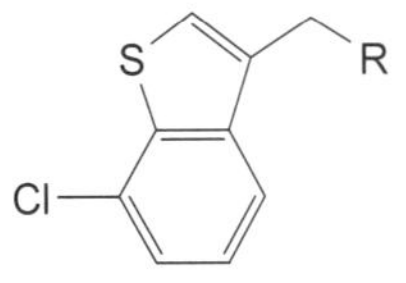

B. R = Br: 3-(bromomethyl)-7-chloro-1-benzothiophen,

C. R = OH: (7-chloro-1-benzothiophen-3-yl)methanol.

04/2008:1705

SERTRALINE HYDROCHLORIDE

Sertralini hydrochloridum

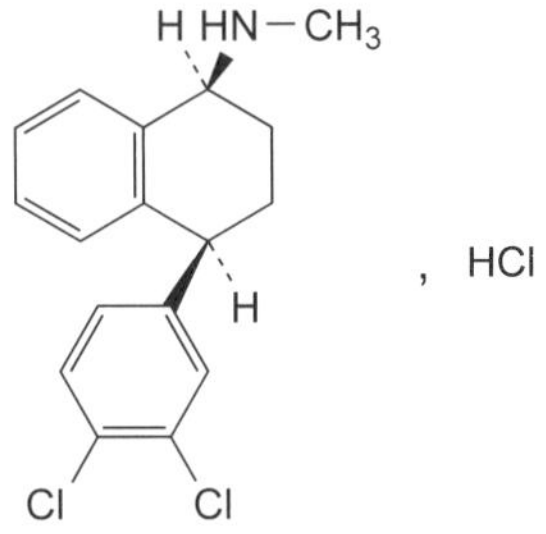

$C_{17}H_{18}Cl_3N$ M_r 342.7
[79559-97-0]

DEFINITION

(1*S*,4*S*)-4-(3,4-Dichlorophenyl)-*N*-methyl-1,2,3,4-tetrahydronaphthalen-1-amine hydrochloride.

Content: 97.5 per cent to 102.0 per cent (anhydrous substance).

CHARACTERS

Appearance: white or almost white, crystalline powder.

Solubility: slightly soluble in water, freely soluble in anhydrous ethanol, slightly soluble in acetone and in isopropanol.

It shows polymorphism (*5.9*).

IDENTIFICATION

A. Specific optical rotation (*2.2.7*): + 38.8 to + 43.0 (anhydrous substance), measured at 25 °C.

Solvent mixture. Dilute 1 volume of a 103 g/l solution of *hydrochloric acid R* to 20 volumes with *methanol R*.

Dissolve 0.250 g in the solvent mixture and dilute to 25.0 ml with the solvent mixture.

B. Infrared absorption spectrophotometry (*2.2.24*).

Comparison: *sertraline hydrochloride CRS*.

If the spectra obtained in the solid state show differences, record new spectra using 10 g/l solutions in *methylene chloride R*.

C. Dissolve 10 mg in 5 ml of *anhydrous ethanol R* and add 5 ml of *water R*. The solution gives reaction (a) of chlorides (*2.3.1*).

TESTS

Enantiomeric purity. Liquid chromatography (*2.2.29*).

Solvent mixture: *diethylamine R, hexane R, 2-propanol R* (1:40:60 *V/V/V*).

Test solution. Dissolve 60.0 mg of the substance to be examined in the solvent mixture and dilute to 10.0 ml with the solvent mixture.

Reference solution (a). Dissolve the contents of a vial of *sertraline for system suitability CRS* (containing impurity G) in 1.0 ml of solvent mixture.

Reference solution (b). Dilute 0.5 ml of the test solution to 100.0 ml with the solvent mixture.

Column:

- *size*: *l* = 0.25 m, Ø = 4.6 mm;
- *stationary phase*: *silica gel AD for chiral separation R* (5 µm).

Mobile phase: mix 30 volumes of *hexane R* and 70 volumes of a mixture of 1 volume of *diethylamine R*, 25 volumes of *2-propanol R* and 975 volumes of *hexane R*.

Flow rate: 0.4 ml/min.

Detection: spectrophotometer at 275 nm.

Injection: 20 µl.

Run time: 30 min.

Elution order: sertraline, impurity G.

System suitability:

- *resolution*: minimum 1.5 between the peaks due to sertraline and impurity G in the chromatogram obtained with reference solution (a);
- *signal-to-noise ratio*: minimum 10 for the peak due to sertraline in the chromatogram obtained with reference solution (b).

Limit:

- *impurity G*: not more than 3 times the area of the principal peak in the chromatogram obtained with reference solution (b) (1.5 per cent).

Impurity E. Thin-layer chromatography (*2.2.27*).

Solvent mixture: *methanol R, methylene chloride R* (50:50 *V/V*).

Test solution. Dissolve 0.500 g of the substance to be examined in the solvent mixture and dilute to 10.0 ml with the solvent mixture.

Reference solution (a). Dissolve 5.0 mg of *mandelic acid R* (impurity E) in the solvent mixture and dilute to 50.0 ml with the solvent mixture.

Reference solution (b). Dissolve 5 mg of *mandelic acid R* (impurity E) and 5 mg of the substance to be examined with the solvent mixture and dilute to 50.0 ml with the solvent mixture.

Plate: *TLC silica gel F_{254} plate R*.

Mobile phase: *dilute ammonia R2, methanol R, methylene chloride R* (15:50:120 *V/V/V*).

Application: 50 µl as bands of about 4 cm. Allow to dry.

Development: over 2/3 of the plate.

Drying: in air.

Detection: examine in ultraviolet light at 254 nm.

System suitability: reference solution (b):

- the chromatogram shows 2 clearly separated spots.

Limit:

- *impurity E*: any zone due to impurity E is not more intense than the zone in the chromatogram obtained with reference solution (a) (0.2 per cent).

Related substances. Gas chromatography (*2.2.28*): use the normalisation procedure.

Test solution. Introduce 0.250 g of the substance to be examined into a 15 ml stoppered centrifuge tube, add 2.0 ml of *methanol R* and 0.20 ml of a 25 per cent solution of *potassium carbonate R* and mix in a vortex mixer for 30 s. Add 8.0 ml of *methylene chloride R,* stopper the tube and mix in a vortex mixer for 60 s. Add 1 g of *anhydrous sodium sulphate R,* mix well and then centrifuge for about 5 min.

Reference solution (a). Dissolve the contents of a vial of *sertraline for peak identification CRS* (containing impurities A, B, C and F) in 0.2 ml of *methylene chloride R.*

Reference solution (b). Dilute 1.0 ml of the test solution to 100.0 ml with *methylene chloride R.* Dilute 1.0 ml of this solution to 20.0 ml with *methylene chloride R.*

Column:

- *material*: fused silica;
- *size*: l = 30 m, Ø = 0.53 mm;
- *stationary phase*: *polymethylphenylsiloxane R* (film thickness 1.0 μm).

Carrier gas: *helium for chromatography R.*

Flow rate: 9 ml/min.

Split ratio: 1:10.

Temperature:

	Time (min)	Temperature (°C)
Column	0 - 1	200
	1 - 31	200 → 260
	31 - 39	260
Injection port		250
Detector		280

Detection: flame ionisation.

Injection: 1 μl.

Identification of impurities: use the chromatogram supplied with *sertraline for peak identification CRS* and the chromatogram obtained with reference solution (a) to identify the peaks due to impurities A, B, C and F.

Relative retention with reference to sertraline (retention time = about 24 min): impurity B = about 0.5; impurities C and D = about 0.7; impurity A = about 1.05; impurity F = about 1.1.

System suitability: reference solution (a):

- *peak-to-valley ratio*: minimum 15, where H_p = height above the baseline of the peak due to impurity A and H_v = height above the baseline of the lowest point of the curve separating this peak from the peak due to sertraline.

Limits:

- *impurities A, B, F*: for each impurity, maximum 0.2 per cent;
- *sum of impurities C and D*: maximum 0.8 per cent;
- *unspecified impurities*: for each impurity, maximum 0.10 per cent;
- *total*: maximum 1.5 per cent;
- *disregard limit*: the area of the principal peak in the chromatogram obtained with reference solution (b) (0.05 per cent).

Heavy metals (*2.4.8*): maximum 20 ppm.

Dissolve 2.0 g in *ethanol (96 per cent) R* and dilute to 20.0 ml with the same solvent. 12 ml of the solution complies with test B. Prepare the reference solution using lead standard solution (2 ppm Pb) obtained by diluting *lead standard solution (100 ppm Pb) R* with *ethanol (96 per cent) R.*

Water (*2.5.12*): maximum 0.5 per cent, determined on 2.00 g.

Sulphated ash (*2.4.14*): maximum 0.2 per cent, determined on 1.0 g.

ASSAY

Liquid chromatography (*2.2.29*).

Buffer solution. To 28.6 ml of *glacial acetic acid R* slowly add, while stirring and cooling, 34.8 ml of *triethylamine R,* and dilute to 100 ml with *water R.* Dilute 10 ml of this solution to 1000 ml with *water R.*

Test solution. Dissolve 55.0 mg of the substance to be examined in the mobile phase and dilute to 50.0 ml with the mobile phase. Dilute 5.0 ml of this solution to 100.0 ml with the mobile phase.

Reference solution. Dissolve 55.0 mg of *sertraline hydrochloride CRS* in the mobile phase and dilute to 50.0 ml with the mobile phase. Dilute 5.0 ml of this solution to 100.0 ml with the mobile phase.

Column:

- *size*: l = 0.15 m, Ø = 3.9 mm;
- *stationary phase*: *octadecylsilyl silica gel for chromatography R* (4 μm);
- *temperature*: 30 °C.

Mobile phase: *methanol R,* buffer solution, *acetonitrile R* (15:40:45 *V/V/V*).

Flow rate: 1.8 ml/min.

Detection: spectrophotometer at 254 nm.

Injection: 20 μl.

Run time: twice the retention time of sertraline.

Retention time: sertraline = about 1.9 min.

Calculate the percentage content of $C_{17}H_{18}Cl_3N$ from the declared content of *sertraline hydrochloride CRS.*

STORAGE

Protected from light.

IMPURITIES

Specified impurities: A, B, C, D, E, F, G.

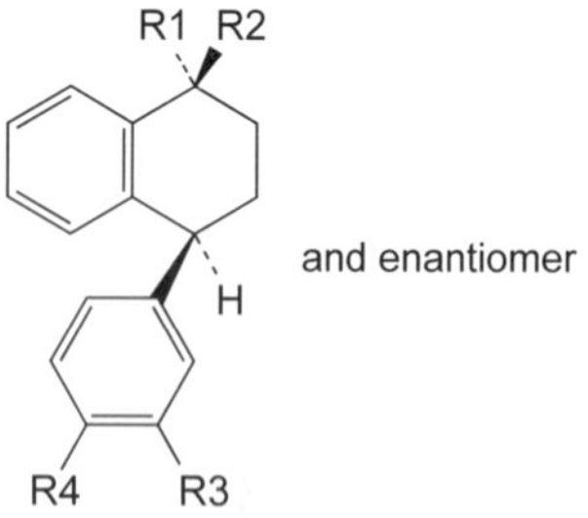

A. R1 = NH-CH_3, R2 = H, R3 = R4 = Cl: (1*RS*,4*SR*)-4-(3,4-dichlorophenyl)-*N*-methyl-1,2,3,4-tetrahydronaphthalen-1-amine,

B. R1 = R3 = R4 = H, R2 = NH-CH_3: (1*RS*,4*RS*)-*N*-methyl-4-phenyl-1,2,3,4-tetrahydronaphthalen-1-amine,

C. R1 = R3 = H, R2 = NH-CH_3, R4 = Cl: (1*RS*,4*RS*)-4-(4-chlorophenyl)-*N*-methyl-1,2,3,4-tetrahydronaphthalen-1-amine,

D. R1 = R4 = H, R2 = NH-CH_3, R3 = Cl: (1*RS*,4*RS*)-4-(3-chlorophenyl)-*N*-methyl-1,2,3,4-tetrahydronaphthalen-1-amine,

Monographs Q-Z

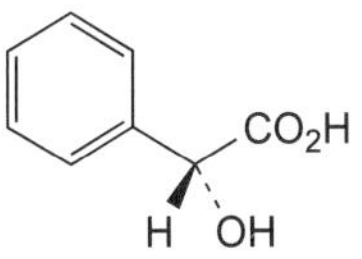

E. (2*R*)-hydroxyphenylacetic acid ((*R*)-mandelic acid),

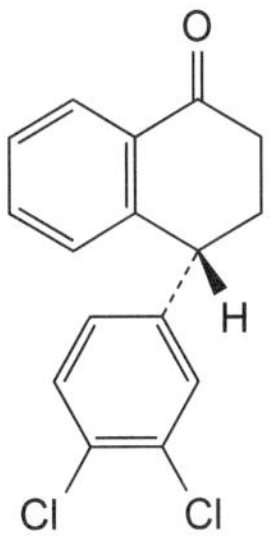

F. (4*R*)-4-(3,4-dichlorophenyl)-3,4-dihydronaphthalen-1(2*H*)-one,

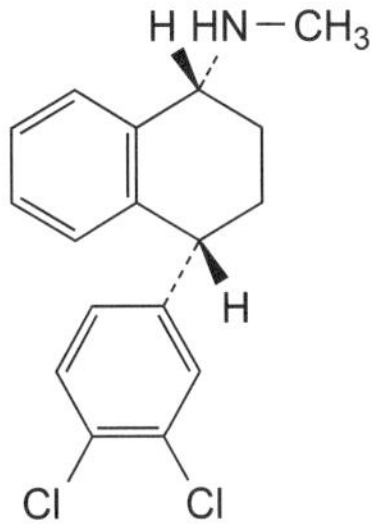

G. (1*R*,4*R*)-4-(3,4-dichlorophenyl)-*N*-methyl-1,2,3,4-tetrahydronaphthalen-1-amine (sertraline enantiomer).

04/2008:2183

SODIUM PHENYLBUTYRATE

Natrii phenylbutyras

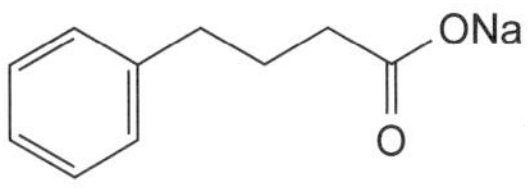

$C_{10}H_{11}NaO_2$ M_r 186.2
[1716-12-7]

DEFINITION

Sodium 4-phenylbutanoate.

Content: 99.0 per cent to 101.0 per cent (anhydrous substance).

CHARACTERS

Appearance: white or yellowish-white powder.

Solubility: freely soluble in water and in methanol, practically insoluble in methylene chloride.

IDENTIFICATION

A. Infrared absorption spectrophotometry (*2.2.24*).
Comparison: *sodium phenylbutyrate CRS.*

B. Dissolve 0.15 g in 2 ml of *water R*. The solution gives reaction (a) of sodium (*2.3.1*).

TESTS

pH (*2.2.3*): 6.5 to 7.5.

Dissolve 0.20 g in *carbon dioxide-free water R* and dilute to 10 ml with the same solvent.

Impurity C. Gas chromatography (*2.2.28*).

Silylation solution. To 2 ml of *N,O-bis(trimethylsilyl)trifluoroacetamide R* add 0.04 ml of *chlorotrimethylsilane R* and mix.

Test solution. Dissolve 50.0 mg of the substance to be examined in 3 ml of *water R* and add 0.5 ml of *hydrochloric acid R*. Extract with 2 quantities, each of 5 ml, of *methylene chloride R*. Evaporate the combined methylene chloride extracts to dryness in a vial with a screw cap and add 0.5 ml of the silylation solution. Seal the vial and heat at 70 ± 5 °C for 20 min.

Reference solution (a). Dissolve 5.0 mg of *sodium phenylbutyrate impurity C CRS* in *methylene chloride R* and dilute to 10.0 ml with the same solvent.

Reference solution (b). Dilute 1.0 ml of reference solution (a) to 10.0 ml with *methylene chloride R*. Place 1.0 ml of this solution in a vial with a screw cap, evaporate to dryness and add 0.5 ml of the silylation solution. Seal the vial and heat at 70 ± 5 °C for 20 min.

Reference solution (c). Dissolve 10 mg of the substance to be examined in 25 ml of *water R*. To 3 ml of this solution add 0.1 ml of *hydrochloric acid R*. Extract with 2 quantities, each of 5 ml, of *methylene chloride R*. Combine the methylene chloride extracts in a vial with a screw cap and add 2 ml of reference solution (a). Evaporate to dryness and add 0.5 ml of the silylation solution. Seal the vial and heat at 70 ± 5 °C for 20 min.

Column:

– *material*: fused silica;
– *size*: l = 25 m, Ø = 0.25 mm;
– *stationary phase*: *poly(dimethyl)(diphenyl)siloxane R* (film thickness 1.0 μm).

Carrier gas: *helium for chromatography R*.

Flow rate: 0.9 ml/min.

Split ratio: 1:100.

Temperature:

	Time (min)	Temperature (°C)
Column	0 - 5	50
	5 - 27	50 → 270
	27 - 32	270
Injection port		270
Detector		270

Detection: flame ionisation.

Injection: 1 μl.

Relative retention with reference to phenylbutyrate (retention time = about 20 min): impurity C = about 0.98.

System suitability: reference solution (c):

– *resolution*: minimum 3.0 between the peaks due to impurity C and phenylbutyrate.

Limit:

– *impurity C*: not more than the area of the corresponding peak in the chromatogram obtained with reference solution (b) (0.1 per cent).

Related substances. Liquid chromatography (*2.2.29*).

Test solution. Dissolve 0.20 g of the substance to be examined in 10 ml of *methanol R* and dilute to 50.0 ml with *water R*.

Reference solution (a). Dissolve 4.0 mg of *α-tetralone R* (impurity B) in 10 ml of *methanol R* and dilute to 200.0 ml with the same solvent.

Reference solution (b). Dissolve 0.20 g of the substance to be examined in 10 ml of *methanol R*, add 1 ml of reference solution (a) and dilute to 50 ml with *water R*.

Reference solution (c). Dilute 1.0 ml of reference solution (a) to 50.0 ml with *water R*.

Reference solution (d). Dissolve 5.0 mg of *3-benzoylpropionic acid R* (impurity A) in 2.5 ml of *methanol R* and dilute to 50.0 ml with the same solvent. Dilute 1.0 ml of this solution to 50.0 ml with *water R*.

Column:

– *size*: l = 0.25 m, Ø = 4.6 mm;
– *stationary phase*: *base-deactivated end-capped octadecylsilyl silica gel for chromatography R* (5 µm).

Mobile phase: *glacial acetic acid R, methanol R, water R* (1:49:50 *V/V/V*).

Flow rate: 1.3 ml/min.

Detection: spectrophotometer at 245 nm.

Injection: 20 µl of the test solution and reference solutions (b), (c) and (d).

Run time: twice the retention time of phenylbutyrate.

Relative retention with reference to phenylbutyrate (retention time = about 17 min): impurity A = about 0.3; impurity B = about 0.7.

System suitability: reference solution (b):

– *resolution*: minimum 6 between the peaks due to impurity B and phenylbutyrate.

Limits:

– *impurity A*: not more than twice the area of the corresponding peak in the chromatogram obtained with reference solution (d) (0.1 per cent);
– *impurity B*: not more than the area of the corresponding peak in the chromatogram obtained with reference solution (c) (0.01 per cent);
– *unspecified impurities*: for each impurity, not more than the area of the principal peak in the chromatogram obtained with reference solution (d) (0.05 per cent);
– *total*: not more than twice the area of the principal peak in the chromatogram obtained with reference solution (d) (0.1 per cent);
– *disregard limit of impurities other than B*: 0.6 times the area of the principal peak in the chromatogram obtained with reference solution (d) (0.03 per cent).

Heavy metals (*2.4.8*): maximum 10 ppm.

Dissolve 2.0 g in a mixture of 25 volumes of *water R* and 75 volumes of *ethanol (96 per cent) R* and dilute to 20 ml with the same mixture of solvents. 12 ml of the solution complies with test B. Prepare the reference solution using lead standard solution (1 ppm Pb) obtained by diluting *lead standard solution (100 ppm Pb) R* with a mixture of 25 volumes of *water R* and 75 volumes of *ethanol (96 per cent) R*.

Water (*2.5.12*): maximum 0.5 per cent, determined on 2.00 g.

ASSAY

Disperse 0.150 g in 50 ml of *anhydrous acetic acid R*. The opalescence of the solution disappears during the titration. Titrate with *0.1 M perchloric acid*, determining the end-point potentiometrically (*2.2.20*).

1 ml of *0.1 M perchloric acid* is equivalent to 18.62 mg of $C_{10}H_{11}NaO_2$.

IMPURITIES

Specified impurities: A, B, C.

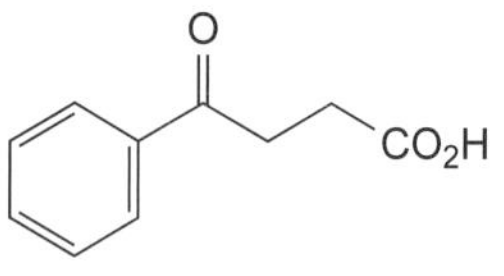

A. 4-oxo-4-phenylbutanoic acid (3-benzoylpropionic acid),

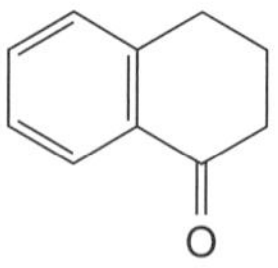

B. 3,4-dihydronaphthalen-1(2*H*)-one (α-tetralone),

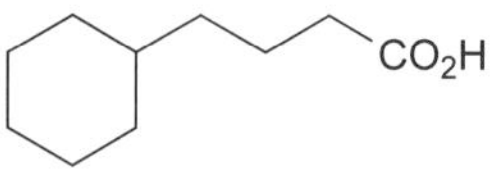

C. 4-cyclohexylbutanoic acid.

04/2008:0293

SPIRAMYCIN

Spiramycinum

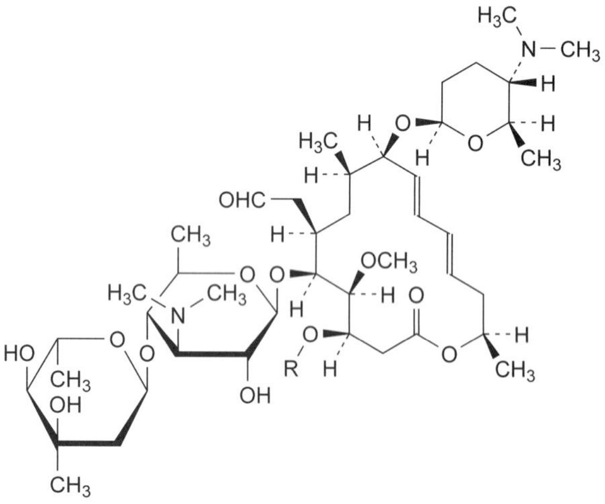

Compound	R	Molec Formula	M_r
Spiramycin I	H	$C_{43}H_{74}N_2O_{14}$	843.1
Spiramycin II	CO-CH3	$C_{45}H_{76}N_2O_{15}$	885.1
Spiramycin III	CO-CH2-CH3	$C_{46}H_{78}N_2O_{15}$	899.1

DEFINITION

Macrolide antibiotic produced by the growth of certain strains of *Streptomyces ambofaciens* or obtained by any other means. The main component is (4*R*,5*S*,6*S*,7*R*,9*R*,10*R*,11*E*,13*E*,16*R*)-6-[[3,6-dideoxy-4-*O*-(2,6-dideoxy-3-*C*-methyl-α-L-*ribo*-hexopyranosyl)-3-(dimethylamino)-β-D-glucopyranosyl]oxy]-4-hydroxy-5-methoxy-9,16-dimethyl-7-(2-oxoethyl)-10-[[2,3,4,6-tetradeoxy-4-(dimethylamino)-D-*erythro*-hexopyranosyl]oxy]oxacyclohexadeca-11,13-dien-2-one (spiramycin I; M_r 843). Spiramycin II (4-*O*-acetylspiramycin I) and spiramycin III (4-*O*-propanoylspiramycin I) are also present.

Potency: minimum 4100 IU/mg (dried substance).

CHARACTERS

Appearance: white or slightly yellowish powder, slightly hygroscopic.

Solubility: slightly soluble in water, freely soluble in acetone, in ethanol (96 per cent) and in methanol.

IDENTIFICATION

A. Ultraviolet and visible absorption spectrophotometry (*2.2.25*).

Test solution. Dissolve 0.10 g of the substance to be examined in *methanol R* and dilute to 100.0 ml with the same solvent. Dilute 1.0 ml of this solution to 100.0 ml with *methanol R*.

Spectral range: 220-350 nm.

Absorption maximum: at 232 nm.

Specific absorbance at the absorption maximum: about 340.

B. Thin-layer chromatography (*2.2.27*).

Test solution. Dissolve 40 mg of the substance to be examined in *methanol R* and dilute to 10 ml with the same solvent.

Reference solution (a). Dissolve 40 mg of *spiramycin CRS* in *methanol R* and dilute to 10 ml with the same solvent.

Reference solution (b). Dissolve 40 mg of *erythromycin A CRS* in *methanol R* and dilute to 10 ml with the same solvent.

Plate: *TLC silica gel G plate R*.

Mobile phase: the upper layer of a mixture of 4 volumes of *2-propanol R*, 8 volumes of a 150 g/l solution of *ammonium acetate R* previously adjusted to pH 9.6 with *strong sodium hydroxide solution R*, and 9 volumes of *ethyl acetate R*.

Application: 5 µl.

Development: over 3/4 of the plate.

Drying: in air.

Detection: spray with *anisaldehyde solution R1* and heat at 110 °C for 5 min.

Results: the principal spot in the chromatogram obtained with the test solution is similar in position, colour and size to the principal spot in the chromatogram obtained with reference solution (a). If in the chromatogram obtained with the test solution 1 or 2 spots occur with R_F values slightly higher than that of the principal spot, these spots are similar in position and colour to the secondary spots in the chromatogram obtained with reference solution (a) and differ from the spots in the chromatogram obtained with reference solution (b).

C. Dissolve 0.5 g in 10 ml of *0.05 M sulphuric acid* and add 25 ml of *water R*. Adjust to about pH 8 with *0.1 M sodium hydroxide* and dilute to 50 ml with *water R*. To 5 ml of this solution add 2 ml of a mixture of 1 volume of *water R* and 2 volumes of *sulphuric acid R*. A brown colour develops.

TESTS

pH (*2.2.3*): 8.5 to 10.5.

Dissolve 0.5 g in 5 ml of *methanol R* and dilute to 100 ml with *carbon dioxide-free water R*.

Specific optical rotation (*2.2.7*): − 80 to − 85 (dried substance).

Dissolve 1.00 g in a 10 per cent *V/V* solution of *dilute acetic acid R* and dilute to 50.0 ml with the same acid solution.

Composition. Liquid chromatography (*2.2.29*) as described in the test for related substances.

Injection: test solution and reference solution (a).

Calculate the percentage content using the declared content of spiramycins I, II and III in *spiramycin CRS*.

Composition of spiramycins (dried substance):

- *spiramycin I*: minimum 80.0 per cent,
- *spiramycin II*: maximum 5.0 per cent,
- *spiramycin III*: maximum 10.0 per cent,
- *sum of spiramycins I, II and III*: minimum 90.0 per cent.

Related substances. Liquid chromatography (*2.2.29*). *Prepare the solutions immediately before use.*

Solvent mixture: *methanol R*, *water R* (30:70 *V/V*).

Test solution. Dissolve 25.0 mg of the substance to be examined in the solvent mixture and dilute to 25.0 ml with the solvent mixture.

Reference solution (a). Dissolve 25.0 mg of *spiramycin CRS* in the solvent mixture and dilute to 25.0 ml with the solvent mixture.

Reference solution (b). Dilute 2.0 ml of reference solution (a) to 100.0 ml with the solvent mixture.

Reference solution (c). Dissolve 5 mg of *spiramycin CRS* in 15 ml of *buffer solution pH 2.2 R* and dilute to 25 ml with *water R*, then heat in a water-bath at 60 °C for 5 min and cool under cold water.

Blank solution. The solvent mixture.

Column:

- *size*: *l* = 0.25 m, Ø = 4.6 mm;
- *stationary phase*: *end-capped polar-embedded octadecylsilyl amorphous organosilica polymer R* (5 µm) (polar-embedded octadecylsilyl methylsilica gel), with a pore size of 12.5 nm and a carbon loading of 15 per cent;
- *temperature*: 70 °C.

Mobile phase: mix 5 volumes of a 34.8 g/l solution of *dipotassium hydrogen phosphate R* adjusted to pH 6.5 with a 27.2 g/l solution of *potassium dihydrogen phosphate R*, 40 volumes of *acetonitrile R* and 55 volumes of *water R*.

Flow rate: 1.0 ml/min.

Detection: spectrophotometer at 232 nm.

Injection: 20 µl of the blank solution, the test solution and reference solutions (b) and (c).

Run time: 3 times the retention time of spiramycin I.

Identification of spiramycins: use the chromatogram supplied with *spiramycin CRS* and the chromatogram obtained with reference solution (a) to identify the peaks due to spiramycins I, II and III.

Relative retention with reference to spiramycin I (retention time = 20 min to 30 min): impurity F = about 0.41; impurity A = about 0.45; impurity D = about 0.50; impurity G = about 0.66; impurity B = about 0.73; impurity H = about 0.87; spiramycin II = about 1.4; spiramycin III = about 2.0; impurity E = about 2.5.

If necessary adjust the composition of the mobile phase by changing the amount of acetonitrile.

System suitability: reference solution (c):

- *resolution*: minimum 10.0 between the peaks due to impurity A and spiramycin I.

Limits:

- *impurities A, B, D, E, F, G, H*: for each impurity, not more than the area of the principal peak in the chromatogram obtained with reference solution (b) (2.0 per cent);

- *any other impurity*: for each impurity, not more than the area of the principal peak in the chromatogram obtained with reference solution (b) (2.0 per cent);
- *total*: not more than 5 times the area of the principal peak in the chromatogram obtained with reference solution (b) (10.0 per cent);
- *disregard limit*: 0.05 times the area of the principal peak in the chromatogram obtained with reference solution (b) (0.1 per cent); disregard any peak due to the blank and the peaks due to spiramycins I, II and III.

Heavy metals (*2.4.8*): maximum 20 ppm.

1.0 g complies with test F. Prepare the reference solution using 2 ml of *lead standard solution (10 ppm Pb) R*.

Loss on drying (*2.2.32*): maximum 3.5 per cent, determined on 0.500 g by drying at 80 °C over *diphosphorus pentoxide R* at a pressure not exceeding 0.67 kPa for 6 h.

Sulphated ash (*2.4.14*): maximum 0.1 per cent, determined on 1.0 g.

ASSAY

Carry out the microbiological assay of antibiotics (*2.7.2*).

STORAGE

In an airtight container.

IMPURITIES

Specified impurities: A, B, D, E, F, G, H.

Other detectable impurities (the following substances would, if present at a sufficient level, be detected by one or other of the tests in the monograph. They are limited by the general acceptance criterion for other/unspecified impurities and/or by the general monograph *Substances for pharmaceutical use (2034)*. It is therefore not necessary to identify these impurities for demonstration of compliance. See also *5.10. Control of impurities in substances for pharmaceutical use*): *C*.

B. R1 = H, R2 = osyl, R3 = CH_2-CH_2OH: (4*R*,5*S*,6*S*,7*R*,9*R*,10*R*,11*E*,13*E*,16*R*)-6-[[3,6-dideoxy-4-*O*-(2,6-dideoxy-3-*C*-methyl-α-L-*ribo*-hexopyranosyl)-3-(dimethylamino)-β-D-glucopyranosyl]oxy]-4-hydroxy-7-(2-hydroxyethyl)-5-methoxy-9,16-dimethyl-10-[[2,3,4,6-tetradeoxy-4-(dimethylamino)-β-D-*erythro*-hexopyranosyl]oxy]oxacyclohexadeca-11,13-dien-2-one (spiramycin IV),

C. R1 = H, R2 = osyl, R3 = C(=CH_2)-CHO: (4*R*,5*S*,6*S*,7*S*,9*R*,10*R*,11*E*,13*E*,16*R*)-6-[[3,6-dideoxy-4-*O*-(2,6-dideoxy-3-*C*-methyl-α-L-*ribo*-hexopyranosyl)-3-(dimethylamino)-β-D-glucopyranosyl]oxy]-7-(1-formylethenyl)-4-hydroxy-5-methoxy-9,16-dimethyl-10-[[2,3,4,6-tetradeoxy-4-(dimethylamino)-β-D-*erythro*-hexopyranosyl]oxy]oxacyclohexadeca-11,13-dien-2-one (17-methylenespiramycin I),

E. R1 = H, R2 = osyl, R3 = CH_2-CH_3: (4*R*,5*S*,6*S*,7*S*,9*R*,10*R*,11*E*,13*E*,16*R*)-6-[[3,6-dideoxy-4-*O*-(2,6-dideoxy-3-*C*-methyl-α-L-*ribo*-hexopyranosyl)-3-(dimethylamino)-β-D-glucopyranosyl]oxy]-7-ethyl-4-hydroxy-5-methoxy-9,16-dimethyl-10-[[2,3,4,6-tetradeoxy-4-(dimethylamino)-β-D-*erythro*-hexopyranosyl]oxy]oxacyclohexadeca-11,13-dien-2-one (18-deoxy-18-dihydrospiramycin I or DSPM),

G. R1 = CO-CH_3, R2 = OH, R3 = CH_2-CHO: (4*R*,5*S*,6*S*,7*R*,9*R*,10*R*,11*E*,13*E*,16*R*)-6-[[3,6-dideoxy-3-(dimethylamino)-β-D-glucopyranosyl]oxy]-5-methoxy-9,16-dimethyl-2-oxo-7-(2-oxoethyl)-10-[[2,3,4,6-tetradeoxy-4-(dimethylamino)-β-D-*erythro*-hexopyranosyl]oxy]oxacyclohexadeca-11,13-dien-4-yl acetate (neospiramycin II),

H. R1 = CO-C_2H_5, R2 = OH, R3 = CH_2-CHO: (4*R*,5*S*,6*S*,7*R*,9*R*,10*R*,11*E*,13*E*,16*R*)-6-[[3,6-dideoxy-3-(dimethylamino)-β-D-glucopyranosyl]oxy]-5-methoxy-9,16-dimethyl-2-oxo-7-(2-oxoethyl)-10-[[2,3,4,6-tetradeoxy-4-(dimethylamino)-β-D-*erythro*-hexopyranosyl]oxy]oxacyclohexadeca-11,13-dien-4-yl propanoatate (neospiramycin III),

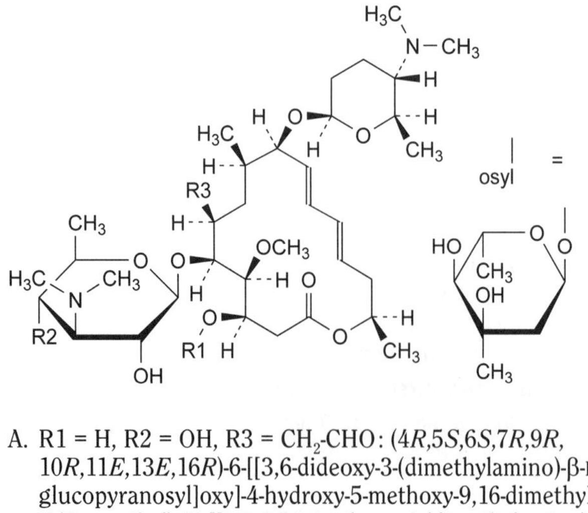

A. R1 = H, R2 = OH, R3 = CH_2-CHO: (4*R*,5*S*,6*S*,7*R*,9*R*,10*R*,11*E*,13*E*,16*R*)-6-[[3,6-dideoxy-3-(dimethylamino)-β-D-glucopyranosyl]oxy]-4-hydroxy-5-methoxy-9,16-dimethyl-7-(2-oxoethyl)-10-[[2,3,4,6-tetradeoxy-4-(dimethylamino)-β-D-*erythro*-hexopyranosyl]oxy]oxacyclohexadeca-11,13-dien-2-one (neospiramycin I),

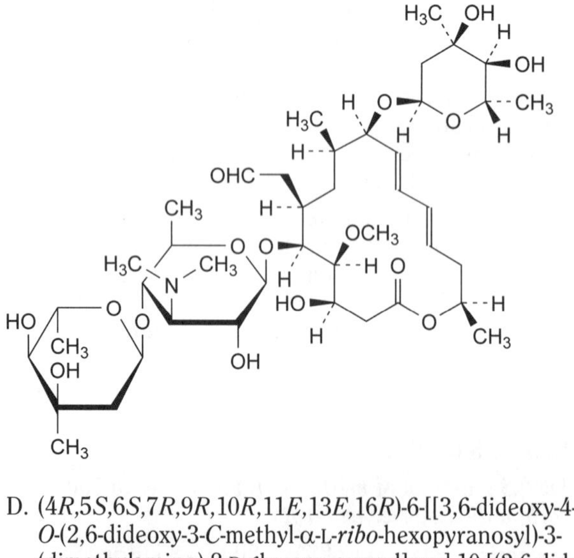

D. (4*R*,5*S*,6*S*,7*R*,9*R*,10*R*,11*E*,13*E*,16*R*)-6-[[3,6-dideoxy-4-*O*-(2,6-dideoxy-3-*C*-methyl-α-L-*ribo*-hexopyranosyl)-3-(dimethylamino)-β-D-glucopyranosyl]oxy]-10-[(2,6-dideoxy-3-*C*-methyl-α-L-*ribo*-hexopyranosyl)oxy]-4-hydroxy-5-methoxy-9,16-dimethyl-7-(2-oxoethyl)oxacyclohexadeca-11,13-dien-2-one (spiramycin V),

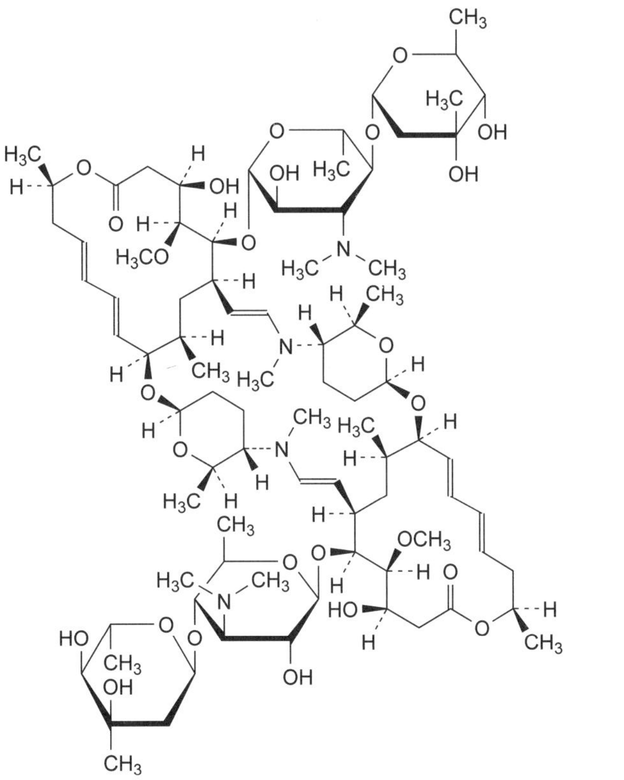

F. spiramycin dimer.

04/2008:2319

SUCROSE MONOPALMITATE

Sacchari monopalmitas

DEFINITION

Mixture of sucrose monoesters, mainly sucrose monopalmitate, obtained by transesterification of palmitic acid methyl esters of vegetable origin with *Sucrose (0204)*. The manufacture of the fatty acid methyl esters includes a distillation step.

It contains variable quantities of mono- and diesters.

Content:

- *monoesters*: minimum 55.0 per cent;
- *diesters*: maximum 40.0 per cent;
- *sum of triesters and polyesters*: maximum 20.0 per cent.

CHARACTERS

Appearance: white or almost white, unctuous powder.

Solubility: very slightly soluble in water, sparingly soluble in ethanol (96 per cent).

IDENTIFICATION

A. Composition of fatty acids (see Tests).

B. It complies with the limits of the assay.

TESTS

Acid value (*2.5.1*): maximum 6.0, determined on 3.00 g.

Use a freshly neutralised mixture of 1 volume of *water R* and 2 volumes of *2-propanol R* as solvent and heat gently.

Composition of fatty acids (*2.4.22, Method C*). Use the mixture of calibrating substances in Table 2.4.22.-1.

Composition of the fatty-acid fraction of the substance:

- *lauric acid*: maximum 3.0 per cent;
- *myristic acid*: maximum 3.0 per cent;
- *palmitic acid*: 70.0 per cent to 85.0 per cent;
- *stearic acid*: 10.0 per cent to 25.0 per cent;
- *sum of the contents of palmitic acid and stearic acid*: minimum 90.0 per cent.

Free sucrose. Liquid chromatography (*2.2.29*).

Solvent mixture: *water for chromatography R, tetrahydrofuran for chromatography R* (12.5:87.5 *V/V*).

Test solution. Dissolve 0.200 g of the substance to be examined in the solvent mixture and dilute to 4.0 ml with the solvent mixture.

Reference solution (a). Dissolve 5.0 mg of *sucrose CRS* in the solvent mixture and dilute to 50.0 ml with the solvent mixture. Dilute 1.0 ml of this solution to 10.0 ml with the solvent mixture.

Reference solution (b). In 4 volumetric flasks, introduce respectively 5.0 mg, 10.0 mg, 20.0 mg and 25.0 mg of *sucrose CRS*, dissolve in the solvent mixture and dilute to 10.0 ml with the solvent mixture.

Column:

- *size*: *l* = 0.25 m, Ø = 4.6 mm;
- *stationary phase*: spherical *aminopropylsilyl silica gel for chromatography R* (4 μm).

Mobile phase:

- *mobile phase A*: 0.01 g/l solution of *ammonium acetate R* in *acetonitrile for chromatography R*;
- *mobile phase B*: 0.01 g/l solution of *ammonium acetate R* in a mixture of 10 volumes of *water for chromatography R* and 90 volumes of *tetrahydrofuran for chromatography R*;

Time (min)	Mobile phase A (per cent *V/V*)	Mobile phase B (per cent *V/V*)	Flow rate (ml/min)
0 - 1	100	0	1.0
1 - 9	100 → 0	0 → 100	1.0
9 - 16	0	100	1.0
16 - 16.01	0	100	1.0 → 2.5
16.01 - 32	0	100	2.5
32 - 33	0 → 100	100 → 0	2.5
33 - 36	100	0	2.5 → 1.0

Detection: evaporative light-scattering detector; the following settings have been found to be suitable; if the detector has different setting parameters, adjust the detector settings so as to comply with the system suitability criterion:

- *carrier gas*: *nitrogen R*;
- *flow rate*: 1.0 ml/min;
- *evaporator temperature*: 45 °C;
- *nebuliser temperature*: 40 °C.

Injection: 20 μl.

Retention time: about 26 min.

System suitability: reference solution (a):

- *signal-to-noise ratio*: minimum 10.

Limit: maximum 4.0 per cent.

Water (*2.5.12*): maximum 4.0 per cent, determined on 0.20 g.

Total ash (*2.4.16*): maximum 1.5 per cent.

ASSAY

Size-exclusion chromatography (*2.2.30*): use the normalisation procedure.

Test solution. Dissolve 60.0 mg of the substance to be examined in *tetrahydrofuran R* and dilute to 4.0 ml with the same solvent.

Monographs Q-Z

Column:

- *size*: l = 0.6 m, Ø = 7 mm;
- *stationary phase*: *styrene-divinylbenzene copolymer R* (5 μm) with a pore size of 10 nm.

Mobile phase: *tetrahydrofuran R.*

Flow rate: 1.2 ml/min.

Detection: differential refractometer.

Injection: 20 μl.

Relative retention with reference to monoesters (retention time = about 10 min): diesters = about 0.92; triesters and polyesters = about 0.90.

Calculations:

- *disregard limit*: disregard the peaks having a signal-to-noise ratio less than 10;
- *free fatty acids*: calculate the percentage content (D) of free fatty acids, using the following expression:

$$\frac{I_A \times 256}{561.1}$$

I_A = acid value.

- *monoesters*: calculate the percentage content of monoesters using the following expression:

$$\frac{A \times (100 - D - S - E)}{100}$$

- *diesters*: calculate the percentage content of diesters using the following expression:

$$\frac{B \times (100 - D - S - E)}{100}$$

- *sum of triesters and polyesters*: calculate the sum of the percentage contents of triesters and polyesters using the following expression:

$$\frac{C \times (100 - D - S - E)}{100}$$

A = percentage content of monoesters determined by the normalisation procedure;

S = percentage content of free sucrose (see Tests);

E = percentage content of water (see Tests);

B = percentage content of diesters determined by the normalisation procedure;

C = sum of the percentage contents of triesters and polyesters determined by the normalisation procedure.

STORAGE

Protected from humidity.

04/2008:2318

SUCROSE STEARATE

Sacchari stearas

DEFINITION

Mixture of sucrose esters, mainly sucrose stearate, obtained by transesterification of stearic acid methyl esters of vegetable origin with *sucrose (0204).* The manufacture of the fatty acid methyl esters includes a distillation step.

It contains variable quantities of mono- and diesters.

Content:

Sucrose stearate type I:

- *monoesters*: minimum 50.0 per cent;
- *diesters*: maximum 40.0 per cent;
- *sum of triesters and polyesters*: maximum 25.0 per cent;

Sucrose stearate type II:

- *monoesters*: 20.0 per cent to 45.0 per cent;
- *diesters*: 30.0 per cent to 40.0 per cent;
- *sum of triesters and polyesters*: maximum 30.0 per cent.

CHARACTERS

Appearance: white or almost white, unctuous powder.

Solubility: very slightly soluble in water, sparingly soluble in ethanol (96 per cent).

IDENTIFICATION

A. Composition of fatty acids (see Tests).

B. It complies with the limits of the assay.

TESTS

Acid value (*2.5.1*): maximum 6.0, determined on 3.00 g.

Use a freshly neutralised mixture of 1 volume of *water R* and 2 volumes of *2-propanol R* as solvent and heat gently.

Composition of fatty acids (*2.4.22, Method C*). Use the mixture of calibrating substances in Table 2.4.22.-1.

Composition of the fatty-acid fraction of the substance:

- *lauric acid*: maximum 3.0 per cent;
- *myristic acid*: maximum 3.0 per cent;
- *palmitic acid*: 25.0 per cent to 40.0 per cent;
- *stearic acid*: 55.0 per cent to 75.0 per cent;
- *sum of the contents of palmitic acid and stearic acid*: minimum 90.0 per cent.

Free sucrose. Liquid chromatography (*2.2.29*).

Solvent mixture: *water for chromatography R, tetrahydrofuran for chromatography R* (12.5:87.5 *V/V*).

Test solution. Dissolve 0.200 g of the substance to be examined in the solvent mixture and dilute to 4.0 ml with the solvent mixture.

Reference solution (a). Dissolve 5.0 mg of *sucrose CRS* in the solvent mixture and dilute to 50.0 ml with the solvent mixture. Dilute 1.0 ml of this solution to 10.0 ml with the solvent mixture.

Reference solution (b). In 4 volumetric flasks, introduce respectively 5.0 mg, 10.0 mg, 20.0 mg and 25.0 mg of *sucrose CRS,* dissolve in the solvent mixture and dilute to 10.0 ml with the solvent mixture.

Column:

- *size*: l = 0.25 m, Ø = 4.6 mm;
- *stationary phase*: spherical *aminopropylsilyl silica gel for chromatography R* (4 μm).

Mobile phase:

- *mobile phase A*: 0.01 g/l solution of *ammonium acetate R* in *acetonitrile for chromatography R*;
- *mobile phase B*: 0.01 g/l solution of *ammonium acetate R* in a mixture of 10 volumes of *water for chromatography R* and 90 volumes of *tetrahydrofuran for chromatography R*;

Time (min)	Mobile phase A (per cent *V/V*)	Mobile phase B (per cent *V/V*)	Flow rate (ml/min)
0 - 1	100	0	1.0
1 - 9	100 → 0	0 → 100	1.0
9 - 16	0	100	1.0
16 - 16.01	0	100	1.0 → 2.5
16.01 - 32	0	100	2.5
32 - 33	0 → 100	100 → 0	2.5
33 - 36	100	0	2.5 → 1.0

Detection: evaporative light-scattering detector; the following settings have been found to be suitable; if the detector has different setting parameters, adjust the detector settings so as to comply with the system suitability criterion:
- *carrier gas*: *nitrogen R*;
- *flow rate*: 1.0 ml/min;
- *evaporator temperature*: 45 °C;
- *nebuliser temperature*: 40 °C.

Injection: 20 µl.

Retention time: about 26 min.

System suitability: reference solution (a):
- *signal-to-noise ratio*: minimum 10.

Limit: maximum 4.0 per cent.

Water (*2.5.12*): maximum 4.0 per cent, determined on 0.20 g.

Total ash (*2.4.16*): maximum 1.5 per cent.

ASSAY

Size-exclusion chromatography (*2.2.30*): use the normalisation procedure.

Test solution. Dissolve 60.0 mg of the substance to be examined in *tetrahydrofuran R* and dilute to 4.0 ml with the same solvent.

Column:
- *size*: l = 0.6 m, Ø = 7 mm;
- *stationary phase*: *styrene-divinylbenzene copolymer R* (5 µm) with a pore size of 10 nm.

Mobile phase: *tetrahydrofuran R*.

Flow rate: 1.2 ml/min.

Detection: differential refractometer.

Injection: 20 µl.

Relative retention with reference to monoesters (retention time = about 10 min): diesters = about 0.92; triesters and polyesters = about 0.90.

Calculations:
- *disregard limit*: disregard the peaks having a signal-to-noise ratio less than 10;
- *free fatty acids*: calculate the percentage content (D) of free fatty acids, using the following expression:

$$\frac{I_A \times 284.5}{561.1}$$

I_A = acid value;

- *monoesters*: calculate the percentage content of monoesters using the following expression:

$$\frac{A \times (100 - D - S - E)}{100}$$

- *diesters*: calculate the percentage content of diesters using the following expression:

$$\frac{B \times (100 - D - S - E)}{100}$$

- *sum of triesters and polyesters*: calculate the sum of the percentage contents of triesters and polyesters using the following expression:

$$\frac{C \times (100 - D - S - E)}{100}$$

A = percentage content of monoesters determined by the normalisation procedure;

S = percentage content of free sucrose (see Tests);

E = percentage content of water (see Tests);

B = percentage content of diesters determined by the normalisation procedure;

C = sum of the percentage contents of triesters and polyesters determined by the normalisation procedure.

LABELLING

The label states the type of sucrose stearate (type I or II).

STORAGE

Protected from humidity.

04/2008:2211

SULTAMICILLIN

Sultamicillinum

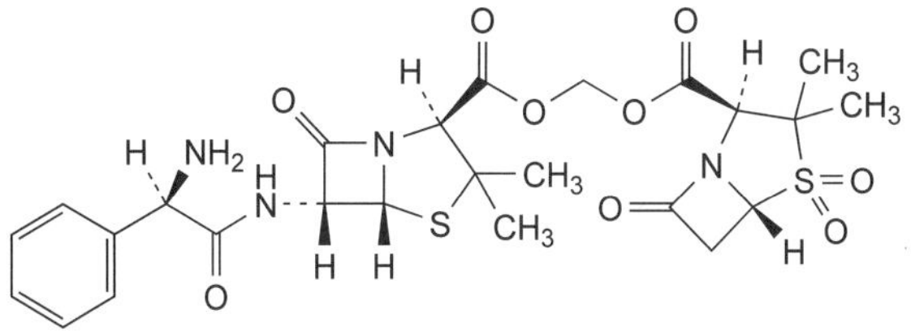

$C_{25}H_{30}N_4O_9S_2$ M_r 594.7

[76497-13-7]

DEFINITION

Methylene (2*S*,5*R*,6*R*)-6-[[(2*R*)-aminophenylacetyl]amino]-3,3-dimethyl-7-oxo-4-thia-1-azabicyclo[3.2.0]heptane-2-carboxylate (2*S*,5*R*)-3,3-dimethyl-4,4,7-trioxo-4λ^6-thia-1-azabicyclo[3.2.0]heptane-2-carboxylate.

Semi-synthetic product derived from a fermentation product.

Content: 96.0 per cent to 102.0 per cent (anhydrous substance).

CHARACTERS

Appearance: white or almost white, slightly hygroscopic, crystalline powder.

Solubility: practically insoluble in water, very slightly soluble in methanol, practically insoluble in ethanol (96 per cent).

IDENTIFICATION

Infrared absorption spectrophotometry (*2.2.24*).

Comparison: *sultamicillin CRS*.

TESTS

Specific optical rotation (*2.2.7*): + 190 to + 210 (anhydrous substance).

Dissolve 0.500 g in *dimethylformamide R* and dilute to 50.0 ml with the same solvent.

Related substances. Liquid chromatography (*2.2.29*). *Prepare the solutions immediately before use or keep at 2-8 °C for not more than 6 h.*

Solution A: *methanol R1, acetonitrile R1* (20:80 *V/V*).

Solution B. Dissolve 1.56 g of *sodium dihydrogen phosphate R* in 900 ml of *water R*. Add 7.0 ml of *phosphoric acid R* and dilute to 1000 ml with *water R*.

Blank solution: solution B, solution A (30:70 *V/V*).

Test solution. Dissolve 50.0 mg of the substance to be examined in 35 ml of solution A and sonicate for about 1 min. Add 13 ml of solution B, mix and sonicate for about 1 min. Dilute to 50.0 ml with solution B and mix.

Reference solution (a). Dissolve 70.0 mg of *sultamicillin tosilate CRS* in 35 ml of solution A and sonicate for about 1 min. Add 13 ml of solution B, mix and sonicate for about 1 min. Dilute to 50.0 ml with solution B and mix.

Reference solution (b). Suspend 15 mg of *sultamicillin tosilate CRS* in 20 ml of a 0.4 g/l solution of *sodium hydroxide R* and sonicate in an ultrasonic bath for about 5 min. Add 20 ml of a 0.36 g/l solution of *hydrochloric acid R* and dilute to 100 ml with *water R*.

Reference solution (c). Dilute 1.0 ml of reference solution (a) to 100.0 ml with the blank solution.

Reference solution (d). Dissolve 17.3 mg of *ampicillin trihydrate CRS* (impurity C) and 15.0 mg of *sulbactam CRS* (impurity A) in *water R* and dilute to 50.0 ml with the same solvent. Dilute 1.0 ml of this solution to 100.0 ml with *water R*.

Reference solution (e). Dissolve 5 mg of *sultamicillin for peak identification CRS* (containing impurity G) in 7.0 ml of solution A and sonicate for about 1 min. Dilute to 10.0 ml with solution B, mix and sonicate for about 1 min.

Column:

– *size*: *l* = 0.10 m, Ø = 4.6 mm;
– *stationary phase*: *octadecylsilyl silica gel for chromatography R* (3.5 μm);
– *temperature*: 25 °C.

Mobile phase:

– *mobile phase A*: 4.68 g/l solution of *sodium dihydrogen phosphate R* adjusted to pH 3.0 with *phosphoric acid R*;
– *mobile phase B*: *acetonitrile R1*;

Time (min)	Mobile phase A (per cent *V/V*)	Mobile phase B (per cent *V/V*)
0 - 15	95 → 30	5 → 70
15 - 16	30	70
16 - 16.5	30 → 95	70 → 5
16.5 - 20	95	5

Flow rate: 1.0 ml/min.

Detection: spectrophotometer at 215 nm.

Injection: 5 μl of the blank solution, the test solution and reference solutions (b), (c), (d) and (e).

Identification of impurities: use the chromatogram supplied with *sultamicillin for peak identification CRS* and the chromatogram obtained with reference solution (e) to identify the peak due to impurity G.

Relative retention with reference to sultamicillin (retention time = about 9.3 min): impurity A = about 0.41; ampicillin penicilloic acid = about 0.47; impurity B = about 0.50; impurity C = about 0.55; impurity D = about 0.94; impurity E = about 1.09; impurity F = about 1.26; impurity G = about 1.42.

System suitability: reference solution (b):

– *resolution*: minimum 2.5 between the peaks due to ampicillin penicilloic acid and impurity B and minimum 2.5 between the peaks due to impurities B and C.

Limits:

– *impurity G*: not more than the area of the peak due to sultamicillin in the chromatogram obtained with reference solution (c) (1.0 per cent);
– *impurity A*: not more than the area of the corresponding peak in the chromatogram obtained with reference solution (d) (0.3 per cent);
– *impurity B*: not more than the area of the corresponding peak in the chromatogram obtained with reference solution (c) (0.3 per cent);
– *impurity C*: not more than the area of the corresponding peak in the chromatogram obtained with reference solution (d) (0.3 per cent);
– *impurities D, E, F*: for each impurity, not more than 0.3 times the area of the peak due to sultamicillin in the chromatogram obtained with reference solution (c) (0.3 per cent);
– *any other impurity*: for each impurity, not more than 0.3 times the area of the peak due to sultamicillin in the chromatogram obtained with reference solution (c) (0.3 per cent);
– *total*: not more than 3 times the area of the peak due to sultamicillin in the chromatogram obtained with reference solution (c) (3.0 per cent);
– *disregard limit*: 0.1 times the area of the peak due to sultamicillin in the chromatogram obtained with reference solution (c) (0.1 per cent).

Ethyl acetate. Head-space gas chromatography (*2.2.28*).

Test solution. Dissolve 0.200 g in 7.0 ml of a mixture of 1 volume of *water R* and 99 volumes of *dimethylformamide R*.

Reference solution. Dissolve 0.200 g of *ethyl acetate R* in 240 ml of a mixture of 1 volume of *water R* and 99 volumes of *dimethylformamide R* and dilute to 250.0 ml with the same mixture of solvents. Dilute 5.0 ml of this solution to 7.0 ml with a mixture of 1 volume of *water R* and 99 volumes of *dimethylformamide R*.

Close the vials immediately with a tight rubber membrane stopper coated with polytetrafluoroethylene and secure with an aluminium crimped cap. Shake to obtain a homogeneous solution.

Column:

– *material*: fused silica;
– *size*: *l* = 50 m, Ø = 0.32 mm;
– *stationary phase*: *poly(dimethyl)siloxane R* (film thickness: 1.8 μm or 3 μm).

Carrier gas: *helium for chromatography R*.

Linear velocity: 35 cm/s.

Split ratio: 1:5.

Static head-space conditions that may be used:

– *equilibration temperature*: 105 °C;
– *equilibration time*: 45 min;
– *transfer-line temperature*: 110 °C;
– *pressurisation time*: 30 s.

Temperature:

	Time (min)	Temperature (°C)
Column	0 - 6	70
	6 - 16	70 → 220
	16 - 18	220
Injection port		140
Detector		250

Detection: flame ionisation.

Injection: 1 ml.

Relative retention with reference to dimethylformamide (retention time = about 14 min): ethyl acetate = about 0.7.

Limit:

– *ethyl acetate*: maximum 2.5 per cent.

Heavy metals (*2.4.8*): maximum 20 ppm.

Dissolve 2.0 g in a mixture of 40 volumes of *methanol R* and 60 volumes of *acetonitrile R* and dilute to 20.0 ml with the same mixture of solvents. 12 ml of the solution complies with test B. Prepare the reference solution using lead standard solution (2 ppm Pb) obtained by diluting *lead standard solution (100 ppm Pb) R* with a mixture of 40 volumes of *methanol R* and 60 volumes of *acetonitrile R*.

Water (*2.5.12*): maximum 1.0 per cent, determined on 0.50 g.

Sulphated ash (*2.4.14*): maximum 0.1 per cent, determined on 1.0 g.

ASSAY

Liquid chromatography (*2.2.29*) as described in the test for related substances with the following modifications.

Injection: test solution and reference solution (a).

Calculate the percentage content of sultamicillin ($C_{25}H_{30}N_4O_9S_2$) from the declared content of $C_{25}H_{30}N_4O_9S_2$ in *sultamicillin tosilate CRS* and by multiplying the sultamicillin tosilate content by 0.7752.

STORAGE

In an airtight container.

IMPURITIES

Specified impurities: A, B, C, D, E, F, G.

A. sulbactam,

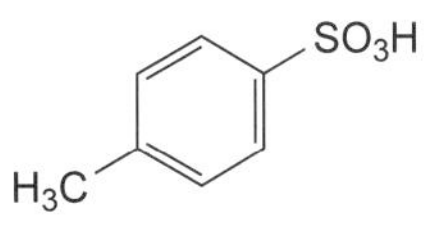

B. 4-methylbenzenesulphonic acid (*p*-toluenesulphonic acid),

C. ampicillin,

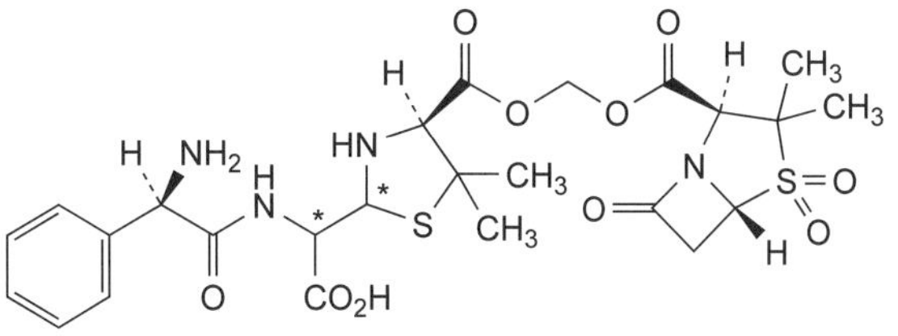

D. [[(2*R*)-aminophenylacetyl]amino][(4*S*)-4-[[[[(2*S*,5*R*)-3,3-dimethyl-4,4,7-trioxo-4λ[6]-thia-1-azabicyclo[3.2.0]hept-2-yl]carbonyl]oxy]methoxy]carbonyl]-5,5-dimethylthiazolidin-2-yl]acetic acid (penicilloic acids of sultamicillin),

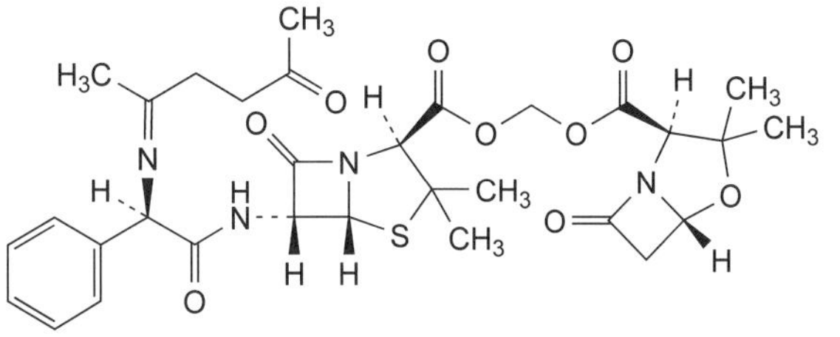

E. methylene (2*S*,5*R*,6*R*)-3,3-dimethyl-6-[[(2*R*)-[(1-methyl-4-oxopentylidene)amino]phenylacetyl]amino]-7-oxo-4-thia-1-azabicyclo[3.2.0]heptane-2-carboxylate (2*S*,5*R*)-3,3-dimethyl-7-oxo-4-oxa-1-azabicyclo[3.2.0]heptane-2-carboxylate,

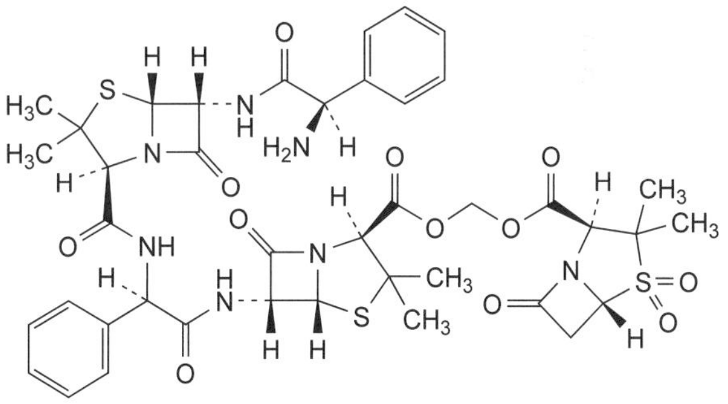

F. methylene (2*S*,5*R*,6*R*)-6-[[(2*R*)-[[[(2*S*,5*R*,6*R*)-6-[[(2*R*)-aminophenylacetyl]amino]-3,3-dimethyl-7-oxo-4-thia-1-azabicyclo[3.2.0]hept-2-yl]carbonyl]amino]phenylacetyl]amino]-3,3-dimethyl-7-oxo-4-thia-1-azabicyclo[3.2.0]heptane-2-carboxylate (2*S*,5*R*)-3,3-dimethyl-4,4,7-trioxo-4λ[6]-thia-1-azabicyclo-[3.2.0]heptane-2-carboxylate (ampicillin sultamicillin amide),

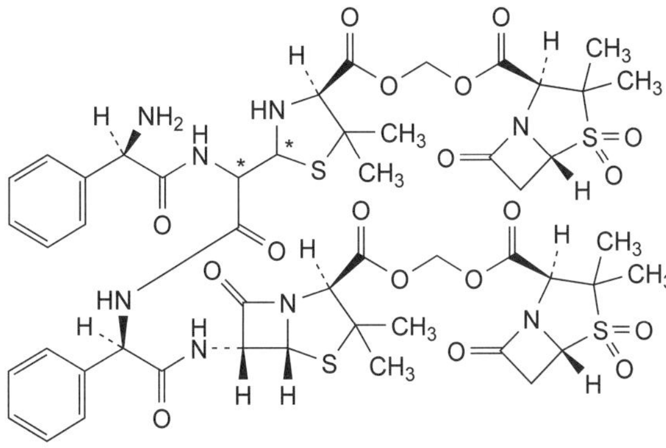

G. methylene (2*S*,5*R*,6*R*)-6-[[(2*R*)-[[[(2*R*)-aminophenylacetyl]amino][(4*S*)-4-[[[[(2*S*,5*R*)-3,3-dimethyl-4,4,7-trioxo-4λ[6]-thia-1-azabicyclo[3.2.0]hept-2-yl]carbonyl]oxy]methoxy]carbonyl]-5,5-dimethylthiazolidin-2-yl]acetyl]amino]phenylacetyl]amino]-3,3-dimethyl-7-oxo-4-thia-1-azabicyclo[3.2.0]heptane-2-carboxylate (2*S*,5*R*)-3,3-dimethyl-4,4,7-trioxo-4λ[6]-thia-1-azabicyclo-[3.2.0]heptane-2-carboxylate (sultamicillin dimer).

Monographs Q-Z

01/2008:2212
corrected 6.1

SULTAMICILLIN TOSILATE DIHYDRATE

Sultamicillini tosilas dihydricus

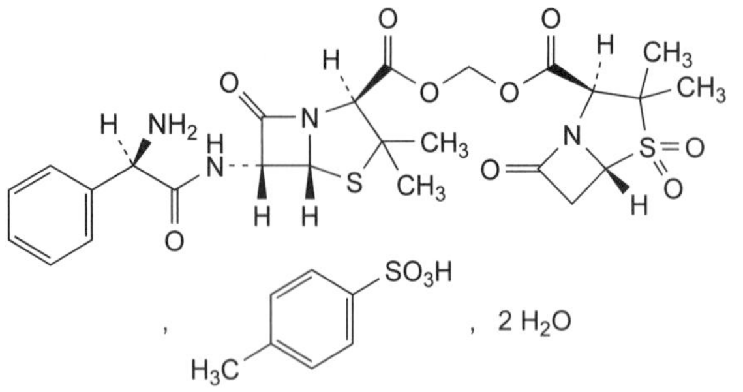

$C_{32}H_{38}N_4O_{12}S_3,2H_2O$ M_r 803

DEFINITION

4-Methylbenzenesulphonate of methylene (2*S*,5*R*,6*R*)-6-[[(2*R*)-aminophenylacetyl]amino]-3,3-dimethyl-7-oxo-4-thia-1-azabicyclo[3.2.0]heptane-2-carboxylate (2*S*,5*R*)-3,3-dimethyl-4,4,7-trioxo-4λ^6-thia-1-azabicyclo[3.2.0]heptane-2-carboxylate dihydrate.

Semi-synthetic product derived from a fermentation product.

Content: 95.0 per cent to 102.0 per cent (anhydrous substance).

CHARACTERS

Appearance: white or almost white, crystalline powder.

Solubility: practically insoluble in water, sparingly soluble in ethanol (96 per cent).

IDENTIFICATION

Infrared absorption spectrophotometry (*2.2.24*).

Comparison: *sultamicillin tosilate CRS*.

TESTS

Specific optical rotation (*2.2.7*): + 178 to + 195 (anhydrous substance).

Dissolve 1.000 g in *dimethylformamide R* and dilute to 50.0 ml with the same solvent.

Related substances. Liquid chromatography (*2.2.29*). *Prepare the solutions immediately before use or keep at 2-8 °C for not more than 6 h.*

Solution A: *methanol R1, acetonitrile R1* (20:80 *V/V*).

Solution B. Dissolve 1.56 g of *sodium dihydrogen phosphate R* in 900 ml of *water R*. Add 7.0 ml of *phosphoric acid R* and dilute to 1000 ml with *water R*.

Blank solution: solution B, solution A (30:70 *V/V*).

Test solution. Dissolve 70.0 mg of the substance to be examined in 35 ml of solution A and sonicate for about 1 min. Add 13 ml of solution B, mix and sonicate for about 1 min. Dilute to 50.0 ml with solution B and mix.

Reference solution (a). Dissolve 70.0 mg of *sultamicillin tosilate CRS* in 35 ml of solution A and sonicate for about 1 min. Add 13 ml of solution B, mix and sonicate for about 1 min. Dilute to 50.0 ml with solution B and mix.

Reference solution (b). Suspend 15 mg of the substance to be examined in 20 ml of a 0.4 g/l solution of *sodium hydroxide R* and sonicate in an ultrasonic bath for about 5 min. Add 20 ml of a 0.36 g/l solution of *hydrochloric acid R* and dilute to 100.0 ml with *water R*.

Reference solution (c). Dissolve 0.200 g of the substance to be examined in 70.0 ml of solution A and sonicate for about 1 min. Add 25.0 ml of solution B, mix and sonicate for about 1 min. Dilute to 100.0 ml with solution B and mix. Dilute 1.0 ml of this solution to 100.0 ml with the blank solution.

Reference solution (d). Dissolve 32.3 mg of *ampicillin trihydrate CRS* (impurity B) and 7.0 mg of *sulbactam CRS* (impurity A) in *water R* and dilute to 1000 ml with the same solvent.

Column:

- *size*: *l* = 0.10 m, Ø = 4.6 mm;
- *stationary phase*: *octadecylsilyl silica gel for chromatography R* (3.5 μm);
- *temperature*: 25 °C.

Mobile phase:

- *mobile phase A*: 4.68 g/l solution of *sodium dihydrogen phosphate R* adjusted to pH 3.0 with *phosphoric acid R*;
- *mobile phase B*: *acetonitrile R1*;

Time (min)	Mobile phase A (per cent *V/V*)	Mobile phase B (per cent *V/V*)
0 - 15	95 → 30	5 → 70
15 - 16	30	70
16 - 16.5	30 → 95	70 → 5
16.5 - 20	95	5

Flow rate: 1.0 ml/min.

Detection: spectrophotometer at 215 nm.

Injection: 5 μl of the blank solution, the test solution and reference solutions (b), (c) and (d).

Relative retention with reference to sultamicillin (retention time = about 9.3 min): impurity A = about 0.41; ampicillin penicilloic acid = about 0.47; tosilate = about 0.50; impurity B = about 0.55; impurity C = about 0.94; impurity D = about 1.09; impurity E = about 1.23; impurity F = about 1.26; impurity G = about 1.42.

System suitability: reference solution (b):

- *resolution*: minimum 2.5 between the peaks due to ampicillin penicilloic acid and tosilate and minimum 2.5 between the peaks due to tosilate and impurity B.

Limits:

- *impurity B*: not more than the area of the corresponding peak in the chromatogram obtained with reference solution (d) (2.0 per cent);
- *impurity A*: not more than the area of the corresponding peak in the chromatogram obtained with reference solution (d) (0.5 per cent);
- *impurities C, D, E, F, G*: for each impurity, not more than 0.5 times the area of the peak due to sultamicillin in the chromatogram obtained with reference solution (c) (0.5 per cent);
- *any other impurity*: for each impurity, not more than 0.5 times the area of the peak due to sultamicillin in the chromatogram obtained with reference solution (c) (0.5 per cent);
- *total*: not more than 4 times the area of the peak due to sultamicillin in the chromatogram obtained with reference solution (c) (4.0 per cent);
- *disregard limit*: 0.1 times the area of the peak due to sultamicillin in the chromatogram obtained with reference solution (c) (0.1 per cent).

Ethyl acetate. Head space gas chromatography (*2.2.28*).

Test solution. Dissolve 0.200 g in 7.0 ml of a mixture of 1 volume of *water R* and 99 volumes of *dimethylformamide R*.

Reference solution. Dissolve 0.200 g of *ethyl acetate R* in 240 ml of a mixture of 1 volume of *water R* and 99 volumes of *dimethylformamide R* and dilute to 250.0 ml with the same mixture of solvents. Dilute 5.0 ml of this solution to 7.0 ml with a mixture of 1 volume of *water R* and 99 volumes of *dimethylformamide R*.

Immediately close the vials with a tight rubber membrane stopper coated with polytetrafluoroethylene and secure with an aluminium crimped cap. Shake to obtain a homogeneous solution.

Column:

- *material*: fused silica;
- *size*: *l* = 50 m, Ø = 0.32 mm;
- *stationary phase*: *poly(dimethyl)siloxane R* (film thickness: 1.8 µm or 3 µm).

Carrier gas: *helium for chromatography R*.

Linear velocity: 35 cm/s.

Split ratio: 1:5.

Static head-space conditions that may be used:

- *equilibration temperature*: 105 °C;
- *equilibration time*: 45 min;
- *transfer-line temperature*: 110 °C;
- *pressurisation time*: 30 s.

Temperature:

	Time (min)	Temperature (°C)
Column	0 - 6	70
	6 - 16	70 → 220
	16 - 18	220
Injection port		140
Detector		250

Detection: flame ionisation.

Injection: 1 ml.

Relative retention with reference to dimethylformamide (retention time = about 14 min): ethyl acetate = about 0.7.

Limit:

- *ethyl acetate*: maximum 2.0 per cent.

Heavy metals (*2.4.8*): maximum 20 ppm.

Dissolve 2.0 g in a mixture of 40 volumes of *methanol R* and 60 volumes of *acetonitrile R* and dilute to 20.0 ml with the same mixture of solvents. 12 ml of the solution complies with test B. Prepare the reference solution using lead standard solution (2 ppm Pb) obtained by diluting *lead standard solution (100 ppm Pb) R* with a mixture of 40 volumes of *methanol R* and 60 volumes of *acetonitrile R*.

Water (*2.5.12*): 4.0 per cent to 6.0 per cent, determined on 0.200 g.

Sulphated ash (*2.4.14*): maximum 0.2 per cent, determined on 1.0 g.

ASSAY

Liquid chromatography (*2.2.29*) as described in the test for related substances with the following modification.

Injection: test solution and reference solution (a).

Calculate the percentage content of sultamicillin tosilate ($C_{32}H_{38}N_4O_{12}S_3$) from the declared content of *sultamicillin tosilate CRS*.

STORAGE

In an airtight container.

IMPURITIES

Specified impurities: A, B, C, D, E, F, G.

A. sulbactam,

B. ampicillin,

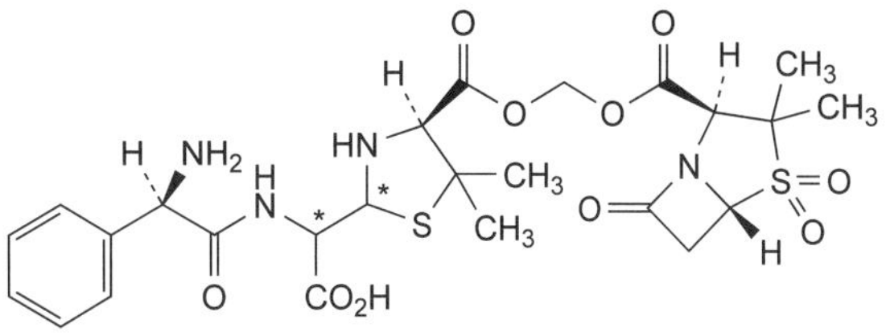

C. [[(2*R*)-aminophenylacetyl]amino][(4*S*)-4-[[[[(2*S*,5*R*)-3,3-dimethyl-4,4,7-trioxo-4λ^6-thia-1-azabicyclo[3.2.0]hept-2-yl]carbonyl]oxy]methoxy]carbonyl]-5,5-dimethylthiazolidin-2-yl]acetic acid (penicilloic acids of sultamicillin),

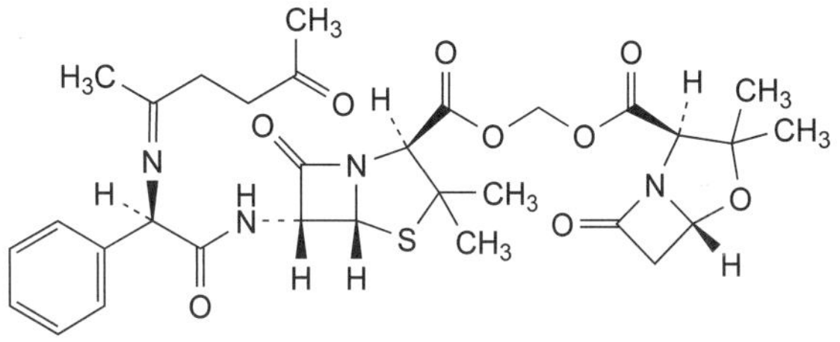

D. methylene (2*S*,5*R*,6*R*)-3,3-dimethyl-6-[[(2*R*)-[(1-methyl-4-oxopentylidene)amino]phenylacetyl]amino]-7-oxo-4-thia-1-azabicyclo[3.2.0]heptane-2-carboxylate (2*S*,5*R*)-3,3-dimethyl-7-oxo-4-oxa-1-azabicyclo[3.2.0]heptane-2-carboxylate,

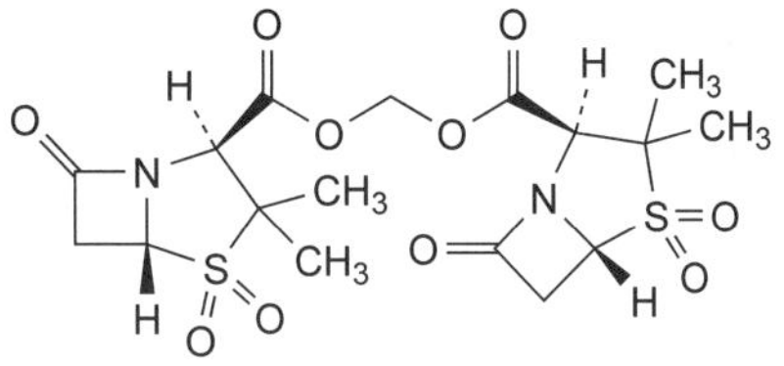

E. methylene bis[(2*S*,5*R*)-3,3-dimethyl-4,4,7-trioxo-4λ^6-thia-1-azabicyclo[3.2.0]heptane-2-carboxylate] (sulbactam methylene ester),

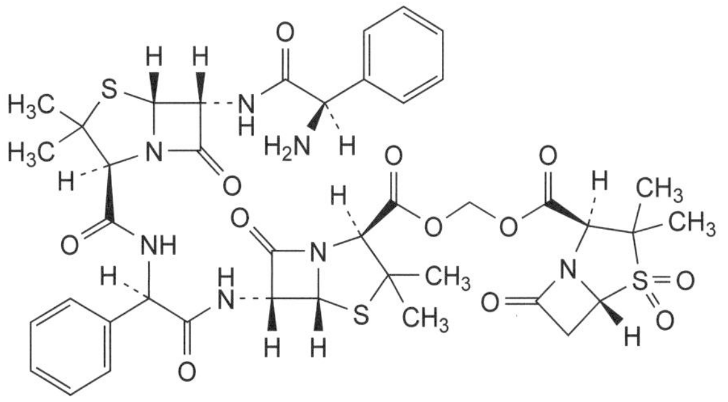

F. methylene (2*S*,5*R*,6*R*)-6-[[(2*R*)-[[[(2*S*,5*R*,6*R*)-6-[[(2*R*)-aminophenylacetyl]amino]-3,3-dimethyl-7-oxo-4-thia-1-azabicyclo[3.2.0]hept-2-yl]carbonyl]amino]phenylacetyl]amino]-3,3-dimethyl-7-oxo-4-thia-1-azabicyclo[3.2.0]heptane-2-carboxylate (2*S*,5*R*)-3,3-dimethyl-4,4,7-trioxo-4λ^6-thia-1-azabicyclo[3.2.0]heptane-2-carboxylate (ampicillin sultamicillin amide),

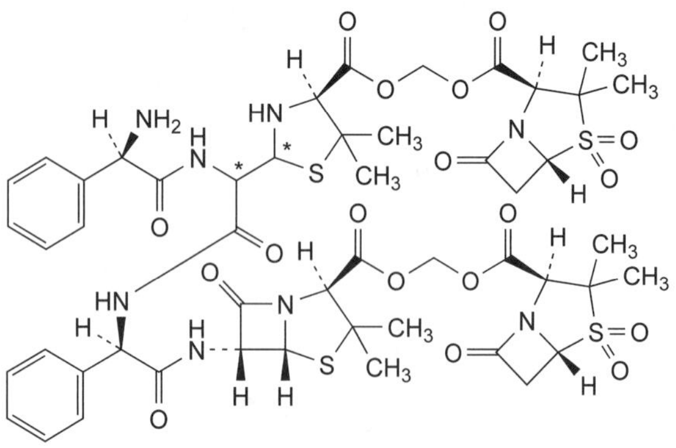

G. methylene (2*S*,5*R*,6*R*)-6-[[(2*R*)-[[[(2*R*)-amino-phenylacetyl]amino][(4*S*)-4-[[[[(2*S*,5*R*)-3,3-dimethyl-4,4,7-trioxo-4λ^6-thia-1-azabicyclo[3.2.0]hept-2-yl]carbonyl]oxy]methoxy]carbonyl]-5,5-dimethylthiazolidin-2-yl]acetyl]amino]phenylacetyl]amino]-3,3-dimethyl-7-oxo-4-thia-1-azabicyclo[3.2.0]heptane-2-carboxylate (2*S*,5*R*)-3,3-dimethyl-4,4,7-trioxo-4λ^6-thia-1-aza-bicyclo[3.2.0]heptane-2-carboxylate (sultamicillin dimer).

T

01/2008:1270
corrected 6.1

TERCONAZOLE

Terconazolum

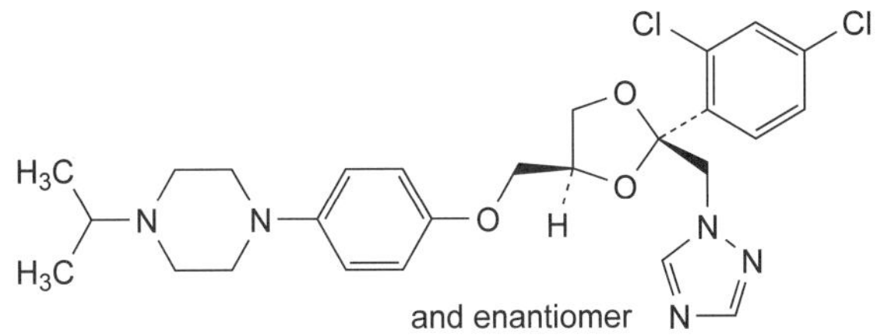

$C_{26}H_{31}Cl_2N_5O_3$ M_r 532.5

[67915-31-5]

DEFINITION

1-[4-[[(2*RS*,4*SR*)-2-(2,4-Dichlorophenyl)-2-[(1*H*-1,2,4-triazol-1-yl)methyl]-1,3-dioxolan-4-yl]methoxy]phenyl]-4-(1-methylethyl)piperazine.

Content: 99.0 per cent to 101.0 per cent (dried substance).

CHARACTERS

Appearance: white or almost white powder.

Solubility: practically insoluble in water, freely soluble in methylene chloride, soluble in acetone, sparingly soluble in ethanol (96 per cent).

It shows polymorphism (*5.9*).

IDENTIFICATION

First identification: A.

Second identification: B, C.

A. Infrared absorption spectrophotometry (*2.2.24*).

Comparison: *terconazole CRS.*

If the spectra obtained in the solid state show differences, dissolve the substance to be examined and the reference substance separately in the minimum volume of *acetone R*, evaporate to dryness in a current of air and record new spectra using the residues.

B. Thin-layer chromatography (*2.2.27*).

Test solution. Dissolve 30 mg of the substance to be examined in *methanol R* and dilute to 5 ml with the same solvent.

Reference solution (a). Dissolve 30 mg of *terconazole CRS* in *methanol R* and dilute to 5 ml with the same solvent.

Reference solution (b). Dissolve 30 mg of *terconazole CRS* and 30 mg of *ketoconazole CRS* in *methanol R* and dilute to 5 ml with the same solvent.

Plate: *TLC octadecylsilyl silica gel plate R.*

Mobile phase: *ammonium acetate solution R, dioxan R, methanol R* (20:40:40 *V/V/V*).

Application: 5 µl.

Development: in an unsaturated tank over a path of 10 cm.

Drying: in a current of warm air for 15 min.

Detection: expose to iodine vapour until the spots appear and examine in daylight.

System suitability: reference solution (b):

– the chromatogram shows 2 clearly separated spots.

Results: the principal spot in the chromatogram obtained with the test solution is similar in position, colour and size to the principal spot in the chromatogram obtained with reference solution (a).

C. To 30 mg in a porcelain crucible add 0.3 g of *anhydrous sodium carbonate R*. Heat over an open flame for 10 min. Allow to cool. Take up the residue with 5 ml of *dilute nitric acid R* and filter. To 1 ml of the filtrate add 1 ml of *water R*. The solution gives reaction (a) of chlorides (*2.3.1*).

TESTS

Optical rotation (*2.2.7*): – 0.10° to + 0.10°.

Dissolve 1.0 g in *methylene chloride R* and dilute to 10 ml with the same solvent.

Related substances. Liquid chromatography (*2.2.29*).

Test solution. Dissolve 0.100 g of the substance to be examined in *methanol R* and dilute to 10.0 ml with the same solvent.

Reference solution (a). Dissolve 2.5 mg of *terconazole CRS* and 2.0 mg of *ketoconazole CRS* in *methanol R* and dilute to 100.0 ml with the same solvent.

Reference solution (b). Dilute 1.0 ml of the test solution to 100.0 ml with *methanol R*. Dilute 5.0 ml of this solution to 20.0 ml with *methanol R*.

Column:

– *size*: *l* = 0.1 m, Ø = 4.6 mm;

– *stationary phase*: *base-deactivated octadecylsilyl silica gel for chromatography R* (3 µm).

Mobile phase:

– *mobile phase A*: 3.4 g/l solution of *tetrabutylammonium hydrogen sulphate R*;

– *mobile phase B*: *acetonitrile R1*;

Time (min)	Mobile phase A (per cent *V/V*)	Mobile phase B (per cent *V/V*)
0 - 10	95 → 50	5 → 50
10 - 15	50	50

Flow rate: 2 ml/min.

Detection: spectrophotometer at 220 nm.

Equilibration: with *acetonitrile R1* for at least 30 min and then with the mobile phase at the initial composition for at least 5 min.

Injection: 10 µl; inject *methanol R* as a blank.

Retention time: ketoconazole = about 6 min; terconazole = about 7.5 min.

System suitability: reference solution (a):

– *resolution*: minimum 13 between the peaks due to ketoconazole and terconazole; if necessary, adjust the concentration of acetonitrile in the mobile phase or adjust the time programme for the linear gradient elution.

Limits:

– *impurities A, B*: for each impurity, not more than the area of the principal peak in the chromatogram obtained with reference solution (b) (0.25 per cent);

– *total*: not more than twice the area of the principal peak in the chromatogram obtained with reference solution (b) (0.5 per cent);

– *disregard limit*: 0.2 times the area of the principal peak in the chromatogram obtained with reference solution (b) (0.05 per cent).

Loss on drying (*2.2.32*): maximum 0.5 per cent, determined on 1.000 g by drying in an oven at 105 °C.

Sulphated ash (*2.4.14*): maximum 0.1 per cent, determined on 1.0 g.

ASSAY

Dissolve 0.150 g in 70 ml of a mixture of 1 volume of *anhydrous acetic acid R* and 7 volumes of *methyl ethyl ketone R*. Titrate with *0.1 M perchloric acid*, determining the end-point potentiometrically at the 2nd point of inflexion (*2.2.20*).

1 ml of *0.1 M perchloric acid* is equivalent to 17.75 mg of $C_{26}H_{31}Cl_2N_5O_3$.

STORAGE

Protected from light.

IMPURITIES

Specified impurities: A, B.

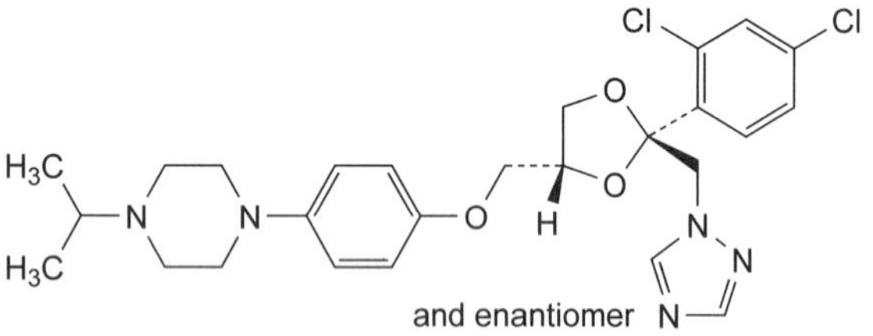

A. 1-[4-[[(2*RS*,4*RS*)2-(2,4-dichlorophenyl)-2-[(1*H*-1,2,4-triazol-1-yl)methyl]-1,3-dioxolan-4-yl]methoxy]phenyl]-4-(1-methylethyl)piperazine,

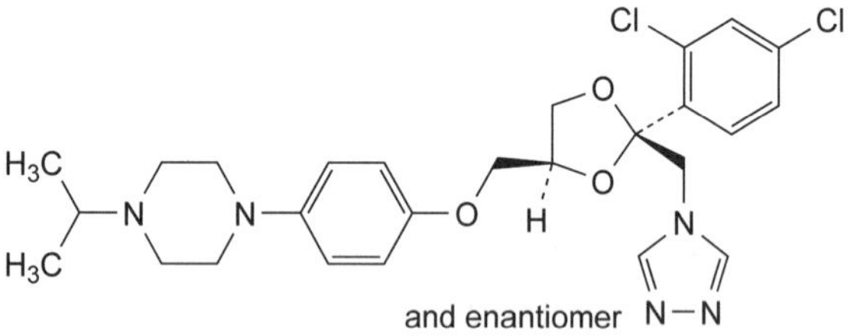

B. 1-[4-[[(2*RS*,4*SR*)-2-(2,4-dichlorophenyl)-2-[(4*H*-1,2,4-triazol-4-yl)methyl]-1,3-dioxolan-4-yl]methoxy]phenyl]-4-(1-methylethyl)piperazine.

01/2008:0955
corrected 6.1

TERFENADINE

Terfenadinum

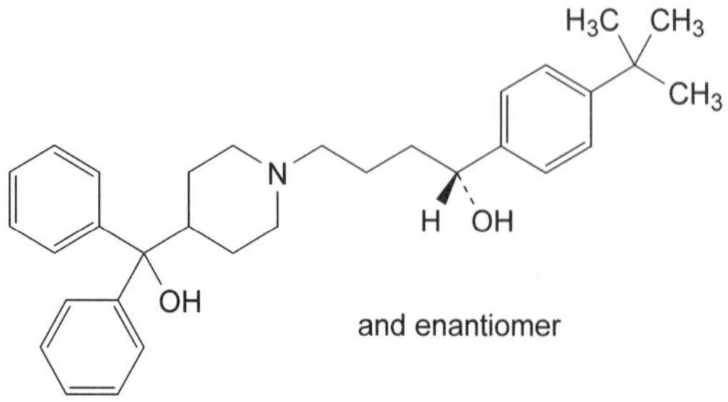

$C_{32}H_{41}NO_2$ M_r 471.7
[50679-08-8]

DEFINITION

(1*RS*)-1-[4-(1,1-Dimethylethyl)phenyl]-4-[4-(hydroxydiphenylmethyl)piperidin-1-yl]butan-1-ol.

Content: 98.5 per cent to 101.0 per cent (dried substance).

CHARACTERS

Appearance: white or almost white, crystalline powder.

Solubility: very slightly soluble in water, freely soluble in methylene chloride, soluble in methanol. It is very slightly soluble in dilute hydrochloric acid.

It shows polymorphism (*5.9*).

IDENTIFICATION

First identification: C.

Second identification: A, B, D.

A. Melting point (*2.2.14*): 146 °C to 152 °C.

B. Ultraviolet and visible absorption spectrophotometry (*2.2.25*).

Test solution. Dissolve 50.0 mg in *methanol R* and dilute to 100.0 ml with the same solvent.

Spectral range: 230-350 nm.

Absorption maximum: at 259 nm.

Shoulders: at 253 nm and 270 nm.

Specific absorbance at the absorption maximum: 13.5 to 14.9.

C. Infrared absorption spectrophotometry (*2.2.24*).

Comparison: *terfenadine CRS.*

D. Thin-layer chromatography (*2.2.27*).

Test solution. Dissolve 50 mg of the substance to be examined in *methylene chloride R* and dilute to 10 ml with the same solvent.

Reference solution. Dissolve 50 mg of *terfenadine CRS* in *methylene chloride R* and dilute to 10 ml with the same solvent.

Plate: *TLC silica gel F_{254} plate R.*

Mobile phase: *methanol R, methylene chloride R* (10:90 *V/V*).

Application: 10 μl.

Development: over a path of 15 cm.

Drying: in air.

Detection: examine in ultraviolet light at 254 nm.

Results: the principal spot in the chromatogram obtained with the test solution is similar in position and size to the principal spot in the chromatogram obtained with the reference solution.

TESTS

Related substances. Liquid chromatography (*2.2.29*).

Test solution. Dissolve 15 mg of the substance to be examined in the mobile phase and dilute to 10.0 ml with the mobile phase.

Reference solution (a). Dilute 1.0 ml of the test solution to 10.0 ml with the mobile phase. Dilute 1.0 ml of this solution to 20.0 ml with the mobile phase.

Reference solution (b). Dissolve 15 mg of *terfenadine impurity A CRS* in the mobile phase and dilute to 10.0 ml with the mobile phase. To 5.0 ml of this solution, add 5.0 ml of the test solution and dilute to 50.0 ml with the mobile phase.

Reference solution (c). Dilute 10.0 ml of reference solution (a) to 25.0 ml with the mobile phase.

Reference solution (d). Dissolve 0.1 g of *potassium iodide R* in the mobile phase and dilute to 100 ml with the mobile phase. Dilute 1 ml of this solution to 100 ml with the mobile phase.

Column:

– *size*: *l* = 0.25 m, Ø = 4.6 mm;

– *stationary phase*: *octylsilyl silica gel for chromatography R* (5 µm).

Mobile phase: dilute 600 ml of *acetonitrile R1* to 1 litre with *diethylammonium phosphate buffer solution pH 6.0 R*.

Flow rate: 1 ml/min.

Detection: spectrophotometer at 217 nm.

Injection: 20 µl.

Run time: 5 times the retention time of terfenadine.

System suitability: reference solution (b):

– *resolution*: minimum 5.0 between the peaks due to terfenadine and impurity A;
– *mass distribution ratio*: minimum 2.0 for the peak due to terfenadine; use *potassium iodide R* as the unretained compound (reference solution (d)).

Limits:

– *impurities A, B, C, D, E, F, G, H, I, J*: for each impurity, not more than the area of the principal peak in the chromatogram obtained with reference solution (c) (0.2 per cent);
– *total*: not more than the area of the principal peak in the chromatogram obtained with reference solution (a) (0.5 per cent);
– *disregard limit*: 0.025 times the area of the principal peak in the chromatogram obtained with reference solution (c) (0.005 per cent).

Loss on drying (*2.2.32*): maximum 0.5 per cent, determined on 1.000 g by drying at 60 °C at a pressure not exceeding 0.5 kPa.

Sulphated ash (*2.4.14*): maximum 0.1 per cent, determined on 1.0 g.

ASSAY

Dissolve 0.400 g in 50 ml of *anhydrous acetic acid R*. Titrate with *0.1 M perchloric acid*, determining the end-point potentiometrically (*2.2.20*).

1 ml of *0.1 M perchloric acid* is equivalent to 47.17 mg of $C_{32}H_{41}NO_2$.

STORAGE

Protected from light.

IMPURITIES

Specified impurities: A, B, C, D, E, F, G, H, I, J.

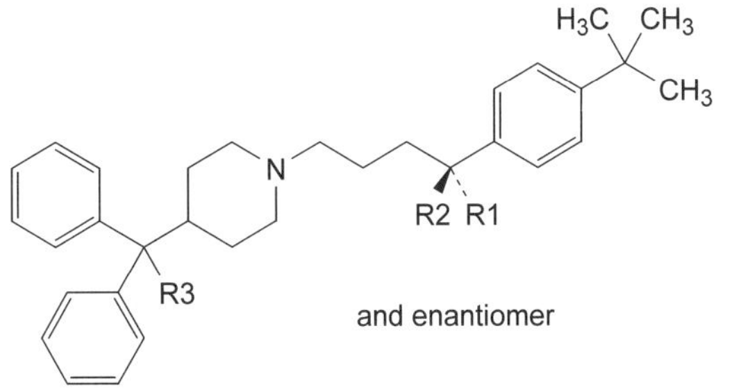

A. R1 + R2 = O, R3 = OH: 1-[4-(1,1-dimethylethyl)phenyl]-4-[4-(hydroxydiphenylmethyl)piperidin-1-yl]butan-1-one,

B. R1 = OH, R2 = R3 = H: (1*RS*)-1-[4-(1,1-dimethylethyl)-phenyl]-4-[4-(diphenylmethyl)piperidin-1-yl]butan-1-ol,

H. R1 = R2 = H, R3 = OH: [1-[4-[4-(1,1-dimethylethyl)-phenyl]butyl]piperidin-4-yl]diphenylmethanol,

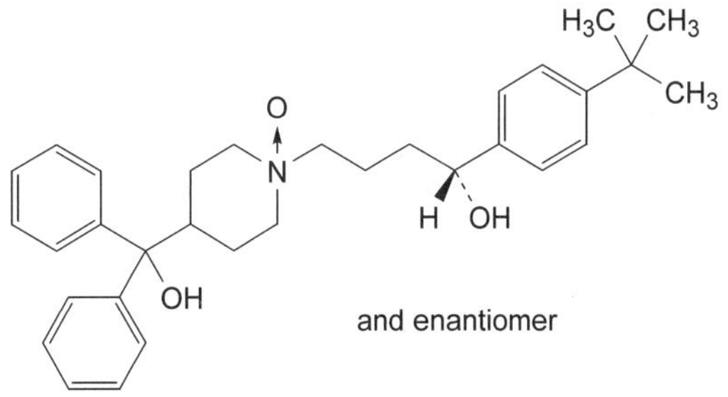

C. 1-[(4*RS*)-4-[4-(1,1-dimethylethyl)phenyl]-4-hydroxybutyl]-4-(hydroxydiphenylmethyl)piperidine 1-oxide,

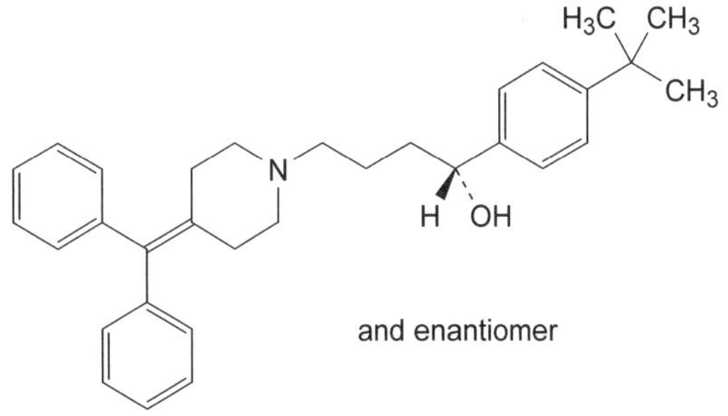

D. (1*RS*)-1-[4-(1,1-dimethylethyl)phenyl]-4-[4-(diphenylmethylene)piperidin-1-yl]butan-1-ol,

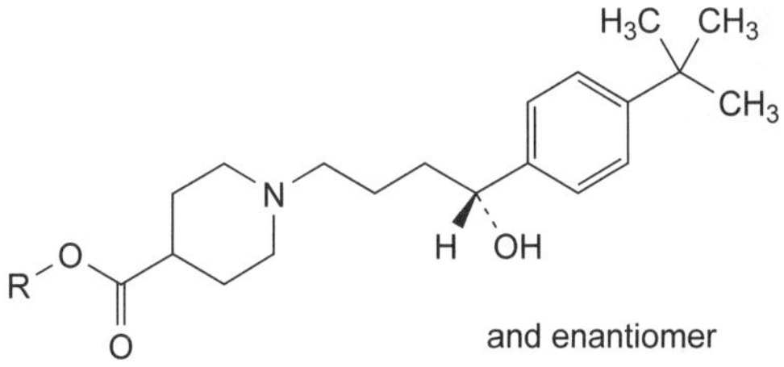

E. R = H: 1-[(4*RS*)-4-[4-(1,1-dimethylethyl)phenyl]-4-hydroxybutyl]piperidine-4-carboxylic acid,

J. R = C_2H_5: ethyl 1-[(4*RS*)-4-[4-(1,1-dimethylethyl)phenyl]-4-hydroxybutyl]piperidine-4-carboxylate,

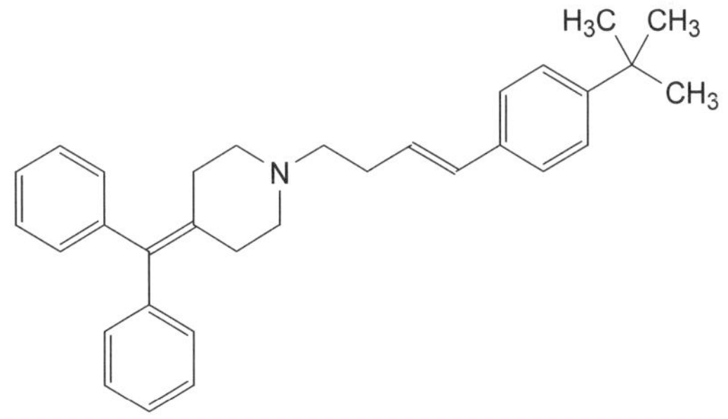

F. 1-[4-[4-(1,1-dimethylethyl)phenyl]but-3-enyl]-4-(diphenylmethylene)piperidine,

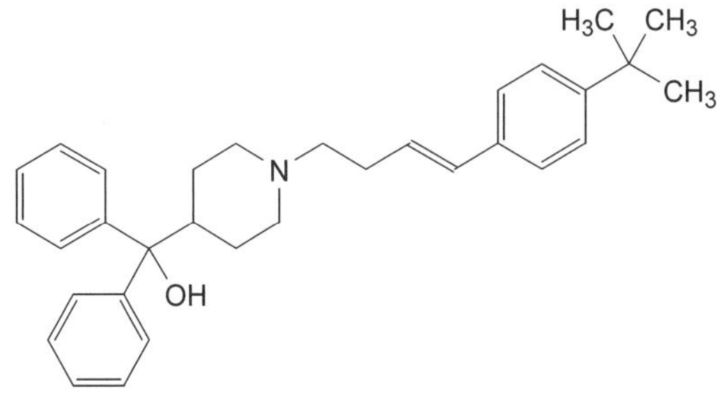

G. [1-[4-[4-(1,1-dimethylethyl)phenyl]but-3-enyl]piperidin-4-yl]diphenylmethanol,

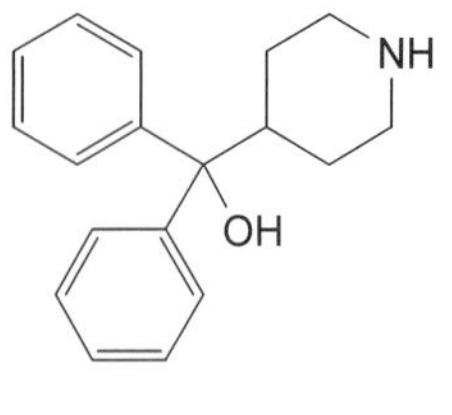

I. diphenyl(piperidin-4-yl)methanol.

04/2008:0057

TETRACAINE HYDROCHLORIDE

Tetracaini hydrochloridum

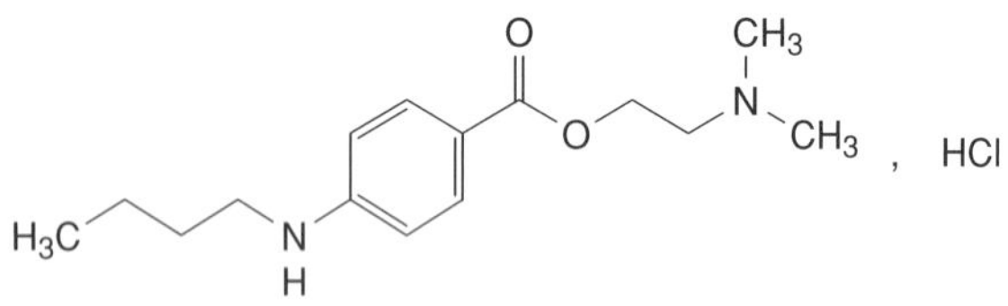

$C_{15}H_{25}ClN_2O_2$ M_r 300.8
[136-47-0]

DEFINITION

2-(Dimethylamino)ethyl 4-(butylamino)benzoate hydrochloride.

Content: 99.0 per cent to 101.0 per cent (dried substance).

CHARACTERS

Appearance: white or almost white, slightly hygroscopic, crystalline powder.

Solubility: freely soluble in water, soluble in ethanol (96 per cent).

It melts at about 148 °C or it may occur in either of 2 other crystalline forms which melt respectively at about 134 °C and 139 °C. Mixtures of these forms melt within the range 134 °C to 147 °C.

IDENTIFICATION

First identification: A, B, D.

Second identification: B, C, D.

A. Infrared absorption spectrophotometry (*2.2.24*).

Comparison: *tetracaine hydrochloride CRS.*

B. To 10 ml of solution S (see Tests) add 1 ml of *ammonium thiocyanate solution R*. A white, crystalline precipitate is formed which, after recrystallisation from *water R* and drying at 80 °C for 2 h, melts (*2.2.14*) at about 131 °C.

C. To about 5 mg add 0.5 ml of *fuming nitric acid R*. Evaporate to dryness on a water-bath, allow to cool and dissolve the residue in 5 ml of *acetone R*. Add 1 ml of *0.1 M alcoholic potassium hydroxide*. A violet colour develops.

D. Solution S gives reaction (a) of chlorides (*2.3.1*).

TESTS

Solution S. Dissolve 5.0 g in *carbon dioxide-free water R* and dilute to 50 ml with the same solvent.

Appearance of solution. The solution is clear (*2.2.1*) and colourless (*2.2.2, Method II*).

Dilute 2 ml of solution S to 10 ml with *water R*.

pH (*2.2.3*): 4.5 to 6.5.

Dilute 1 ml of solution S to 10 ml with *carbon dioxide-free water R*.

Related substances. Liquid chromatography (*2.2.29*). *Prepare the solutions immediately before use or store them at a temperature of 2 °C to 8 °C.*

Solvent mixture: *acetonitrile R, water R* (20:80 *V/V*).

Test solution. Dissolve 50 mg of the substance to be examined in the solvent mixture and dilute to 50 ml with the solvent mixture.

Reference solution (a). Dilute 1.0 ml of the test solution to 100.0 ml with the solvent mixture. Dilute 1.0 ml of this solution to 10.0 ml with the solvent mixture.

Reference solution (b). Dissolve the contents of a vial of *tetracaine for system suitability CRS* (containing impurities A, B and C) in 2 ml of the solvent mixture.

Column:

– *size*: *l* = 0.15 m, Ø = 4.6 mm;
– *stationary phase*: *octadecylsilyl silica gel for chromatography R* (5 µm);
– *temperature*: 30 °C.

Mobile phase:

– *mobile phase A*: dissolve 1.36 g of *potassium dihydrogen phosphate R* in *water R*, add 0.5 ml of *phosphoric acid R* and dilute to 1000 ml with *water R*;
– *mobile phase B*: *acetonitrile R*;

Time (min)	Mobile phase A (per cent *V/V*)	Mobile phase B (per cent *V/V*)
0 - 3	80	20
3 - 18	80 → 40	20 → 60
18 - 23	40	60

Flow rate: 1.5 ml/min.

Detection: spectrophotometer at 300 nm.

Injection: 10 µl.

Identification of impurities: use the chromatogram supplied with *tetracaine for system suitability CRS* and the chromatogram obtained with reference solution (b) to identify the peaks due to impurities A, B and C.

Relative retention with reference to tetracaine (retention time = about 8 min): impurity A = about 0.3; impurity B = about 1.7; impurity C = about 2.1.

System suitability: reference solution (b):

– *resolution*: minimum 5.0 between the peaks due to tetracaine and impurity B.

Limits:

– *correction factors*: for the calculation of content, multiply the peak areas of the following impurities by the corresponding correction factor: impurity B = 0.6; impurity C = 0.7;
– *impurity A*: not more than 0.5 times the area of the principal peak in the chromatogram obtained with reference solution (a) (0.05 per cent);
– *impurities B, C*: for each impurity, not more than the area of the principal peak in the chromatogram obtained with reference solution (a) (0.1 per cent);
– *unspecified impurities*: for each impurity, not more than the area of the principal peak in the chromatogram obtained with reference solution (a) (0.10 per cent);

- *total*: not more than 5 times the area of the principal peak in the chromatogram obtained with reference solution (a) (0.5 per cent);
- *disregard limit*: 0.5 times the area of the principal peak in the chromatogram obtained with reference solution (a) (0.05 per cent).

Heavy metals (*2.4.8*): maximum 10 ppm.

12 ml of solution S complies with test A. Prepare the reference solution using *lead standard solution (1 ppm Pb) R*.

Loss on drying (*2.2.32*): maximum 1.0 per cent, determined on 1.000 g by drying in an oven at 105 °C.

Sulphated ash (*2.4.14*): maximum 0.1 per cent, determined on 1.0 g.

ASSAY

Dissolve 0.250 g in 50 ml of *ethanol (96 per cent) R* and add 5.0 ml of *0.01 M hydrochloric acid*. Carry out a potentiometric titration (*2.2.20*), using *0.1 M sodium hydroxide*. Read the volume added between the 2 points of inflexion.

1 ml of *0.1 M sodium hydroxide* is equivalent to 30.08 mg of $C_{15}H_{25}ClN_2O_2$.

STORAGE

In an airtight container, protected from light.

IMPURITIES

Specified impurities: A, B, C.

A. 4-aminobenzoic acid,

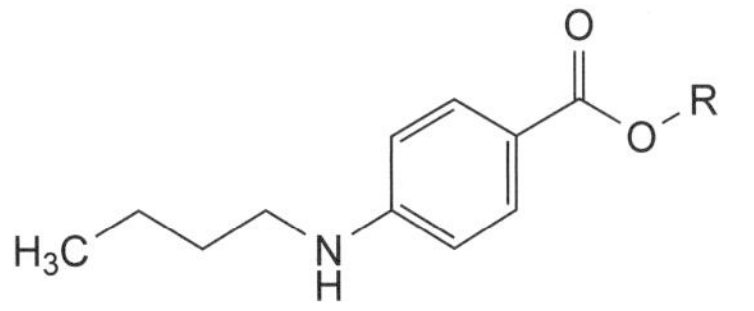

B. R =H: 4-(butylamino)benzoic acid,

C. R = CH_3: methyl 4-(butylamino)benzoate.

04/2008:0058

TRIAMTERENE

Triamterenum

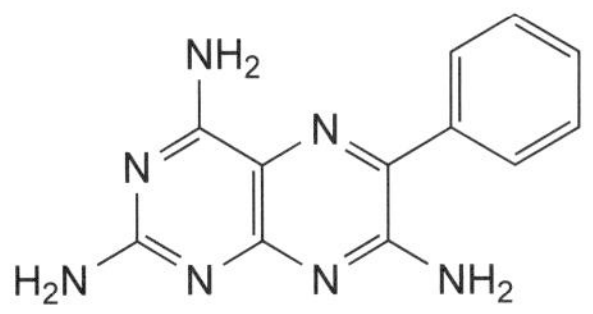

$C_{12}H_{11}N_7$ M_r 253.3

[396-01-0]

DEFINITION

6-Phenylpteridine-2,4,7-triamine.

Content: 99.0 per cent to 101.0 per cent (dried substance).

CHARACTERS

Appearance: yellow, crystalline powder.

Solubility: very slightly soluble in water and in ethanol (96 per cent).

IDENTIFICATION

Infrared absorption spectrophotometry (*2.2.24*).

Comparison: *triamterene CRS*.

TESTS

Acidity. Boil 1.0 g with 20 ml of *water R* for 5 min, cool, filter and wash the filter with 3 quantities, each of 10 ml, of *water R*. Combine the filtrate and washings and add 0.3 ml of *phenolphthalein solution R*. Not more than 1.5 ml of *0.01 M sodium hydroxide* is required to change the colour of the indicator.

Impurity D. Gas chromatography (*2.2.28*).

Internal standard solution. Dilute 0.1 ml of *nitrobenzene R* to 100 ml with *methanol R*. Dilute 1 ml of this solution to 50 ml with *methanol R*.

Test solution. Introduce 0.800 g of the substance to be examined into a suitable vial, add 5 ml of *dimethyl sulphoxide R* and heat until the sample is dissolved (do not heat to boiling). Allow to cool. Add 5 ml of cold *methanol R* to enhance the precipitation of triamterene. Filter and wash the filter with 5 ml of *methanol R*. Combine the filtrate and washing, add 2.0 ml of the internal standard solution and dilute to 20.0 ml with *methanol R*.

Reference solution. Dissolve 20.0 mg of *benzyl cyanide R* (impurity D) in *methanol R* and dilute to 100.0 ml with the same solvent. Dilute 5.0 ml of the solution to 50.0 ml with *methanol R*. To 2.0 ml of this solution add 2.0 ml of the internal standard solution and 5 ml of *dimethyl sulphoxide R* and dilute to 20.0 ml with *methanol R*.

Blank solution. Dilute 5 ml of *dimethyl sulphoxide R* to 20 ml with *methanol R*.

Column:
- *material*: fused silica;
- *size*: l = 30 m, Ø = 0.25 mm;
- *stationary phase*: *macrogol 20 000 R* (0.5 µm).

Carrier gas: *helium for chromatography R*.

Flow rate: 1.5 ml/min.

Split ratio: 1:15.

Temperature:
- *column*: 170 °C;
- *injection port*: 210 °C;
- *detector*: 230 °C.

Detection: flame ionisation.

Injection: 1 µl.

Run time: twice the retention time of the internal standard.

Relative retention with reference to the internal standard (retention time = about 6 min): impurity D = about 1.6.

System suitability: reference solution:
- *resolution*: minimum 2.0 between the peak due to impurity D and the nearest peak due to the solvent (blank solution);
- *signal-to-noise ratio*: minimum 10 for the peak due to impurity D.

Limit:
- *impurity D*: calculate the ratio (R) of the area of the peak due to impurity D to the area of the peak due to the internal standard from the chromatogram obtained with the reference solution; from the chromatogram obtained with the test solution, calculate the ratio of the area of

the peak due to impurity D to the area of the peak due to the internal standard: this ratio is not greater than *R* (50 ppm).

Related substances. Liquid chromatography (*2.2.29*).

Test solution. Dissolve 10.0 mg of the substance to be examined in the mobile phase and dilute to 10.0 ml with the mobile phase.

Reference solution (a). Dilute 1.0 ml of the test solution to 100.0 ml with the mobile phase. Dilute 1.0 ml of this solution to 10.0 ml with the mobile phase.

Reference solution (b). Dissolve 5.0 mg of *nitrosotriaminopyrimidine CRS* (impurity A) in the mobile phase and dilute to 100.0 ml with the mobile phase. Dilute 1.0 ml of the solution to 100.0 ml with the mobile phase. Dilute 1.0 ml of this solution to 10.0 ml with the mobile phase.

Reference solution (c). Dissolve the contents of a vial of *triamterene impurity B CRS* in 0.5 ml of the mobile phase with the aid of ultrasound. To this solution, add 0.5 ml of the test solution.

Column:

- *size*: *l* = 0.25 m, Ø = 4.0 mm;
- *stationary phase*: spherical *end-capped octylsilyl silica gel for chromatography R* (5 μm).

Mobile phase: *butylamine R, acetonitrile R, methanol R, water R* (2:200:200:600 *V/V/V/V*), adjusted to pH 5.3 with *acetic acid R*.

Flow rate: 1 ml/min.

Detection: spectrophotometer at 320 nm and at 355 nm.

Injection: 50 μl.

Relative retention with reference to triamterene (retention time = about 5 min): impurity A = about 0.6; impurity B = about 0.8; impurity C = about 1.7.

System suitability:

- *resolution*: minimum 1.5 between the peaks due to impurity B and triamterene in the chromatogram obtained with reference solution (c) at 355 nm; if necessary, increase the quantity of *water R* in the mobile phase;
- *signal-to-noise ratio*: minimum 10 for the principal peak in the chromatogram obtained with reference solution (b) at 320 nm.

Limits:

- *correction factors*: for the calculation of content, multiply the peak areas of the following impurities by the corresponding correction factor: impurity B = 1.8; impurity C = 1.5;
- *impurity A at 320 nm*: not more than the area of the corresponding peak in the chromatogram obtained with reference solution (b) (50 ppm);
- *impurities B, C at 355 nm*: for each impurity, not more than the area of the principal peak in the chromatogram obtained with reference solution (a) (0.1 per cent);
- *unspecified impurities at 355 nm*: for each impurity, not more than the area of the principal peak in the chromatogram obtained with reference solution (a) (0.10 per cent);
- *total at 355 nm*: not more than twice the area of the principal peak in the chromatogram obtained with reference solution (a) (0.2 per cent);
- *disregard limit at 355 nm*: 0.5 times the area of the principal peak in the chromatogram obtained with reference solution (a) (0.05 per cent).

Loss on drying (*2.2.32*): maximum 1.0 per cent, determined on 1.000 g by drying in an oven at 105 °C.

Sulphated ash (*2.4.14*): maximum 0.1 per cent, determined on 1.0 g.

ASSAY

Dissolve 0.150 g in 5 ml of *anhydrous formic acid R* and add 100 ml of *anhydrous acetic acid R*. Titrate with *0.1 M perchloric acid*, determining the end-point potentiometrically (*2.2.20*).

1 ml of *0.1 M perchloric acid* is equivalent to 25.33 mg of $C_{12}H_{11}N_7$.

STORAGE

Protected from light.

IMPURITIES

Specified impurities: A, B, C, D.

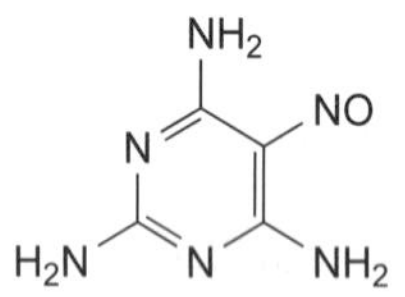

A. 5-nitrosopyrimidine-2,4,6-triamine (nitrosotriaminopyrimidine),

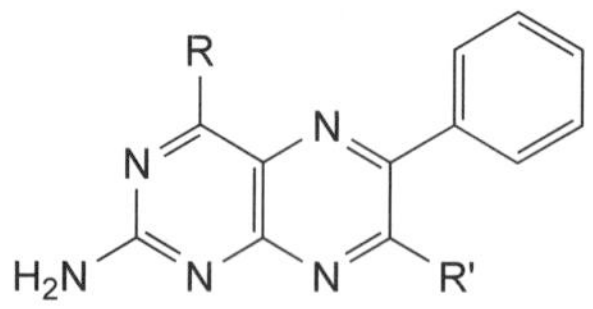

B. R = OH, R′ = NH_2: 2,7-diamino-6-phenylpteridin-4-ol,

C. R = NH_2, R′ = OH: 2,4-diamino-6-phenylpteridin-7-ol,

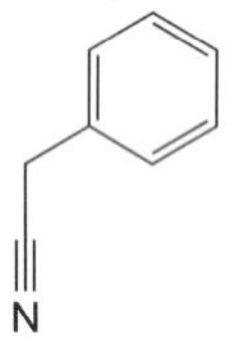

D. phenylacetonitrile (benzyl cyanide).

04/2008:2032

TRIGLYCEROL DIISOSTEARATE

Triglyceroli diisostearas

DEFINITION

Mixture of polyglycerol diesters of mainly isostearic acid, obtained by esterification of polyglycerol and isostearic acid. The polyglycerol consists mainly of triglycerol.

CHARACTERS

Appearance: clear, yellowish, viscous liquid.

Solubility: practically insoluble in water, miscible with ethanol (96 per cent) and with fatty oils.

IDENTIFICATION

A. Infrared absorption spectrophotometry (*2.2.24*).

Preparation: film between 2 plates of *sodium chloride R*.

Comparison: *triglycerol diisostearate CRS*.

B. Composition of fatty acids (see Tests).

TESTS

Appearance of solution. The solution is not more intensely coloured than reference solution BY_3 (*2.2.2, Method I*).

Mix 10 ml with 10 ml of *ethanol (96 per cent) R*.

Acid value (*2.5.1*): maximum 3.0, determined on 1.0 g.

Hydroxyl value (*2.5.3, Method A*): 180 to 230, determined on 0.25 g.

Iodine value (*2.5.4, Method B*): maximum 3.0.

Peroxide value (*2.5.5, Method B*): maximum 6.0.

Saponification value (*2.5.6*): 128 to 160.

Composition of fatty acids (*2.4.22, Method B*). Use the mixture of calibrating substances in Table 2.4.22.-1.

Composition of the fatty-acid fraction of the substance:

- *sum of the contents of the fatty acids eluting between palmitic acid and stearic acid*: minimum 60.0 per cent;
- *sum of the contents of myristic acid, palmitic acid and stearic acid*: maximum 11.0 per cent.

Water (*2.5.12*): maximum 0.5 per cent, determined on 2.00 g.

Sulphated ash: maximum 0.5 per cent, determined on 1.0 g.

Heat a silica crucible to redness for 30 min, allow to cool in a desiccator and weigh. Evenly distribute 1.00 g of the substance to be examined in the crucible and weigh. Dry at 100-105 °C for 1 h and ignite in a muffle furnace at 600 °C ± 25 °C, until the substance is thoroughly charred. Carry out the test for sulphated ash (*2.4.14*) on the residue obtained, starting with "Moisten the substance to be examined...".

STORAGE

In an airtight container, protected from light.

W

04/2008:1583

WILLOW BARK

Salicis cortex

DEFINITION

Whole or fragmented dried bark of young branches or whole dried pieces of current-year twigs of various species of genus *Salix* including *S. purpurea* L., *S. daphnoides* Vill. and *S. fragilis* L.

Content: minimum 1.5 per cent of total salicylic derivatives, expressed as salicin ($C_{13}H_{18}O_7$; M_r 286.3) (dried drug).

IDENTIFICATION

A. The bark is 1-2 mm thick and occurs in flexible, elongated, quilled or curved pieces. The outer surface is smooth or slightly wrinkled longitudinally and greenish-yellow or brownish-grey. The inner surface is smooth or finely striated longitudinally and white, pale yellow or reddish-brown, depending on the species. The fracture is short in the outer part and coarsely fibrous in the inner region. The diameter of current-year twigs is not greater than 10 mm. The wood is white or pale yellow.

B. Reduce to a powder (355) (*2.9.12*). The powder is pale yellow, greenish-yellow or light brown. Examine under a microscope using *chloral hydrate solution R*. The powder shows the following diagnostic characters: bundles of narrow fibres, up to about 600 µm long, with very thick walls and surrounded by a crystal sheath containing prism crystals of calcium oxalate; parenchyma of the cortex with thick, pitted and deeply beaded walls, and containing large cluster crystals of calcium oxalate; uniseriate medullary rays; thickened cork cells. Groups of brownish collenchyma from the bud may be present. Twigs show, additionally, fragments of lignified fibres and vessels.

C. Thin-layer chromatography (*2.2.27*).

Test solution (a). To 1.0 g of the powdered drug (355) (*2.9.12*) add 10 ml of *methanol R*. Heat in a water-bath at about 50 °C, with frequent shaking, for 10 min. Cool and filter.

Test solution (b). To 5.0 ml of test solution (a) add 1.0 ml of a 50 g/l solution of *anhydrous sodium carbonate R* and heat in a water-bath at about 60 °C for 10 min. Cool and filter if necessary.

Reference solution. Dissolve 2 mg of *salicin R* and 2 mg of *chlorogenic acid R* in 1.0 ml of *methanol R*.

Plate: *TLC silica gel plate R* (5-40 µm) [or *TLC silica gel plate R* (2-10 µm)].

Mobile phase: *water R, methanol R, ethyl acetate R* (8:15:77 *V/V/V*).

Application: 10 µl [or 2 µl], as bands.

Development: over a path of 15 cm [or 6 cm].

Drying: in a current of warm air.

Detection: spray with a mixture of 5 volumes of *sulphuric acid R* and 95 volumes of *methanol R*. Heat at 100-105 °C for 5 min and examine in daylight.

Results: see below the sequence of zones present in the chromatograms obtained with the reference solution and test solutions (a) and (b). Furthermore, other zones may be present in the chromatograms obtained with test solutions (a) and (b).

Top of the plate		
_______		_______
	Several reddish-violet zones may be present	
Salicin: a reddish-violet zone	A weak reddish-violet zone (salicin)	A reddish-violet zone (salicin)
_______		_______
Chlorogenic acid: a brown zone		
Reference solution	**Test solution (a)**	**Test solution (b)**

TESTS

Foreign matter (*2.8.2*): maximum 3 per cent of twigs with a diameter greater than 10 mm and maximum 2 per cent of other foreign matter.

Loss on drying (*2.2.32*): maximum 11 per cent, determined on 1.000 g of the powdered drug (355) (*2.9.12*) by drying in an oven at 105 °C for 2 h.

Total ash (*2.4.16*): maximum 10 per cent.

ASSAY

Liquid chromatography (*2.2.29*).

Test solution. To 1.000 g of the powdered drug (355) (*2.9.12*) add 40 ml of *methanol R* and 40.0 ml of a 4.2 g/l solution of *sodium hydroxide R*. Heat in a water-bath at about 60 °C under a reflux condenser, with frequent shaking, for about 1 h. After cooling, add 4.0 ml of a 103.0 g/l solution of *hydrochloric acid R*. Filter the suspension into a 100 ml volumetric flask, wash and dilute to 100.0 ml with a mixture of 50 volumes of *methanol R* and 50 volumes of *water R*. Filter through a membrane filter (nominal pore size 0.45 µm).

Reference solution. Dissolve 5.0 mg of *picein R* in 25.0 ml of a mixture of 20 volumes of *water R* and 80 volumes of *methanol R* (solution A). Dissolve 15.0 mg of *salicin CRS* in 25 ml of a mixture of 20 volumes of *water R* and 80 volumes of *methanol R*; add 5.0 ml of solution A and dilute to 50.0 ml with *water R*.

Column:
- *size*: *l* = 0.10 m, Ø = 4.6 mm;
- *stationary phase*: *octadecylsilyl silica gel for chromatography R* (3 µm).

Mobile phase:
- *mobile phase A*: *tetrahydrofuran R*, 0.5 per cent *V/V* solution of *phosphoric acid R* (1.8:98.2 *V/V*);
- *mobile phase B*: *tetrahydrofuran R*;

Time (min)	Mobile phase A (per cent *V/V*)	Mobile phase B (per cent *V/V*)
0 - 15	100	0
15 - 17	100 → 90	0 → 10
17 - 23	90	10
23 - 25	90 → 100	10 → 0
25 - 40	100	0

Flow rate: 1.0 ml/min.

Detection: spectrophotometer at 270 nm.

Injection: 10 µl.

Retention time: salicin = about 6.4 min; picein = about 7.7 min.

System suitability: reference solution:
- *resolution*: minimum 1.5 between the peaks due to salicin and picein.

Monographs Q-Z

Calculate the percentage content of total salicylic derivatives, expressed as salicin, using the following expression:

$$\frac{A_1 \times m_2 \times p \times 2}{A_2 \times m_1}$$

A_1 = area of the peak due to salicin in the chromatogram obtained with the test solution;

A_2 = area of the peak due to salicin in the chromatogram obtained with the reference solution;

m_1 = mass of the drug to be examined used to prepare the test solution, in grams;

m_2 = mass of *salicin CRS* used to prepare the reference solution, in grams;

p = percentage content of salicin in *salicin CRS*.

04/2008:2312

WILLOW BARK DRY EXTRACT

Salicis corticis extractum siccum

DEFINITION

Dry extract produced from *Willow bark (1583)*.

Content: minimum 5.0 per cent of total salicylic derivatives, expressed as salicin ($C_{13}H_{18}O_7$; M_r 286.3) (dried extract).

PRODUCTION

The extract is produced from the herbal drug by a suitable procedure using either water or a hydroalcoholic solvent equivalent in strength to a maximum of 80 per cent *V/V* ethanol.

CHARACTERS

Appearance: yellowish-brown amorphous powder.

IDENTIFICATION

Thin-layer chromatography (*2.2.27*).

Test solution (a). To 0.200 g of the extract to be examined add 5 ml of *methanol R*. Sonicate for 5 min, filter and dilute to 10 ml with *methanol R*.

Test solution (b). To 5.0 ml of test solution (a) add 1.0 ml of a 50 g/l solution of *anhydrous sodium carbonate R* and heat in a water-bath at about 60 °C for 10 min. Cool and filter if necessary.

Reference solution. Dissolve 2.0 mg of *salicin R* and 2.0 mg of *chlorogenic acid R* in 1.0 ml of *methanol R*.

Plate: *TLC silica gel plate R* (5-40 μm) [or *TLC silica gel plate R* (2-10 μm)].

Mobile phase: *water R, methanol R, ethyl acetate R* (8:15:77 *V/V/V*).

Application: 10 μl [or 2 μl] as bands.

Development: over a path of 15 cm [or 6 cm].

Drying: in a current of warm air.

Detection: spray with a mixture of 5 volumes of *sulphuric acid R* and 95 volumes of *methanol R*. Heat at 100-105 °C for 5 min and examine in daylight.

Results: see below the sequence of the zones present in the chromatograms obtained with the reference solution and test solutions (a) and (b). Furthermore, other zones may be present in the chromatogram obtained with test solutions (a) and (b).

Top of the plate		
———		———
	Several reddish-violet zones may be present	
Salicin: a reddish-violet zone	A weak reddish-violet zone (salicin)	A reddish-violet zone (salicin)
———		———
Chlorogenic acid: a brown zone		
Reference solution	**Test solution (a)**	**Test solution (b)**

ASSAY

Liquid chromatography (*2.2.29*).

Test solution. To 0.300 g of the extract to be examined add 40 ml of *methanol R* and 40.0 ml of *0.1 M sodium hydroxide*. Heat in a water-bath at about 60 °C under a reflux condenser, with frequent shaking, for about 1 h. After cooling, add 4.0 ml of *1 M hydrochloric acid*. Filter the suspension into a 100 ml volumetric flask, then wash and dilute to 100.0 ml with a mixture of equal volumes of *water R* and *methanol R*. Filter through a membrane filter (nominal pore size 0.45 μm).

Reference solution. Dissolve 5.0 mg of *picein R* in 25.0 ml of a mixture of 20 volumes of *water R* and 80 volumes of *methanol R* (solution A). Dissolve 15.0 mg of *salicin CRS* in 25 ml of a mixture of 20 volumes of *water R* and 80 volumes of *methanol R*. Add 5.0 ml of solution A and dilute to 50.0 ml with *water R*.

Column:

– *size*: *l* = 0.10 m, Ø = 4.6 mm;

– *stationary phase*: *octadecylsilyl silica gel for chromatography R* (3 μm).

Mobile phase:

– *mobile phase A*: *tetrahydrofuran R*, 0.5 per cent *V/V* solution of *phosphoric acid R* (1.8:98.2 *V/V*);

– *mobile phase B*: *tetrahydrofuran R*;

Time (min)	Mobile phase A (per cent *V/V*)	Mobile phase B (per cent *V/V*)
0 - 15	100	0
15 - 17	100 → 90	0 → 10
17 - 23	90	10
23 - 25	90 → 100	10 → 0
25 - 40	100	0

Flow rate: 1.0 ml/min.

Detection: spectrophotometer at 270 nm.

Injection: 10 μl.

Retention time: salicin = about 6.4 min; picein = about 7.7 min.

System suitability: reference solution:

– *resolution*: minimum 1.5 between the peaks due to salicin and picein.

Calculate the percentage content of total salicylic derivatives, expressed as salicin, from the following expression:

$$\frac{A_1 \times m_2 \times p \times 2}{A_2 \times m_1}$$

A_1 = area of the peak due to salicin in the chromatogram obtained with the test solution;

A_2 = area of the peak due to salicin in the chromatogram obtained with the reference solution;

m_1 = mass of the extract to be examined used to prepare the test solution, in grams;

m_2 = mass of *salicin CRS* used to prepare the reference solution, in grams;

p = percentage content of salicin in *salicin CRS*.

X

01/2008:1277
corrected 6.1

XANTHAN GUM

Xanthani gummi

DEFINITION

High-molecular-mass anionic polysaccharide produced by fermentation of carbohydrates with *Xanthomonas campestris*. It consists of a principal chain of β(1→4)-linked D-glucose units with trisaccharide side chains, on alternating anhydroglucose units, consisting of 1 glucuronic acid unit included between 2 mannose units. Most of the terminal units contain a pyruvate moiety and the mannose unit adjacent to the principal chain may be acetylated at C-6.

Xanthan gum has a relative molecular mass of approximately 1×10^6. It exists as the sodium, potassium or calcium salt.

Content: minimum 1.5 per cent of pyruvoyl groups ($C_3H_3O_2$; M_r 71.1) (dried substance).

CHARACTERS

Appearance: white or yellowish-white, free-flowing powder.

Solubility: soluble in water giving a highly viscous solution, practically insoluble in organic solvents.

IDENTIFICATION

A. In a flask, suspend 1 g in 15 ml of *0.1 M hydrochloric acid*. Close the flask with a fermentation bulb containing *barium hydroxide solution R* and heat carefully for 5 min. The barium hydroxide solution shows a white turbidity.

B. To 300 ml of *water R*, previously heated to 80 °C and stirred rapidly with a mechanical stirrer in a 400 ml beaker, add, at the point of maximum agitation, a dry blend of 1.5 g of *carob bean gum R* and 1.5 g of the substance to be examined. Stir until the mixture forms a solution, and then continue stirring for 30 min or longer. Do not allow the water temperature to drop below 60 °C during stirring. Discontinue stirring and allow the mixture to stand for at least 2 h. A firm rubbery gel forms after the temperature drops below 40 °C but no such gel forms in a 1 per cent control solution of the sample prepared in the same manner but omitting the carob bean gum.

TESTS

pH (*2.2.3*): 6.0 to 8.0 for a 10.0 g/l solution.

Viscosity (*2.2.10*): minimum 600 mPa·s.

Add 3.0 g within 45-90 s into 250 ml of a 12 g/l solution of *potassium chloride R* in a 500 ml beaker stirring with a low-pitch propeller-type stirrer rotating at 800 r/min. When adding the substance take care that agglomerates are destroyed. Add an additional quantity of 44 ml of *water R*, to rinse any adhering residue from the walls of the beaker. Stir the preparation at 800 r/min for 2 h whilst maintaining the temperature at 24 ± 1 °C. Determine the viscosity within 15 min at 24 ± 1 °C using a rotating viscosimeter set at 60 r/min and equipped with a rotating spindle 12.7 mm in diameter and 1.6 mm high which is attached to a shaft 3.2 mm in diameter. The distance from the top of the cylinder to the lower tip of the shaft being 25.4 mm, and the immersion depth being 50.0 mm.

2-Propanol. Gas chromatography (*2.2.28*).

Internal standard solution. Dilute 0.50 g of *2-methyl-2-propanol R* to 500 ml with *water R*.

Test solution. To 200 ml of *water R* in a 1000 ml round-bottomed flask, add 5.0 g of the substance to be examined and 1 ml of a 10 g/l emulsion of *dimeticone R* in *liquid paraffin R*, stopper the flask and shake for 1 h. Distil about 90.0 ml, mix the distillate with 4.0 ml of the internal standard solution and dilute to 100.0 ml with *water R*.

Reference solution. Dilute a suitable quantity of *2-propanol R*, accurately weighed, with *water R* to obtain a solution having a known concentration of 2-propanol of about 1 mg/ml. To 4.0 ml of this solution add 4.0 ml of the internal standard solution and dilute to 100.0 ml with *water R*.

Column:
- *size*: l = 1.8 m, Ø = 4.0 mm;
- *stationary phase*: *styrene-divinylbenzene copolymer R* (149-177 μm).

Carrier gas: *helium for chromatography R*.

Flow rate: 30 ml/min.

Temperature:
- *column*: 165 °C;
- *injection port and detector*: 200 °C.

Detection: flame ionisation.

Injection: 5 μl.

Relative retention with reference to 2-propanol: 2-methyl-2-propanol = about 1.5.

Limit:
- *2-propanol*: maximum 750 ppm.

Other polysaccharides. Thin-layer chromatography (*2.2.27*).

Test solution. To 10 mg of the substance to be examined in a thick-walled centrifuge test tube add 2 ml of a 230 g/l solution of *trifluoroacetic acid R*, shake vigorously to dissolve the forming gel, stopper the test tube, and heat the mixture at 120 °C for 1 h. Centrifuge the hydrolysate, transfer the clear supernatant liquid carefully into a 50 ml flask, add 10 ml of *water R* and evaporate the solution to dryness under reduced pressure. Take up the residue thus obtained in 10 ml of *water R* and evaporate to dryness under reduced pressure. Wash 3 times with 20 ml of *methanol R* and evaporate under reduced pressure. To the resulting clear film which has no odour of acetic acid, add 0.1 ml of *water R* and 1 ml of *methanol R*. Centrifuge to separate the amorphous precipitate. Dilute the supernatant liquid, if necessary, to 1 ml with *methanol R*.

Reference solution. Dissolve 10 mg of *glucose R* and 10 mg of *mannose R* in 2 ml of *water R* and dilute to 10 ml with *methanol R*.

Plate: *TLC silica gel plate R*.

Mobile phase: 16 g/l solution of *sodium dihydrogen phosphate R*, *butanol R*, *acetone R* (10:40:50 *V/V/V*).

Application: 5 μl, as bands.

Development: over a path of 15 cm.

Detection: spray with a solution of 0.5 g of *diphenylamine R* in 25 ml of *methanol R* to which 0.5 ml of *aniline R* and 2.5 ml of *phosphoric acid R* have been added. Heat for 5 min at 120 °C and examine in daylight.

System suitability: reference solution:
- the chromatogram shows 2 clearly separated greyish-brown zones due to glucose and mannose in the middle third.

Results: the chromatogram obtained with the test solution shows 2 zones corresponding to the zones due to glucose and mannose in the chromatogram obtained with the reference solution. In addition, 1 weak reddish and 2 faint bluish-grey bands may be visible just above the starting line. 1 or 2 bluish-grey bands may also be seen in the upper quarter of the chromatogram. No other bands are visible.

Loss on drying (*2.2.32*): maximum 15.0 per cent, determined on 1.000 g by drying in an oven at 105 °C for 2.5 h.

Total ash (*2.4.16*): 6.5 per cent to 16.0 per cent.

Microbial contamination. Total viable aerobic count (*2.6.12*) not more than 10^3 bacteria and 10^2 fungi per gram, determined by plate count. It complies with the test for *Escherichia coli* (*2.6.13*).

ASSAY

Test solution. Dissolve a quantity of the substance to be examined corresponding to 120.0 mg of the dried substance in *water R* and dilute to 20.0 ml with the same solvent.

Reference solution. Dissolve 45.0 mg of *pyruvic acid R* in *water R* and dilute to 500.0 ml with the same solvent.

Place 10.0 ml of the test solution in a 50 ml round-bottomed flask, add 20.0 ml of *0.1 M hydrochloric acid* and weigh. Boil on a water-bath under a reflux condenser for 3 h. Weigh and adjust to the initial mass with *water R*. In a separating funnel mix 2.0 ml of the solution with 1.0 ml of *dinitrophenylhydrazine-hydrochloric solution R*. Allow to stand for 5 min and add 5.0 ml of *ethyl acetate R*. Shake and allow the solids to settle. Collect the upper layer and shake with 3 quantities, each of 5.0 ml, of *sodium carbonate solution R*. Combine the aqueous layers and dilute to 50.0 ml with *sodium carbonate solution R*. Mix. Treat 10.0 ml of the reference solution at the same time and in the same manner as for the test solution.

Immediately measure the absorbance (*2.2.25*) of the 2 solutions at 375 nm, using *sodium carbonate solution R* as the compensation liquid.

The absorbance of the test solution is not less than that of the reference solution, which corresponds to a content of pyruvic acid of not less than 1.5 per cent.

INDEX

To aid users the index includes a reference to the supplement where the latest version of a text can be found.

For example: Amikacin...**6.1**-3396

means the monograph Amikacin can be found on page 3396 of Supplement 6.1.

Note that where no reference to a supplement is made, the text can be found in the principal volume.

Monographs deleted from the 6th Edition are not included in the index; a list of deleted texts is found in the Contents of this supplement, page xxxii.

Numerics

1. General notices ... 3
2.1.1. Droppers ... 15
2.1.2. Comparative table of porosity of sintered-glass filters ... 15
2.1.3. Ultraviolet ray lamps for analytical purposes ... 15
2.1.4. Sieves ... 16
2.1.5. Tubes for comparative tests ... 17
2.1.6. Gas detector tubes ... 17
2.1. Apparatus ... 15
2.2.10. Viscosity - Rotating viscometer method ... 28
2.2.11. Distillation range ... 30
2.2.12. Boiling point ... 31
2.2.13. Determination of water by distillation ... 31
2.2.14. Melting point - capillary method ... 32
2.2.15. Melting point - open capillary method ... 32
2.2.16. Melting point - instantaneous method ... 33
2.2.17. Drop point ... 33
2.2.18. Freezing point ... 35
2.2.19. Amperometric titration ... 35
2.2.1. Clarity and degree of opalescence of liquids ... 21
2.2.20. Potentiometric titration ... 35
2.2.21. Fluorimetry ... 36
2.2.22. Atomic emission spectrometry ... 36
2.2.23. Atomic absorption spectrometry ... 37
2.2.24. Absorption spectrophotometry, infrared ... 39
2.2.25. Absorption spectrophotometry, ultraviolet and visible ... 41
2.2.26. Paper chromatography ... 43
2.2.27. Thin-layer chromatography ... 43
2.2.28. Gas chromatography ... 45
2.2.29. Liquid chromatography ... 46
2.2.2. Degree of coloration of liquids ... 22
2.2.30. Size-exclusion chromatography ... 47
2.2.31. Electrophoresis ... 48
2.2.32. Loss on drying ... 53
2.2.33. Nuclear magnetic resonance spectrometry ... 54
2.2.34. Thermal analysis ... **6.1**-3311
2.2.35. Osmolality ... 57
2.2.36. Potentiometric determination of ionic concentration using ion-selective electrodes ... 58
2.2.37. X-ray fluorescence spectrometry ... 59
2.2.38. Conductivity ... 59
2.2.39. Molecular mass distribution in dextrans ... 60
2.2.3. Potentiometric determination of pH ... 24
2.2.40. Near-infrared spectrophotometry ... 62
2.2.41. Circular dichroism ... 66
2.2.42. Density of solids ... 67
2.2.43. Mass spectrometry ... 68
2.2.44. Total organic carbon in water for pharmaceutical use ... 71
2.2.45. Supercritical fluid chromatography ... 71
2.2.46. Chromatographic separation techniques ... 72
2.2.47. Capillary electrophoresis ... 77
2.2.48. Raman spectrometry ... 82
2.2.49. Falling ball viscometer method ... 84
2.2.4. Relationship between reaction of solution, approximate pH and colour of certain indicators ... 25
2.2.54. Isoelectric focusing ... 84
2.2.55. Peptide mapping ... 86
2.2.56. Amino acid analysis ... 89
2.2.57. Inductively coupled plasma-atomic emission spectrometry ... 96
2.2.58. Inductively coupled plasma-mass spectrometry ... 98
2.2.5. Relative density ... 25
2.2.60. Melting point - instrumental method ... **6.1**-3313
2.2.6. Refractive index ... 26
2.2.7. Optical rotation ... 26
2.2.8. Viscosity ... 27
2.2.9. Capillary viscometer method ... 27
2.2. Physical and physicochemical methods ... 21
2.3.1. Identification reactions of ions and functional groups ... 103
2.3.2. Identification of fatty oils by thin-layer chromatography ... 106
2.3.3. Identification of phenothiazines by thin-layer chromatography ... 107
2.3.4. Odour ... 107
2.3. Identification ... 103
2.4.10. Lead in sugars ... 115
2.4.11. Phosphates ... 116
2.4.12. Potassium ... 116
2.4.13. Sulphates ... 116
2.4.14. Sulphated ash ... 116
2.4.15. Nickel in polyols ... 116
2.4.16. Total ash ... 116
2.4.17. Aluminium ... 117
2.4.18. Free formaldehyde ... 117
2.4.19. Alkaline impurities in fatty oils ... 117
2.4.1. Ammonium ... 111
2.4.21. Foreign oils in fatty oils by thin-layer chromatography ... 117
2.4.22. Composition of fatty acids by gas chromatography ... 118
2.4.23. Sterols in fatty oils ... 120
2.4.24. Identification and control of residual solvents ... 121
2.4.25. Ethylene oxide and dioxan ... 126
2.4.26. *N,N*-Dimethylaniline ... 127
2.4.27. Heavy metals in herbal drugs and fatty oils ... 128
2.4.28. 2-Ethylhexanoic acid ... 129
2.4.29. Composition of fatty acids in oils rich in omega-3 acids ... 130
2.4.2. Arsenic ... 111
2.4.30. Ethylene glycol and diethylene glycol in ethoxylated substances ... 131
2.4.31. Nickel in hydrogenated vegetable oils ... 131
2.4.32. Total cholesterol in oils rich in omega-3 acids ... 132
2.4.3. Calcium ... 111
2.4.4. Chlorides ... 112
2.4.5. Fluorides ... 112
2.4.6. Magnesium ... 112
2.4.7. Magnesium and alkaline-earth metals ... 112
2.4.8. Heavy metals ... 112
2.4.9. Iron ... 115
2.4. Limit tests ... 111
2.5.10. Oxygen-flask method ... 140
2.5.11. Complexometric titrations ... 140
2.5.12. Water: semi-micro determination ... 141
2.5.13. Aluminium in adsorbed vaccines ... 141
2.5.14. Calcium in adsorbed vaccines ... 142
2.5.15. Phenol in immunosera and vaccines ... 142
2.5.16. Protein in polysaccharide vaccines ... 142
2.5.17. Nucleic acids in polysaccharide vaccines ... 142
2.5.18. Phosphorus in polysaccharide vaccines ... 142
2.5.19. *O*-Acetyl in polysaccharide vaccines ... 143
2.5.1. Acid value ... 137
2.5.20. Hexosamines in polysaccharide vaccines ... 143
2.5.21. Methylpentoses in polysaccharide vaccines ... 143
2.5.22. Uronic acids in polysaccharide vaccines ... 144
2.5.23. Sialic acid in polysaccharide vaccines ... 144
2.5.24. Carbon dioxide in gases ... 144
2.5.25. Carbon monoxide in gases ... 145
2.5.26. Nitrogen monoxide and nitrogen dioxide in gases ... 146
2.5.27. Oxygen in gases ... 146
2.5.28. Water in gases ... 146
2.5.29. Sulphur dioxide ... 146
2.5.2. Ester value ... 137

2.5.30. Oxidising substances ... 147
2.5.31. Ribose in polysaccharide vaccines ... 147
2.5.32. Water: micro determination ... 147
2.5.33. Total protein ... 148
2.5.34. Acetic acid in synthetic peptides ... 151
2.5.35. Nitrous oxide in gases ... 152
2.5.36. Anisidine value ... 152
2.5.3. Hydroxyl value ... 137
2.5.4. Iodine value ... 137
2.5.5. Peroxide value ... 138
2.5.6. Saponification value ... 139
2.5.7. Unsaponifiable matter ... 139
2.5.8. Determination of primary aromatic amino-nitrogen ... 139
2.5.9. Determination of nitrogen by sulphuric acid digestion ... 139
2.5. Assays ... 137
2.6.10. Histamine ... 165
2.6.11. Depressor substances ... 166
2.6.12. Microbiological examination of non-sterile products: total viable aerobic count ... 166
2.6.13. Microbiological examination of non-sterile products: test for specified micro-organisms ... 173
2.6.14. Bacterial endotoxins ... 182
2.6.15. Prekallikrein activator ... 189
2.6.16. Tests for extraneous agents in viral vaccines for human use ... 190
2.6.17. Test for anticomplementary activity of immunoglobulin ... 191
2.6.18. Test for neurovirulence of live virus vaccines ... 193
2.6.19. Test for neurovirulence of poliomyelitis vaccine (oral) ... 193
2.6.1. Sterility ... 155
2.6.20. Anti-A and anti-B haemagglutinins (indirect method) ... 195
2.6.21. Nucleic acid amplification techniques ... 195
2.6.22. Activated coagulation factors ... 198
2.6.24. Avian viral vaccines: tests for extraneous agents in seed lots ... 198
2.6.25. Avian live virus vaccines: tests for extraneous agents in batches of finished product ... 202
2.6.26. Test for anti-D antibodies in human immunoglobulin for intravenous administration ... 205
2.6.27. Microbiological control of cellular products ... 205
2.6.2. Mycobacteria ... 159
2.6.7. Mycoplasmas ... **6.1**-3317
2.6.8. Pyrogens ... 164
2.6.9. Abnormal toxicity ... 165
2.6. Biological tests ... 155
2.7.10. Assay of human coagulation factor VII ... 228
2.7.11. Assay of human coagulation factor IX ... 229
2.7.12. Assay of heparin in coagulation factors ... 230
2.7.13. Assay of human anti-D immunoglobulin ... 230
2.7.14. Assay of hepatitis A vaccine ... 232
2.7.15. Assay of hepatitis B vaccine (rDNA) ... 233
2.7.16. Assay of pertussis vaccine (acellular) ... 233
2.7.17. Assay of human antithrombin III ... 234
2.7.18. Assay of human coagulation factor II ... 234
2.7.19. Assay of human coagulation factor X ... 235
2.7.19. Assay of human coagulation factor X (2.7.19.) ... 235
2.7.1. Immunochemical methods ... 209
2.7.20. *In vivo* assay of poliomyelitis vaccine (inactivated) ... 235
2.7.21. Assay of human von Willebrand factor ... 237
2.7.22. Assay of human coagulation factor XI ... 238
2.7.23. Numeration of CD34/CD45+ cells in haematopoietic products ... 238
2.7.24. Flow cytometry ... 240
2.7.27. Flocculation value (Lf) of diphtheria and tetanus toxins and toxoids (Ramon assay) ... 241
2.7.28. Colony-forming cell assay for human haematopoietic progenitor cells ... 242
2.7.29. Nucleated cell count and viability ... 243
2.7.2. Microbiological assay of antibiotics ... 210
2.7.4. Assay of human coagulation factor VIII ... 216
2.7.5. Assay of heparin ... 217
2.7.6. Assay of diphtheria vaccine (adsorbed) ... 217
2.7.7. Assay of pertussis vaccine ... 222
2.7.8. Assay of tetanus vaccine (adsorbed) ... 223
2.7.9. Test for Fc function of immunoglobulin ... 227
2.7. Biological assays ... 209
2.8.10. Solubility in alcohol of essential oils ... 250
2.8.11. Assay of 1,8-cineole in essential oils ... 250
2.8.12. Determination of essential oils in herbal drugs ... 251
2.8.13. Pesticide residues ... 252
2.8.14. Determination of tannins in herbal drugs ... 255
2.8.15. Bitterness value ... 255
2.8.16. Dry residue of extracts ... 256
2.8.17. Loss on drying of extracts ... 256
2.8.18. Determination of aflatoxin B_1 in herbal drugs ... 256
2.8.1. Ash insoluble in hydrochloric acid ... 249
2.8.20. Herbal drugs: sampling and sample preparation ... 258
2.8.2. Foreign matter ... 249
2.8.3. Stomata and stomatal index ... 249
2.8.4. Swelling index ... 249
2.8.5. Water in essential oils ... 249
2.8.6. Foreign esters in essential oils ... 250
2.8.7. Fatty oils and resinified essential oils in essential oils ... 250
2.8.8. Odour and taste of essential oils ... 250
2.8.9. Residue on evaporation of essential oils ... 250
2.8. Methods in pharmacognosy ... 249
2.9.10. Ethanol content and alcoholimetric tables ... 281
2.9.11. Test for methanol and 2-propanol ... 282
2.9.12. Sieve test ... 283
2.9.14. Specific surface area by air permeability ... 283
2.9.15. Apparent volume ... 285
2.9.16. Flowability ... 286
2.9.17. Test for extractable volume of parenteral preparations ... 287
2.9.18. Preparations for inhalation: aerodynamic assessment of fine particles ... 287
2.9.19. Particulate contamination: sub-visible particles ... 300
2.9.1. Disintegration of tablets and capsules ... 263
2.9.20. Particulate contamination: visible particles ... 302
2.9.22. Softening time determination of lipophilic suppositories ... 302
2.9.23. Pycnometric density of solids ... 304
2.9.25. Dissolution test for medicated chewing gums ... 304
2.9.26. Specific surface area by gas adsorption ... 306
2.9.27. Uniformity of mass of delivered doses from multidose containers ... 309
2.9.29. Intrinsic dissolution ... 309
2.9.2. Disintegration of suppositories and pessaries ... 265
2.9.31. Particle size analysis by laser light diffraction ... 311
2.9.33. Characterisation of crystalline and partially crystalline solids by X-ray powder diffraction (XRPD) ... 314
2.9.36. Powder flow ... 320
2.9.37. Optical microscopy ... 323
2.9.38. Particle-size distribution estimation by analytical sieving ... 325
2.9.3. Dissolution test for solid dosage forms ... 266
2.9.40. Uniformity of dosage units ... **6.1**-3325
2.9.41. Friability of granules and spheroids ... 330
2.9.42. Dissolution test for lipophilic solid dosage forms ... 332
2.9.43. Apparent dissolution ... **6.1**-3327
2.9.4. Dissolution test for transdermal patches ... 275

2.9.5. Uniformity of mass of single-dose preparations....... 278
2.9.6. Uniformity of content of single-dose preparations.. 278
2.9.7. Friability of uncoated tablets 278
2.9.8. Resistance to crushing of tablets........ 279
2.9.9. Measurement of consistency by penetrometry 279
2.9. Pharmaceutical technical procedures 263
3.1.10. Materials based on non-plasticised poly(vinyl chloride) for containers for non-injectable, aqueous solutions 360
3.1.11. Materials based on non-plasticised poly(vinyl chloride) for containers for dry dosage forms for oral administration 362
3.1.1.1. Materials based on plasticised poly(vinyl chloride) for containers for human blood and blood components....... 339
3.1.1.2. Materials based on plasticised poly(vinyl chloride) for tubing used in sets for the transfusion of blood and blood components 342
3.1.13. Plastic additives 364
3.1.14. Materials based on plasticised poly(vinyl chloride) for containers for aqueous solutions for intravenous infusion 366
3.1.15. Polyethylene terephthalate for containers for preparations not for parenteral use 369
3.1.1. Materials for containers for human blood and blood components 339
3.1.3. Polyolefines 344
3.1.4. Polyethylene without additives for containers for parenteral preparations and for ophthalmic preparations 348
3.1.5. Polyethylene with additives for containers for parenteral preparations and for ophthalmic preparations 349
3.1.6. Polypropylene for containers and closures for parenteral preparations and ophthalmic preparations ... 352
3.1.7. Poly(ethylene - vinyl acetate) for containers and tubing for total parenteral nutrition preparations 356
3.1.8. Silicone oil used as a lubricant 358
3.1.9. Silicone elastomer for closures and tubing 358
3.1. Materials used for the manufacture of containers 339
3.2.1. Glass containers for pharmaceutical use 373
3.2.2.1. Plastic containers for aqueous solutions for infusion 379
3.2.2. Plastic containers and closures for pharmaceutical use 378
3.2.3. Sterile plastic containers for human blood and blood components 379
3.2.4. Empty sterile containers of plasticised poly(vinyl chloride) for human blood and blood components.......... 381
3.2.5. Sterile containers of plasticised poly(vinyl chloride) for human blood containing anticoagulant solution 382
3.2.6. Sets for the transfusion of blood and blood components 383
3.2.8. Sterile single-use plastic syringes 384
3.2.9. Rubber closures for containers for aqueous parenteral preparations, for powders and for freeze-dried powders 386
3.2. Containers 373
4.1.1. Reagents 391
4.1.1. Reagents **6.1**-3331
4.1.2. Standard solutions for limit tests 504
4.1.3. Buffer solutions 508
4.1.3. Buffer solutions **6.1**-3331
4.1. Reagents, standard solutions, buffer solutions 391
4.2.1. Primary standards for volumetric solutions 514
4.2.2. Volumetric solutions 514
4.2. Volumetric analysis 514
4-Aminobenzoic acid 1164
4. Reagents 391
5.10. Control of impurities in substances for pharmaceutical use 653
5.11. Characters section in monographs 659
5.1.1. Methods of preparation of sterile products 525
5.1.2. Biological indicators of sterilisation 527
5.12. Reference standards 663
5.1.3. Efficacy of antimicrobial preservation 528
5.14. Gene transfer medicinal products for human use 669
5.1.4. Microbiological quality of pharmaceutical preparations 529
5.1.5. Application of the F_0 concept to steam sterilisation of aqueous preparations 531
5.15. Functionality-related characteristics of excipients **6.1**-3339
5.1.6. Alternative methods for control of microbiological quality 532
5.1.7. Viral safety 543
5.1. General texts on microbiology 525
5.2.1. Terminology used in monographs on biological products 547
5.2.2. Chicken flocks free from specified pathogens for the production and quality control of vaccines 547
5.2.3. Cell substrates for the production of vaccines for human use 550
5.2.4. Cell cultures for the production of veterinary vaccines 553
5.2.5. Substances of animal origin for the production of veterinary vaccines 555
5.2.6. Evaluation of safety of veterinary vaccines and immunosera 556
5.2.7. Evaluation of efficacy of veterinary vaccines and immunosera **6.1**-3335
5.2.8. Minimising the risk of transmitting animal spongiform encephalopathy agents via human and veterinary medicinal products 558
5.2.9. Evaluation of safety of each batch of veterinary vaccines and immunosera 567
5.2. General texts on biological products 547
5.3. Statistical analysis of results of biological assays and tests 571
5.4. Residual solvents 603
5.5. Alcoholimetric tables 613
5.6. Assay of interferons 627
5.7. Table of physical characteristics of radionuclides mentioned in the European Pharmacopoeia 633
5.8. Pharmacopoeial harmonisation 645
5.9. Polymorphism 649

A

Abbreviations and symbols (1.) 3
Abnormal toxicity (2.6.9.) 165
Absorption spectrophotometry, infrared (2.2.24.) 39
Absorption spectrophotometry, ultraviolet and visible (2.2.25.) 41
Acacia 1087
Acacia, spray-dried 1087
Acamprosate calcium 1088
Acarbose 1089
Acebutolol hydrochloride 1091
Aceclofenac 1093
Acemetacin **6.1**-3393
Acesulfame potassium 1095
Acetazolamide 1096
Acetic acid, glacial 1097
Acetic acid in synthetic peptides (2.5.34.) 151
Acetone 1098
Acetylcholine chloride 1099
Acetylcysteine 1100
β-Acetyldigoxin 1101
Acetylsalicylic acid 1103
Acetyltryptophan, *N*- 1104

Acetyltyrosine, *N*- 1106
Aciclovir 1107
Acid value (2.5.1.) 137
Acitretin 1109
Actinobacillosis vaccine (inactivated), porcine 943
Activated charcoal 1488
Activated coagulation factors (2.6.22.) 198
Additives, plastic (3.1.13.) 364
Adenine 1110
Adenosine 1111
Adenovirus vectors for human use 670
Adipic acid 1113
Adrenaline tartrate 1114
Aerodynamic assessment of fine particles in preparations for inhalation (2.9.18.) 287
Aflatoxin B_1 in herbal drugs, determination of (2.8.18.) 256
Agar 1115
Agnus castus fruit 1116
Agrimony 1117
Air, medicinal 1118
Air, synthetic medicinal 1121
Alanine 1121
Albendazole 1122
Albumin solution, human 2057
Alchemilla 1123
Alcoholimetric tables (2.9.10.) 281
Alcoholimetric tables (5.5.) 613
Alcuronium chloride 1124
Alexandrian senna pods 2870
Alfacalcidol 1126
Alfadex 1127
Alfentanil hydrochloride 1128
Alfuzosin hydrochloride **6.1**-3394
Alginic acid 1131
Alkaline-earth metals and magnesium (2.4.7.) 112
Alkaline impurities in fatty oils (2.4.19.) 117
Allantoin 1131
Allergen products 679
Allopurinol 1132
all-*rac*-α-Tocopherol 3086
all-*rac*-α-Tocopheryl acetate 3089
Almagate 1134
Almond oil, refined 1136
Almond oil, virgin 1136
Aloes, Barbados 1137
Aloes, Cape 1138
Aloes dry extract, standardised 1139
Alphacyclodextrin 1127
Alprazolam 1139
Alprenolol hydrochloride 1141
Alprostadil 1143
Alteplase for injection 1145
Alternative methods for control of microbiological quality (5.1.6.) 532
Alum 1149
Aluminium (2.4.17.) 117
Aluminium chloride hexahydrate 1149
Aluminium hydroxide, hydrated, for adsorption **6.1**-3395
Aluminium in adsorbed vaccines (2.5.13.) 141
Aluminium magnesium silicate 1151
Aluminium oxide, hydrated 1152
Aluminium phosphate gel 1152
Aluminium phosphate, hydrated 1153
Aluminium sulphate 1154
Alverine citrate 1154
Amantadine hydrochloride 1156
Ambroxol hydrochloride 1156
Amfetamine sulphate 1158
Amidotrizoic acid dihydrate 1158
Amikacin **6.1**-3396
Amikacin sulphate **6.1**-3398
Amiloride hydrochloride 1163
Amino acid analysis (2.2.56.) 89
Aminobenzoic acid, 4- 1164
Aminocaproic acid 1166
Aminoglutethimide 1167
Amiodarone hydrochloride 1168
Amisulpride 1170
Amitriptyline hydrochloride 1172
Amlodipine besilate 1173
Ammonia (^{13}N) injection 981
Ammonia solution, concentrated 1175
Ammonio methacrylate copolymer (type A) 1175
Ammonio methacrylate copolymer (type B) 1176
Ammonium (2.4.1.) 111
Ammonium bromide 1177
Ammonium chloride 1178
Ammonium glycyrrhizate 1179
Ammonium hydrogen carbonate 1180
Amobarbital 1180
Amobarbital sodium 1181
Amoxicillin sodium 1182
Amoxicillin trihydrate 1184
Amperometric titration (2.2.19.) 35
Amphotericin B 1187
Ampicillin, anhydrous 1188
Ampicillin sodium 1190
Ampicillin trihydrate 1193
Anaesthetic ether 1834
Analysis, thermal (2.2.34.) **6.1**-3311
Analytical sieving, particle-size distribution estimation by (2.9.38.) 325
Angelica root 1196
Animal anti-T lymphocyte immunoglobulin for human use 1203
Animal immunosera for human use 685
Animal spongiform encephalopathies, products with risk of transmitting agents of 694
Animal spongiform encephalopathy agents, minimising the risk of transmitting via human and veterinary medicinal products (5.2.8.) 558
Aniseed 1199
Anise oil 1197
Anisidine value (2.5.36.) 152
Antazoline hydrochloride 1199
Anthrax spore vaccine (live) for veterinary use 859
Anthrax vaccine for human use (adsorbed, prepared from culture filtrates) 757
Anti-A and anti-B haemagglutinins (indirect method) (2.6.20.) 195
Antibiotics, microbiological assay of (2.7.2.) 210
Antibodies for human use, monoclonal 690
Anticoagulant and preservative solutions for human blood 1200
Anticomplementary activity of immunoglobulin (2.6.17.) 191
Anti-D antibodies in human immunoglobulins for intravenous administration, test for (2.6.26.) 205
Anti-D immunoglobulin for intravenous administration, human 2059
Anti-D immunoglobulin, human 2058
Anti-D immunoglobulin, human, assay of (2.7.13.) 230
Antimicrobial preservation, efficacy of (5.1.3.) 528
Antiserum, European viper venom 970
Antithrombin III concentrate, human 2060
Antithrombin III, human, assay of (2.7.17.) 234
Anti-T lymphocyte immunoglobulin for human use, animal 1203
Apomorphine hydrochloride 1207

Apparatus (2.1.) 15
Apparent dissolution (2.9.43.) **6.1**-3327
Apparent volume (2.9.15.) 285
Application of the F_0 concept to steam sterilisation of aqueous preparations (5.1.5.) 531
Aprotinin 1208
Aprotinin concentrated solution 1209
Arachis oil, hydrogenated 1211
Arachis oil, refined 1211
Arginine 1212
Arginine aspartate 1213
Arginine hydrochloride 1214
Arnica flower **6.1**-3400
Arnica tincture 1216
Arsenic (2.4.2.) 111
Arsenious trioxide for homoeopathic preparations 1073
Articaine hydrochloride 1217
Artichoke leaf 1219
Ascorbic acid 1221
Ascorbyl palmitate 1222
Ash insoluble in hydrochloric acid (2.8.1.) 249
Ash leaf 1222
Asparagine monohydrate 1223
Aspartame 1224
Aspartic acid 1225
Assay of 1,8-cineole in essential oils (2.8.11.) 250
Assay of diphtheria vaccine (adsorbed) (2.7.6.) 217
Assay of heparin (2.7.5.) 217
Assay of heparin in coagulation factors (2.7.12.) 230
Assay of hepatitis A vaccine (2.7.14.) 232
Assay of hepatitis B vaccine (rDNA) (2.7.15.) 233
Assay of human anti-D immunoglobulin (2.7.13.) 230
Assay of human antithrombin III (2.7.17.) 234
Assay of human coagulation factor II (2.7.18.) 234
Assay of human coagulation factor IX (2.7.11.) 229
Assay of human coagulation factor VII (2.7.10.) 228
Assay of human coagulation factor VIII (2.7.4.) 216
Assay of human coagulation factor X (2.7.19.) 235
Assay of human coagulation factor XI (2.7.22.) 238
Assay of human von Willebrand factor (2.7.21.) 237
Assay of interferons (5.6.) 627
Assay of pertussis vaccine (2.7.7.) 222
Assay of pertussis vaccine (acellular) (2.7.16.) 233
Assay of poliomyelitis vaccine (inactivated), *in vivo* (2.7.20.) 235
Assay of tetanus vaccine (adsorbed) (2.7.8.) 223
Assays (2.5.) 137
Astemizole 1226
Atenolol 1228
Atomic absorption spectrometry (2.2.23.) 37
Atomic emission spectrometry (2.2.22.) 36
Atomic emission spectrometry, inductively coupled plasma- (2.2.57.) 96
Atracurium besilate 1230
Atropine **6.1**-3403
Atropine sulphate **6.1**-3404
Aujeszky's disease vaccine (inactivated) for pigs 859
Aujeszky's disease vaccine (live) for pigs for parenteral administration 861
Avian infectious bronchitis vaccine (inactivated) 864
Avian infectious bronchitis vaccine (live) **6.1**-3371
Avian infectious bursal disease vaccine (inactivated) 867
Avian infectious bursal disease vaccine (live) 869
Avian infectious encephalomyelitis vaccine (live) 871
Avian infectious laryngotracheitis vaccine (live) 872
Avian live virus vaccines: tests for extraneous agents in batches of finished product (2.6.25.) 202
Avian paramyxovirus 1 (Newcastle disease) vaccine (inactivated) 937
Avian paramyxovirus 3 vaccine (inactivated) 874
Avian tuberculin purified protein derivative 3146
Avian viral tenosynovitis vaccine (live) 875
Avian viral vaccines: tests for extraneous agents in seed lots (2.6.24.) 198
Azaperone for veterinary use 1234
Azathioprine 1236
Azelastine hydrochloride 1236
Azithromycin 1238

B

Bacampicillin hydrochloride **6.1**-3409
Bacitracin 1245
Bacitracin zinc 1247
Baclofen 1250
Bacterial cells used for the manufacture of plasmid vectors for human use 676
Bacterial endotoxins (2.6.14.) 182
Bambuterol hydrochloride 1251
Barbados aloes 1137
Barbital 1252
Barium chloride dihydrate for homoeopathic preparations 1073
Barium sulphate 1253
Basic butylated methacrylate copolymer 1254
BCG for immunotherapy 758
BCG vaccine, freeze-dried 759
Bearberry leaf **6.1**-3410
Beclometasone dipropionate, anhydrous 1256
Beclometasone dipropionate monohydrate 1258
Bee for homoeopathic preparations, honey 1079
Beeswax, white 1260
Beeswax, yellow 1261
Belladonna leaf 1261
Belladonna leaf dry extract, standardised 1263
Belladonna leaf tincture, standardised 1264
Belladonna, prepared 1265
Bendroflumethiazide 1266
Benfluorex hydrochloride 1267
Benperidol 1269
Benserazide hydrochloride 1270
Bentonite 1271
Benzalkonium chloride 1272
Benzalkonium chloride solution 1273
Benzathine benzylpenicillin 1283
Benzbromarone 1273
Benzethonium chloride 1275
Benzocaine 1276
Benzoic acid 1276
Benzoin, Siam 1277
Benzoin, Sumatra 1278
Benzoin tincture, Siam 1278
Benzoin tincture, Sumatra 1279
Benzoyl peroxide, hydrous 1280
Benzyl alcohol 1281
Benzyl benzoate 1283
Benzylpenicillin, benzathine 1283
Benzylpenicillin potassium 1285
Benzylpenicillin, procaine 1287
Benzylpenicillin sodium 1288
Betacarotene 1290
Betacyclodextrin 1291
Betadex 1291
Betahistine dihydrochloride 1292
Betahistine mesilate 1293
Betamethasone 1295
Betamethasone acetate 1297
Betamethasone dipropionate 1298
Betamethasone sodium phosphate 1300

Betamethasone valerate ... 1301
Betaxolol hydrochloride ... 1303
Bezafibrate ... 1304
Bifonazole ... 1306
Bilberry fruit, dried ... 1307
Bilberry fruit, fresh ... **6.1**-3412
Biological assays (2.7.) ... 209
Biological assays and tests, statistical analysis of results of (5.3.) ... 571
Biological indicators of sterilisation (5.1.2.) ... 527
Biological products, general texts on (5.2.) ... 547
Biological products, terminology used in monographs on (5.2.1.) ... 547
Biological tests (2.6.) ... 155
Biotin ... 1308
Biperiden hydrochloride ... 1309
Biphasic insulin injection ... 2140
Biphasic isophane insulin injection ... 2140
Birch leaf ... 1311
Bisacodyl ... 1312
Bismuth subcarbonate ... 1313
Bismuth subgallate ... 1314
Bismuth subnitrate, heavy ... 1315
Bismuth subsalicylate ... 1316
Bisoprolol fumarate ... **6.1**-3412
Bistort rhizome ... 1317
Bitter fennel ... 1873
Bitter-fennel fruit oil ... 1318
Bitterness value (2.8.15.) ... 255
Bitter-orange epicarp and mesocarp ... 1319
Bitter-orange-epicarp and mesocarp tincture ... 1320
Bitter-orange flower ... 1320
Bitter-orange-flower oil ... 2490
Black horehound ... 1321
Bleomycin sulphate ... 1322
Blood and blood components, empty sterile containers of plasticised poly(vinyl chloride) for (3.2.4.) ... 381
Blood and blood components, materials for containers for (3.1.1.) ... 339
Blood and blood components, sets for the transfusion of (3.2.6.) ... 383
Blood and blood components, sterile plastic containers for (3.2.3.) ... 379
Blood, anticoagulant and preservative solutions for ... 1200
Blood, sterile containers of plasticised poly(vinyl chloride) containing anticoagulant solution (3.2.5.) ... 382
Bogbean leaf ... 1323
Boiling point (2.2.12.) ... 31
Boldo leaf ... 1324
Boldo leaf dry extract ... **6.1**-3415
Borage (starflower) oil, refined ... 1326
Borax ... 1326
Boric acid ... 1327
Botulinum antitoxin ... 965
Botulinum toxin type A for injection ... 1327
Bovine infectious rhinotracheitis vaccine (live) ... 924
Bovine insulin ... 2135
Bovine leptospirosis vaccine (inactivated) ... 876
Bovine parainfluenza virus vaccine (live) ... 878
Bovine respiratory syncytial virus vaccine (live) ... 879
Bovine serum ... 1329
Bovine tuberculin purified protein derivative ... 3147
Bovine viral diarrhoea vaccine (inactivated) ... 880
Bromazepam ... 1331
Bromhexine hydrochloride ... 1332
Bromocriptine mesilate ... 1333
Bromperidol ... 1335
Bromperidol decanoate ... 1337
Brompheniramine maleate ... 1339
Brotizolam ... 1340
Brucellosis vaccine (live) (Brucella melitensis Rev. 1 strain) for veterinary use ... 881
Buccal tablets and sublingual tablets ... 734
Buckwheat herb ... 1341
Budesonide ... 1342
Bufexamac ... 1344
Buffer solutions (4.1.3.) ... 508
Buffer solutions (4.1.3.) ... **6.1**-3331
Buflomedil hydrochloride ... 1345
Bumetanide ... 1346
Bupivacaine hydrochloride ... 1347
Buprenorphine ... 1349
Buprenorphine hydrochloride ... 1350
Buserelin ... 1351
Buspirone hydrochloride ... 1353
Busulfan ... 1355
Butcher's broom ... **6.1**-3416
Butylated methacrylate copolymer, basic ... 1254
Butylhydroxyanisole ... 1357
Butylhydroxytoluene ... 1357
Butyl parahydroxybenzoate ... 1358

C

Cabergoline ... 1363
Cachets ... 719
Cadmium sulphate hydrate for homoeopathic preparations ... 1074
Caffeine ... **6.1**-3421
Caffeine monohydrate ... 1365
Calcifediol ... 1366
Calcipotriol, anhydrous ... 1367
Calcipotriol monohydrate ... 1370
Calcitonin (salmon) ... 1372
Calcitriol ... 1375
Calcium (2.4.3.) ... 111
Calcium acetate ... 1376
Calcium ascorbate ... 1377
Calcium carbonate ... 1378
Calcium carboxymethylcellulose ... 1422
Calcium chloride dihydrate ... 1378
Calcium chloride hexahydrate ... 1379
Calcium dobesilate monohydrate ... 1380
Calcium folinate ... 1380
Calcium glucoheptonate ... 1383
Calcium gluconate ... 1384
Calcium gluconate for injection ... 1385
Calcium glycerophosphate ... 1386
Calcium hydrogen phosphate, anhydrous ... 1387
Calcium hydrogen phosphate dihydrate ... 1388
Calcium hydroxide ... 1389
Calcium in adsorbed vaccines (2.5.14.) ... 142
Calcium iodide tetrahydrate for homoeopathic preparations ... 1074
Calcium lactate, anhydrous ... 1389
Calcium lactate monohydrate ... 1390
Calcium lactate pentahydrate ... 1390
Calcium lactate trihydrate ... 1391
Calcium levofolinate pentahydrate ... 1392
Calcium levulinate dihydrate ... 1394
Calcium pantothenate ... 1395
Calcium phosphate ... 1396
Calcium stearate ... 1397
Calcium sulphate dihydrate ... 1398
Calendula flower ... 1398
Calf coronavirus diarrhoea vaccine (inactivated) ... 882
Calf rotavirus diarrhoea vaccine (inactivated) ... 884
Calicivirosis vaccine (inactivated), feline ... 909
Calicivirosis vaccine (live), feline ... 910

Camphor, D- 1400
Camphor, racemic 1401
Canine adenovirus vaccine (inactivated) 885
Canine adenovirus vaccine (live) 886
Canine distemper vaccine (live) 887
Canine leptospirosis vaccine (inactivated) 888
Canine parainfluenza virus vaccine (live) 890
Canine parvovirosis vaccine (inactivated) 891
Canine parvovirosis vaccine (live) 892
Cape aloes 1138
Capillary electrophoresis (2.2.47.) 77
Capillary viscometer method (2.2.9.) 27
Caprylic acid 1402
Caprylocaproyl macrogolglycerides 1403
Capsicum 1404
Capsicum oleoresin, refined and quantified 1405
Capsicum tincture, standardised 1406
Capsules 717
Capsules and tablets, disintegration of (2.9.1.) 263
Capsules, gastro-resistant 718
Capsules, hard 718
Capsules, intrauterine 726
Capsules, modified-release 718
Capsules, oromucosal 734
Capsules, rectal 745
Capsules, soft 718
Capsules, vaginal 752
Captopril 1407
Caraway fruit 1408
Caraway oil 1408
Carbachol 1410
Carbamazepine 1411
Carbasalate calcium 1412
Carbidopa 1413
Carbimazole 1414
Carbocisteine 1415
Carbomers **6.1**-3422
Carbon dioxide 1417
Carbon dioxide in gases (2.5.24.) 144
Carbon monoxide (^{15}O) 982
Carbon monoxide in gases (2.5.25.) 145
Carboplatin 1419
Carboprost trometamol 1420
Carboxymethylcellulose calcium 1422
Carboxymethylcellulose sodium 1423
Carboxymethylcellulose sodium, cross-linked 1626
Carboxymethylcellulose sodium, low-substituted 1424
Carisoprodol 1421
Carmellose calcium 1422
Carmellose sodium 1423
Carmellose sodium and microcrystalline cellulose 2422
Carmellose sodium, low-substituted 1424
Carmustine 1425
Carnauba wax 1425
Carteolol hydrochloride 1426
Carvedilol 1427
Cascara 1429
Cascara dry extract, standardised 1430
Cassia oil 1431
Castor oil, hydrogenated 1432
Castor oil, polyoxyl 2304
Castor oil, polyoxyl hydrogenated 2303
Castor oil, refined 1433
Castor oil, virgin 1434
Catgut, sterile 1045
Catgut, sterile, in distributor for veterinary use 1057
CD34/CD45+ cells in haematopoietic products, numeration of (2.7.23.) 238
Cefaclor 1435
Cefadroxil monohydrate **6.1**-3423
Cefalexin monohydrate **6.1**-3425
Cefalotin sodium 1440
Cefamandole nafate 1441
Cefapirin sodium 1443
Cefatrizine propylene glycol 1444
Cefazolin sodium 1445
Cefepime dihydrochloride monohydrate 1448
Cefixime 1450
Cefoperazone sodium 1451
Cefotaxime sodium 1453
Cefoxitin sodium 1455
Cefradine 1457
Ceftazidime 1459
Ceftriaxone sodium 1461
Cefuroxime axetil 1462
Cefuroxime sodium 1464
Celiprolol hydrochloride 1465
Cell count and viability, nucleated (2.7.29.) 243
Cell cultures for the production of veterinary vaccines (5.2.4.) 553
Cell substrates for the production of vaccines for human use (5.2.3.) 550
Cellular products, microbiological control of (2.6.27.) 205
Cellulose acetate 1467
Cellulose acetate butyrate 1468
Cellulose acetate phthalate 1468
Cellulose, microcrystalline 1469
Cellulose (microcrystalline) and carmellose sodium 2422
Cellulose, powdered 1473
Centaury 1477
Centella 1477
Cetirizine dihydrochloride 1479
Cetostearyl alcohol 1480
Cetostearyl alcohol (type A), emulsifying 1481
Cetostearyl alcohol (type B), emulsifying 1482
Cetostearyl isononanoate 1484
Cetrimide 1484
Cetyl alcohol 1485
Cetyl palmitate 1486
Cetylpyridinium chloride 1486
Ceylon cinnamon bark oil 1543
Ceylon cinnamon leaf oil 1544
CFC assay for human haematopoietic progenitor cells (2.7.28.) 242
Chamomile flower, Roman 1487
Characterisation of crystalline and partially crystalline solids by X-ray powder diffraction (XRPD) (2.9.33.) 314
Characters section in monographs (5.11.) 659
Charcoal, activated 1488
Chenodeoxycholic acid 1489
Chewing gum, medicated (2.9.25.) 304
Chewing gums, medicated 719
Chicken flocks free from specified pathogens for the production and quality control of vaccines (5.2.2.) 547
Chicken infectious anaemia vaccine (live) 925
Chitosan hydrochloride 1490
Chlamydiosis vaccine (inactivated), feline 911
Chloral hydrate 1491
Chlorambucil 1492
Chloramine 3103
Chloramphenicol 1492
Chloramphenicol palmitate 1493
Chloramphenicol sodium succinate 1495
Chlorcyclizine hydrochloride 1496
Chlordiazepoxide 1497
Chlordiazepoxide hydrochloride 1498
Chlorhexidine diacetate 1499
Chlorhexidine digluconate solution 1500

Chlorhexidine dihydrochloride 1502
Chlorides (2.4.4.) 112
Chlorobutanol, anhydrous 1503
Chlorobutanol hemihydrate 1504
Chlorocresol 1504
Chloroquine phosphate 1505
Chloroquine sulphate 1506
Chlorothiazide 1507
Chlorphenamine maleate **6.1**-3427
Chlorpromazine hydrochloride 1509
Chlorpropamide 1510
Chlorprothixene hydrochloride 1511
Chlortalidone 1513
Chlortetracycline hydrochloride 1514
Cholecalciferol 1516
Cholecalciferol concentrate (oily form) 1517
Cholecalciferol concentrate (powder form) 1519
Cholecalciferol concentrate (water-dispersible form) 1521
Cholera vaccine 761
Cholera vaccine, freeze-dried 761
Cholera vaccine (inactivated, oral) 762
Cholesterol 1524
Cholesterol in oils rich in omega-3 acids, total (2.4.32.) 132
Chondroitin sulphate sodium 1525
Chromatographic separation techniques (2.2.46.) 72
Chromatography, gas (2.2.28.) 45
Chromatography, liquid (2.2.29.) 46
Chromatography, paper (2.2.26.) 43
Chromatography, size-exclusion (2.2.30.) 47
Chromatography, supercritical fluid (2.2.45.) 71
Chromatography, thin-layer (2.2.27.) 43
Chromium (^{51}Cr) edetate injection 983
Chymotrypsin 1527
Ciclopirox 1528
Ciclopirox olamine 1530
Ciclosporin 1531
Cilastatin sodium **6.1**-3428
Cilazapril 1534
Cimetidine 1536
Cimetidine hydrochloride 1537
Cinchocaine hydrochloride 1538
Cinchona bark 1539
Cinchona liquid extract, standardised 1540
Cineole 1541
Cineole in essential oils, 1,8-, assay of (2.8.11.) 250
Cinnamon 1542
Cinnamon bark oil, Ceylon 1543
Cinnamon leaf oil, Ceylon 1544
Cinnamon tincture 1545
Cinnarizine 1545
Ciprofibrate 1547
Ciprofloxacin 1548
Ciprofloxacin hydrochloride 1550
Circular dichroism (2.2.41.) 66
Cisapride monohydrate 1551
Cisapride tartrate 1552
Cisplatin 1554
Citric acid, anhydrous 1554
Citric acid monohydrate 1555
Citronella oil 1556
Cladribine 1557
Clarithromycin 1559
Clarity and degree of opalescence of liquids (2.2.1.) 21
Clary sage oil 1561
Clazuril for veterinary use 1562
Clebopride malate 1564
Clemastine fumarate **6.1**-3430
Clenbuterol hydrochloride 1567
Clindamycin hydrochloride 1568
Clindamycin phosphate 1570
Clioquinol 1571
Clobazam 1572
Clobetasol propionate 1573
Clobetasone butyrate 1575
Clofazimine 1577
Clofibrate 1578
Clomifene citrate 1579
Clomipramine hydrochloride 1580
Clonazepam 1582
Clonidine hydrochloride 1583
Clopamide **6.1**-3431
Closantel sodium dihydrate for veterinary use 1584
Clostridium botulinum vaccine for veterinary use 894
Clostridium chauvoei vaccine for veterinary use 894
Clostridium novyi alpha antitoxin for veterinary use 973
Clostridium novyi (type b) vaccine for veterinary use 895
Clostridium perfringens beta antitoxin for veterinary use 974
Clostridium perfringens epsilon antitoxin for veterinary use 975
Clostridium perfringens vaccine for veterinary use 897
Clostridium septicum vaccine for veterinary use 899
Closures and containers for parenteral preparations and ophthalmic preparations, polypropylene for (3.1.6.) 352
Closures and containers for pharmaceutical use, plastic (3.2.2.) 378
Closures and tubing, silicone elastomer for (3.1.9.) 358
Closures for containers for aqueous parenteral preparations, for powders and for freeze-dried powders, rubber (3.2.9.) 386
Clotrimazole **6.1**-3433
Clove 1587
Clove oil 1588
Cloxacillin sodium 1589
Clozapine 1590
Coagulation factor II, assay of (2.7.18.) 234
Coagulation factor IX, human 2064
Coagulation factor IX, human, assay of (2.7.11.) 229
Coagulation factors, activated (2.6.22.) 198
Coagulation factors, assay of heparin (2.7.12.) 230
Coagulation factor VII, human 2061
Coagulation factor VII, human, assay of (2.7.10.) 228
Coagulation factor VIII, human 2062
Coagulation factor VIII, human, assay of (2.7.4.) 216
Coagulation factor VIII (rDNA), human 2063
Coagulation factor X, assay of (2.7.19.) 235
Coagulation factor XI, human 2065
Coagulation factor XI, human, assay of (2.7.22.) 238
Coated granules 724
Coated tablets 749
Cocaine hydrochloride 1592
Coconut oil, refined 1593
Cocoyl caprylocaprate 1594
Codeine **6.1**-3434
Codeine hydrochloride dihydrate 1596
Codeine phosphate hemihydrate 1598
Codeine phosphate sesquihydrate 1599
Codergocrine mesilate 1601
Cod-liver oil (type A) 1603
Cod-liver oil (type B) 1607
Cola 1611
Colchicine 1612
Colestyramine 1613
Colibacillosis vaccine (inactivated), neonatal piglet 934
Colibacillosis vaccine (inactivated), neonatal ruminant 936
Colistimethate sodium 1614
Colistin sulphate 1615
Colloidal anhydrous silica 2877

Colloidal hydrated silica....2877
Colloidal silica, hydrophobic....2878
Colloidal silver, for external use....2879
Colony-forming cell assay for human haematopoietic progenitor cells (2.7.28.)....242
Colophony....1617
Coloration of liquids (2.2.2.)....22
Common stinging nettle for homoeopathic preparations....1075
Comparative table of porosity of sintered-glass filters (2.1.2.)....15
Complexometric titrations (2.5.11.)....140
Composition of fatty acids by gas chromatography (2.4.22.)....118
Composition of fatty acids in oils rich in omega-3 acids (2.4.29.)....130
Compressed lozenges....734
Concentrated solutions for haemodialysis....2022
Concentrates for injections or infusions....736
Concentrates for intrauterine solutions....726
Conductivity (2.2.38.)....59
Coneflower herb, purple....2785
Coneflower root, narrow-leaved....2483
Coneflower root, pale....2602
Coneflower root, purple....2787
Conjugated estrogens....1824
Containers (3.2.)....373
Containers and closures for parenteral preparations and ophthalmic preparations, polypropylene for (3.1.6.)....352
Containers and closures for pharmaceutical use, plastic (3.2.2.)....378
Containers and tubing for total parenteral nutrition preparations, poly(ethylene - vinyl acetate) for (3.1.7.)....356
Containers for aqueous solutions for infusion, plastic (3.2.2.1.)....379
Containers for aqueous solutions for intravenous infusion, materials based on plasticised poly(vinyl chloride) for (3.1.14.)....366
Containers for dry dosage forms for oral administration, materials based on non-plasticised poly(vinyl chloride) for (3.1.11.)....362
Containers for human blood and blood components, materials based on plasticised poly(vinyl chloride) for (3.1.1.1.)....339
Containers for human blood and blood components, materials for (3.1.1.)....339
Containers for human blood and blood components, plastic, sterile (3.2.3.)....379
Containers for non-injectable aqueous solutions, materials based on non-plasticised poly(vinyl chloride) for (3.1.10.)....360
Containers for parenteral preparations and for ophthalmic preparations, polyethylene with additives for (3.1.5.)....349
Containers for parenteral preparations and for ophthalmic preparations, polyethylene without additives for (3.1.4.)....348
Containers for pharmaceutical use, glass (3.2.1.)....373
Containers for preparations not for parenteral use, polyethylene terephthalate for (3.1.15)....369
Containers of plasticised poly(vinyl chloride) for human blood and blood components, empty sterile (3.2.4.)....381
Containers of plasticised poly(vinyl chloride) for human blood containing anticoagulant solution, sterile (3.2.5.)....382
Contamination, microbial: test for specified micro-organisms (2.6.13.)....173
Contamination, microbial: total viable aerobic count (2.6.12.)....166
Content uniformity of single-dose preparations (2.9.6.)....278
Control of impurities in substances for pharmaceutical use (5.10.)....653
Control of microbiological quality, alternative methods for (5.1.6.)....532
Copolymer, basic butylated methacrylate....1254
Copolymer, methacrylic acid - ethyl acrylate (1:1)....2371
Copolymer (type A), ammonio methacrylate....1175
Copolymer (type B), ammonio methacrylate....1176
Copovidone....1617
Copper acetate monohydrate for homoeopathic preparations....1075
Copper for homoeopathic preparations....1076
Copper sulphate, anhydrous....1619
Copper sulphate pentahydrate....1620
Coriander....1620
Coriander oil....1621
Cortisone acetate....1622
Cotton, absorbent....1624
Cottonseed oil, hydrogenated....1625
Couch grass rhizome....1625
Creams....747
Cresol, crude....1626
Croscarmellose sodium....1626
Crospovidone....1628
Crotamiton....1629
Crystalline and partially crystalline solids, characterisation by X-ray powder diffraction (XRPD) of (2.9.33.)....314
Cutaneous application, liquid preparations for....728
Cutaneous application, powders for....738
Cutaneous application, semi-solid preparations for....746
Cutaneous application, veterinary liquid preparations for....752
Cutaneous foams....728
Cyanocobalamin....1630
Cyanocobalamin (^{57}Co) capsules....983
Cyanocobalamin (^{57}Co) solution....984
Cyanocobalamin (^{58}Co) capsules....985
Cyanocobalamin (^{58}Co) solution....986
Cyclizine hydrochloride....1631
Cyclopentolate hydrochloride....1632
Cyclophosphamide....1633
Cyproheptadine hydrochloride....1634
Cyproterone acetate....1635
Cysteine hydrochloride monohydrate....1636
Cystine....1637
Cytarabine....1638

D

Dacarbazine....1641
Dalteparin sodium....1642
Danaparoid sodium....1644
Dapsone....1646
Daunorubicin hydrochloride....1647
D-Camphor....1400
Decyl oleate....1648
Deferoxamine mesilate....1649
Degree of coloration of liquids (2.2.2.)....22
Dembrexine hydrochloride monohydrate for veterinary use....1650
Demeclocycline hydrochloride....1651
Density of solids (2.2.42.)....67
Density, relative (2.2.5.)....25
Dental type silica....2878
Depressor substances (2.6.11.)....166
Deptropine citrate....1653
Dequalinium chloride....1654
Desflurane....**6.1**-3439
Desipramine hydrochloride....1655
Deslanoside....1656

Desmopressin ... 1657
Desogestrel ... 1658
Desoxycortone acetate ... 1659
Detector tubes, gas (2.1.6.) ... 17
Determination of aflatoxin B_1 in herbal drugs (2.8.18.) ... 256
Determination of essential oils in herbal drugs (2.8.12.) .. 251
Determination of nitrogen by sulphuric acid digestion (2.5.9.) ... 139
Determination of primary aromatic amino-nitrogen (2.5.8.) ... 139
Determination of tannins in herbal drugs (2.8.14.) ... 255
Determination of water by distillation (2.2.13.) ... 31
Detomidine hydrochloride for veterinary use ... 1660
Devil's claw dry extract ... 1662
Devil's claw root ... **6.1**-3440
Dexamethasone ... 1663
Dexamethasone acetate ... 1665
Dexamethasone isonicotinate ... 1666
Dexamethasone sodium phosphate ... 1667
Dexchlorpheniramine maleate ... 1669
Dexpanthenol ... 1670
Dextran 1 for injection ... 1671
Dextran 40 for injection ... 1672
Dextran 60 for injection ... 1673
Dextran 70 for injection ... 1674
Dextranomer ... 1675
Dextrans, molecular mass distribution in (2.2.39.) ... 60
Dextrin ... 1675
Dextromethorphan hydrobromide ... 1676
Dextromoramide tartrate ... 1677
Dextropropoxyphene hydrochloride ... 1678
Diazepam ... 1679
Diazoxide ... 1680
Dibrompropamidine diisetionate ... 1681
Dibutyl phthalate ... 1682
Dichloromethane ... 2387
Diclazuril for veterinary use ... 1683
Diclofenac potassium ... 1685
Diclofenac sodium ... 1686
Dicloxacillin sodium ... 1687
Dicycloverine hydrochloride ... 1689
Didanosine ... 1689
Dienestrol ... 1691
Diethylcarbamazine citrate ... 1693
Diethylene glycol and ethylene glycol in ethoxylated substances (2.4.30.) ... 131
Diethylene glycol monoethyl ether ... 1694
Diethylene glycol palmitostearate ... 1695
Diethyl phthalate ... **6.1**-3441
Diethylstilbestrol ... 1696
Diffraction, laser light, particle size analysis by (2.9.31.) .. 311
Diflunisal ... 1697
Digitalis leaf ... 1698
Digitoxin ... 1700
Digoxin ... 1701
Dihydralazine sulphate, hydrated ... **6.1**-3442
Dihydrocodeine hydrogen tartrate ... 1704
Dihydroergocristine mesilate ... 1705
Dihydroergotamine mesilate ... **6.1**-3444
Dihydroergotamine tartrate ... 1709
Dihydrostreptomycin sulphate for veterinary use ... 1710
Dihydrotachysterol ... 1712
Diltiazem hydrochloride ... **6.1**-3446
Dimenhydrinate ... 1715
Dimercaprol ... 1716
Dimethylacetamide ... 1717
Dimethylaniline, *N,N*- (2.4.26.) ... 127
Dimethyl sulfoxide ... 1716
Dimeticone ... 1718
Dimetindene maleate ... 1719
Dinoprostone ... 1722
Dinoprost trometamol ... 1720
Diosmin ... 1723
Dioxan and ethylene oxide (2.4.25.) ... 126
Dip concentrates ... 753
Diphenhydramine hydrochloride ... 1725
Diphenoxylate hydrochloride ... 1726
Diphtheria and tetanus toxins and toxoids, flocculation value (Lf) of, (Ramon assay) (2.7.27.) ... 241
Diphtheria and tetanus vaccine (adsorbed) ... 763
Diphtheria and tetanus vaccine (adsorbed, reduced antigen(s) content) ... 764
Diphtheria antitoxin ... 965
Diphtheria, tetanus and hepatitis B (rDNA) vaccine (adsorbed) ... 765
Diphtheria, tetanus and pertussis (acellular, component) vaccine (adsorbed) ... 767
Diphtheria, tetanus and pertussis vaccine (adsorbed) ... 768
Diphtheria, tetanus and poliomyelitis (inactivated) vaccine (adsorbed, reduced antigen(s) content) ... 770
Diphtheria, tetanus, pertussis (acellular, component) and haemophilus type b conjugate vaccine (adsorbed) ... 771
Diphtheria, tetanus, pertussis (acellular, component) and hepatitis B (rDNA) vaccine (adsorbed) ... 774
Diphtheria, tetanus, pertussis (acellular, component) and poliomyelitis (inactivated) vaccine (adsorbed) ... 775
Diphtheria, tetanus, pertussis (acellular, component) and poliomyelitis (inactivated) vaccine (adsorbed, reduced antigen(s) content) ... 778
Diphtheria, tetanus, pertussis (acellular, component), hepatitis B (rDNA), poliomyelitis (inactivated) and haemophilus type b conjugate vaccine (adsorbed) ... 780
Diphtheria, tetanus, pertussis (acellular, component), poliomyelitis (inactivated) and haemophilus type b conjugate vaccine (adsorbed) ... 783
Diphtheria, tetanus, pertussis and poliomyelitis (inactivated) vaccine (adsorbed) ... 785
Diphtheria, tetanus, pertussis, poliomyelitis (inactivated) and haemophilus type b conjugate vaccine (adsorbed) ... 787
Diphtheria vaccine (adsorbed) ... 789
Diphtheria vaccine (adsorbed), assay of (2.7.6.) ... 217
Diphtheria vaccine (adsorbed, reduced antigen content) .. 791
Dipivefrine hydrochloride ... 1727
Dipotassium clorazepate ... 1728
Dipotassium phosphate ... 1729
Diprophylline ... 1730
Dipyridamole ... 1731
Dirithromycin ... **6.1**-3447
Disintegration of suppositories and pessaries (2.9.2.) ... 265
Disintegration of tablets and capsules (2.9.1.) ... 263
Disodium edetate ... 1734
Disodium phosphate, anhydrous ... 1735
Disodium phosphate dihydrate ... 1735
Disodium phosphate dodecahydrate ... **6.1**-3449
Disopyramide ... 1737
Disopyramide phosphate ... 1738
Dispersible tablets ... 750
Dissolution, apparent (2.9.43.) ... **6.1**-3327
Dissolution, intrinsic (2.9.29.) ... 309
Dissolution test for lipophilic solid dosage forms (2.9.42.) ... 332
Dissolution test for solid dosage forms (2.9.3.) ... 266
Dissolution test for transdermal patches (2.9.4.) ... 275
Distemper vaccine (live), canine ... 887
Distemper vaccine (live) for mustelids ... 900
Distillation range (2.2.11.) ... 30
Distribution estimation by analytical sieving, particle-size (2.9.38.) ... 325

Disulfiram ... 1739
Dithranol ... 1740
DL-Methionine ... 2380
DL-α-Tocopheryl hydrogen succinate ... 3093
Dobutamine hydrochloride ... 1741
Docusate sodium ... 1743
Dodecyl gallate ... 1744
Dog rose ... 1744
Domperidone ... 1745
Domperidone maleate ... 1747
Dopamine hydrochloride ... 1749
Dopexamine dihydrochloride ... 1750
Dorzolamide hydrochloride ... 1752
Dosage units, uniformity of (2.9.40.) ... **6.1**-3325
Dosulepin hydrochloride ... 1753
Doxapram hydrochloride ... 1754
Doxazosin mesilate ... 1756
Doxepin hydrochloride ... **6.1**-3449
Doxorubicin hydrochloride ... 1759
Doxycycline hyclate ... 1760
Doxycycline monohydrate ... 1762
Doxylamine hydrogen succinate ... **6.1**-3451
Droperidol ... 1765
Droppers (2.1.1.) ... 15
Drop point (2.2.17.) ... 33
Drops (nasal) and sprays (liquid nasal) ... 731
Drops, oral ... 730
Dry extracts ... **6.1**-3344
Dry residue of extracts (2.8.16.) ... 256
Duck plague vaccine (live) ... 901
Duck viral hepatitis type I vaccine (live) ... 902
Dwarf pine oil ... 1766

E

Ear drops and ear sprays ... 720
Ear powders ... 720
Ear preparations ... 719
Ear preparations, semi-solid ... 720
Ear sprays and ear drops ... 720
Ear tampons ... 720
Ear washes ... 720
Ebastine ... 1771
Econazole ... 1772
Econazole nitrate ... 1773
Edetic acid ... 1774
Edrophonium chloride ... 1775
Effervescent granules ... 724
Effervescent powders ... 739
Effervescent tablets ... 749
Efficacy of antimicrobial preservation (5.1.3.) ... 528
Efficacy of veterinary vaccines and immunosera, evaluation of (5.2.7.) ... **6.1**-3335
Egg drop syndrome '76 vaccine (inactivated) ... 904
Elder flower ... 1776
Electrophoresis (2.2.31.) ... 48
Electrophoresis, capillary (2.2.47.) ... 77
Eleutherococcus ... 1777
Emedastine difumarate ... 1779
Emetine hydrochloride heptahydrate ... 1780
Emetine hydrochloride pentahydrate ... 1781
Empty sterile containers of plasticised poly(vinyl chloride) for human blood and blood components (3.2.4.) ... 381
Emulsifying cetostearyl alcohol (type A) ... 1481
Emulsifying cetostearyl alcohol (type B) ... 1482
Emulsions, solutions and suspensions, oral ... 729
Enalaprilat dihydrate ... 1784
Enalapril maleate ... 1782
Encephalitis vaccine (inactivated), tick-borne ... 845
Endotoxins, bacterial (2.6.14.) ... 182
Enilconazole for veterinary use ... 1785
Enoxaparin sodium ... 1787
Enoxolone ... 1788
Ephedrine, anhydrous ... 1789
Ephedrine hemihydrate ... 1790
Ephedrine hydrochloride ... 1791
Ephedrine hydrochloride, racemic ... 1792
Epinephrine tartrate ... 1114
Epirubicin hydrochloride ... 1793
Equine herpesvirus vaccine (inactivated) ... 905
Equine influenza vaccine (inactivated) ... 907
Equisetum stem ... 1794
Ergocalciferol ... 1795
Ergometrine maleate ... 1797
Ergotamine tartrate ... 1798
Erysipelas vaccine (inactivated), swine ... 955
Erythritol ... 1800
Erythromycin ... 1801
Erythromycin estolate ... 1803
Erythromycin ethylsuccinate ... 1806
Erythromycin lactobionate ... 1808
Erythromycin stearate ... 1810
Erythropoietin concentrated solution ... 1813
Eserine salicylate ... 2677
Eserine sulphate ... 2678
Esketamine hydrochloride ... 1817
Essential oils ... 680
Essential oils, assay of 1,8-cineole in (2.8.11.) ... 250
Essential oils, fatty oils and resinified essential oils in (2.8.7.) ... 250
Essential oils, foreign esters in (2.8.6.) ... 250
Essential oils in herbal drugs, determination of (2.8.12.).. 251
Essential oils, odour and taste (2.8.8.) ... 250
Essential oils, residue on evaporation (2.8.9.) ... 250
Essential oils, solubility in alcohol (2.8.10.) ... 250
Essential oils, water in (2.8.5.) ... 249
Ester value (2.5.2.) ... 137
Estradiol benzoate ... **6.1**-3455
Estradiol hemihydrate ... 1819
Estradiol valerate ... 1821
Estriol ... 1822
Estrogens, conjugated ... 1824
Etacrynic acid ... 1826
Etamsylate ... 1827
Ethacridine lactate monohydrate ... 1828
Ethambutol hydrochloride ... **6.1**-3456
Ethanol (96 per cent) ... 1829
Ethanol, anhydrous ... 1831
Ethanol content and alcoholimetric tables (2.9.10.) ... 281
Ether ... 1833
Ether, anaesthetic ... 1834
Ethinylestradiol ... 1834
Ethionamide ... 1835
Ethosuximide ... 1836
Ethoxylated substances, ethylene glycol and diethylene glycol in (2.4.30.) ... 131
Ethyl acetate ... 1838
Ethyl acrylate - methacrylic acid copolymer (1:1) ... 2371
Ethylcellulose ... 1841
Ethylenediamine ... 1843
Ethylene glycol and diethylene glycol in ethoxylated substances (2.4.30.) ... 131
Ethylene glycol monopalmitostearate ... 1842
Ethylene glycol monostearate ... 1842
Ethylene oxide and dioxan (2.4.25.) ... 126
Ethylhexanoic acid, 2- (2.4.28.) ... 129
Ethylmorphine hydrochloride ... 1843
Ethyl oleate ... 1838
Ethyl parahydroxybenzoate ... 1839

Ethyl parahydroxybenzoate sodium 1840
Etidronate disodium 1844
Etilefrine hydrochloride 1845
Etodolac 1847
Etofenamate 1849
Etofylline 1850
Etomidate 1851
Etoposide 1852
Eucalyptus leaf 1857
Eucalyptus oil 1858
Eugenol 1859
European goldenrod 2000
European viper venom antiserum 970
Evaluation of efficacy of veterinary vaccines and immunosera (5.2.7.) **6.1**-3335
Evaluation of safety of each batch of veterinary vaccines and immunosera (5.2.9.) 567
Evaluation of safety of veterinary vaccines and immunosera (5.2.6.) 556
Evening primrose oil, refined 1860
Extractable volume of parenteral preparations, test for (2.9.17.) 287
Extracts **6.1**-3343
Extracts, dry **6.1**-3344
Extracts, dry residue of (2.8.16.) 256
Extracts, liquid **6.1**-3343
Extracts, loss on drying of (2.8.17.) 256
Extracts, soft **6.1**-3344
Extraneous agents in viral vaccines for human use, tests for (2.6.16.) 190
Extraneous agents: tests in batches of finished product of avian live virus vaccines (2.6.25.) 202
Extraneous agents: tests in seed lots of avian viral vaccines (2.6.24.) 198
Eye drops 721
Eye lotions 721
Eye preparations 721
Eye preparations, semi-solid 722

F

F_0 concept to steam sterilisation of aqueous preparations, application of (5.1.5.) 531
Factor II, human coagulation, assay of (2.7.18.) 234
Factor IX, human coagulation 2064
Factor IX, human coagulation, assay of (2.7.11.) 229
Factor VII, human coagulation 2061
Factor VII, human coagulation, assay of (2.7.10.) 228
Factor VIII, human coagulation 2062
Factor VIII, human coagulation, assay of (2.7.4.) 216
Factor VIII (rDNA), human coagulation 2063
Factor X, human coagulation, assay of (2.7.19.) 235
Factor XI, human coagulation 2065
Factor XI, human coagulation, assay of (2.7.22.) 238
Falling ball viscometer method (2.2.49.) 84
Famotidine 1865
Fatty acids, composition by gas chromatography (2.4.22.) 118
Fatty oils, alkaline impurities in (2.4.19.) 117
Fatty oils and herbal drugs, heavy metals in (2.4.27.) 128
Fatty oils and resinified essential oils in essential oils (2.8.7.) 250
Fatty oils, foreign oils in, by thin-layer chromatography (2.4.21.) 117
Fatty oils, identification by thin-layer chromatography (2.3.2.) 106
Fatty oils, sterols in (2.4.23.) 120
Fatty oils, vegetable 712
Fc function of immunoglobulin, test for (2.7.9.) 227
Febantel for veterinary use 1870
Felbinac 1866
Feline calicivirosis vaccine (inactivated) 909
Feline calicivirosis vaccine (live) 910
Feline chlamydiosis vaccine (inactivated) 911
Feline infectious enteritis (feline panleucopenia) vaccine (inactivated) 912
Feline infectious enteritis (feline panleucopenia) vaccine (live) 913
Feline leukaemia vaccine (inactivated) 914
Feline panleucopenia vaccine (inactivated) 912
Feline panleucopenia vaccine (live) 913
Feline viral rhinotracheitis vaccine (inactivated) 916
Feline viral rhinotracheitis vaccine (live) 917
Felodipine 1867
Felypressin 1869
Fenbendazole for veterinary use 1871
Fenbufen 1872
Fennel, bitter 1873
Fennel, sweet 1874
Fenofibrate 1875
Fenoterol hydrobromide 1876
Fentanyl 1878
Fentanyl citrate 1879
Fenticonazole nitrate 1880
Fenugreek 1882
Fermentation, products of 693
Ferric chloride hexahydrate 1882
Ferrous fumarate 1883
Ferrous gluconate 1884
Ferrous sulphate, dried 1885
Ferrous sulphate heptahydrate 1886
Feverfew 1887
Fexofenadine hydrochloride 1888
Fibrinogen, human 2066
Fibrin sealant kit 1890
Finasteride 1891
Fish oil, rich in omega-3 acids 1893
Flavoxate hydrochloride 1895
Flecainide acetate 1896
Flocculation value (Lf) of diphtheria and tetanus toxins and toxoids (Ramon assay) (2.7.27.) 241
Flowability (2.9.16.) 286
Flow cytometry (2.7.24.) 240
Flubendazole 1898
Flucloxacillin sodium 1899
Fluconazole 1900
Flucytosine 1902
Fludarabine phosphate 1903
Fludeoxyglucose (^{18}F) injection 986
Fludrocortisone acetate 1906
Flumazenil 1908
Flumazenil (*N*-[^{11}C]methyl) injection 989
Flumequine 1909
Flumetasone pivalate 1910
Flunarizine dihydrochloride 1911
Flunitrazepam 1913
Flunixin meglumine for veterinary use 1914
Fluocinolone acetonide 1915
Fluocortolone pivalate 1916
Fluorescein 1918
Fluorescein sodium 1919
Fluorides (2.4.5.) 112
Fluorimetry (2.2.21.) 36
Fluorodopa (^{18}F) (prepared by electrophilic substitution) injection 990
Fluorouracil 1920
Fluoxetine hydrochloride 1922
Flupentixol dihydrochloride 1924
Fluphenazine decanoate 1926

Fluphenazine dihydrochloride 1928
Fluphenazine enantate 1927
Flurazepam monohydrochloride 1930
Flurbiprofen 1931
Fluspirilene 1932
Flutamide 1933
Fluticasone propionate 1934
Flutrimazole 1936
Foams, cutaneous 728
Foams, intrauterine 726
Foams, medicated 723
Foams, rectal 746
Foams, vaginal 752
Folic acid 1938
Foot-and-mouth disease (ruminants) vaccine (inactivated) 918
Foreign esters in essential oils (2.8.6.) 250
Foreign matter (2.8.2.) 249
Foreign oils in fatty oils by thin-layer chromatography (2.4.21.) 117
Formaldehyde, free (2.4.18.) 117
Formaldehyde solution (35 per cent) 1939
Formoterol fumarate dihydrate 1940
Foscarnet sodium hexahydrate 1942
Fosfomycin calcium 1943
Fosfomycin sodium 1945
Fosfomycin trometamol 1946
Fowl cholera vaccine (inactivated) 920
Fowl-pox vaccine (live) 921
Framycetin sulphate 1947
Frangula bark 1949
Frangula bark dry extract, standardised 1950
Frankincense, Indian 2128
Free formaldehyde (2.4.18.) 117
Freezing point (2.2.18.) 35
Friability of granules and spheroids (2.9.41.) 330
Friability of uncoated tablets (2.9.7.) 278
Fructose 1951
Fucus 2213
Fumitory 1952
Functional groups and ions, identification reactions of (2.3.1.) 103
Furosemide 1953
Furunculosis vaccine (inactivated, oil-adjuvanted, injectable) for salmonids 922
Fusidic acid 1954

G

Galactose 1959
Gallamine triethiodide 1959
Gallium (^{67}Ga) citrate injection 992
Gargles 733
Garlic for homoeopathic preparations 1077
Garlic powder 1961
Gas chromatography (2.2.28.) 45
Gas detector tubes (2.1.6.) 17
Gases, carbon dioxide in (2.5.24.) 144
Gases, carbon monoxide in (2.5.25.) 145
Gases, nitrogen monoxide and nitrogen dioxide in (2.5.26.) 146
Gases, nitrous oxide in (2.5.35.) 152
Gases, oxygen in (2.5.27.) 146
Gases, water in (2.5.28.) 146
Gas-gangrene antitoxin, mixed 966
Gas-gangrene antitoxin (novyi) 966
Gas-gangrene antitoxin (perfringens) 967
Gas-gangrene antitoxin (septicum) 968
Gastro-resistant capsules 718
Gastro-resistant granules 724
Gastro-resistant tablets 750
Gelatin 1961
Gels 747
Gels for injections 737
Gemcitabine hydrochloride 1963
Gemfibrozil 1964
General notices (1.) 3
General texts on biological products (5.2.) 547
General texts on microbiology (5.1.) 525
Gene transfer medicinal products for human use (5.14.) 669
Gentamicin sulphate 1965
Gentian root 1967
Gentian tincture 1968
Ginger 1969
Gingival solutions 733
Ginkgo dry extract, refined and quantified **6.1**-3461
Ginkgo leaf 1969
Ginseng 1971
Glass containers for pharmaceutical use (3.2.1.) 373
Glibenclamide 1972
Gliclazide 1974
Glimepiride 1975
Glipizide 1977
Glossary 717
Glossary (dosage forms) 717
Glucagon, human 1979
Glucose, anhydrous 1981
Glucose, liquid 1982
Glucose, liquid, spray-dried 1982
Glucose monohydrate 1983
Glutamic acid 1984
Glutathione **6.1**-3463
Glycerol 1987
Glycerol (85 per cent) 1988
Glycerol dibehenate 1990
Glycerol distearate 1991
Glycerol monocaprylate 1992
Glycerol monocaprylocaprate 1993
Glycerol monolinoleate 1994
Glycerol mono-oleate 1995
Glycerol monostearate 40-55 1996
Glycerol triacetate 3112
Glyceryl trinitrate solution **6.1**-3465
Glycine 1998
Glycyrrhizate ammonium 1179
Goldenrod 1999
Goldenrod, European 2000
Goldenseal rhizome **6.1**-3467
Gonadorelin acetate 2003
Gonadotrophin, chorionic 2004
Gonadotrophin, equine serum, for veterinary use 2005
Goserelin 2005
Gramicidin 2007
Granisetron hydrochloride 2009
Granules 723
Granules and powders for oral solutions and suspensions 729
Granules and powders for syrups 730
Granules and spheroids, friability of (2.9.41.) 330
Granules, coated 724
Granules, effervescent 724
Granules, gastro-resistant 724
Granules, modified-release 724
Greater celandine 2010
Griseofulvin 2011
Guaiacol 2012
Guaifenesin 2014
Guanethidine monosulphate 2015
Guar 2016

Guar galactomannan ... 2016

H

Haematopoietic products, numeration of CD34/CD45+ cells in (2.7.23.) ... 238
Haematopoietic progenitor cells, human, colony-forming cell assay for (2.7.28.) ... 242
Haematopoietic stem cells, human ... 2067
Haemodiafiltration and for haemofiltration, solutions for ... 2025
Haemodialysis, concentrated solutions for ... 2022
Haemodialysis solutions, concentrated, water for diluting ... 2021
Haemodialysis, solutions for ... 2022
Haemofiltration and for haemodiafiltration, solutions for ... 2025
Haemophilus type b (conjugate), diphtheria, tetanus and pertussis (acellular, component) vaccine (adsorbed) ... 771
Haemophilus type b (conjugate), diphtheria, tetanus, pertussis (acellular, component) and poliomyelitis (inactivated) vaccine (adsorbed) ... 783
Haemophilus type b (conjugate), diphtheria, tetanus, pertussis (acellular, component), hepatitis B (rDNA) and poliomyelitis (inactivated) vaccine (adsorbed) ... 780
Haemophilus type b (conjugate), diphtheria, tetanus, pertussis and poliomyelitis (inactivated) vaccine (adsorbed) ... 787
Haemophilus type b conjugate vaccine ... 792
Haemorrhagic disease vaccine (inactivated), rabbit ... 949
Halofantrine hydrochloride ... 2027
Haloperidol ... 2028
Haloperidol decanoate ... 2030
Halothane ... 2031
Hamamelis leaf ... **6.1**-3471
Hard capsules ... 718
Hard fat ... 2034
Hard paraffin ... 2612
Hawthorn berries ... 2034
Hawthorn leaf and flower ... 2035
Hawthorn leaf and flower dry extract ... 2036
Hawthorn leaf and flower liquid extract, quantified ... 2037
Heavy bismuth subnitrate ... 1315
Heavy kaolin ... 2213
Heavy magnesium carbonate ... 2315
Heavy magnesium oxide ... 2320
Heavy metals (2.4.8.) ... 112
Heavy metals in herbal drugs and fatty oils (2.4.27.) ... 128
Hedera helix for homoeopathic preparations ... 1078
Helium ... 2038
Heparin, assay of (2.7.5.) ... 217
Heparin calcium ... 2039
Heparin in coagulation factors, assay of (2.7.12.) ... 230
Heparins, low-molecular-mass ... 2041
Heparin sodium ... 2040
Hepatitis A immunoglobulin, human ... 2068
Hepatitis A (inactivated) and hepatitis B (rDNA) vaccine (adsorbed) ... 794
Hepatitis A vaccine, assay of (2.7.14.) ... 232
Hepatitis A vaccine (inactivated, adsorbed) ... 795
Hepatitis A vaccine (inactivated, virosome) ... 797
Hepatitis B immunoglobulin for intravenous administration, human ... 2069
Hepatitis B immunoglobulin, human ... 2069
Hepatitis B (rDNA), diphtheria and tetanus vaccine (adsorbed) ... 765
Hepatitis B (rDNA), diphtheria, tetanus and pertussis (acellular, component) vaccine (adsorbed) ... 774
Hepatitis B (rDNA), diphtheria, tetanus, pertussis (acellular, component), poliomyelitis (inactivated) and haemophilus type b conjugate vaccine (adsorbed) ... 780
Hepatitis B vaccine (rDNA) ... 800
Hepatitis B vaccine (rDNA), assay of (2.7.15.) ... 233
Hepatitis C virus (HCV), validation of nucleic acid amplification techniques for the detection of HCV RNA in plasma pools: Guidelines ... 195
Heptaminol hydrochloride ... 2043
Herbal drug preparations ... 684
Herbal drugs ... 684
Herbal drugs and fatty oils, heavy metals in (2.4.27.) ... 128
Herbal drugs, determination of aflatoxin B_1 in (2.8.18.) ... 256
Herbal drugs, determination of essential oils in herbal drugs (2.8.12.) ... 251
Herbal drugs, determination of tannins (2.8.14.) ... 255
Herbal drugs for homoeopathic preparations ... 1065
Herbal teas ... 685
Hexamidine diisetionate ... 2044
Hexetidine ... 2045
Hexobarbital ... 2047
Hexosamines in polysaccharide vaccines (2.5.20.) ... 143
Hexylresorcinol ... 2047
Highly purified water ... 3212
Histamine (2.6.10.) ... 165
Histamine dihydrochloride ... 2049
Histamine phosphate ... 2049
Histidine ... 2050
Histidine hydrochloride monohydrate ... 2051
Homatropine hydrobromide ... 2052
Homatropine methylbromide ... 2053
Homoeopathic preparations ... 1065
Homoeopathic preparations, arsenious trioxide for ... 1073
Homoeopathic preparations, calcium iodide tetrahydrate for ... 1074
Homoeopathic preparations, common stinging nettle for ... 1075
Homoeopathic preparations, copper acetate monohydrate for ... 1075
Homoeopathic preparations, copper for ... 1076
Homoeopathic preparations, garlic for ... 1077
Homoeopathic preparations, hedera helix for ... 1078
Homoeopathic preparations, herbal drugs for ... 1065
Homoeopathic preparations, honey bee for ... 1079
Homoeopathic preparations, hyoscyamus for ... 1079
Homoeopathic preparations, hypericum for ... 1080
Homoeopathic preparations, iron for ... 1081
Homoeopathic preparations, mother tinctures for ... 1072
Homoeopathic preparations, oriental cashew for ... 1082
Homoeopathic preparations, saffron for ... 1084
Homoeopathic stocks (methods of preparation of) and potentisation ... **6.1**-3385
Honey ... 2055
Honey bee for homoeopathic preparations ... 1079
Hop strobile ... **6.1**-3472
Human albumin injection, iodinated (^{125}I) ... 993
Human albumin solution ... 2057
Human anti-D immunoglobulin ... 2058
Human anti-D immunoglobulin, assay of (2.7.13.) ... 230
Human anti-D immunoglobulin for intravenous administration ... 2059
Human antithrombin III, assay of (2.7.17.) ... 234
Human antithrombin III concentrate ... 2060
Human coagulation factor II, assay of (2.7.18.) ... 234
Human coagulation factor IX ... 2064
Human coagulation factor IX, assay of (2.7.11.) ... 229
Human coagulation factor VII ... 2061
Human coagulation factor VII, assay of (2.7.10.) ... 228
Human coagulation factor VIII ... 2062

Human coagulation factor VIII, assay of (2.7.4.)....216
Human coagulation factor VIII (rDNA)....2063
Human coagulation factor X, assay of (2.7.19.)....235
Human coagulation factor XI....2065
Human coagulation factor XI, assay of (2.7.22.)....238
Human fibrinogen....2066
Human haematopoietic progenitor cells, colony-forming cell assay for (2.7.28.)....242
Human haematopoietic stem cells....2067
Human hepatitis A immunoglobulin....2068
Human hepatitis B immunoglobulin....2069
Human hepatitis B immunoglobulin for intravenous administration....2069
Human insulin....2137
Human measles immunoglobulin....2069
Human normal immunoglobulin....2070
Human normal immunoglobulin for intravenous administration....2072
Human plasma for fractionation....2073
Human plasma (pooled and treated for virus inactivation)....2075
Human prothrombin complex....2076
Human rabies immunoglobulin....2078
Human rubella immunoglobulin....2079
Human tetanus immunoglobulin....2079
Human varicella immunoglobulin....2080
Human varicella immunoglobulin for intravenous administration....2081
Human von Willebrand factor....2081
Human von Willebrand factor, assay of (2.7.21.)....237
Hyaluronidase....2082
Hydralazine hydrochloride....2083
Hydrochloric acid, concentrated....2085
Hydrochloric acid, dilute....2085
Hydrochlorothiazide....2086
Hydrocodone hydrogen tartrate 2.5-hydrate....2087
Hydrocortisone....2089
Hydrocortisone acetate....2091
Hydrocortisone hydrogen succinate....2092
Hydrogenated arachis oil....1211
Hydrogenated castor oil....1432
Hydrogenated cottonseed oil....1625
Hydrogenated soya-bean oil....2946
Hydrogenated vegetable oils, nickel in (2.4.31.)....131
Hydrogenated wool fat....3226
Hydrogen peroxide solution (30 per cent)....2094
Hydrogen peroxide solution (3 per cent)....2094
Hydromorphone hydrochloride....2095
Hydrophobic colloidal silica....2878
Hydrous wool fat....3227
Hydroxocobalamin acetate....2096
Hydroxocobalamin chloride....2098
Hydroxocobalamin sulphate....2099
Hydroxycarbamide....2100
Hydroxyethylcellulose....2102
Hydroxyethylmethylcellulose....2390
Hydroxyethyl salicylate....2101
Hydroxyl value (2.5.3.)....137
Hydroxypropylbetadex....2103
Hydroxypropylcellulose....2105
Hydroxypropylmethylcellulose....**6.1**-3473
Hydroxypropylmethylcellulose phthalate....**6.1**-3475
Hydroxyzine hydrochloride....2106
Hymecromone....2107
Hyoscine....2108
Hyoscine butylbromide....2109
Hyoscine hydrobromide....2110
Hyoscyamine sulphate....2112
Hyoscyamus for homoeopathic preparations....1079
Hypericum....2958
Hypericum for homoeopathic preparations....1080
Hypromellose....**6.1**-3473
Hypromellose phthalate....**6.1**-3475

I

Ibuprofen....**6.1**-3479
Iceland moss....2121
ICH (5.8.)....645
Ichthammol....2122
Identification (2.3.)....103
Identification and control of residual solvents (2.4.24.)....121
Identification of fatty oils by thin-layer chromatography (2.3.2.)....106
Identification of phenothiazines by thin-layer chromatography (2.3.3.)....107
Identification reactions of ions and functional groups (2.3.1.)....103
Idoxuridine....2122
Ifosfamide....2123
Imipenem....2125
Imipramine hydrochloride....2126
Immunochemical methods (2.7.1.)....209
Immunoglobulin for human use, anti-T lymphocyte, animal....1203
Immunoglobulin for intravenous administration, human anti-D....2059
Immunoglobulin for intravenous administration, human hepatitis B....2069
Immunoglobulin for intravenous administration, human normal....2072
Immunoglobulin for intravenous administration, human varicella....2081
Immunoglobulin, human anti-D....2058
Immunoglobulin, human anti-D, assay of (2.7.13.)....230
Immunoglobulin, human hepatitis A....2068
Immunoglobulin, human hepatitis B....2069
Immunoglobulin, human measles....2069
Immunoglobulin, human normal....2070
Immunoglobulin, human rabies....2078
Immunoglobulin, human rubella....2079
Immunoglobulin, human tetanus....2079
Immunoglobulin, human varicella....2080
Immunoglobulin, test for anticomplementary activity of (2.6.17.)....191
Immunoglobulin, test for Fc function of (2.7.9.)....227
Immunosera and vaccines, phenol in (2.5.15.)....142
Immunosera and vaccines, veterinary, evaluation of efficacy of (5.2.7.)....**6.1**-3335
Immunosera and vaccines, veterinary, evaluation of safety (5.2.6.)....556
Immunosera and vaccines, veterinary, evaluation of the safety of each batch (5.2.9.)....567
Immunosera for human use, animal....685
Immunosera for veterinary use....687
Implants....737
Impurities in substances for pharmaceutical use, control of (5.10.)....653
Indapamide....2127
Indian frankincense....2128
Indicators, relationship between approximate pH and colour (2.2.4.)....25
Indinavir sulphate....2130
Indium (^{111}In) chloride solution....994
Indium (^{111}In) oxine solution....995
Indium (^{111}In) pentetate injection....996
Indometacin....2132
Inductively coupled plasma-atomic emission spectrometry (2.2.57.)....96

Inductively coupled plasma-mass spectrometry (2.2.58.).... 98
Infectious bovine rhinotracheitis vaccine (live)....924
Infectious bronchitis vaccine (inactivated), avian....864
Infectious bronchitis vaccine (live), avian....**6.1**-3371
Infectious bursal disease vaccine (inactivated), avian....867
Infectious bursal disease vaccine (live), avian....869
Infectious chicken anaemia vaccine (live)....925
Infectious encephalomyelitis vaccine (live), avian....871
Infectious laryngotracheitis vaccine (live), avian....872
Influenza vaccine (split virion, inactivated)....801
Influenza vaccine (surface antigen, inactivated)....803
Influenza vaccine (surface antigen, inactivated, prepared in cell cultures)....804
Influenza vaccine (surface antigen, inactivated, virosome)....806
Influenza vaccine (whole virion, inactivated)....808
Influenza vaccine (whole virion, inactivated, prepared in cell cultures)....810
Infrared absorption spectrophotometry (2.2.24.)....39
Infusions....736
Inhalation gas, krypton (^{81M}Kr)....1000
Inhalation, preparations for....739
Inhalation, preparations for: aerodynamic assessment of fine particles (2.9.18.)....287
Injectable insulin preparations....2146
Injections....736
Injections, gels for....737
Injections or infusions, concentrates for....736
Injections or infusions, powders for....736
Inositol, *myo*-....2460
Inserts, ophthalmic....722
Insulin aspart....2133
Insulin, bovine....2135
Insulin, human....2137
Insulin injection, biphasic....2140
Insulin injection, biphasic isophane....2140
Insulin injection, isophane....2141
Insulin injection, soluble....2141
Insulin lispro....2141
Insulin, porcine....2144
Insulin preparations, injectable....2146
Insulin zinc injectable suspension....2148
Insulin zinc injectable suspension (amorphous)....2149
Insulin zinc injectable suspension (crystalline)....2149
Interferon alfa-2 concentrated solution....2150
Interferon gamma-1b concentrated solution....2153
Interferons, assay of (5.6.)....627
International System (SI) units (1.)....3
Intramammary preparations for veterinary use....725
Intraruminal devices....725
Intrauterine capsules....726
Intrauterine foams....726
Intrauterine preparations for veterinary use....726
Intrauterine solutions, suspensions....726
Intrauterine sticks....726
Intrauterine tablets....726
Intrinsic dissolution (2.9.29.)....309
In vivo assay of poliomyelitis vaccine (inactivated) (2.7.20.)....235
Iobenguane (^{123}I) injection....997
Iobenguane (^{131}I) injection for diagnostic use....998
Iobenguane (^{131}I) injection for therapeutic use....999
Iobenguane sulphate for radiopharmaceutical preparations....**6.1**-3381
Iodinated (^{125}I) human albumin injection....993
Iodinated povidone....2734
Iodine....2156
Iodine value (2.5.4.)....137
Iohexol....2157
Ionic concentration, potentiometric determination of using ion-selective electrodes (2.2.36.)....58
Ions and functional groups, identification reactions of (2.3.1.)....103
Ion-selective electrodes, potentiometric determination of ionic concentration (2.2.36.)....58
Iopamidol....2160
Iopanoic acid....2162
Iotalamic acid....2163
Iotrolan....2164
Ioxaglic acid....2167
Ipecacuanha liquid extract, standardised....2168
Ipecacuanha, prepared....2169
Ipecacuanha root....2170
Ipecacuanha tincture, standardised....2171
Ipratropium bromide....2172
Iron (2.4.9.)....115
Iron for homoeopathic preparations....1081
Irrigation, preparations for....743
Isoconazole....2173
Isoconazole nitrate....2175
Isoelectric focusing (2.2.54.)....84
Isoflurane....2176
Isoleucine....2177
Isomalt....2178
Isoniazid....2180
Isophane insulin injection....2141
Isoprenaline hydrochloride....2181
Isoprenaline sulphate....2182
Isopropyl alcohol....2182
Isopropyl myristate....2183
Isopropyl palmitate....2184
Isosorbide dinitrate, diluted....2185
Isosorbide mononitrate, diluted....2186
Isotretinoin....2188
Isoxsuprine hydrochloride....2189
Ispaghula husk....2191
Ispaghula seed....2192
Isradipine....2192
Itraconazole....2194
Ivermectin....2196
Ivy leaf....2198

J

Javanese turmeric....3150
Java tea....2203
Josamycin....2204
Josamycin propionate....2205
Juniper....2206
Juniper oil....2207

K

Kanamycin acid sulphate....2211
Kanamycin monosulphate....2212
Kaolin, heavy....2213
Kelp....2213
Ketamine hydrochloride....2214
Ketobemidone hydrochloride....2215
Ketoconazole....2216
Ketoprofen....2218
Ketorolac trometamol....2220
Ketotifen hydrogen fumarate....2221
Knotgrass....2223
Krypton (^{81m}Kr) inhalation gas....1000

L

Labetalol hydrochloride....2227
Lactic acid....2228

Lactic acid, (*S*)-........2229
Lactitol monohydrate........2229
Lactobionic acid........2231
Lactose, anhydrous........2232
Lactose monohydrate........2233
Lactulose........2234
Lactulose, liquid........2236
Lamivudine........2238
Lansoprazole........2240
Laser light diffraction, particle size analysis by (2.9.31.)........311
Lauroyl macrogolglycerides........2242
Lavender flower........2243
Lavender oil........2244
Lead in sugars (2.4.10.)........115
Leflunomide........2245
Lemon oil........2246
Lemon verbena leaf........2248
Leptospirosis vaccine (inactivated), bovine........876
Leptospirosis vaccine (inactivated), canine........888
Letrozole........2249
Leucine........2250
Leuprorelin........2251
Levamisole for veterinary use........2253
Levamisole hydrochloride........2254
Levocabastine hydrochloride........2255
Levocarnitine........2257
Levodopa........2258
Levodropropizine........2260
Levomenthol........2261
Levomepromazine hydrochloride........2262
Levomepromazine maleate........2263
Levomethadone hydrochloride........2264
Levonorgestrel........2266
Levothyroxine sodium........2267
Lidocaine........**6.1**-3485
Lidocaine hydrochloride........2269
Light liquid paraffin........2612
Light magnesium carbonate........2316
Light magnesium oxide........2321
Lime flower........2270
Limit tests (2.4.)........111
Limit tests, standard solutions for (4.1.2.)........504
Lincomycin hydrochloride........2271
Lindane........2272
Linen thread, sterile, in distributor for veterinary use........1058
Linoleoyl macrogolglycerides........2273
Linseed........2273
Linseed oil, virgin........2274
Liothyronine sodium........**6.1**-3486
Lipophilic solid dosage forms, dissolution test for (2.9.42.)........332
Liquid chromatography (2.2.29.)........46
Liquid extracts........**6.1**-3343
Liquid glucose........1982
Liquid glucose, spray-dried........1982
Liquid lactulose........2236
Liquid maltitol........2332
Liquid paraffin........2613
Liquid preparations for cutaneous application........728
Liquid preparations for cutaneous application, veterinary........752
Liquid preparations for inhalation........740
Liquid preparations for oral use........728
Liquids, clarity and degree of opalescence of (2.2.1.)........21
Liquid sorbitol (crystallising)........2942
Liquid sorbitol (non-crystallising)........2943
Liquid sorbitol, partially dehydrated........2944
Liquorice dry extract for flavouring purposes........**6.1**-3488
Liquorice ethanolic liquid extract, standardised........2275
Liquorice root........2276
Lisinopril dihydrate........2277
Lithium carbonate........2279
Lithium citrate........2279
L-Methionine ([^{11}C]methyl) injection........1001
Lobeline hydrochloride........2280
Lomustine........2281
Loosestrife........2283
Loperamide hydrochloride........2283
Loperamide oxide monohydrate........2285
Loratadine........2286
Lorazepam........2288
Loss on drying (2.2.32.)........53
Loss on drying of extracts (2.8.17.)........256
Lovage root........2290
Lovastatin........2291
Low-molecular-mass heparins........2041
Lozenges and pastilles........734
Lozenges, compressed........734
Lubricant, silicone oil (3.1.8.)........358
Lymecycline........**6.1**-3489
Lynestrenol........2294
Lyophilisates, oral........748
Lysine acetate........2295
Lysine hydrochloride........2296

M

Macrogol 15 hydroxystearate........2305
Macrogol 20 glycerol monostearate........2304
Macrogol 40 sorbitol heptaoleate........2310
Macrogol 6 glycerol caprylocaprate........2302
Macrogol cetostearyl ether........2301
Macrogolglycerol cocoates........2302
Macrogolglycerol hydroxystearate........2303
Macrogolglycerol ricinoleate........2304
Macrogol lauryl ether........2306
Macrogol oleate........2307
Macrogol oleyl ether........2308
Macrogols........2308
Macrogol stearate........2311
Macrogol stearyl ether........2312
Magaldrate........2312
Magnesium (2.4.6.)........112
Magnesium acetate tetrahydrate........2313
Magnesium and alkaline-earth metals (2.4.7.)........112
Magnesium aspartate dihydrate........2314
Magnesium carbonate, heavy........2315
Magnesium carbonate, light........2316
Magnesium chloride 4.5-hydrate........2317
Magnesium chloride hexahydrate........2316
Magnesium citrate, anhydrous........2318
Magnesium gluconate........**6.1**-3495
Magnesium glycerophosphate........2318
Magnesium hydroxide........2319
Magnesium lactate dihydrate........2320
Magnesium oxide, heavy........2320
Magnesium oxide, light........2321
Magnesium peroxide........2321
Magnesium pidolate........2322
Magnesium stearate........2323
Magnesium sulphate heptahydrate........2325
Magnesium trisilicate........2325
Maize oil, refined........2326
Maize starch........2326
Malathion........2327
Maleic acid........2328
Malic acid........2329
Mallow flower........2330
Maltitol........2330

Maltitol, liquid 2332
Maltodextrin 2333
Mandarin oil 2333
Manganese gluconate **6.1**-3495
Manganese glycerophosphate, hydrated 2334
Manganese sulphate monohydrate 2335
Mannheimia vaccine (inactivated) for cattle 927
Mannheimia vaccine (inactivated) for sheep 928
Mannitol 2336
Maprotiline hydrochloride 2337
Marbofloxacin for veterinary use **6.1**-3496
Marek's disease vaccine (live) 930
Marshmallow leaf 2338
Marshmallow root 2339
Mass spectrometry (2.2.43.) 68
Mass spectrometry, inductively coupled plasma- (2.2.58.) 98
Mass uniformity of delivered doses from multidose containers (2.9.27.) 309
Mass uniformity of single-dose preparations (2.9.5.) 278
Mastic 2340
Materials based on non-plasticised poly(vinyl chloride) for containers for dry dosage forms for oral administration (3.1.11.) 362
Materials based on non-plasticised poly(vinyl chloride) for containers for non-injectable, aqueous solutions (3.1.10.) 360
Materials based on plasticised poly(vinyl chloride) for containers for aqueous solutions for intravenous infusion (3.1.14.) 366
Materials based on plasticised poly(vinyl chloride) for containers for human blood and blood components (3.1.1.1.) 339
Materials based on plasticised poly(vinyl chloride) for tubing used in sets for the transfusion of blood and blood components (3.1.1.2.) 342
Materials for containers for human blood and blood components (3.1.1.) 339
Materials used for the manufacture of containers (3.1.) 339
Matricaria flower 2340
Matricaria liquid extract 2341
Matricaria oil 2342
Meadowsweet 2344
Measles immunoglobulin, human 2069
Measles, mumps and rubella vaccine (live) **6.1**-3347
Measles vaccine (live) **6.1**-3348
Measurement of consistency by penetrometry (2.9.9.) 279
Mebendazole 2345
Meclozine hydrochloride 2346
Medicated chewing gum (2.9.25.) 304
Medicated chewing gums 719
Medicated feeding stuffs for veterinary use, premixes for 739
Medicated foams 723
Medicated plasters 747
Medicated tampons 751
Medicated vaginal tampons 752
Medicinal air 1118
Medicinal air, synthetic 1121
Medium-chain triglycerides 3122
Medroxyprogesterone acetate 2347
Mefenamic acid 2349
Mefloquine hydrochloride 2350
Megestrol acetate 2352
Meglumine 2353
Melilot 2354
Melissa leaf 2355
Melting point - capillary method (2.2.14.) 32
Melting point - instantaneous method (2.2.16.) 33
Melting point - open capillary method (2.2.15.) 32
Menadione 2356
Meningococcal group C conjugate vaccine 814
Meningococcal polysaccharide vaccine 816
Menthol, racemic 2356
Mepivacaine hydrochloride 2357
Meprobamate 2359
Mepyramine maleate 2360
Mercaptopurine 2361
Mercuric chloride 2361
Mesalazine 2362
Mesna 2364
Mesterolone 2366
Mestranol 2367
Metacresol 2368
Metamizole sodium 2369
Metformin hydrochloride 2370
Methacrylate copolymer, basic butylated 1254
Methacrylic acid - ethyl acrylate copolymer (1:1) 2371
Methacrylic acid - ethyl acrylate copolymer (1:1) dispersion 30 per cent 2372
Methacrylic acid - methyl methacrylate copolymer (1:1) 2373
Methacrylic acid - methyl methacrylate copolymer (1:2) 2374
Methadone hydrochloride 2374
Methanol 2376
Methanol and 2-propanol, test for (2.9.11.) 282
Methaqualone 2377
Methenamine 2378
Methionine 2379
Methionine ([^{11}C]methyl) injection, L- 1001
Methionine, DL- 2380
Methods in pharmacognosy (2.8.) 249
Methods of preparation of homoeopathic stocks and potentisation **6.1**-3385
Methods of preparation of sterile products (5.1.1.) 525
Methotrexate 2380
Methylatropine bromide 2383
Methylatropine nitrate 2383
Methylcellulose **6.1**-3497
Methyldopa 2386
Methylene blue 2402
Methylene chloride 2387
Methylergometrine maleate 2388
Methylhydroxyethylcellulose 2390
Methyl nicotinate 2390
Methyl parahydroxybenzoate 2391
Methylpentoses in polysaccharide vaccines (2.5.21.) 143
Methylphenobarbital 2392
Methylprednisolone 2393
Methylprednisolone acetate 2395
Methylprednisolone hydrogen succinate 2397
Methylpyrrolidone, *N*- 2399
Methylrosanilinium chloride 2400
Methyl salicylate 2401
Methyltestosterone 2402
Methylthioninium chloride 2402
Metixene hydrochloride 2404
Metoclopramide 2405
Metoclopramide hydrochloride 2407
Metolazone 2407
Metoprolol succinate 2409
Metoprolol tartrate 2410
Metrifonate 2412
Metronidazole 2414
Metronidazole benzoate 2415
Mexiletine hydrochloride 2416
Mianserin hydrochloride 2417
Miconazole 2418
Miconazole nitrate 2420
Microbial enumeration tests (microbiological examination of non-sterile products) (2.6.12.) 166

Microbiological assay of antibiotics (2.7.2.) 210
Microbiological control of cellular products (2.6.27.) 205
Microbiological examination of non-sterile products: test for specified micro-organisms (2.6.13.) 173
Microbiological examination of non-sterile products: total viable aerobic count (2.6.12.) 166
Microbiological quality, alternative methods for control of (5.1.6.) 532
Microbiological quality of pharmaceutical preparations (5.1.4.) 529
Microbiology, general texts on (5.1.) 525
Microcrystalline cellulose 1469
Microcrystalline cellulose and carmellose sodium 2422
Micro determination of water (2.5.32.) 147
Microscopy, optical (2.9.37.) 323
Midazolam 2422
Milk thistle dry extract, refined and standardised 2426
Milk-thistle fruit 2425
Minimising the risk of transmitting animal spongiform encephalopathy agents via human and veterinary medicinal products (5.2.8.) 558
Minocycline hydrochloride dihydrate 2427
Minoxidil 2429
Mint oil, partly dementholised 2430
Mirtazapine 2431
Misoprostol 2433
Mitomycin 2434
Mitoxantrone hydrochloride 2436
Modafinil 2437
Modified-release capsules 718
Modified-release granules 724
Modified-release tablets 750
Molecular mass distribution in dextrans (2.2.39.) 60
Molgramostim concentrated solution 2438
Molsidomine **6.1**-3499
Mometasone furoate 2441
Monoclonal antibodies for human use 690
Morantel hydrogen tartrate for veterinary use 2443
Morphine hydrochloride **6.1**-3501
Morphine sulphate **6.1**-3503
Moss, Iceland 2121
Mother tinctures for homoeopathic preparations 1072
Motherwort 2447
Mouthwashes 733
Moxidectin for veterinary use 2448
Moxifloxacin hydrochloride 2451
Moxonidine 2453
Mucoadhesive preparations 735
Mullein flower 2454
Multidose containers, uniformity of mass of delivered doses (2.9.27.) 309
Mumps, measles and rubella vaccine (live) **6.1**-3347
Mumps vaccine (live) **6.1**-3349
Mupirocin 2454
Mupirocin calcium 2456
Mycobacteria (2.6.2.) 159
Mycophenolate mofetil 2458
Mycoplasma gallisepticum vaccine (inactivated) 932
Mycoplasmas (2.6.7.) **6.1**-3317
myo-Inositol 2460
Myrrh 2461
Myrrh tincture 2461
Myxomatosis vaccine (live) for rabbits 933

N

Nabumetone 2465
N-Acetyltryptophan 1104
N-Acetyltyrosine 1106
Nadolol 2466
Nadroparin calcium 2467
Naftidrofuryl hydrogen oxalate 2470
Nalidixic acid 2472
Naloxone hydrochloride dihydrate 2473
Naltrexone hydrochloride 2474
Nandrolone decanoate 2476
Naphazoline hydrochloride 2478
Naphazoline nitrate 2479
Naproxen 2480
Naproxen sodium **6.1**-3507
Narrow-leaved coneflower root 2483
Nasal drops and liquid nasal sprays 731
Nasal powders 732
Nasal preparations 730
Nasal preparations, semi-solid 732
Nasal sprays (liquid) and nasal drops 730
Nasal sticks 732
Nasal washes 732
Near-infrared spectrophotometry (2.2.40.) 62
Neohesperidin-dihydrochalcone 2485
Neomycin sulphate 2487
Neonatal piglet colibacillosis vaccine (inactivated) 934
Neonatal ruminant colibacillosis vaccine (inactivated) 936
Neostigmine bromide 2489
Neostigmine metilsulfate 2490
Neroli oil 2490
Netilmicin sulphate 2492
Nettle leaf 2493
Neurovirulence test for poliomyelitis vaccine (oral) (2.6.19.) 193
Neurovirulence test of live viral vaccines (2.6.18.) 193
Nevirapine, anhydrous 2495
Newcastle disease vaccine (inactivated) 937
Newcastle disease vaccine (live) 939
Nicergoline 2496
Nickel in hydrogenated vegetable oils (2.4.31.) 131
Nickel in polyols (2.4.15.) 116
Niclosamide, anhydrous 2497
Niclosamide monohydrate 2498
Nicotinamide 2499
Nicotine 2500
Nicotine resinate 2501
Nicotinic acid 2502
Nifedipine 2503
Niflumic acid **6.1**-3508
Nifuroxazide **6.1**-3510
Nikethamide 2505
Nimesulide 2506
Nimodipine 2507
Nitrazepam 2508
Nitrendipine 2509
Nitric acid 2510
Nitric oxide 2511
Nitrofural 2512
Nitrofurantoin 2513
Nitrogen 2513
Nitrogen determination by sulphuric acid digestion (2.5.9.) 139
Nitrogen determination, primary aromatic amino (2.5.8.) 139
Nitrogen, low-oxygen 2514
Nitrogen monoxide and nitrogen dioxide in gases (2.5.26.) 146
Nitrous oxide 2515
Nitrous oxide in gases (2.5.35.) 152
Nizatidine 2516
N-Methylpyrrolidone 2399
N,N-Dimethylaniline (2.4.26.) 127
Nomegestrol acetate 2518

Nonoxinol 9 2519
Non-sterile products, microbiological examination of (test for specified micro-organisms) (2.6.13.) 173
Non-sterile products, microbiological examination of (total viable aerobic count) (2.6.12.) 166
Noradrenaline hydrochloride 2520
Noradrenaline tartrate 2521
Norcholesterol injection, iodinated (^{131}I) 1003
Norepinephrine hydrochloride 2520
Norepinephrine tartrate 2521
Norethisterone 2523
Norethisterone acetate 2524
Norfloxacin 2525
Norgestimate 2526
Norgestrel 2527
Normal immunoglobulin for intravenous administration, human 2072
Normal immunoglobulin, human 2070
Nortriptyline hydrochloride 2528
Noscapine 2529
Noscapine hydrochloride 2530
Notoginseng root 2531
Nuclear magnetic resonance spectrometry (2.2.33.) 54
Nucleated cell count and viability (2.7.29.) 243
Nucleic acid amplification techniques (2.6.21.) 195
Nucleic acids in polysaccharide vaccines (2.5.17.) 142
Numeration of CD34/CD45+ cells in haematopoietic products (2.7.23.) 238
Nutmeg oil 2533
Nystatin 2534

O

O-Acetyl in polysaccharide vaccines (2.5.19.) 143
Oak bark 2539
Octoxinol 10 2539
Octyldodecanol 2540
Octyl gallate 2539
Odour (2.3.4.) 107
Odour and taste of essential oils (2.8.8.) 250
Ofloxacin 2541
Oils, essential 680
Oils, fatty, vegetable 712
Oils rich in omega-3 acids, composition of fatty acids in (2.4.29.) 130
Oils rich in omega-3 acids, total cholesterol in (2.4.32.) ... 132
Ointments 747
Oleic acid 2543
Oleoresins **6.1**-3344
Oleoyl macrogolglycerides 2543
Oleyl alcohol 2544
Olive leaf 2545
Olive oil, refined 2546
Olive oil, virgin 2547
Olsalazine sodium 2548
Omega-3 acid ethyl esters 60 2550
Omega-3-acid ethyl esters 90 2552
Omega-3 acids, composition of fatty acids in oils rich in (2.4.29.) 130
Omega-3 acids, fish oil rich in 1893
Omega-3 acids, total cholesterol in oils rich in (2.4.32.) ... 132
Omega-3 acid triglycerides 2554
Omeprazole 2557
Omeprazole sodium 2558
Ondansetron hydrochloride dihydrate 2560
Opalescence of liquids, clarity and degree of (2.2.1.) 21
Ophthalmic inserts 722
Opium dry extract, standardised 2562
Opium, prepared 2563
Opium, raw 2564
Opium tincture, standardised 2565
Optical microscopy (2.9.37.) 323
Optical rotation (2.2.7.) 26
Oral drops 730
Oral lyophilisates 748
Oral powders 738
Oral solutions, emulsions and suspensions 729
Oral use, liquid preparations for 728
Orciprenaline sulphate 2567
Oregano 2568
Organ preservation, solutions for 2929
Oriental cashew for homoeopathic preparations 1082
Orodispersible tablets 750
Oromucosal capsules 734
Oromucosal drops, oromucosal sprays and sublingual sprays 733
Oromucosal preparations 732
Oromucosal preparations, semi-solid 733
Oromucosal solutions and oromucosal suspensions 733
Oromucosal sprays, oromucosal drops and sublingual sprays 732
Oromucosal suspensions and oromucosal solutions 732
Orphenadrine citrate 2569
Orphenadrine hydrochloride 2570
Osmolality (2.2.35.) 57
Ouabain 2571
Oxacillin sodium monohydrate 2572
Oxaliplatin 2574
Oxazepam 2577
Oxeladin hydrogen citrate 2578
Oxfendazole for veterinary use 2580
Oxidising substances (2.5.30.) 147
Oxitropium bromide 2581
Oxolinic acid 2582
Oxprenolol hydrochloride 2583
Oxybuprocaine hydrochloride 2584
Oxybutynin hydrochloride 2585
Oxycodone hydrochloride 2587
Oxygen 2588
Oxygen (^{15}O) 1004
Oxygen-flask method (2.5.10.) 140
Oxygen in gases (2.5.27.) 146
Oxymetazoline hydrochloride 2589
Oxytetracycline dihydrate 2590
Oxytetracycline hydrochloride 2591
Oxytocin 2593
Oxytocin concentrated solution 2594

P

Paclitaxel **6.1**-3515
Pale coneflower root 2602
Palmitic acid 2604
Pamidronate disodium pentahydrate 2604
Pancreas powder 2605
Pancuronium bromide 2608
Pansy, wild (flowering aerial parts) 3217
Pantoprazole sodium sesquihydrate **6.1**-3518
Papaverine hydrochloride 2609
Paper chromatography (2.2.26.) 43
Paracetamol 2611
Paraffin, hard 2612
Paraffin, light liquid 2612
Paraffin, liquid 2613
Paraffin, white soft 2614
Paraffin, yellow soft 2615
Parainfluenza virus vaccine (live), bovine 878
Parainfluenza virus vaccine (live), canine 890
Paraldehyde 2615

Paramyxovirus 1 (Newcastle disease) vaccine (inactivated), avian ... 937
Parenteral preparations ... 735
Parenteral preparations, test for extractable volume of (2.9.17.) ... 287
Parnaparin sodium ... 2616
Paroxetine hydrochloride, anhydrous ... 2616
Paroxetine hydrochloride hemihydrate ... 2619
Particles, fine, aerodynamic assessment of in preparations for inhalation (2.9.18.) ... 287
Particle size analysis by laser light diffraction (2.9.31.) ... 311
Particle-size distribution estimation by analytical sieving (2.9.38.) ... 325
Particulate contamination: sub-visible particles (2.9.19.) ... 300
Particulate contamination: visible particles (2.9.20.) ... 302
Parvovirosis vaccine (inactivated), canine ... 891
Parvovirosis vaccine (inactivated), porcine ... 946
Parvovirosis vaccine (live), canine ... 892
Passion flower ... 2621
Passion flower dry extract ... 2622
Pastes ... 747
Pasteurella vaccine (inactivated) for sheep ... 941
Pastilles and lozenges ... 734
Patches, transdermal ... 737
Patches, transdermal, dissolution test for (2.9.4.) ... 275
Pefloxacin mesilate dihydrate ... 2623
Pelargonium root ... 2625
Penbutolol sulphate ... 2625
Penetrometry, measurement of consistency (2.9.9.) ... 279
Penicillamine ... 2626
Pentaerythrityl tetranitrate, diluted ... 2628
Pentamidine diisetionate ... 2630
Pentazocine ... 2631
Pentazocine hydrochloride ... 2632
Pentazocine lactate ... 2632
Pentobarbital ... 2633
Pentobarbital sodium ... 2634
Pentoxifylline ... 2635
Pentoxyverine hydrogen citrate ... 2637
Peppermint leaf ... 2638
Peppermint oil ... 2639
Pepsin powder ... 2640
Peptide mapping (2.2.55.) ... 86
Peptides, synthetic, acetic acid in (2.5.34.) ... 151
Pergolide mesilate ... 2641
Perindopril *tert*-butylamine ... 2643
Peritoneal dialysis, solutions for ... 2646
Peroxide value (2.5.5.) ... 138
Perphenazine ... 2648
Pertussis (acellular, component), diphtheria and tetanus vaccine (adsorbed) ... 767
Pertussis (acellular, component), diphtheria, tetanus and haemophilus type b conjugate vaccine (adsorbed) ... 771
Pertussis (acellular, component), diphtheria, tetanus and hepatitis B (rDNA) vaccine (adsorbed) ... 774
Pertussis (acellular, component), diphtheria, tetanus and poliomyelitis (inactivated) vaccine (adsorbed) ... 775
Pertussis (acellular, component), diphtheria, tetanus and poliomyelitis (inactivated) vaccine (adsorbed, reduced antigen(s) content) ... 778
Pertussis (acellular, component), diphtheria, tetanus, hepatitis B (rDNA), poliomyelitis (inactivated) and haemophilus type b conjugate vaccine (adsorbed) ... 780
Pertussis (acellular, component), diphtheria, tetanus, poliomyelitis (inactivated) and haemophilus type b conjugate vaccine (adsorbed) ... 783
Pertussis, diphtheria, tetanus and poliomyelitis (inactivated) vaccine (adsorbed) ... 785
Pertussis, diphtheria, tetanus, poliomyelitis (inactivated) and haemophilus type b conjugate vaccine (adsorbed) ... 787
Pertussis vaccine (acellular), assay of (2.7.16.) ... 233
Pertussis vaccine (acellular, component, adsorbed) ... 820
Pertussis vaccine (acellular, co-purified, adsorbed) ... 822
Pertussis vaccine (adsorbed) ... 824
Pertussis vaccine, assay of (2.7.7.) ... 222
Peru balsam ... 2649
Pessaries ... 751
Pessaries and suppositories, disintegration of (2.9.2.) ... 265
Pesticide residues (2.8.13.) ... 252
Pethidine hydrochloride ... 2650
Pharmaceutical technical procedures (2.9.) ... 263
Pharmacognosy, methods in (2.8.) ... 249
Pharmacopoeial harmonisation (5.8.) ... 645
Phenazone ... 2651
Pheniramine maleate ... 2652
Phenobarbital ... 2653
Phenobarbital sodium ... 2654
Phenol ... 2655
Phenol in immunosera and vaccines (2.5.15.) ... 142
Phenolphthalein ... 2656
Phenolsulfonphthalein ... 2657
Phenothiazines, identification by thin-layer chromatography (2.3.3.) ... 107
Phenoxyethanol ... 2657
Phenoxymethylpenicillin ... **6.1**-3520
Phenoxymethylpenicillin potassium ... **6.1**-3521
Phentolamine mesilate ... 2662
Phenylalanine ... 2663
Phenylbutazone ... 2664
Phenylephrine ... 2665
Phenylephrine hydrochloride ... 2667
Phenylmercuric acetate ... 2668
Phenylmercuric borate ... 2669
Phenylmercuric nitrate ... 2669
Phenylpropanolamine hydrochloride ... 2670
Phenytoin ... 2671
Phenytoin sodium ... 2672
Phloroglucinol, anhydrous ... 2672
Phloroglucinol dihydrate ... 2673
Pholcodine ... 2674
Phosphates (2.4.11.) ... 116
Phosphoric acid, concentrated ... 2675
Phosphoric acid, dilute ... 2676
Phosphorus in polysaccharide vaccines (2.5.18.) ... 142
pH, potentiometric determination of (2.2.3.) ... 24
Phthalylsulfathiazole ... 2676
Physical and physicochemical methods (2.2.) ... 21
Physostigmine salicylate ... 2677
Physostigmine sulphate ... 2678
Phytomenadione ... 2679
Phytosterol ... 2680
Picotamide monohydrate ... 2682
Pilocarpine hydrochloride ... 2682
Pilocarpine nitrate ... 2684
Pimobendan ... 2685
Pimozide ... 2686
Pindolol ... 2688
Pine (dwarf) oil ... 1766
Pine sylvestris oil ... 2689
Pinus pinaster type turpentine oil ... 3151
Pipemidic acid trihydrate ... 2690
Piperacillin ... 2691
Piperacillin sodium ... 2692
Piperazine adipate ... 2694
Piperazine citrate ... 2695
Piperazine hydrate ... 2696
Piracetam ... 2697

Pirenzepine dihydrochloride monohydrate 2698
Piretanide 2699
Piroxicam 2700
Pivampicillin 2702
Pivmecillinam hydrochloride 2704
Plasma for fractionation, human 2073
Plasma (pooled and treated for virus inactivation), human 2075
Plasmid vectors for human use 674
Plasmid vectors for human use, bacterial cells used for the manufacture of 676
Plasters, medicated 746
Plastic additives (3.1.13.) 364
Plastic containers and closures for pharmaceutical use (3.2.2.) 378
Plastic containers for aqueous solutions for infusion (3.2.2.1.) 379
Plastic containers for human blood and blood components, sterile (3.2.3.) 379
Plastic syringes, single-use, sterile (3.2.8.) 384
Pneumococcal polysaccharide conjugate vaccine (adsorbed) 825
Pneumococcal polysaccharide vaccine 827
Poliomyelitis (inactivated), diphtheria and tetanus vaccine (adsorbed, reduced antigen(s) content) 770
Poliomyelitis (inactivated), diphtheria, tetanus and pertussis (acellular, component) vaccine (adsorbed) 775
Poliomyelitis (inactivated), diphtheria, tetanus and pertussis (acellular, component) vaccine (adsorbed, reduced antigen(s) content) 778
Poliomyelitis (inactivated), diphtheria, tetanus and pertussis vaccine (adsorbed) 785
Poliomyelitis (inactivated), diphtheria, tetanus, pertussis (acellular, component) and haemophilus type b conjugate vaccine (adsorbed) 783
Poliomyelitis (inactivated), diphtheria, tetanus, pertussis (acellular, component), hepatitis B (rDNA) and haemophilus type b conjugate vaccine (adsorbed) 780
Poliomyelitis (inactivated), diphtheria, tetanus, pertussis and haemophilus type b conjugate vaccine (adsorbed) 787
Poliomyelitis vaccine (inactivated) 829
Poliomyelitis vaccine (inactivated), *in vivo* assay of (2.7.20.) 235
Poliomyelitis vaccine (oral) **6.1**-3351
Poliomyelitis vaccine (oral), test for neurovirulence (2.6.19.) 193
Poloxamers 2705
Polyacrylate dispersion 30 per cent 2706
Polyamide 6/6 suture, sterile, in distributor for veterinary use 1059
Polyamide 6 suture, sterile, in distributor for veterinary use 1058
Polyethyleneglycols 2308
Polyethylene terephthalate for containers for preparations not for parenteral use (3.1.15.) 369
Poly(ethylene terephthalate) suture, sterile, in distributor for veterinary use 1059
Poly(ethylene - vinyl acetate) for containers and tubing for total parenteral nutrition preparations (3.1.7.) 356
Polyethylene with additives for containers for parenteral preparations and for ophthalmic preparations (3.1.5.) ... 349
Polyethylene without additives for containers for parenteral preparations and for ophthalmic preparations (3.1.4.) ... 348
Polymorphism (5.9.) 649
Polymyxin B sulphate 2707
Polyolefines (3.1.3.) 344
Polyoxyl castor oil 2304
Polyoxyl hydrogenated castor oil 2303
Polypropylene for containers and closures for parenteral preparations and ophthalmic preparations (3.1.6.) 352
Polysaccharide vaccines, hexosamines in (2.5.20.) 143
Polysaccharide vaccines, methylpentoses in (2.5.21.) 143
Polysaccharide vaccines, nucleic acids in (2.5.17.) 142
Polysaccharide vaccines, *O*-acetyl in (2.5.19.) 143
Polysaccharide vaccines, phosphorus in (2.5.18.) 142
Polysaccharide vaccines, protein in (2.5.16.) 142
Polysaccharide vaccines, ribose in (2.5.31.) 147
Polysaccharide vaccines, sialic acid in (2.5.23.) 144
Polysaccharide vaccines, uronic acids in (2.5.22.) 144
Polysorbate 20 2709
Polysorbate 40 2710
Polysorbate 60 2710
Polysorbate 80 2711
Poly(vinyl acetate) 2712
Poly(vinyl acetate) dispersion 30 per cent 2713
Poly(vinyl alcohol) 2715
Poly(vinyl chloride), non-plasticised, materials based on for containers for dry dosage forms for oral administration (3.1.11.) 362
Poly(vinyl chloride), non-plasticised, materials based on for containers for non-injectable aqueous solutions (3.1.10.) 360
Poly(vinyl chloride), plasticised, empty sterile containers of for human blood and blood components (3.2.4.) 381
Poly(vinyl chloride), plasticised, materials based on for containers for aqueous solutions for intravenous infusion (3.1.14.) 366
Poly(vinyl chloride), plasticised, materials based on for containers for human blood and blood components (3.1.1.1.) 339
Poly(vinyl chloride), plasticised, materials based on for tubing used in sets for the transfusion of blood and blood components (3.1.1.2.) 342
Poly(vinyl chloride), plasticised, sterile containers of for human blood containing anticoagulant solution (3.2.5.) 382
Poppy petals, red 2811
Porcine actinobacillosis vaccine (inactivated) 943
Porcine influenza vaccine (inactivated) 944
Porcine insulin 2144
Porcine parvovirosis vaccine (inactivated) 946
Porcine progressive atrophic rhinitis vaccine (inactivated) **6.1**-3373
Porosity of sintered-glass filters (2.1.2.) 15
Potassium (2.4.12.) 116
Potassium acetate 2716
Potassium bromide 2716
Potassium carbonate 2717
Potassium chloride 2717
Potassium citrate 2718
Potassium clavulanate 2719
Potassium clavulanate, diluted 2721
Potassium dihydrogen phosphate 2723
Potassium hydrogen aspartate hemihydrate 2723
Potassium hydrogen carbonate 2724
Potassium hydrogen tartrate 2725
Potassium hydroxide 2726
Potassium iodide 2726
Potassium metabisulphite 2727
Potassium nitrate 2728
Potassium perchlorate 2728
Potassium permanganate 2729
Potassium sodium tartrate tetrahydrate 2729
Potassium sorbate 2730
Potassium sulphate 2731
Potato starch 2731

Potentiometric determination of ionic concentration using ion-selective electrodes (2.2.36.) 58
Potentiometric determination of pH (2.2.3.) 24
Potentiometric titration (2.2.20.) 35
Potentisation, methods of preparation of homoeopathic stocks and **6.1**-3385
Poultices 747
Pour-on preparations 753
Povidone **6.1**-3523
Povidone, iodinated 2734
Powdered cellulose 1473
Powder flow (2.9.36.) 320
Powders and granules for oral solutions and suspensions 729
Powders and granules for syrups 730
Powders and tablets for rectal solutions and suspensions 746
Powders, ear 720
Powders, effervescent 739
Powders for cutaneous application 738
Powders for eye drops and powders for eye lotions 722
Powders for inhalation 742
Powders for injections or infusions 736
Powders for oral drops 730
Powders, nasal 732
Powders, oral 738
Poxvirus vectors for human use 672
Pravastatin sodium 2735
Prazepam 2736
Praziquantel 2737
Prazosin hydrochloride 2738
Prednicarbate 2740
Prednisolone 2741
Prednisolone acetate 2742
Prednisolone pivalate 2744
Prednisolone sodium phosphate 2745
Prednisone 2746
Prekallikrein activator (2.6.15.) 189
Premixes for medicated feeding stuffs for veterinary use 739
Preparations for inhalation 739
Preparations for inhalation: aerodynamic assessment of fine particles (2.9.18.) 287
Preparations for irrigation 743
Pressurised pharmaceutical preparations 744
Prilocaine 2748
Prilocaine hydrochloride 2750
Primaquine diphosphate 2751
Primary aromatic amino-nitrogen, determination of (2.5.8.) 139
Primary standards for volumetric solutions (4.2.1.) 514
Primidone 2752
Primula root 2753
Probenecid 2754
Procainamide hydrochloride 2755
Procaine benzylpenicillin 1287
Procaine hydrochloride 2756
Prochlorperazine maleate 2756
Products of fermentation 693
Products of recombinant DNA technology 701
Products with risk of transmitting agents of animal spongiform encephalopathies 694
Progenitor cells, human haematopoietic, colony-forming cell assay for (2.7.28.) 242
Progesterone 2757
Progressive atrophic rhinitis vaccine (inactivated), porcine **6.1**-3373
Proguanil hydrochloride 2758
Proline 2760
Promazine hydrochloride 2761
Promethazine hydrochloride 2761
Propacetamol hydrochloride 2763
Propafenone hydrochloride 2764
Propanol 2766
Propanol and methanol, 2-, test for (2.9.11.) 282
Propantheline bromide 2767
Propofol 2768
Propranolol hydrochloride 2770
Propylene glycol 2773
Propylene glycol dicaprylocaprate 2774
Propylene glycol dilaurate 2774
Propylene glycol monolaurate 2775
Propylene glycol monopalmitostearate 2776
Propylene glycol monostearate 2776
Propyl gallate 2771
Propyl parahydroxybenzoate 2772
Propylthiouracil 2777
Propyphenazone 2778
Protamine hydrochloride 2779
Protamine sulphate 2780
Protein in polysaccharide vaccines (2.5.16.) 142
Protein, total (2.5.33.) 148
Prothrombin complex, human 2076
Protirelin 2781
Proxyphylline 2783
Pseudoephedrine hydrochloride 2784
Psyllium seed 2785
Purified water 3213
Purified water, highly 3212
Purple coneflower herb 2785
Purple coneflower root 2787
Pycnometric density of solids (2.9.23.) 304
Pygeum africanum bark 2789
Pyrantel embonate 2790
Pyrazinamide 2791
Pyridostigmine bromide 2792
Pyridoxine hydrochloride 2793
Pyrimethamine 2794
Pyrogens (2.6.8.) 164
Pyrrolidone 2794

Q

Quality of pharmaceutical preparations, microbiological (5.1.4.) 529
Quantified hawthorn leaf and flower liquid extract 2037
Quinidine sulphate 2799
Quinine hydrochloride 2800
Quinine sulphate 2802

R

Rabbit haemorrhagic disease vaccine (inactivated) 949
Rabies immunoglobulin, human 2078
Rabies vaccine for human use prepared in cell cultures **6.1**-3355
Rabies vaccine (inactivated) for veterinary use **6.1**-3375
Rabies vaccine (live, oral) for foxes 952
Racemic camphor 1401
Racemic ephedrine hydrochloride 1792
Racemic menthol 2356
Raclopride ([^{11}C]methoxy) injection 1005
Radionuclides, table of physical characteristics (5.7.) 633
Radiopharmaceutical preparations 695
Radiopharmaceutical preparations, iobenguane sulphate for **6.1**-3381
Raman spectrometry (2.2.48.) 82
Ramipril 2807
Ramon assay, flocculation value (Lf) of diphtheria and tetanus toxins and toxoids (2.7.27.) 241
Ranitidine hydrochloride 2809

Rapeseed oil, refined ... 2811
Reagents (4.) ... 391
Reagents (4.1.1.) ... 391
Reagents (4.1.1.) ... **6.1**-3331
Reagents, standard solutions, buffer solutions (4.1.) ... 391
Recombinant DNA technology, products of ... 701
Rectal capsules ... 745
Rectal foams ... 746
Rectal preparations ... 744
Rectal preparations, semi-solid ... 746
Rectal solutions and suspensions, powders and tablets for ... 744
Rectal solutions, emulsions and suspensions ... 745
Rectal tampons ... 746
Red poppy petals ... 2811
Reference standards (5.12.) ... 663
Refractive index (2.2.6.) ... 26
Relationship between reaction of solution, approximate pH and colour of certain indicators (2.2.4.) ... 25
Relative density (2.2.5.) ... 25
Repaglinide ... 2812
Reserpine ... 2814
Residual solvents (5.4.) ... 603
Residual solvents, identification and control (2.4.24.) ... 121
Residue on evaporation of essential oils (2.8.9.) ... 250
Resistance to crushing of tablets (2.9.8.) ... 279
Resorcinol ... 2815
Restharrow root ... 2815
Rhatany root ... 2816
Rhatany tincture ... 2817
Rhinotracheitis vaccine (inactivated), viral, feline ... 916
Rhinotracheitis vaccine (live), viral, feline ... 917
Rhubarb ... 2817
Ribavirin ... 2818
Riboflavin ... 2820
Riboflavin sodium phosphate ... 2821
Ribose in polysaccharide vaccines (2.5.31.) ... 147
Ribwort plantain ... 2823
Rice starch ... 2824
Rifabutin ... 2825
Rifampicin ... 2826
Rifamycin sodium ... 2827
Rilmenidine dihydrogen phosphate ... 2829
Risperidone ... 2830
Ritonavir ... 2832
Rocuronium bromide ... 2835
Roman chamomile flower ... 1487
Ropivacaine hydrochloride monohydrate ... 2837
Roselle ... **6.1**-3529
Rosemary leaf ... 2839
Rosemary oil ... 2840
Rotating viscometer method - viscosity (2.2.10.) ... 28
Rotation, optical (2.2.7.) ... 26
Roxithromycin ... 2842
RRR-α-Tocopherol ... 3088
RRR-α-Tocopheryl acetate ... 3090
RRR-α-Tocopheryl hydrogen succinate ... 3095
Rubber closures for containers for aqueous parenteral preparations, for powders and for freeze-dried powders (3.2.9.) ... 386
Rubella immunoglobulin, human ... 2079
Rubella, measles and mumps vaccine (live) ... **6.1**-3347
Rubella vaccine (live) ... **6.1**-3358
Rutoside trihydrate ... 2844

S

Saccharin ... 2849
Saccharin sodium ... 2850
Safety, viral (5.1.7.) ... 543
Safflower flower ... 2851
Safflower oil, refined ... 2852
Saffron for homoeopathic preparations ... 1084
Sage leaf (salvia officinalis) ... 2853
Sage leaf, three-lobed ... 2854
Sage tincture ... 2854
Salbutamol ... 2855
Salbutamol sulphate ... 2857
Salicylic acid ... 2859
Salmeterol xinafoate ... 2860
Salmonella Enteritidis vaccine (inactivated) for chickens ... 953
Salmonella Typhimurium vaccine (inactivated) for chickens ... 954
Salmon oil, farmed ... 2862
Sanguisorba root ... **6.1**-3533
Saponification value (2.5.6.) ... 139
Saw palmetto fruit ... 2864
Scopolamine ... 2108
Scopolamine butylbromide ... 2109
Scopolamine hydrobromide ... 2110
Selamectin for veterinary use ... **6.1**-3534
Selegiline hydrochloride ... 2866
Selenium disulphide ... 2867
Semi-micro determination of water (2.5.12.) ... 141
Semi-solid ear preparations ... 720
Semi-solid eye preparations ... 722
Semi-solid intrauterine preparations ... 726
Semi-solid nasal preparations ... 732
Semi-solid oromucosal preparations ... 733
Semi-solid preparations for cutaneous application ... 746
Semi-solid rectal preparations ... 746
Semi-solid vaginal preparations ... 752
Senega root ... 2867
Senna leaf ... 2868
Senna leaf dry extract, standardised ... 2869
Senna pods, Alexandrian ... 2870
Senna pods, Tinnevelly ... 2871
Separation techniques, chromatographic (2.2.46.) ... 72
Serine ... 2872
Sertaconazole nitrate ... **6.1**-3535
Sertraline hydrochloride ... **6.1**-3537
Sesame oil, refined ... 2874
Sets for the transfusion of blood and blood components (3.2.6.) ... 383
Shampoos ... 728
Shellac ... 2876
Sialic acid in polysaccharide vaccines (2.5.23.) ... 144
Siam benzoin tincture ... 1278
Sieves (2.1.4.) ... 16
Sieve test (2.9.12.) ... 283
Sieving, analytical, particle-size distribution estimation by (2.9.38.) ... 325
SI (International System) units (1.) ... 3
Silica, colloidal anhydrous ... 2877
Silica, colloidal hydrated ... 2877
Silica, dental type ... 2878
Silica, hydrophobic colloidal ... 2878
Silicone elastomer for closures and tubing (3.1.9.) ... 358
Silicone oil used as a lubricant (3.1.8.) ... 358
Silk suture, sterile, braided, in distributor for veterinary use ... 1059
Silver, colloidal, for external use ... 2879
Silver nitrate ... 2880
Simeticone ... 2880
Simvastatin ... 2881
Single-dose preparations, uniformity of content (2.9.6.) ... 278
Single-dose preparations, uniformity of mass (2.9.5.) ... 278
Sintered-glass filters (2.1.2.) ... 15
Size-exclusion chromatography (2.2.30.) ... 47

(*S*)-Lactic acid....2229
Smallpox vaccine (live)....**6.1**-3359
Sodium acetate ([1-^{11}C]) injection....1006
Sodium acetate trihydrate....2883
Sodium alendronate....2884
Sodium alginate....2885
Sodium amidotrizoate....2886
Sodium aminosalicylate dihydrate....2887
Sodium ascorbate....2888
Sodium aurothiomalate....2889
Sodium benzoate....2890
Sodium bromide....2891
Sodium calcium edetate....2892
Sodium caprylate....2893
Sodium carbonate, anhydrous....2894
Sodium carbonate decahydrate....2894
Sodium carbonate monohydrate....2895
Sodium carboxymethylcellulose....1423
Sodium carboxymethylcellulose, cross-linked....1626
Sodium carboxymethylcellulose, low-substituted....1424
Sodium cetostearyl sulphate....2895
Sodium chloride....2897
Sodium chromate (^{51}Cr) sterile solution....1007
Sodium citrate....2898
Sodium cromoglicate....2899
Sodium cyclamate....2900
Sodium dihydrogen phosphate dihydrate....2901
Sodium fluoride....2902
Sodium fluoride (^{18}F) injection....1008
Sodium fusidate....2902
Sodium glycerophosphate, hydrated....2903
Sodium hyaluronate....2904
Sodium hydrogen carbonate....2906
Sodium hydroxide....2907
Sodium iodide....2907
Sodium iodide (^{123}I) injection....1009
Sodium iodide (^{123}I) solution for radiolabelling....1010
Sodium iodide (^{131}I) capsules for diagnostic use....1011
Sodium iodide (^{131}I) capsules for therapeutic use....1012
Sodium iodide (^{131}I) solution....1013
Sodium iodide (^{131}I) solution for radiolabelling....1014
Sodium iodohippurate (^{123}I) injection....1014
Sodium iodohippurate (^{131}I) injection....1015
Sodium lactate solution....2908
Sodium laurilsulfate....2910
Sodium metabisulphite....2911
Sodium methyl parahydroxybenzoate....2911
Sodium molybdate (^{99}Mo) solution (fission)....1016
Sodium molybdate dihydrate....2912
Sodium nitrite....2913
Sodium nitroprusside....2913
Sodium perborate, hydrated....2914
Sodium pertechnetate (^{99m}Tc) injection (fission)....1018
Sodium pertechnetate (^{99m}Tc) injection (non-fission)....1020
Sodium phenylbutyrate....**6.1**-3539
Sodium phosphate (^{32}P) injection....1020
Sodium picosulfate....2915
Sodium polystyrene sulphonate....2916
Sodium propionate....2917
Sodium propyl parahydroxybenzoate....2918
Sodium salicylate....2919
Sodium selenite pentahydrate....2919
Sodium (*S*)-lactate solution....2909
Sodium starch glycolate (type A)....2920
Sodium starch glycolate (type B)....2921
Sodium starch glycolate (type C)....2922
Sodium stearate....2923
Sodium stearyl fumarate....2924
Sodium sulphate, anhydrous....2924
Sodium sulphate decahydrate....2925
Sodium sulphite, anhydrous....2926
Sodium sulphite heptahydrate....2926
Sodium thiosulphate....2927
Sodium valproate....2927
Soft capsules....718
Softening time determination of lipophilic suppositories (2.9.22.)....302
Soft extracts....**6.1**-3344
Solid dosage forms, dissolution test for (2.9.3.)....266
Solids, density of (2.2.42.)....67
Solids, pycnometric density of (2.9.23.)....304
Solubility in alcohol of essential oils (2.8.10.)....250
Soluble tablets....750
Solutions, emulsions and suspensions, oral....729
Solutions for haemodialysis....2022
Solutions for haemodialysis, concentrated, water for diluting....2021
Solutions for haemofiltration and for haemodiafiltration....2025
Solutions for organ preservation....2929
Solutions for peritoneal dialysis....2646
Solutions, suspensions, intrauterine....726
Solvents, residual (5.4.)....603
Solvents, residual, identification and control (2.4.24.)....121
Somatostatin....2930
Somatropin....2931
Somatropin concentrated solution....2933
Somatropin for injection....2935
Sorbic acid....2937
Sorbitan laurate....2938
Sorbitan oleate....2938
Sorbitan palmitate....2939
Sorbitan sesquioleate....2939
Sorbitan stearate....2940
Sorbitan trioleate....2940
Sorbitol....2941
Sorbitol, liquid (crystallising)....2942
Sorbitol, liquid (non-crystallising)....2943
Sorbitol, liquid, partially dehydrated....2944
Sotalol hydrochloride....2944
Soya-bean oil, hydrogenated....2946
Soya-bean oil, refined....2946
Specific surface area by air permeability (2.9.14.)....283
Specific surface area by gas adsorption (2.9.26.)....306
Spectinomycin dihydrochloride pentahydrate....2947
Spectinomycin sulphate tetrahydrate for veterinary use....2949
Spectrometry, atomic absorption (2.2.23.)....37
Spectrometry, atomic emission (2.2.22.)....36
Spectrometry, mass (2.2.43.)....68
Spectrometry, nuclear magnetic resonance (2.2.33.)....54
Spectrometry, Raman (2.2.48.)....82
Spectrometry, X-ray fluorescence (2.2.37.)....59
Spectrophotometry, infrared absorption (2.2.24.)....39
Spectrophotometry, near-infrared (2.2.40.)....62
Spectrophotometry, ultraviolet and visible absorption (2.2.25.)....41
SPF chicken flocks for the production and quality control of vaccines (5.2.2.)....547
Spheroids and granules, friability of (2.9.41.)....330
Spiramycin....**6.1**-3540
Spirapril hydrochloride monohydrate....2954
Spironolactone....2955
Spot-on preparations....753
Sprays....753
Sprays (liquid nasal) and drops (nasal)....731
Squalane....2956
Standard solutions for limit tests (4.1.2.)....504
Standards, reference (5.12.)....663

Stannous chloride dihydrate....2959
Star anise....2960
Star anise oil....2962
Starch glycolate (type A), sodium....2920
Starch glycolate (type B), sodium....2921
Starch glycolate (type C), sodium....2922
Starch, maize....2326
Starch, potato....2731
Starch, pregelatinised....2964
Starch, rice....2824
Starch, wheat....3215
Starflower (borage) oil, refined....1326
Statistical analysis of results of biological assays and tests (5.3.)....571
Stavudine....2964
Steam sterilisation of aqueous preparations, application of the F_0 concept (5.1.5.)....531
Stearic acid....2966
Stearoyl macrogolglycerides....2967
Stearyl alcohol....2968
Stem cells, human haematopoietic....2067
Sterile braided silk suture in distributor for veterinary use....1059
Sterile catgut....1045
Sterile catgut in distributor for veterinary use....1057
Sterile containers of plasticised poly(vinyl chloride) for human blood containing anticoagulant solution (3.2.5.)....382
Sterile linen thread in distributor for veterinary use....1058
Sterile non-absorbable strands in distributor for veterinary use....1060
Sterile non-absorbable sutures....1046
Sterile plastic containers for human blood and blood components (3.2.3.)....379
Sterile polyamide 6/6 suture in distributor for veterinary use....1059
Sterile polyamide 6 suture in distributor for veterinary use....1058
Sterile poly(ethylene terephthalate) suture in distributor for veterinary use....1059
Sterile products, methods of preparation (5.1.1.)....525
Sterile single-use plastic syringes (3.2.8.)....384
Sterile synthetic absorbable braided sutures....1050
Sterile synthetic absorbable monofilament sutures....1052
Sterilisation procedures, biological indicators (5.1.2.)....527
Sterility (2.6.1.)....155
Sterols in fatty oils (2.4.23.)....120
Sticks....748
Sticks, intrauterine....726
Sticks, nasal....732
St. John's wort....2958
Stomata and stomatal index (2.8.3.)....249
Stramonium leaf....2968
Stramonium, prepared....2970
Strands, sterile non-absorbable, in distributor for veterinary use....1060
Streptokinase bulk solution....2971
Streptomycin sulphate....2972
Strontium (^{89}Sr) chloride injection....1021
Subdivision of tablets....748
Sublingual sprays, oromucosal drops and oromucosal sprays....732
Sublingual tablets and buccal tablets....734
Substances for pharmaceutical use....703
Substances for pharmaceutical use, control of impurities in (5.10.)....653
Substances of animal origin for the production of veterinary vaccines (5.2.5.)....555
Sub-visible particles, particulate contamination (2.9.19.)..300
Succinylsulfathiazole....2974
Sucrose....2975
Sucrose monopalmitate....**6.1**-3543
Sucrose stearate....**6.1**-3544
Sufentanil....2977
Sufentanil citrate....2978
Sugars, lead in (2.4.10.)....115
Sugar spheres....2979
Sulbactam sodium....2980
Sulfacetamide sodium....2982
Sulfadiazine....2983
Sulfadimidine....2984
Sulfadoxine....2984
Sulfafurazole....2985
Sulfaguanidine....2986
Sulfamerazine....2987
Sulfamethizole....2988
Sulfamethoxazole....2989
Sulfamethoxypyridazine for veterinary use....2990
Sulfanilamide....2991
Sulfasalazine....2992
Sulfathiazole....2994
Sulfinpyrazone....2995
Sulfisomidine....2996
Sulindac....2996
Sulphated ash (2.4.14.)....116
Sulphates (2.4.13.)....116
Sulphur dioxide (2.5.29.)....146
Sulphur for external use....2998
Sulphuric acid....2998
Sulpiride....2999
Sultamicillin....**6.1**-3545
Sultamicillin tosilate dihydrate....**6.1**-3548
Sumatra benzoin....1278
Sumatra benzoin tincture....1279
Sumatriptan succinate....3005
Sunflower oil, refined....3007
Supercritical fluid chromatography (2.2.45.)....71
Suppositories....745
Suppositories and pessaries, disintegration of (2.9.2.)....265
Suppositories, lipophilic, softening time determination (2.9.22.)....302
Suspensions, solutions and emulsions, oral....729
Suspensions, solutions, intrauterine....726
Sutures, sterile non-absorbable....1046
Sutures, sterile synthetic absorbable braided....1050
Sutures, sterile synthetic absorbable monofilament....1052
Suxamethonium chloride....3007
Suxibuzone....3008
Sweet fennel....1874
Sweet orange oil....3009
Swelling index (2.8.4.)....249
Swine erysipelas vaccine (inactivated)....955
Swine-fever vaccine (live), classical, freeze-dried....956
Symbols and abbreviations (1.)....3
Synthetic absorbable braided sutures, sterile....1050
Synthetic absorbable monofilament sutures, sterile....1052
Syringes, plastic, sterile single-use (3.2.8.)....384
Syrups....730

T

Table of physical characteristics of radionuclides mentioned in the European Pharmacopoeia (5.7.)....633
Tablets....748
Tablets and capsules, disintegration of (2.9.1.)....263
Tablets, buccal....734
Tablets, coated....749
Tablets, dispersible....750
Tablets, effervescent....749

Tablets for intrauterine solutions and suspensions 726
Tablets for use in the mouth 750
Tablets for vaginal solutions and suspensions 752
Tablets, gastro-resistant 750
Tablets, intrauterine 726
Tablets, modified-release 750
Tablets, orodispersible 750
Tablets, resistance to crushing (2.9.8.) 279
Tablets, soluble 750
Tablets, subdivision of 748
Tablets, sublingual 734
Tablets, uncoated 749
Tablets, uncoated, friability of (2.9.7.) 278
Tablets, vaginal 752
Talc 3013
Tamoxifen citrate 3014
Tampons, ear 720
Tampons, medicated 751
Tampons, rectal 746
Tampons, vaginal, medicated 752
Tamsulosin hydrochloride 3016
Tannic acid 3018
Tannins in herbal drugs, determination of (2.8.14.) 255
Tartaric acid 3018
Teat dips 753
Tea tree oil 3019
Teat sprays 753
Technetium (^{99m}Tc) bicisate injection 1022
Technetium (^{99m}Tc) colloidal rhenium sulphide injection 1023
Technetium (^{99m}Tc) colloidal sulphur injection 1024
Technetium (^{99m}Tc) colloidal tin injection 1025
Technetium (^{99m}Tc) etifenin injection 1026
Technetium (^{99m}Tc) exametazime injection 1027
Technetium (^{99m}Tc) gluconate injection 1028
Technetium (^{99m}Tc) human albumin injection 1029
Technetium (^{99m}Tc) macrosalb injection 1030
Technetium (^{99m}Tc) medronate injection 1031
Technetium (^{99m}Tc) mertiatide injection 1033
Technetium (^{99m}Tc) microspheres injection 1034
Technetium (^{99m}Tc) pentetate injection 1035
Technetium (^{99m}Tc) sestamibi injection 1036
Technetium (^{99m}Tc) succimer injection 1037
Technetium (^{99m}Tc) tin pyrophosphate injection 1038
Temazepam 3020
Tenosynovitis avian viral vaccine (live) 875
Tenoxicam 3021
Terazosin hydrochloride dihydrate 3022
Terbinafine hydrochloride 3024
Terbutaline sulphate 3025
Terconazole **6.1**-3553
Terfenadine **6.1**-3554
Terminology used in monographs on biological products (5.2.1.) 547
Test for anticomplementary activity of immunoglobulin (2.6.17.) 191
Test for anti-D antibodies in human immunoglobulin for intravenous administration (2.6.26.) 205
Test for extractable volume of parenteral preparations (2.9.17.) 287
Test for Fc function of immunoglobulin (2.7.9.) 227
Test for methanol and 2-propanol (2.9.11.) 282
Test for neurovirulence of live virus vaccines (2.6.18.) 193
Test for neurovirulence of poliomyelitis vaccine (oral) (2.6.19.) 193
Test for specified micro-organisms (microbiological examination of non-sterile products) (2.6.13.) 173
Testosterone 3030
Testosterone decanoate 3031
Testosterone enantate 3033
Testosterone isocaproate 3034
Testosterone propionate 3035
Tests for extraneous agents in viral vaccines for human use (2.6.16.) 190
Tetanus and diphtheria toxins and toxoids, flocculation value (Lf) of, (Ramon assay) (2.7.27.) 241
Tetanus and diphtheria vaccine (adsorbed, reduced antigen(s) content) 764
Tetanus antitoxin for human use 969
Tetanus antitoxin for veterinary use 976
Tetanus, diphtheria and hepatitis B (rDNA) vaccine (adsorbed) 765
Tetanus, diphtheria and pertussis (acellular, component) vaccine (adsorbed) 767
Tetanus, diphtheria and poliomyelitis (inactivated) vaccine (adsorbed, reduced antigen(s) content) 770
Tetanus, diphtheria, pertussis (acellular, component) and haemophilus type b conjugate vaccine (adsorbed) 771
Tetanus, diphtheria, pertussis (acellular, component) and hepatitis B (rDNA) vaccine (adsorbed) 774
Tetanus, diphtheria, pertussis (acellular, component) and poliomyelitis (inactivated) vaccine (adsorbed) 775
Tetanus, diphtheria, pertussis (acellular, component) and poliomyelitis (inactivated) vaccine (adsorbed, reduced antigen(s) content) 778
Tetanus, diphtheria, pertussis (acellular, component), hepatitis B (rDNA), poliomyelitis (inactivated) and haemophilus type b conjugate vaccine (adsorbed) 780
Tetanus, diphtheria, pertussis (acellular, component), poliomyelitis (inactivated) and haemophilus type b conjugate vaccine (adsorbed) 783
Tetanus, diphtheria, pertussis and poliomyelitis (inactivated) vaccine (adsorbed) 785
Tetanus, diphtheria, pertussis, poliomyelitis (inactivated) and haemophilus type b conjugate vaccine (adsorbed) 787
Tetanus immunoglobulin, human 2079
Tetanus vaccine (adsorbed) 844
Tetanus vaccine (adsorbed), assay of (2.7.8.) 223
Tetanus vaccine for veterinary use 957
Tetracaine hydrochloride **6.1**-3556
Tetracosactide 3037
Tetracycline 3040
Tetracycline hydrochloride 3041
Tetrazepam 3043
Tetryzoline hydrochloride 3044
Thallous (^{201}Tl) chloride injection 1039
Theobromine 3045
Theophylline 3046
Theophylline-ethylenediamine 3048
Theophylline-ethylenediamine hydrate 3049
Theophylline monohydrate 3047
Thermal analysis (2.2.34.) **6.1**-3311
Thermogravimetry (2.2.34.) **6.1**-3311
Thiamazole 3050
Thiamine hydrochloride 3051
Thiamine nitrate 3053
Thiamphenicol 3054
Thin-layer chromatography (2.2.27.) 43
Thioctic acid 3055
Thiomersal 3056
Thiopental sodium and sodium carbonate 3057
Thioridazine 3058
Thioridazine hydrochloride 3059
Three-lobed sage leaf 2854
Threonine 3060
Thyme 3061
Thyme oil 3063
Thyme, wild 3219

Thymol 3064
Tiabendazole 3064
Tiamulin for veterinary use 3065
Tiamulin hydrogen fumarate for veterinary use 3068
Tianeptine sodium 3070
Tiapride hydrochloride 3071
Tiaprofenic acid 3072
Tibolone 3074
Ticarcillin sodium 3075
Tick-borne encephalitis vaccine (inactivated) 845
Ticlopidine hydrochloride 3077
Tilidine hydrochloride hemihydrate 3079
Timolol maleate 3080
Tinctures **6.1**-3344
Tinidazole 3081
Tinnevelly senna pods 2871
Tinzaparin sodium 3082
Tioconazole 3083
Titanium dioxide 3084
Titration, amperometric (2.2.19.) 35
Titration, potentiometric (2.2.20.) 35
Titrations, complexometric (2.5.11.) 140
Tobramycin 3085
Tocopherol, all-*rac*-α- 3086
Tocopherol, *RRR*-α- 3088
Tocopheryl acetate, all-*rac*-α- 3089
α-Tocopheryl acetate concentrate (powder form) 3091
Tocopheryl acetate, *RRR*-α- 3090
Tocopheryl hydrogen succinate, DL-α- 3093
Tocopheryl hydrogen succinate, *RRR*-α- 3095
Tolbutamide 3097
Tolfenamic acid 3097
Tolnaftate 3099
Tolu balsam 3099
Torasemide, anhydrous 3100
Tormentil 3101
Tormentil tincture 3102
Tosylchloramide sodium 3103
Total ash (2.4.16.) 116
Total cholesterol in oils rich in omega-3 acids (2.4.32.) 132
Total organic carbon in water for pharmaceutical use (2.2.44.) 71
Total protein (2.5.33.) 148
Total viable aerobic count (microbiological examination of non-sterile products) (2.6.12.) 166
Toxicity, abnormal (2.6.9.) 165
Toxin, botulinum type A for injection 1327
Tragacanth 3103
Tramadol hydrochloride 3104
Tramazoline hydrochloride monohydrate 3106
Trandolapril 3107
Tranexamic acid 3108
Transdermal patches 737
Transdermal patches, dissolution test for (2.9.4.) 275
Trapidil 3110
Tretinoin 3111
Triacetin 3112
Triamcinolone 3112
Triamcinolone acetonide 3114
Triamcinolone hexacetonide 3115
Triamterene **6.1**-3557
Tribenoside 3117
Tributyl acetylcitrate 3118
Trichloroacetic acid 3119
Triethanolamine 3133
Triethyl citrate 3120
Trifluoperazine hydrochloride 3121
Triflusal 3121
Triglycerides, medium-chain 3122
Triglycerides, omega-3 acid 2554
Triglycerol diisostearate **6.1**-3558
Trihexyphenidyl hydrochloride 3125
Trimetazidine dihydrochloride 3126
Trimethadione 3127
Trimethoprim 3128
Trimipramine maleate 3130
Tri-*n*-butyl phosphate 3132
Tritiated (^{3}H) water injection 1040
Trolamine 3133
Trometamol 3135
Tropicamide 3135
Tropisetron hydrochloride 3136
Trospium chloride 3138
Troxerutin 3139
Trypsin 3141
Tryptophan 3142
TSE, animal, minimising the risk of transmitting via human and veterinary medicinal products (5.2.8.) 558
TSE, animal, products with risk of transmitting agents of 694
Tuberculin for human use, old 3144
Tuberculin purified protein derivative, avian 3146
Tuberculin purified protein derivative, bovine 3147
Tuberculin purified protein derivative for human use 3147
Tubes for comparative tests (2.1.5.) 17
Tubing and closures, silicone elastomer for (3.1.9.) 358
Tubing and containers for total parenteral nutrition preparations, poly(ethylene - vinyl acetate) for (3.1.7.) 356
Tubing used in sets for the transfusion of blood and blood components, materials based on plasticised poly(vinyl chloride) for (3.1.1.2.) 342
Tubocurarine chloride 3150
Turmeric, Javanese 3150
Turpentine oil, Pinus pinaster type 3151
Tylosin for veterinary use 3152
Tylosin phosphate bulk solution for veterinary use 3154
Tylosin tartrate for veterinary use 3156
Typhoid polysaccharide vaccine 847
Typhoid vaccine 849
Typhoid vaccine, freeze-dried 849
Typhoid vaccine (live, oral, strain Ty 21a) 849
Tyrosine 3157
Tyrothricin 3158

U

Ubidecarenone 3163
Udder-washes 753
Ultraviolet and visible absorption spectrophotometry (2.2.25.) 41
Ultraviolet ray lamps for analytical purposes (2.1.3.) 15
Uncoated tablets 749
Undecylenic acid 3164
Uniformity of content of single-dose preparations (2.9.6.) 278
Uniformity of dosage units (2.9.40.) **6.1**-3325
Uniformity of mass of delivered doses from multidose containers (2.9.27.) 309
Uniformity of mass of single-dose preparations (2.9.5.) 278
Units of the International System (SI) used in the Pharmacopoeia and equivalence with other units (1.) 3
Unsaponifiable matter (2.5.7.) 139
Urea 3165
Urofollitropin 3166
Urokinase 3167
Uronic acids in polysaccharide vaccines (2.5.22.) 144
Ursodeoxycholic acid 3168

V

Vaccines, adsorbed, aluminium in (2.5.13.) 141
Vaccines, adsorbed, calcium in (2.5.14.) 142
Vaccines and immunosera, phenol in (2.5.15.) 142
Vaccines and immunosera, veterinary, evaluation of efficacy of (5.2.7.) **6.1**-3335
Vaccines and immunosera, veterinary, evaluation of safety (5.2.6.) 556
Vaccines and immunosera, veterinary, evaluation of the safety of each batch (5.2.9.) 567
Vaccines for human use 705
Vaccines for human use, cell substrates for the production of (5.2.3.) 550
Vaccines for human use, viral, extraneous agents in (2.6.16.) 190
Vaccines for veterinary use 707
Vaccines, polysaccharide, hexosamines in (2.5.20.) 143
Vaccines, polysaccharide, methylpentoses in (2.5.21.) 143
Vaccines, polysaccharide, nucleic acids in (2.5.17.) 142
Vaccines, polysaccharide, *O*-acetyl in (2.5.19.) 143
Vaccines, polysaccharide, phosphorus in (2.5.18.) 142
Vaccines, polysaccharide, protein in (2.5.16.) 142
Vaccines, polysaccharide, ribose in (2.5.31.) 147
Vaccines, polysaccharide, sialic acid in (2.5.23.) 144
Vaccines, polysaccharide, uronic acids in (2.5.22.) 144
Vaccines, SPF chicken flocks for the production and quality control of (5.2.2.) 547
Vaccines, veterinary, cell cultures for the production of (5.2.4.) 553
Vaccines, veterinary, substances of animal origin for the production of (5.2.5.) 555
Vaccines, viral live, test for neurovirulence (2.6.18.) 193
Vaginal capsules 752
Vaginal foams 752
Vaginal preparations 751
Vaginal preparations, semi-solid 752
Vaginal solutions and suspensions, tablets for 752
Vaginal solutions, emulsions and suspensions 752
Vaginal tablets 752
Vaginal tampons, medicated 752
Valerian dry hydroalcoholic extract 3173
Valerian root 3174
Valerian tincture 3175
Valine 3176
Valnemulin hydrochloride for veterinary use 3177
Valproic acid 3178
Vancomycin hydrochloride 3180
Vanillin 3182
Varicella immunoglobulin for intravenous administration, human 2081
Varicella immunoglobulin, human 2080
Varicella vaccine (live) **6.1**-3364
Vectors for human use, adenovirus 670
Vectors for human use, plasmid 674
Vectors for human use, plasmid, bacterial cells used for the manufacture of 676
Vectors for human use, poxvirus 672
Vecuronium bromide 3183
Vegetable fatty oils 712
Venlafaxine hydrochloride 3184
Verapamil hydrochloride 3186
Verbena herb 3188
Veterinary liquid preparations for cutaneous application 752
Veterinary vaccines and immunosera, evaluation of efficacy of (5.2.7.) **6.1**-3335
Viability, nucleated cell count and (2.7.29.) 243
Vibriosis (cold-water) vaccine (inactivated) for salmonids 959
Vibriosis vaccine (inactivated) for salmonids 960
VICH (5.8.) 645
Vinblastine sulphate 3189
Vincristine sulphate 3190
Vindesine sulphate 3192
Vinorelbine tartrate 3194
Vinpocetine 3196
Viper venom antiserum, European 970
Viral rhinotracheitis vaccine (inactivated), feline 916
Viral rhinotracheitis vaccine (live), feline 917
Viral safety (5.1.7.) 543
Viscometer method, capillary (2.2.9.) 27
Viscometer method, falling ball (2.2.49.) 84
Viscose wadding, absorbent 3197
Viscosity (2.2.8.) 27
Viscosity - rotating viscometer method (2.2.10.) 28
Visible and ultraviolet absorption spectrophotometry (2.2.25.) 41
Visible particles, particulate contamination (2.9.20.) 302
Vitamin A 3199
Vitamin A concentrate (oily form), synthetic 3200
Vitamin A concentrate (powder form), synthetic 3201
Vitamin A concentrate (solubilisate/emulsion), synthetic 3203
Volumetric analysis (4.2.) 514
Volumetric solutions (4.2.2.) 514
Volumetric solutions, primary standards for (4.2.1.) 514
von Willebrand factor, human 2081
von Willebrand factor, human, assay of (2.7.21.) 237

W

Warfarin sodium 3207
Warfarin sodium clathrate 3208
Washes, nasal 732
Water (^{15}O) injection 1040
Water, determination by distillation (2.2.13.) 31
Water for diluting concentrated haemodialysis solutions 2021
Water for injections 3209
Water for pharmaceutical use, total organic carbon in (2.2.44.) 71
Water, highly purified 3212
Water in essential oils (2.8.5.) 249
Water in gases (2.5.28.) 146
Water: micro determination (2.5.32.) 147
Water, purified 3213
Water: semi-micro determination (2.5.12.) 141
Wheat-germ oil, refined 3215
Wheat-germ oil, virgin 3216
Wheat starch 3215
White beeswax 1260
White horehound 3216
White soft paraffin 2614
Wild pansy (flowering aerial parts) 3217
Wild thyme 3219
Willow bark **6.1**-3563
Willow bark dry extract **6.1**-3564
Wool alcohols 3221
Wool fat 3222
Wool fat, hydrogenated 3226
Wool fat, hydrous 3227
Wormwood 3228

X

Xanthan gum **6.1**-3569
Xenon (^{133}Xe) injection 1042
X-ray fluorescence spectrometry (2.2.37.) 59
X-ray powder diffraction (XRPD), characterisation of crystalline and partially crystalline solids by (2.9.33.) 314
Xylazine hydrochloride for veterinary use 3234

Xylitol 3235
Xylometazoline hydrochloride 3237
Xylose 3238

Y

Yarrow 3243
Yellow beeswax 1261
Yellow fever vaccine (live) **6.1**-3365
Yellow soft paraffin 2615
Yohimbine hydrochloride 3244

Z

Zidovudine 3249
Zinc acetate dihydrate 3250
Zinc acexamate 3251
Zinc chloride 3253
Zinc oxide 3253
Zinc stearate 3254
Zinc sulphate heptahydrate 3254
Zinc sulphate hexahydrate 3255
Zinc sulphate monohydrate 3255
Zinc undecylenate 3256
Zolpidem tartrate 3256
Zopiclone 3257
Zuclopenthixol decanoate 3259

A

Absinthii herba 3228
Acaciae gummi 1087
Acaciae gummi dispersione desiccatum 1087
Acamprosatum calcicum 1088
Acarbosum 1089
Acebutololi hydrochloridum 1091
Aceclofenacum 1093
Acemetacinum **6.1**-3393
Acesulfamum kalicum 1095
Acetazolamidum 1096
Acetonum 1098
Acetylcholini chloridum 1099
Acetylcysteinum 1100
β-Acetyldigoxinum 1101
Aciclovirum 1107
Acidi methacrylici et ethylis acrylatis polymerisati 1:1 dispersio 30 per centum 2372
Acidi methacrylici et ethylis acrylatis polymerisatum 1:1 2371
Acidi methacrylici et methylis methacrylatis polymerisatum 1:1 2373
Acidi methacrylici et methylis methacrylatis polymerisatum 1:2 2374
Acidum 4-aminobenzoicum 1164
Acidum aceticum glaciale 1097
Acidum acetylsalicylicum 1103
Acidum adipicum 1113
Acidum alginicum 1131
Acidum amidotrizoicum dihydricum 1158
Acidum aminocaproicum 1166
Acidum ascorbicum 1221
Acidum asparticum 1225
Acidum benzoicum 1276
Acidum boricum 1327
Acidum caprylicum 1402
Acidum chenodeoxycholicum 1489
Acidum citricum anhydricum 1554
Acidum citricum monohydricum 1555
Acidum edeticum 1774
Acidum etacrynicum 1826
Acidum folicum 1938
Acidum fusidicum 1954
Acidum glutamicum 1984
Acidum hydrochloridum concentratum 2085
Acidum hydrochloridum dilutum 2085
Acidum iopanoicum 2162
Acidum iotalamicum 2163
Acidum ioxaglicum 2167
Acidum lacticum 2228
Acidum lactobionicum 2231
Acidum maleicum 2328
Acidum malicum 2329
Acidum mefenamicum 2349
Acidum nalidixicum 2472
Acidum nicotinicum 2502
Acidum niflumicum **6.1**-3508
Acidum nitricum 2510
Acidum oleicum 2543
Acidum oxolinicum 2582
Acidum palmiticum 2604
Acidum phosphoricum concentratum 2675
Acidum phosphoricum dilutum 2676
Acidum pipemidicum trihydricum 2690
Acidum salicylicum 2859
Acidum (S)-lacticum 2229
Acidum sorbicum 2937
Acidum stearicum 2966
Acidum sulfuricum 2998
Acidum tartaricum 3018
Acidum thiocticum 3055
Acidum tiaprofenicum 3072
Acidum tolfenamicum 3097
Acidum tranexamicum 3108
Acidum trichloraceticum 3119
Acidum undecylenicum 3164
Acidum ursodeoxycholicum 3168
Acidum valproicum 3178
Acitretinum 1109
Adeninum 1110
Adenosinum 1111
Adeps lanae 3222
Adeps lanae cum aqua 3227
Adeps lanae hydrogenatus 3226
Adeps solidus 2034
Adrenalini tartras 1114
Aer medicinalis 1118
Aer medicinalis artificiosus 1121
Aether 1833
Aether anaestheticus 1834
Aetherolea 680
Agar 1115
Agni casti fructus 1116
Agrimoniae herba 1117
Alaninum 1121
Albendazolum 1122
Albumini humani solutio 2057
Alchemillae herba 1123
Alcohol benzylicus 1281
Alcohol cetylicus 1485
Alcohol cetylicus et stearylicus 1480
Alcohol cetylicus et stearylicus emulsificans A 1481
Alcohol cetylicus et stearylicus emulsificans B 1482
Alcoholes adipis lanae 3221
Alcohol isopropylicus 2182
Alcohol oleicus 2544
Alcohol stearylicus 2968
Alcuronii chloridum 1124
Alfacalcidolum 1126
Alfadexum 1127
Alfentanili hydrochloridum 1128
Alfuzosini hydrochloridum **6.1**-3394
Allantoinum 1131
Allii sativi bulbi pulvis 1961
Allium sativum ad praeparationes homoeopathicas 1077
Allopurinolum 1132
Almagatum 1134
Aloe barbadensis 1137
Aloe capensis 1138
Aloes extractum siccum normatum 1139
Alprazolamum 1139
Alprenololi hydrochloridum 1141
Alprostadilum 1143
Alteplasum ad iniectabile 1145
Althaeae folium 2338
Althaeae radix 2339
Alumen 1149
Aluminii chloridum hexahydricum 1149
Aluminii hydroxidum hydricum ad adsorptionem **6.1**-3395
Aluminii magnesii silicas 1151
Aluminii oxidum hydricum 1152
Aluminii phosphas hydricus 1153
Aluminii phosphatis liquamen 1152
Aluminii sulfas 1154
Alverini citras 1154
Amantadini hydrochloridum 1156
Ambroxoli hydrochloridum 1156
Amfetamini sulfas 1158

Amikacini sulfas **6.1**-3398
Amikacinum **6.1**-3396
Amiloridi hydrochloridum 1163
Aminoglutethimidum 1167
Amiodaroni hydrochloridum 1168
Amisulpridum 1170
Amitriptylini hydrochloridum 1172
Amlodipini besilas 1173
Ammoniae (^{13}N) solutio iniectabilis 981
Ammoniae solutio concentrata 1175
Ammonii bromidum 1177
Ammonii chloridum 1178
Ammonii glycyrrhizas 1179
Ammonii hydrogenocarbonas 1180
Ammonio methacrylatis copolymerum A 1175
Ammonio methacrylatis copolymerum B 1176
Amobarbitalum 1180
Amobarbitalum natricum 1181
Amoxicillinum natricum 1182
Amoxicillinum trihydricum 1184
Amphotericinum B 1187
Ampicillinum anhydricum 1188
Ampicillinum natricum 1190
Ampicillinum trihydricum 1193
Amygdalae oleum raffinatum 1136
Amygdalae oleum virginale 1136
Amylum pregelificatum 2964
Angelicae radix 1196
Anisi aetheroleum 1197
Anisi fructus 1199
Anisi stellati aetheroleum 2962
Anisi stellati fructus 2960
Antazolini hydrochloridum 1199
Anticorpora monoclonalia ad usum humanum 690
Antithrombinum III humanum densatum 2060
Apis mellifera ad praeparationes homoeopathicas 1079
Apomorphini hydrochloridum 1207
Aprotinini solutio concentrata 1209
Aprotininum 1208
Aqua ad dilutionem solutionum concentratarum ad haemodialysim 2021
Aqua ad iniectabilia 3209
Aquae (^{15}O) solutio iniectabilis 1040
Aquae tritiatae (^{3}H) solutio iniectabilis 1040
Aqua purificata 3213
Aqua valde purificata 3212
Arachidis oleum hydrogenatum 1211
Arachidis oleum raffinatum 1211
Argenti nitras 2880
Argentum colloidale ad usum externum 2879
Arginini aspartas 1213
Arginini hydrochloridum 1214
Argininum 1212
Arnicae flos **6.1**-3400
Arnicae tinctura 1216
Arsenii trioxidum ad praeparationes homoeopathicas 1073
Articaini hydrochloridum 1217
Ascorbylis palmitas 1222
Asparaginum monohydricum 1223
Aspartamum 1224
Astemizolum 1226
Atenololum 1228
Atracurii besilas 1230
Atropini sulfas **6.1**-3404
Atropinum **6.1**-3403
Aurantii amari epicarpii et mesocarpii tinctura 1320
Aurantii amari epicarpium et mesocarpium 1319
Aurantii amari flos 1320
Aurantii dulcis aetheroleum 3009
Auricularia 719
Azaperonum ad usum veterinarium 1234
Azathioprinum 1236
Azelastini hydrochloridum 1236
Azithromycinum 1238

B

Bacampicillini hydrochloridum **6.1**-3409
Bacitracinum 1245
Bacitracinum zincum 1247
Baclofenum 1250
Ballotae nigrae herba 1321
Balsamum peruvianum 2649
Balsamum tolutanum 3099
Bambuteroli hydrochloridum 1251
Barbitalum 1252
Barii chloridum dihydricum ad praeparationes homoeopathicas 1073
Barii sulfas 1253
BCG ad immunocurationem 758
Beclometasoni dipropionas anhydricus 1256
Beclometasoni dipropionas monohydricus 1258
Belladonnae folii extractum siccum normatum 1263
Belladonnae folii tinctura normata 1264
Belladonnae folium 1261
Belladonnae pulvis normatus 1265
Bendroflumethiazidum 1266
Benfluorexi hydrochloridum 1267
Benperidolum 1269
Benserazidi hydrochloridum 1270
Bentonitum 1271
Benzalkonii chloridi solutio 1273
Benzalkonii chloridum 1272
Benzbromaronum 1273
Benzethonii chloridum 1275
Benzocainum 1276
Benzoe sumatranus 1278
Benzoe tonkinensis 1277
Benzois sumatrani tinctura 1279
Benzois tonkinensis tinctura 1278
Benzoylis peroxidum cum aqua 1280
Benzylis benzoas 1283
Benzylpenicillinum benzathinum 1283
Benzylpenicillinum kalicum 1285
Benzylpenicillinum natricum 1288
Benzylpenicillinum procainum 1287
Betacarotenum 1290
Betadexum 1291
Betahistini dihydrochloridum 1292
Betahistini mesilas 1293
Betamethasoni acetas 1297
Betamethasoni dipropionas 1298
Betamethasoni natrii phosphas 1300
Betamethasoni valeras 1301
Betamethasonum 1295
Betaxololi hydrochloridum 1303
Betulae folium 1311
Bezafibratum 1304
Bifonazolum 1306
Biotinum 1308
Biperideni hydrochloridum 1309
Bisacodylum 1312
Bismuthi subcarbonas 1313
Bismuthi subgallas 1314
Bismuthi subnitras ponderosus 1315
Bismuthi subsalicylas 1316
Bisoprololi fumaras **6.1**-3412
Bistortae rhizoma 1317
Bleomycini sulfas 1322

Boldi folii extractum siccum **6.1**-3415
Boldi folium 1324
Boragonis officinalis oleum raffinatum 1326
Borax 1326
Bromazepamum 1331
Bromhexini hydrochloridum 1332
Bromocriptini mesilas 1333
Bromperidoli decanoas 1337
Bromperidolum 1335
Brompheniramini maleas 1339
Brotizolamum 1340
Budesonidum 1342
Bufexamacum 1344
Buflomedili hydrochloridum 1345
Bumetanidum 1346
Bupivacaini hydrochloridum 1347
Buprenorphini hydrochloridum 1350
Buprenorphinum 1349
Buserelinum 1351
Buspironi hydrochloridum 1353
Busulfanum 1355
Butylhydroxyanisolum 1357
Butylhydroxytoluenum 1357
Butylis parahydroxybenzoas 1358

C

Cabergolinum 1363
Cadmii sulfas hydricus ad praeparationes homoeopathicas 1074
Calcifediolum 1366
Calcii acetas 1376
Calcii ascorbas 1377
Calcii carbonas 1378
Calcii chloridum dihydricum 1378
Calcii chloridum hexahydricum 1379
Calcii dobesilas monohydricus 1380
Calcii folinas 1380
Calcii glucoheptonas 1383
Calcii gluconas 1384
Calcii gluconas ad iniectabile 1385
Calcii glycerophosphas 1386
Calcii hydrogenophosphas anhydricus 1387
Calcii hydrogenophosphas dihydricus 1388
Calcii hydroxidum 1389
Calcii iodidum tetrahydricum ad praeparationes homoeopathicas 1074
Calcii lactas anhydricus 1389
Calcii lactas monohydricus 1390
Calcii lactas pentahydricus 1390
Calcii lactas trihydricus 1391
Calcii laevulinas dihydricus 1394
Calcii levofolinas pentahydricus 1392
Calcii pantothenas 1395
Calcii stearas 1397
Calcii sulfas dihydricus 1398
Calcipotriolum anhydricum 1367
Calcipotriolum monohydricum 1370
Calcitoninum salmonis 1372
Calcitriolum 1375
Calendulae flos 1398
Camphora racemica 1401
Capsici fructus 1404
Capsici oleoresina raffinata et quantificata 1405
Capsici tinctura normata 1406
Capsulae 717
Captoprilum 1407
Carbacholum 1410
Carbamazepinum 1411
Carbasalatum calcicum 1412
Carbidopum 1413
Carbimazolum 1414
Carbo activatus 1488
Carbocisteinum 1415
Carbomera **6.1**-3422
Carbonei dioxidum 1417
Carbonei monoxidum (^{15}O) 982
Carboplatinum 1419
Carboprostum trometamolum 1420
Carboxymethylamylum natricum A 2920
Carboxymethylamylum natricum B 2921
Carboxymethylamylum natricum C 2922
Carisoprodolum 1421
Carmellosum calcicum 1422
Carmellosum natricum 1423
Carmellosum natricum conexum 1626
Carmellosum natricum, substitutum humile 1424
Carmustinum 1425
Carteololi hydrochloridum 1426
Carthami flos 2851
Carthami oleum raffinatum 2852
Carvedilolum 1427
Carvi aetheroleum 1408
Carvi fructus 1408
Caryophylli floris aetheroleum 1588
Caryophylli flos 1587
Cefaclorum 1435
Cefadroxilum monohydricum **6.1**-3423
Cefalexinum monohydricum **6.1**-3425
Cefalotinum natricum 1440
Cefamandoli nafas 1441
Cefapirinum natricum 1443
Cefatrizinum propylen glycolum 1444
Cefazolinum natricum 1445
Cefepimi dihydrochloridum monohydricum 1448
Cefiximum 1450
Cefoperazonum natricum 1451
Cefotaximum natricum 1453
Cefoxitinum natricum 1455
Cefradinum 1457
Ceftazidimum 1459
Ceftriaxonum natricum 1461
Cefuroximum axetili 1462
Cefuroximum natricum 1464
Celiprololi hydrochloridum 1465
Cellulae stirpes haematopoieticae humanae 2067
Cellulosi acetas 1467
Cellulosi acetas butyras 1468
Cellulosi acetas phthalas 1468
Cellulosi pulvis 1473
Cellulosum microcristallinum 1469
Cellulosum microcristallinum et carmellosum natricum 2422
Centaurii herba 1477
Centellae asiaticae herba 1477
Cera alba 1260
Cera carnauba 1425
Cera flava 1261
Cetirizini dihydrochloridum 1479
Cetobemidoni hydrochloridum 2215
Cetostearylis isononanoas 1484
Cetrimidum 1484
Cetylis palmitas 1486
Cetylpyridinii chloridum 1486
Chamomillae romanae flos 1487
Chelidonii herba 2010
Chinidini sulfas 2799
Chinini hydrochloridum 2800
Chinini sulfas 2802

Chitosani hydrochloridum 1490
Chlorali hydras 1491
Chlorambucilum 1492
Chloramphenicoli natrii succinas 1495
Chloramphenicoli palmitas 1493
Chloramphenicolum 1492
Chlorcyclizini hydrochloridum 1496
Chlordiazepoxidi hydrochloridum 1498
Chlordiazepoxidum 1497
Chlorhexidini diacetas 1499
Chlorhexidini digluconatis solutio 1500
Chlorhexidini dihydrochloridum 1502
Chlorobutanolum anhydricum 1503
Chlorobutanolum hemihydricum 1504
Chlorocresolum 1504
Chloroquini phosphas 1505
Chloroquini sulfas 1506
Chlorothiazidum 1507
Chlorphenamini maleas **6.1**-3427
Chlorpromazini hydrochloridum 1509
Chlorpropamidum 1510
Chlorprothixeni hydrochloridum 1511
Chlortalidonum 1513
Chlortetracyclini hydrochloridum 1514
Cholecalciferoli pulvis 1519
Cholecalciferolum 1516
Cholecalciferolum densatum oleosum 1517
Cholecalciferolum in aqua dispergibile 1521
Cholesterolum 1524
Chondroitini natrii sulfas 1525
Chorda resorbilis sterilis 1045
Chorda resorbilis sterilis in fuso ad usum veterinarium 1057
Chromii (^{51}Cr) edetatis solutio iniectabilis 983
Chymotrypsinum 1527
Ciclopirox olaminum 1530
Ciclopiroxum 1528
Ciclosporinum 1531
Cilastatinum natricum **6.1**-3428
Cilazaprilum 1534
Cimetidini hydrochloridum 1537
Cimetidinum 1536
Cinchocaini hydrochloridum 1538
Cinchonae cortex 1539
Cinchonae extractum fluidum normatum 1540
Cineolum 1541
Cinnamomi cassiae aetheroleum 1431
Cinnamomi cortex 1542
Cinnamomi corticis tinctura 1545
Cinnamomi zeylanici folii aetheroleum 1544
Cinnamomi zeylanicii corticis aetheroleum 1543
Cinnarizinum 1545
Ciprofibratum 1547
Ciprofloxacini hydrochloridum 1550
Ciprofloxacinum 1548
Cisapridi tartras 1552
Cisapridum monohydricum 1551
Cisplatinum 1554
Citri reticulatae aetheroleum 2333
Citronellae aetheroleum 1556
Cladribinum 1557
Clarithromycinum 1559
Clazurilum ad usum veterinarium 1562
Clebopridi malas 1564
Clemastini fumaras **6.1**-3430
Clenbuteroli hydrochloridum 1567
Clindamycini hydrochloridum 1568
Clindamycini phosphas 1570
Clioquinolum 1571
Clobazamum 1572
Clobetasoli propionas 1573
Clobetasoni butyras 1575
Clofaziminum 1577
Clofibratum 1578
Clomifeni citras 1579
Clomipramini hydrochloridum 1580
Clonazepamum 1582
Clonidini hydrochloridum 1583
Clopamidum **6.1**-3431
Closantelum natricum dihydricum ad usum veterinarium 1584
Clotrimazolum **6.1**-3433
Cloxacillinum natricum 1589
Clozapinum 1590
Cocaini hydrochloridum 1592
Cocois oleum raffinatum 1593
Cocoylis caprylocapras 1594
Codeini hydrochloridum dihydricum 1596
Codeini phosphas hemihydricus 1598
Codeini phosphas sesquihydricus 1599
Codeinum **6.1**-3434
Codergocrini mesilas 1601
Coffeinum **6.1**-3421
Coffeinum monohydricum 1365
Colae semen 1611
Colchicinum 1612
Colestyraminum 1613
Colistimethatum natricum 1614
Colistini sulfas 1615
Colophonium 1617
Compressi 748
Copolymerum methacrylatis butylati basicum 1254
Copovidonum 1617
Coriandri aetheroleum 1621
Coriandri fructus 1620
Corpora ad usum pharmaceuticum 703
Cortisoni acetas 1622
Crataegi folii cum flore extractum fluidum quantificatum 2037
Crataegi folii cum flore extractum siccum 2036
Crataegi folium cum flore 2035
Crataegi fructus 2034
Cresolum crudum 1626
Croci stigma ad praeparationes homoeopathicas 1084
Crospovidonum 1628
Crotamitonum 1629
Cupri acetas monohydricus ad praeparationes homoeopathicas 1075
Cupri sulfas anhydricus 1619
Cupri sulfas pentahydricus 1620
Cuprum ad praeparationes homoeopathicas 1076
Curcumae xanthorrhizae rhizoma 3150
Cyamopsidis seminis pulvis 2016
Cyanocobalamini (^{57}Co) capsulae 983
Cyanocobalamini (^{57}Co) solutio 984
Cyanocobalamini (^{58}Co) capsulae 985
Cyanocobalamini (^{58}Co) solutio 986
Cyanocobalaminum 1630
Cyclizini hydrochloridum 1631
Cyclopentolati hydrochloridum 1632
Cyclophosphamidum 1633
Cynarae folium 1219
Cyproheptadini hydrochloridum 1634
Cyproteroni acetas 1635
Cysteini hydrochloridum monohydricum 1636
Cystinum 1637
Cytarabinum 1638

D

Dacarbazinum 1641
Dalteparinum natricum 1642
Danaparoidum natricum 1644
Dapsonum 1646
Daunorubicini hydrochloridum 1647
D-Camphora 1400
Decylis oleas 1648
Deferoxamini mesilas 1649
Dembrexini hydrochloridum monohydricum ad usum veterinarium 1650
Demeclocyclini hydrochloridum 1651
Deptropini citras 1653
Dequalinii chloridum 1654
Desfluranum **6.1**-3439
Desipramini hydrochloridum 1655
Deslanosidum 1656
Desmopressinum 1657
Desogestrelum 1658
Desoxycortoni acetas 1659
Detomidini hydrochloridum ad usum veterinarium 1660
Dexamethasoni acetas 1665
Dexamethasoni isonicotinas 1666
Dexamethasoni natrii phosphas 1667
Dexamethasonum 1663
Dexchlorpheniramini maleas 1669
Dexpanthenolum 1670
Dextranomerum 1675
Dextranum 1 ad iniectabile 1671
Dextranum 40 ad iniectabile 1672
Dextranum 60 ad iniectabile 1673
Dextranum 70 ad iniectabile 1674
Dextrinum 1675
Dextromethorphani hydrobromidum 1676
Dextromoramidi tartras 1677
Dextropropoxypheni hydrochloridum 1678
Diazepamum 1679
Diazoxidum 1680
Dibrompropamidini diisetionas 1681
Dibutylis phthalas 1682
Diclazurilum ad usum veterinarium 1683
Diclofenacum kalicum 1685
Diclofenacum natricum 1686
Dicloxacillinum natricum 1687
Dicycloverini hydrochloridum 1689
Didanosinum 1689
Dienestrolum 1691
Diethylcarbamazini citras 1693
Diethylenglycoli aether monoethilicus 1694
Diethylenglycoli palmitostearas 1695
Diethylis phthalas **6.1**-3441
Diethylstilbestrolum 1696
Diflunisalum 1697
Digitalis purpureae folium 1698
Digitoxinum 1700
Digoxinum 1701
Dihydralazini sulfas hydricus **6.1**-3442
Dihydrocodeini hydrogenotartras 1704
Dihydroergocristini mesilas 1705
Dihydroergotamini mesilas **6.1**-3444
Dihydroergotamini tartras 1709
Dihydrostreptomycini sulfas ad usum veterinarium 1710
Dihydrotachysterolum 1712
Dikalii clorazepas 1728
Dikalii phosphas 1729
Diltiazemi hydrochloridum **6.1**-3446
Dimenhydrinatum 1715
Dimercaprolum 1716
Dimethylacetamidum 1717
Dimethylis sulfoxidum 1716
Dimeticonum 1718
Dimetindeni maleas 1719
Dinatrii edetas 1734
Dinatrii etidronas 1844
Dinatrii pamidronas pentahydricus 2604
Dinatrii phosphas anhydricus 1735
Dinatrii phosphas dihydricus 1735
Dinatrii phosphas dodecahydricus **6.1**-3449
Dinitrogenii oxidum 2515
Dinoprostonum 1722
Dinoprostum trometamolum 1720
Diosminum 1723
Diphenhydramini hydrochloridum 1725
Diphenoxylati hydrochloridum 1726
Dipivefrini hydrochloridum 1727
Diprophyllinum 1730
Dipyridamolum 1731
Dirithromycinum **6.1**-3447
Disopyramidi phosphas 1738
Disopyramidum 1737
Disulfiramum 1739
Dithranolum 1740
DL-Methioninum 2380
DL-α-Tocopherylis hydrogenosuccinas 3093
Dobutamini hydrochloridum 1741
Dodecylis gallas 1744
Domperidoni maleas 1747
Domperidonum 1745
Dopamini hydrochloridum 1749
Dopexamini dihydrochloridum 1750
Dorzolamidi hydrochloridum 1752
Dosulepini hydrochloridum 1753
Doxaprami hydrochloridum 1754
Doxazosini mesilas 1756
Doxepini hydrochloridum **6.1**-3449
Doxorubicini hydrochloridum 1759
Doxycyclini hyclas 1760
Doxycyclinum monohydricum 1762
Doxylamini hydrogenosuccinas **6.1**-3451
Droperidolum 1765

E

Ebastinum 1771
Echinaceae angustifoliae radix 2483
Echinaceae pallidae radix 2602
Echinaceae purpureae herba 2785
Echinaceae purpureae radix 2787
Econazoli nitras 1773
Econazolum 1772
Edrophonii chloridum 1775
Eleutherococci radix 1777
Emedastini difumaras 1779
Emetini hydrochloridum heptahydricum 1780
Emetini hydrochloridum pentahydricum 1781
Emplastra transcutanea 737
Enalaprilatum dihydricum 1784
Enalaprili maleas 1782
Enilconazolum ad usum veterinarium 1785
Enoxaparinum natricum 1787
Enoxolonum 1788
Ephedrini hydrochloridum 1791
Ephedrini racemici hydrochloridum 1792
Ephedrinum anhydricum 1789
Ephedrinum hemihydricum 1790
Epirubicini hydrochloridum 1793
Equiseti herba 1794
Ergocalciferolum 1795
Ergometrini maleas 1797

Ergotamini tartras 1798
Erythritolum 1800
Erythromycini estolas 1803
Erythromycini ethylsuccinas 1806
Erythromycini lactobionas 1808
Erythromycini stearas 1810
Erythromycinum 1801
Erythropoietini solutio concentrata 1813
Eserini salicylas 2677
Eserini sulfas 2678
Esketamini hydrochloridum 1817
Estradioli benzoas **6.1**-3455
Estradioli valeras 1821
Estradiolum hemihydricum 1819
Estriolum 1822
Estrogeni coniuncti 1824
Etamsylatum 1827
Ethacridini lactas monohydricus 1828
Ethambutoli hydrochloridum **6.1**-3456
Ethanolum (96 per centum) 1829
Ethanolum anhydricum 1831
Ethinylestradiolum 1834
Ethionamidum 1835
Ethosuximidum 1836
Ethylcellulosum 1841
Ethylendiaminum 1843
Ethylenglycoli monopalmitostearas 1842
Ethylis acetas 1838
Ethylis oleas 1838
Ethylis parahydroxybenzoas 1839
Ethylis parahydroxybenzoas natricus 1840
Ethylmorphini hydrochloridum 1843
Etilefrini hydrochloridum 1845
Etodolacum 1847
Etofenamatum 1849
Etofyllinum 1850
Etomidatum 1851
Etoposidum 1852
Eucalypti aetheroleum 1858
Eucalypti folium 1857
Eugenolum 1859
Extracta **6.1**-3343

F

Factor humanus von Willebrandi 2081
Factor IX coagulationis humanus 2064
Factor VII coagulationis humanus 2061
Factor VIII coagulationis humanus 2062
Factor VIII coagulationis humanus (ADNr) 2063
Factor XI coagulationis humanus 2065
Fagopyri herba 1341
Famotidinum 1865
Febantelum ad usum veterinarium 1870
Felbinacum 1866
Felodipinum 1867
Felypressinum 1869
Fenbendazolum ad usum veterinarium 1871
Fenbufenum 1872
Fenofibratum 1875
Fenoteroli hydrobromidum 1876
Fentanyli citras 1879
Fentanylum 1878
Fenticonazoli nitras 1880
Ferri chloridum hexahydricum 1882
Ferrosi fumaras 1883
Ferrosi gluconas 1884
Ferrosi sulfas desiccatus 1885
Ferrosi sulfas heptahydricus 1886
Ferrum ad praeparationes homoeopathicas 1081
Fexofenadini hydrochloridum 1888
Fibrini glutinum 1890
Fibrinogenum humanum 2066
Fila non resorbilia sterilia 1046
Fila non resorbilia sterilia in fuso ad usum veterinarium 1060
Fila resorbilia synthetica monofilamenta sterilia 1052
Fila resorbilia synthetica torta sterilia 1050
Filipendulae ulmariae herba 2344
Filum bombycis tortum sterile in fuso ad usum veterinarium 1059
Filum ethyleni polyterephthalici sterile in fuso ad usum veterinarium 1059
Filum lini sterile in fuso ad usum veterinarium 1058
Filum polyamidicum-6/6 sterile in fuso ad usum veterinarium 1059
Filum polyamidicum-6 sterile in fuso ad usum veterinarium 1058
Finasteridum 1891
Flavoxati hydrochloridum 1895
Flecainidi acetas 1896
Flubendazolum 1898
Flucloxacillinum natricum 1899
Fluconazolum 1900
Flucytosinum 1902
Fludarabini phosphas 1903
Fludeoxyglucosi (^{18}F) solutio iniectabilis 986
Fludrocortisoni acetas 1906
Flumazenili (N-[^{11}C]methyl) solutio iniectabilis 989
Flumazenilum 1908
Flumequinum 1909
Flumetasoni pivalas 1910
Flunarizini dihydrochloridum 1911
Flunitrazepamum 1913
Flunixini megluminum ad usum veterinarium 1914
Fluocinoloni acetonidum 1915
Fluocortoloni pivalas 1916
Fluoresceinum 1918
Fluoresceinum natricum 1919
Fluorodopae (^{18}F) ab electrophila substitutione solutio iniectabilis 990
Fluorouracilum 1920
Fluoxetini hydrochloridum 1922
Flupentixoli dihydrochloridum 1924
Fluphenazini decanoas 1926
Fluphenazini dihydrochloridum 1928
Fluphenazini enantas 1927
Flurazepami monohydrochloridum 1930
Flurbiprofenum 1931
Fluspirilenum 1932
Flutamidum 1933
Fluticasoni propionas 1934
Flutrimazolum 1936
Foeniculi amari fructus 1873
Foeniculi amari fructus aetheroleum 1318
Foeniculi dulcis fructus 1874
Formaldehydi solutio (35 per centum) 1939
Formoteroli fumaras dihydricus 1940
Foscarnetum natricum hexahydricum 1942
Fosfomycinum calcicum 1943
Fosfomycinum natricum 1945
Fosfomycinum trometamolum 1946
Framycetini sulfas 1947
Frangulae cortex 1949
Frangulae corticis extractum siccum normatum 1950
Fraxini folium 1222
Fructosum 1951
Fucus vel Ascophyllum 2213
Fumariae herba 1952

Furosemidum 1953

G
Galactosum 1959
Gallamini triethiodidum 1959
Gallii (^{67}Ga) citratis solutio iniectabilis 992
Gelatina 1961
Gemcitabini hydrochloridum 1963
Gemfibrozilum 1964
Gentamicini sulfas 1965
Gentianae radix 1967
Gentianae tinctura 1968
Ginkgonis extractum siccum raffinatum et quantificatum **6.1**-3461
Ginkgonis folium 1969
Ginseng radix 1971
Glibenclamidum 1972
Gliclazidum 1974
Glimepiridum 1975
Glipizidum 1977
Glucagonum humanum 1979
Glucosum anhydricum 1981
Glucosum liquidum 1982
Glucosum liquidum dispersione desiccatum 1982
Glucosum monohydricum 1983
Glutathionum **6.1**-3463
Glyceroli dibehenas 1990
Glyceroli distearas 1991
Glyceroli monocaprylas 1992
Glyceroli monocaprylocapras 1993
Glyceroli monolinoleas 1994
Glyceroli mono-oleas 1995
Glyceroli monostearas 40-55 1996
Glyceroli trinitratis solutio **6.1**-3465
Glycerolum 1987
Glycerolum (85 per centum) 1988
Glycinum 1998
Gonadorelini acetas 2003
Gonadotropinum chorionicum 2004
Gonadotropinum sericum equinum ad usum veterinarium 2005
Goserelinum 2005
Gossypii oleum hydrogenatum 1625
Gramicidinum 2007
Graminis rhizoma 1625
Granisetroni hydrochloridum 2009
Granulata 723
Griseofulvinum 2011
Guaiacolum 2012
Guaifenesinum 2014
Guanethidini monosulfas 2015
Guar galactomannanum 2016

H
Halofantrini hydrochloridum 2027
Haloperidoli decanoas 2030
Haloperidolum 2028
Halothanum 2031
Hamamelidis folium **6.1**-3471
Harpagophyti extractum siccum 1662
Harpagophyti radix **6.1**-3440
Hederae folium 2198
Hedera helix ad praeparationes homoeopathicas 1078
Helianthi annui oleum raffinatum 3007
Helium 2038
Heparina massae molecularis minoris 2041
Heparinum calcicum 2039
Heparinum natricum 2040
Heptaminoli hydrochloridum 2043
Hexamidini diisetionas 2044
Hexetidinum 2045
Hexobarbitalum 2047
Hexylresorcinolum 2047
Hibisci sabdariffae flos **6.1**-3529
Histamini dihydrochloridum 2049
Histamini phosphas 2049
Histidini hydrochloridum monohydricum 2051
Histidinum 2050
Homatropini hydrobromidum 2052
Homatropini methylbromidum 2053
Hyaluronidasum 2082
Hydralazini hydrochloridum 2083
Hydrargyri dichloridum 2361
Hydrastis rhizoma **6.1**-3467
Hydrochlorothiazidum 2086
Hydrocodoni hydrogenotartras 2.5-hydricus 2087
Hydrocortisoni acetas 2091
Hydrocortisoni hydrogenosuccinas 2092
Hydrocortisonum 2089
Hydrogenii peroxidum 30 per centum 2094
Hydrogenii peroxidum 3 per centum 2094
Hydromorphoni hydrochloridum 2095
Hydroxocobalamini acetas 2096
Hydroxocobalamini chloridum 2098
Hydroxocobalamini sulfas 2099
Hydroxycarbamidum 2100
Hydroxyethylcellulosum 2102
Hydroxyethylis salicylas 2101
Hydroxypropylbetadexum 2103
Hydroxypropylcellulosum 2105
Hydroxyzini hydrochloridum 2106
Hymecromonum 2107
Hyoscini butylbromidum 2109
Hyoscini hydrobromidum 2110
Hyoscinum 2108
Hyoscyamini sulfas 2112
Hyoscyamus niger ad praeparationes homoeopathicas 1079
Hyperici herba 2958
Hypericum perforatum ad praeparationes homoeopathicas 1080
Hypromellosi phthalas **6.1**-3475
Hypromellosum **6.1**-3473

I
Ibuprofenum **6.1**-3479
Ichthammolum 2122
Idoxuridinum 2122
Iecoris aselli oleum A 1603
Iecoris aselli oleum B 1607
Ifosfamidum 2123
Imipenemum 2125
Imipramini hydrochloridum 2126
Immunoglobulinum anti-T lymphocytorum ex animale ad usum humanum 1203
Immunoglobulinum humanum anti-D 2058
Immunoglobulinum humanum anti-D ad usum intravenosum 2059
Immunoglobulinum humanum hepatitidis A 2068
Immunoglobulinum humanum hepatitidis B 2069
Immunoglobulinum humanum hepatitidis B ad usum intravenosum 2069
Immunoglobulinum humanum morbillicum 2069
Immunoglobulinum humanum normale 2070
Immunoglobulinum humanum normale ad usum intravenosum 2072
Immunoglobulinum humanum rabicum 2078

Immunoglobulinum humanum rubellae 2079
Immunoglobulinum humanum tetanicum 2079
Immunoglobulinum humanum varicellae 2080
Immunoglobulinum humanum varicellae ad usum intravenosum 2081
Immunosera ad usum veterinarium 687
Immunosera ex animali ad usum humanum 685
Immunoserum botulinicum 965
Immunoserum Clostridii novyi alpha ad usum veterinarium 973
Immunoserum Clostridii perfringentis beta ad usum veterinarium 974
Immunoserum Clostridii perfringentis epsilon ad usum veterinarium 975
Immunoserum contra venena viperarum europaearum 970
Immunoserum diphthericum 965
Immunoserum gangraenicum (Clostridium novyi) 966
Immunoserum gangraenicum (Clostridium perfringens) 967
Immunoserum gangraenicum (Clostridium septicum) 968
Immunoserum gangraenicum mixtum 966
Immunoserum tetanicum ad usum humanum 969
Immunoserum tetanicum ad usum veterinarium 976
Indapamidum 2127
Indii (^{111}In) chloridi solutio 994
Indii (^{111}In) oxini solutio 995
Indii (^{111}In) pentetatis solutio iniectabilis 996
Indinaviri sulfas 2130
Indometacinum 2132
Inhalanda 739
Insulini zinci amorphi suspensio iniectabilis 2149
Insulini zinci cristallini suspensio iniectabilis 2149
Insulini zinci suspensio iniectabilis 2148
Insulinum aspartum 2133
Insulinum biphasicum iniectabile 2140
Insulinum bovinum 2135
Insulinum humanum 2137
Insulinum isophanum biphasicum iniectabile 2140
Insulinum isophanum iniectabile 2141
Insulinum lisprum 2141
Insulinum porcinum 2144
Insulinum solubile iniectabile 2141
Interferoni alfa-2 solutio concentrata 2150
Interferoni gamma-1b solutio concentrata 2153
int-rac-α-Tocopherolum 3086
int-rac-α-Tocopherylis acetas 3089
Iobenguani (^{123}I) solutio iniectabilis 997
Iobenguani (^{131}I) solutio iniectabilis ad usum diagnosticum 998
Iobenguani (^{131}I) solutio iniectabilis ad usum therapeuticum 999
Iobenguani sulfas ad radiopharmaceutica **6.1**-3381
Iodinati (^{125}I) humani albumini solutio iniectabilis 993
Iodum 2156
Iohexolum 2157
Iopamidolum 2160
Iotrolanum 2164
Ipecacuanhae extractum fluidum normatum 2168
Ipecacuanhae pulvis normatus 2169
Ipecacuanhae radix 2170
Ipecacuanhae tinctura normata 2171
Ipratropii bromidum 2172
Isoconazoli nitras 2175
Isoconazolum 2173
Isofluranum 2176
Isoleucinum 2177
Isomaltum 2178
Isoniazidum 2180
Isoprenalini hydrochloridum 2181
Isoprenalini sulfas 2182
Isopropylis myristas 2183
Isopropylis palmitas 2184
Isosorbidi dinitras dilutus 2185
Isosorbidi mononitras dilutus 2186
Isotretinoinum 2188
Isoxsuprini hydrochloridum 2189
Isradipinum 2192
Itraconazolum 2194
Iuniperi aetheroleum 2207
Iuniperi pseudo-fructus 2206
Ivermectinum 2196

J

Josamycini propionas 2205
Josamycinum 2204

K

Kalii acetas 2716
Kalii bromidum 2716
Kalii carbonas 2717
Kalii chloridum 2717
Kalii citras 2718
Kalii clavulanas 2719
Kalii clavulanas dilutus 2721
Kalii dihydrogenophosphas 2723
Kalii hydrogenoaspartas hemihydricus 2723
Kalii hydrogenocarbonas 2724
Kalii hydrogenotartras 2725
Kalii hydroxidum 2726
Kalii iodidum 2726
Kalii metabisulfis 2727
Kalii natrii tartras tetrahydricus 2729
Kalii nitras 2728
Kalii perchloras 2728
Kalii permanganas 2729
Kalii sorbas 2730
Kalii sulfas 2731
Kanamycini monosulfas 2212
Kanamycini sulfas acidus 2211
Kaolinum ponderosum 2213
Ketamini hydrochloridum 2214
Ketoconazolum 2216
Ketoprofenum 2218
Ketorolacum trometamolum 2220
Ketotifeni hydrogenofumaras 2221
Kryptonum (^{81m}Kr) ad inhalationem 1000

L

Labetaloli hydrochloridum 2227
Lacca 2876
Lactitolum monohydricum 2229
Lactosum anhydricum 2232
Lactosum monohydricum 2233
Lactulosum 2234
Lactulosum liquidum 2236
Lamivudinum 2238
Lansoprazolum 2240
Lanugo cellulosi absorbens 3197
Lanugo gossypii absorbens 1624
Lavandulae aetheroleum 2244
Lavandulae flos 2243
Leflunomidum 2245
Leonuri cardiacae herba 2447
Letrozolum 2249
Leucinum 2250
Leuprorelinum 2251

Levamisoli hydrochloridum 2254
Levamisolum ad usum veterinarium 2253
Levistici radix 2290
Levocabastini hydrochloridum 2255
Levocarnitinum 2257
Levodopum 2258
Levodropropizinum 2260
Levomentholum 2261
Levomepromazini hydrochloridum 2262
Levomepromazini maleas 2263
Levomethadoni hydrochloridum 2264
Levonorgestrelum 2266
Levothyroxinum natricum 2267
Lichen islandicus 2121
Lidocaini hydrochloridum 2269
Lidocainum **6.1**-3485
Limonis aetheroleum 2246
Lincomycini hydrochloridum 2271
Lindanum 2272
Lini oleum virginale 2274
Lini semen 2273
Liothyroninum natricum **6.1**-3486
Liquiritiae extractum fluidum ethanolicum normatum 2275
Liquiritiae extractum siccum ad saporandum **6.1**-3488
Liquiritiae radix 2276
Lisinoprilum dihydricum 2277
Lithii carbonas 2279
Lithii citras 2279
L-Methionini ([^{11}C]methyl) solutio iniectabilis 1001
Lobelini hydrochloridum 2280
Lomustinum 2281
Loperamidi hydrochloridum 2283
Loperamidi oxidum monohydricum 2285
Loratadinum 2286
Lorazepamum 2288
Lovastatinum 2291
Lupuli flos **6.1**-3472
Lymecyclinum **6.1**-3489
Lynestrenolum 2294
Lysini acetas 2295
Lysini hydrochloridum 2296
Lythri herba 2283

M

Macrogol 20 glyceroli monostearas 2304
Macrogol 40 sorbitoli heptaoleas 2310
Macrogol 6 glyceroli caprylocapras 2302
Macrogola 2308
Macrogolglyceridorum caprylocaprates 1403
Macrogolglyceridorum laurates 2242
Macrogolglyceridorum linoleates 2273
Macrogolglyceridorum oleates 2543
Macrogolglyceridorum stearates 2967
Macrogolglyceroli cocoates 2302
Macrogolglyceroli hydroxystearas 2303
Macrogolglyceroli ricinoleas 2304
Macrogoli 15 hydroxystearas 2305
Macrogoli aether cetostearylicus 2301
Macrogoli aether laurilicus 2306
Macrogoli aether oleicus 2308
Macrogoli aether stearylicus 2312
Macrogoli oleas 2307
Macrogoli stearas 2311
Magaldratum 2312
Magnesii acetas tetrahydricus 2313
Magnesii aspartas dihydricus 2314
Magnesii chloridum 4.5-hydricum 2317
Magnesii chloridum hexahydricum 2316
Magnesii citras anhydricus 2318
Magnesii gluconas **6.1**-3495
Magnesii glycerophosphas 2318
Magnesii hydroxidum 2319
Magnesii lactas dihydricus 2320
Magnesii oxidum leve 2321
Magnesii oxidum ponderosum 2320
Magnesii peroxidum 2321
Magnesii pidolas 2322
Magnesii stearas 2323
Magnesii subcarbonas levis 2316
Magnesii subcarbonas ponderosus 2315
Magnesii sulfas heptahydricus 2325
Magnesii trisilicas 2325
Malathionum 2327
Maltitolum 2330
Maltitolum liquidum 2332
Maltodextrinum 2333
Malvae sylvestris flos 2330
Mangani gluconas **6.1**-3495
Mangani glycerophosphas hydricus 2334
Mangani sulfas monohydricus 2335
Mannitolum 2336
Maprotilini hydrochloridum 2337
Marbofloxacinum ad usum veterinarium **6.1**-3496
Marrubii herba 3216
Masticabilia gummis medicata 719
Mastix 2340
Matricariae aetheroleum 2342
Matricariae extractum fluidum 2341
Matricariae flos 2340
Maydis amylum 2326
Maydis oleum raffinatum 2326
Mebendazolum 2345
Meclozini hydrochloridum 2346
Medroxyprogesteroni acetas 2347
Mefloquini hydrochloridum 2350
Megestroli acetas 2352
Megluminum 2353
Mel 2055
Melaleucae aetheroleum 3019
Meliloti herba 2354
Melissae folium 2355
Menadionum 2356
Menthae arvensis aetheroleum partim mentholum depletum 2430
Menthae piperitae aetheroleum 2639
Menthae piperitae folium 2638
Mentholum racemicum 2356
Menyanthidis trifoliatae folium 1323
Mepivacaini hydrochloridum 2357
Meprobamatum 2359
Mepyramini maleas 2360
Mercaptopurinum 2361
Mesalazinum 2362
Mesnum 2364
Mesterolonum 2366
Mestranolum 2367
Metacresolum 2368
Metamizolum natricum 2369
Metformini hydrochloridum 2370
Methadoni hydrochloridum 2374
Methanolum 2376
Methaqualonum 2377
Methenaminum 2378
Methioninum 2379
Methotrexatum 2380
Methylatropini bromidum 2383
Methylatropini nitras 2383

Methylcellulosum ... **6.1**-3497
Methyldopum ... 2386
Methyleni chloridum ... 2387
Methylergometrini maleas ... 2388
Methylhydroxyethylcellulosum ... 2390
Methylis nicotinas ... 2390
Methylis parahydroxybenzoas ... 2391
Methylis parahydroxybenzoas natricus ... 2911
Methylis salicylas ... 2401
Methylphenobarbitalum ... 2392
Methylprednisoloni acetas ... 2395
Methylprednisoloni hydrogenosuccinas ... 2397
Methylprednisolonum ... 2393
Methylrosanilinii chloridum ... 2400
Methyltestosteronum ... 2402
Methylthioninii chloridum ... 2402
Metixeni hydrochloridum ... 2404
Metoclopramidi hydrochloridum ... 2407
Metoclopramidum ... 2405
Metolazonum ... 2407
Metoprololi succinas ... 2409
Metoprololi tartras ... 2410
Metrifonatum ... 2412
Metronidazoli benzoas ... 2415
Metronidazolum ... 2414
Mexiletini hydrochloridum ... 2416
Mianserini hydrochloridum ... 2417
Miconazoli nitras ... 2420
Miconazolum ... 2418
Midazolamum ... 2422
Millefolii herba ... 3243
Minocyclini hydrochloridum dihydricum ... 2427
Minoxidilum ... 2429
Mirtazapinum ... 2431
Misoprostolum ... 2433
Mitomycinum ... 2434
Mitoxantroni hydrochloridum ... 2436
Modafinilum ... 2437
Molgramostimi solutio concentrata ... 2438
Molsidominum ... **6.1**-3499
Mometasoni furoas ... 2441
Moranteli hydrogenotartras ad usum veterinarium ... 2443
Morphini hydrochloridum ... **6.1**-3501
Morphini sulfas ... **6.1**-3503
Moxidectinum ad usum veterinarium ... 2448
Moxifloxacini hydrochloridum ... 2451
Moxonidinum ... 2453
Mupirocinum ... 2454
Mupirocinum calcicum ... 2456
Musci medicati ... 723
Mycophenolas mofetil ... 2458
myo-Inositolum ... 2460
Myristicae fragrantis aetheroleum ... 2533
Myrrha ... 2461
Myrrhae tinctura ... 2461
Myrtilli fructus recens ... **6.1**-3412
Myrtilli fructus siccus ... 1307

N

Nabumetonum ... 2465
N-Acetyltryptophanum ... 1104
N-Acetyltyrosinum ... 1106
Nadololum ... 2466
Nadroparinum calcicum ... 2467
Naftidrofuryli hydrogenooxalas ... 2470
Naloxoni hydrochloridum dihydricum ... 2473
Naltrexoni hydrochloridum ... 2474
Nandroloni decanoas ... 2476
Naphazolini hydrochloridum ... 2478
Naphazolini nitras ... 2479
Naproxenum ... 2480
Naproxenum natricum ... **6.1**-3507
Nasalia ... 730
Natrii acetas trihydricus ... 2883
Natrii acetatis ([1-^{11}C]) solutio iniectabilis ... 1006
Natrii alendronas ... 2884
Natrii alginas ... 2885
Natrii amidotrizoas ... 2886
Natrii aminosalicylas dihydricus ... 2887
Natrii ascorbas ... 2888
Natrii aurothiomalas ... 2889
Natrii benzoas ... 2890
Natrii bromidum ... 2891
Natrii calcii edetas ... 2892
Natrii caprylas ... 2893
Natrii carbonas anhydricus ... 2894
Natrii carbonas decahydricus ... 2894
Natrii carbonas monohydricus ... 2895
Natrii cetylo- et stearylosulfas. ... 2895
Natrii chloridum ... 2897
Natrii chromatis (^{51}Cr) solutio sterilis ... 1007
Natrii citras ... 2898
Natrii cromoglicas ... 2899
Natrii cyclamas ... 2900
Natrii dihydrogenophosphas dihydricus ... 2901
Natrii docusas ... 1743
Natrii fluoridi (^{18}F) solutio iniectabilis ... 1008
Natrii fluoridum ... 2902
Natrii fusidas ... 2902
Natrii glycerophosphas hydricus ... 2903
Natrii hyaluronas ... 2904
Natrii hydrogenocarbonas ... 2906
Natrii hydroxidum ... 2907
Natrii iodidi (^{123}I) solutioad radio-signandum ... 1010
Natrii iodidi (^{123}I) solutio iniectabilis ... 1009
Natrii iodidi (^{131}I) capsulae ad usum diagnosticum ... 1011
Natrii iodidi (^{131}I) capsulae ad usum therapeuticum ... 1012
Natrii iodidi (^{131}I) solutio ... 1013
Natrii iodidi (^{131}I) solutio ad radio-signandum ... 1014
Natrii iodidum ... 2907
Natrii iodohippurati (^{123}I) solutio iniectabilis ... 1014
Natrii iodohippurati (^{131}I) solutio iniectabilis ... 1015
Natrii lactatis solutio ... 2908
Natrii laurilsulfas ... 2910
Natrii metabisulfis ... 2911
Natrii molybdas dihydricus ... 2912
Natrii molybdatis (^{99}Mo) fissione formati solutio ... 1016
Natrii nitris ... 2913
Natrii nitroprussias ... 2913
Natrii perboras hydricus ... 2914
Natrii pertechnetatis (^{99m}Tc) fissione formati solutio iniectabilis ... 1018
Natrii pertechnetatis (^{99m}Tc) sine fissione formati solutio iniectabilis ... 1020
Natrii phenylbutyras ... **6.1**-3539
Natrii phosphatis (^{32}P) solutio iniectabilis ... 1020
Natrii picosulfas ... 2915
Natrii polystyrenesulfonas ... 2916
Natrii propionas ... 2917
Natrii salicylas ... 2919
Natrii selenis pentahydricus ... 2919
Natrii (S)-lactatis solutio ... 2909
Natrii stearas ... 2923
Natrii stearylis fumaras ... 2924
Natrii sulfas anhydricus ... 2924
Natrii sulfas decahydricus ... 2925
Natrii sulfis anhydricus ... 2926
Natrii sulfis heptahydricus ... 2926

Natrii thiosulfas 2927
Natrii valproas 2927
Neohesperidin-dihydrochalconum 2485
Neomycini sulfas 2487
Neostigmini bromidum 2489
Neostigmini metilsulfas 2490
Neroli aetheroleum 2490
Netilmicini sulfas 2492
Nevirapinum anhydricum 2495
Nicergolinum 2496
Nicethamidum 2505
Niclosamidum anhydricum 2497
Niclosamidum monohydricum 2498
Nicotinamidum 2499
Nicotini resinas 2501
Nicotinum 2500
Nifedipinum 2503
Nifuroxazidum **6.1**-3510
Nimesulidum 2506
Nimodipinum 2507
Nitrazepamum 2508
Nitrendipinum 2509
Nitrofuralum 2512
Nitrofurantoinum 2513
Nitrogenii oxidum 2511
Nitrogenium 2513
Nitrogenium oxygenio depletum 2514
Nizatidinum 2516
N-Methylpyrrolidonum 2399
Nomegestroli acetas 2518
Nonoxinolum 9 2519
Noradrenalini hydrochloridum 2520
Noradrenalini tartras 2521
Norcholesteroli iodinati (^{131}I) solutio iniectabilis 1003
Norethisteroni acetas 2524
Norethisteronum 2523
Norfloxacinum 2525
Norgestimatum 2526
Norgestrelum 2527
Nortriptylini hydrochloridum 2528
Noscapini hydrochloridum 2530
Noscapinum 2529
Notoginseng radix 2531
Nystatinum 2534

O

Octoxinolum 10 2539
Octyldodecanolum 2540
Octylis gallas 2539
Oenotherae oleum raffinatum 1860
Ofloxacinum 2541
Oleae folium 2545
Olea herbaria 712
Olibanum indicum 2128
Olivae oleum raffinatum 2546
Olivae oleum virginale 2547
Olsalazinum natricum 2548
Omega-3 acidorum esteri ethylici 60 2550
Omega-3 acidorum esteri ethylici 90 2552
Omega-3 acidorum triglycerida 2554
Omeprazolum 2557
Omeprazolum natricum 2558
Ondansetroni hydrochloridum dihydricum 2560
Ononidis radix 2815
Ophthalmica 721
Opii extractum siccum normatum 2562
Opii pulvis normatus 2563
Opii tinctura normata 2565
Opium crudum 2564
Orciprenalini sulfas 2567
Origani herba 2568
Orphenadrini citras 2569
Orphenadrini hydrochloridum 2570
Orthosiphonis folium 2203
Oryzae amylum 2824
Ouabainum 2571
Oxacillinum natricum monohydricum 2572
Oxaliplatinum 2574
Oxazepamum 2577
Oxeladini hydrogenocitras 2578
Oxfendazolum ad usum veterinarium 2580
Oxitropii bromidum 2581
Oxprenololi hydrochloridum 2583
Oxybuprocaini hydrochloridum 2584
Oxybutynini hydrochloridum 2585
Oxycodoni hydrochloridum 2587
Oxygenium 2588
Oxygenium (^{15}O) 1004
Oxymetazolini hydrochloridum 2589
Oxytetracyclini hydrochloridum 2591
Oxytetracyclinum dihydricum 2590
Oxytocini solutio concentrata 2594
Oxytocinum 2593

P

Paclitaxelum **6.1**-3515
Pancreatis pulvis 2605
Pancuronii bromidum 2608
Pantoprazolum natricum sesquihydricum **6.1**-3518
Papaverini hydrochloridum 2609
Papaveris rhoeados flos 2811
Paracetamolum 2611
Paraffinum liquidum 2613
Paraffinum perliquidum 2612
Paraffinum solidum 2612
Paraldehydum 2615
Parenteralia 735
Parnaparinum natricum 2616
Paroxetini hydrochloridum anhydricum 2616
Paroxetini hydrochloridum hemihydricum 2619
Passiflorae herba 2621
Passiflorae herbae extractum siccum 2622
Pefloxacini mesilas dihydricus 2623
Pelargonii radix 2625
Penbutololi sulfas 2625
Penicillaminum 2626
Pentaerythrityli tetranitras dilutus 2628
Pentamidini diisetionas 2630
Pentazocini hydrochloridum 2632
Pentazocini lactas 2632
Pentazocinum 2631
Pentobarbitalum 2633
Pentobarbitalum natricum 2634
Pentoxifyllinum 2635
Pentoxyverini hydrogenocitras 2637
Pepsini pulvis 2640
Pergolidi mesilas 2641
Perphenazinum 2648
Pethidini hydrochloridum 2650
Phenazonum 2651
Pheniramini maleas 2652
Phenobarbitalum 2653
Phenobarbitalum natricum 2654
Phenolphthaleinum 2656
Phenolsulfonphthaleinum 2657
Phenolum 2655
Phenoxyethanolum 2657
Phenoxymethylpenicillinum **6.1**-3520

Phenoxymethylpenicillinum kalicum **6.1**-3521
Phentolamini mesilas 2662
Phenylalaninum 2663
Phenylbutazonum 2664
Phenylephrini hydrochloridum 2667
Phenylephrinum 2665
Phenylhydrargyri acetas 2668
Phenylhydrargyri boras 2669
Phenylhydrargyri nitras 2669
Phenylpropanolamini hydrochloridum 2670
Phenytoinum 2671
Phenytoinum natricum 2672
Phloroglucinolum anhydricum 2672
Phloroglucinolum dihydricum 2673
Pholcodinum 2674
Phthalylsulfathiazolum 2676
Physostigmini salicylas 2677
Physostigmini sulfas 2678
Phytomenadionum 2679
Phytosterolum 2680
Picotamidum monohydricum 2682
Pilocarpini hydrochloridum 2682
Pilocarpini nitras 2684
Pimobendanum 2685
Pimozidum 2686
Pindololum 2688
Pini pumilionis aetheroleum 1766
Pini sylvestris aetheroleum 2689
Piperacillinum 2691
Piperacillinum natricum 2692
Piperazini adipas 2694
Piperazini citras 2695
Piperazinum hydricum 2696
Piracetamum 2697
Pirenzepini dihydrochloridum monohydricum 2698
Piretanidum 2699
Piroxicamum 2700
Piscis oleum omega-3 acidis abundans 1893
Pivampicillinum 2702
Pivmecillinami hydrochloridum 2704
Plantae ad ptisanam 685
Plantae medicinales 684
Plantae medicinales ad praeparationes homoeopathicas 1065
Plantae medicinales praeparatae 684
Plantaginis lanceolatae folium 2823
Plantaginis ovatae semen 2192
Plantaginis ovatae seminis tegumentum 2191
Plasma humanum ad separationem 2073
Plasma humanum coagmentatum conditumque ad exstinguendum virum 2075
Poloxamera 2705
Polyacrylatis dispersio 30 per centum 2706
Poly(alcohol vinylicus) 2715
Polygalae radix 2867
Polygoni avicularis herba 2223
Polymyxini B sulfas 2707
Polysorbatum 20 2709
Polysorbatum 40 2710
Polysorbatum 60 2710
Polysorbatum 80 2711
Poly(vinylis acetas) 2712
Poly(vinylis acetas) dispersio 30 per centum 2713
Povidonum **6.1**-3523
Povidonum iodinatum 2734
Praeadmixta ad alimenta medicata ad usum veterinarium 739
Praeparationes ad irrigationem 743
Praeparationes buccales 732
Praeparationes homoeopathicas 1065
Praeparationes insulini iniectabiles 2146
Praeparationes intramammariae ad usum veterinarium 725
Praeparationes intraruminales 725
Praeparationes intra-uterinae ad usum veterinarium 726
Praeparationes liquidae ad usum dermicum 728
Praeparationes liquidae peroraliae 728
Praeparationes liquidae veterinariae ad usum dermicum 752
Praeparationes molles ad usum dermicum 746
Praeparationes pharmaceuticae in vasis cum pressu 744
Pravastatinum natricum 2735
Prazepamum 2736
Praziquantelum 2737
Prazosini hydrochloridum 2738
Prednicarbatum 2740
Prednisoloni acetas 2742
Prednisoloni natrii phosphas 2745
Prednisoloni pivalas 2744
Prednisolonum 2741
Prednisonum 2746
Prilocaini hydrochloridum 2750
Prilocainum 2748
Primaquini diphosphas 2751
Primidonum 2752
Primulae radix 2753
Probenecidum 2754
Procainamidi hydrochloridum 2755
Procaini hydrochloridum 2756
Prochlorperazini maleas 2756
Producta ab arte ADN recombinandorum 701
Producta ab fermentatione 693
Producta allergenica 679
Producta cum possibili transmissione vectorium enkephalopathiarum spongiformium animalium 694
Progesteronum 2757
Proguanili hydrochloridum 2758
Prolinum 2760
Promazini hydrochloridum 2761
Promethazini hydrochloridum 2761
Propacetamoli hydrochloridum 2763
Propafenoni hydrochloridum 2764
Propanolum 2766
Propanthelini bromidum 2767
Propofolum 2768
Propranololi hydrochloridum 2770
Propylenglycoli dicaprylocapras 2774
Propylenglycoli dilauras 2774
Propylenglycoli monolauras 2775
Propylenglycoli monopalmitostearas 2776
Propylenglycolum 2773
Propylis gallas 2771
Propylis parahydroxybenzoas 2772
Propylis parahydroxybenzoas natricus 2918
Propylthiouracilum 2777
Propyphenazonum 2778
Protamini hydrochloridum 2779
Protamini sulfas 2780
Prothrombinum multiplex humanum 2076
Protirelinum 2781
Proxyphyllinum 2783
Pruni africanae cortex 2789
Pseudoephedrini hydrochloridum 2784
Psyllii semen 2785
Pulveres ad usum dermicum 738
Pulveres perorales 738
Pyranteli embonas 2790
Pyrazinamidum 2791

Pyridostigmini bromidum 2792
Pyridoxini hydrochloridum 2793
Pyrimethaminum 2794
Pyrrolidonum 2794

Q

Quercus cortex 2539

R

Raclopridi ([^{11}C]methoxy) solutio iniectabilis 1005
Radiopharmaceutica 695
Ramiprilum 2807
Ranitidini hydrochloridum 2809
Rapae oleum raffinatum 2811
Ratanhiae radix 2816
Ratanhiae tinctura 2817
Rectalia 744
Repaglinidum 2812
Reserpinum 2814
Resorcinolum 2815
Rhamni purshianae cortex 1429
Rhamni purshianae extractum siccum normatum 1430
Rhei radix 2817
Rhenii sulfidi colloidalis et technetii (^{99m}Tc) solutio iniectabilis 1023
Ribavirinum 2818
Riboflavini natrii phosphas 2821
Riboflavinum 2820
Ricini oleum hydrogenatum 1432
Ricini oleum raffinatum 1433
Ricini oleum virginale 1434
Rifabutinum 2825
Rifampicinum 2826
Rifamycinum natricum 2827
Rilmenidini dihydrogenophosphas 2829
Risperidonum 2830
Ritonavirum 2832
Rocuronii bromidum 2835
Ropivacaini hydrochloridum monohydricum 2837
Rosae pseudo-fructus 1744
Rosmarini aetheroleum 2840
Rosmarini folium 2839
Roxithromycinum 2842
RRR-α-Tocopherolum 3088
RRR-α-Tocopherylis acetas 3090
RRR-α-Tocopherylis hydrogenosuccinas 3095
Rusci rhizoma **6.1**-3416
Rutosidum trihydricum 2844

S

Sabalis serrulatae fructus 2864
Sacchari monopalmitas **6.1**-3543
Saccharinum 2849
Saccharinum natricum 2850
Sacchari sphaerae 2979
Sacchari stearas **6.1**-3544
Saccharum 2975
Salbutamoli sulfas 2857
Salbutamolum 2855
Salicis cortex **6.1**-3563
Salicis corticis extractum siccum **6.1**-3564
Salmeteroli xinafoas 2860
Salmonis domestici oleum 2862
Salviae officinalis folium 2853
Salviae sclareae aetheroleum 1561
Salviae tinctura 2854
Salviae trilobae folium 2854
Sambuci flos 1776
Sanguisorbae radix **6.1**-3533
Scopolamini butylbromidum 2109
Scopolamini hydrobromidum 2110
Scopolaminum 2108
Selamectinum ad usum veterinarium **6.1**-3534
Selegilini hydrochloridum 2866
Selenii disulfidum 2867
Semecarpus anacardium ad praeparationes homoeopathicas 1082
Sennae folii extractum siccum normatum 2869
Sennae folium 2868
Sennae fructus acutifoliae 2870
Sennae fructus angustifoliae 2871
Serinum 2872
Serpylli herba 3219
Sertaconazoli nitras **6.1**-3535
Sertralini hydrochloridum **6.1**-3537
Serum bovinum 1329
Sesami oleum raffinatum 2874
Silica ad usum dentalem 2878
Silica colloidalis anhydrica 2877
Silica colloidalis hydrica 2877
Silica hydrophobica colloidalis 2878
Silybi mariani extractum siccum raffinatum et normatum 2426
Silybi mariani fructus 2425
Simeticonum 2880
Simvastatinum 2881
Soiae oleum hydrogenatum 2946
Soiae oleum raffinatum 2946
Solani amylum 2731
Solidaginis herba 1999
Solidaginis virgaureae herba 2000
Solutiones ad conservationem partium corporis 2929
Solutiones ad haemocolaturam haemodiacolaturamque 2025
Solutiones ad haemodialysim 2022
Solutiones ad peritonealem dialysim 2646
Solutiones anticoagulantes et sanguinem humanum conservantes 1200
Somatostatinum 2930
Somatropini solutio concentrata 2933
Somatropinum 2931
Somatropinum iniectabile 2935
Sorbitani lauras 2938
Sorbitani oleas 2938
Sorbitani palmitas 2939
Sorbitani sesquioleas 2939
Sorbitani stearas 2940
Sorbitani trioleas 2940
Sorbitolum 2941
Sorbitolum liquidum cristallisabile 2942
Sorbitolum liquidum non cristallisabile 2943
Sorbitolum liquidum partim deshydricum 2944
Sotaloli hydrochloridum 2944
Spectinomycini dihydrochloridum pentahydricum 2947
Spectinomycini sulfas tetrahydricus ad usum veterinarium 2949
Spiramycinum **6.1**-3540
Spiraprili hydrochloridum monohydricum 2954
Spironolactonum 2955
Squalanum 2956
Stanni colloidalis et technetii (^{99m}Tc) solutio iniectabilis 1025
Stanni pyrophosphatis et technetii (^{99m}Tc) solutio iniectabilis 1038
Stannosi chloridum dihydricum 2959
Stavudinum 2964
Stramonii folium 2968

Stramonii pulvis normatus 2970
Streptokinasi solutio ad praeparationem 2971
Streptomycini sulfas 2972
Strontii (^{89}Sr) chloridi solutio iniectabilis 1021
Styli 748
Succinylsulfathiazolum 2974
Sufentanili citras 2978
Sufentanilum 2977
Sulbactamum natricum 2980
Sulfacetamidum natricum 2982
Sulfadiazinum 2983
Sulfadimidinum 2984
Sulfadoxinum 2984
Sulfafurazolum 2985
Sulfaguanidinum 2986
Sulfamerazinum 2987
Sulfamethizolum 2988
Sulfamethoxazolum 2989
Sulfamethoxypyridazinum ad usum veterinarium 2990
Sulfanilamidum 2991
Sulfasalazinum 2992
Sulfathiazolum 2994
Sulfinpyrazonum 2995
Sulfisomidinum 2996
Sulfur ad usum externum 2998
Sulfuris colloidalis et technetii (^{99m}Tc) solutio iniectabilis 1024
Sulindacum 2996
Sulpiridum 2999
Sultamicillini tosilas dihydricus **6.1**-3548
Sultamicillinum **6.1**-3545
Sumatriptani succinas 3005
Suxamethonii chloridum 3007
Suxibuzonum 3008

T

Talcum 3013
Tamoxifeni citras 3014
Tamponae medicatae 751
Tamsulosini hydrochloridum 3016
Tanaceti parthenii herba 1887
Tanninum 3018
Technetii (^{99m}Tc) bicisati solutio iniectabilis 1022
Technetii (^{99m}Tc) et etifenini solutio iniectabilis 1026
Technetii (^{99m}Tc) exametazimi solutio iniectabilis 1027
Technetii (^{99m}Tc) gluconatis solutio iniectabilis 1028
Technetii (^{99m}Tc) humani albumini solutio iniectabilis 1029
Technetii (^{99m}Tc) macrosalbi suspensio iniectabilis 1030
Technetii (^{99m}Tc) medronati solutio iniectabilis 1031
Technetii (^{99m}Tc) mertiatidi solutio iniectabilis 1033
Technetii (^{99m}Tc) microsphaerarum suspensio iniectabilis 1034
Technetii (^{99m}Tc) pentetatis solutio iniectabilis 1035
Technetii (^{99m}Tc) sestamibi solutio iniectabilis 1036
Technetii (^{99m}Tc) succimeri solutio iniectabilis 1037
Temazepamum 3020
Tenoxicamum 3021
Terazosini hydrochloridum dihydricum 3022
Terbinafini hydrochloridum 3024
Terbutalini sulfas 3025
Terconazolum **6.1**-3553
Terebinthinae aetheroleum a Pino pinastro 3151
Terfenadinum **6.1**-3554
tert-Butylamini perindoprilum 2643
Testosteroni decanoas 3031
Testosteroni enantas 3033
Testosteroni isocaproas 3034
Testosteroni propionas 3035
Testosteronum 3030
Tetracaini hydrochloridum **6.1**-3556
Tetracosactidum 3037
Tetracyclini hydrochloridum 3041
Tetracyclinum 3040
Tetrazepamum 3043
Tetryzolini hydrochloridum 3044
Thallosi (^{201}Tl) chloridi solutio iniectabilis 1039
Theobrominum 3045
Theophyllinum 3046
Theophyllinum et ethylenediaminum 3048
Theophyllinum et ethylenediaminum hydricum 3049
Theophyllinum monohydricum 3047
Thiamazolum 3050
Thiamini hydrochloridum 3051
Thiamini nitras 3053
Thiamphenicolum 3054
Thiomersalum 3056
Thiopentalum natricum et natrii carbonas 3057
Thioridazini hydrochloridum 3059
Thioridazinum 3058
Threoninum 3060
Thymi aetheroleum 3063
Thymi herba 3061
Thymolum 3064
Tiabendazolum 3064
Tiamulini hydrogenofumaras ad usum veterinarium 3068
Tiamulinum ad usum veterinarium 3065
Tianeptinum natricum 3070
Tiapridi hydrochloridum 3071
Tibolonum 3074
Ticarcillinum natricum 3075
Ticlopidini hydrochloridum 3077
Tiliae flos 2270
Tilidini hydrochloridum hemihydricum 3079
Timololi maleas 3080
Tincturae maternae ad praeparationes homoeopathicas 1072
Tinidazolum 3081
Tinzaparinum natricum 3082
Tioconazolum 3083
Titanii dioxidum 3084
Tobramycinum 3085
α-Tocopherylis acetatis pulvis 3091
Tolbutamidum 3097
Tolnaftatum 3099
Torasemidum anhydricum 3100
Tormentillae rhizoma 3101
Tormentillae tinctura 3102
Tosylchloramidum natricum 3103
Toxinum botulinicum typum A ad iniectabile 1327
Tragacantha 3103
Tramadoli hydrochloridum 3104
Tramazolini hydrochloridum monohydricum 3106
Trandolaprilum 3107
Trapidilum 3110
Tretinoinum 3111
Triacetinum 3112
Triamcinoloni acetonidum 3114
Triamcinoloni hexacetonidum 3115
Triamcinolonum 3112
Triamterenum **6.1**-3557
Tribenosidum 3117
Tributylis acetylcitras 3118
Tricalcii phosphas 1396
Triethylis citras 3120
Trifluoperazini hydrochloridum 3121
Triflusalum 3121
Triglycerida saturata media 3122
Triglyceroli diisostearas **6.1**-3558

Trigonellae foenugraeci semen 1882
Trihexyphenidyli hydrochloridum 3125
Trimetazidini dihydrochloridum 3126
Trimethadionum 3127
Trimethoprimum 3128
Trimipramini maleas 3130
Tri-n-butylis phosphas 3132
Tritici aestivi oleum raffinatum 3215
Tritici aestivi oleum virginale 3216
Tritici amylum 3215
Trolaminum 3133
Trometamolum 3135
Tropicamidum 3135
Tropisetroni hydrochloridum 3136
Trospii chloridum 3138
Troxerutinum 3139
Trypsinum 3141
Tryptophanum 3142
Tuberculini aviarii derivatum proteinosum purificatum 3146
Tuberculini bovini derivatum proteinosum purificatum 3147
Tuberculini derivatum proteinosum purificatum ad usum humanum 3147
Tuberculinum pristinum ad usum humanum 3144
Tubocurarini chloridum 3150
Tylosini phosphatis solutio ad usum veterinarium 3154
Tylosini tartras ad usum veterinarium 3156
Tylosinum ad usum veterinarium 3152
Tyrosinum 3157
Tyrothricinum 3158

U

Ubidecarenonum 3163
Ureum 3165
Urofollitropinum 3166
Urokinasum 3167
Urtica dioica ad praeparationes homoeopathicas 1075
Urticae folium 2493
Uvae ursi folium **6.1**-3410

V

Vaccina ad usum humanum 705
Vaccina ad usum veterinarium 707
Vaccinum actinobacillosidis inactivatum ad suem 943
Vaccinum adenovirosidis caninae vivum 886
Vaccinum adenovirosis caninae inactivatum 885
Vaccinum anaemiae infectivae pulli vivum 925
Vaccinum anthracis adsorbatum ab colato culturarum ad usum humanum 757
Vaccinum anthracis vivum ad usum veterinarium 859
Vaccinum aphtharum epizooticarum inactivatum ad ruminantes 918
Vaccinum bronchitidis infectivae aviariae inactivatum 864
Vaccinum bronchitidis infectivae aviariae vivum **6.1**-3371
Vaccinum brucellosis (Brucella melitensis stirpe Rev. 1) vivum ad usum veterinarium 881
Vaccinum bursitidis infectivae aviariae inactivatum 867
Vaccinum bursitidis infectivae aviariae vivum 869
Vaccinum calicivirosis felinae inactivatum 909
Vaccinum calicivirosis felinae vivum 910
Vaccinum chlamydiosidis felinae inactivatum 911
Vaccinum cholerae 761
Vaccinum cholerae aviariae inactivatum 920
Vaccinum cholerae cryodesiccatum 761
Vaccinum cholerae perorale inactivatum 762
Vaccinum Clostridii botulini ad usum veterinarium 894
Vaccinum Clostridii chauvoei ad usum veterinarium 894
Vaccinum Clostridii novyi B ad usum veterinarium 895
Vaccinum Clostridii perfringentis ad usum veterinarium 897
Vaccinum Clostridii septici ad usum veterinarium 899
Vaccinum colibacillosis fetus a partu recentis inactivatum ad ruminantes 936
Vaccinum colibacillosis fetus a partu recentis inactivatum ad suem 934
Vaccinum diarrhoeae viralis bovinae inactivatum 880
Vaccinum diphtheriae adsorbatum 789
Vaccinum diphtheriae, antigeniis minutum, adsorbatum 791
Vaccinum diphtheriae et tetani adsorbatum 763
Vaccinum diphtheriae et tetani, antigeni-o(-is) minutum, adsorbatum 764
Vaccinum diphtheriae, tetani et hepatitidis B (ADNr) adsorbatum 765
Vaccinum diphtheriae, tetani et pertussis adsorbatum 768
Vaccinum diphtheriae, tetani et pertussis sine cellulis ex elementis praeparatum adsorbatum 767
Vaccinum diphtheriae, tetani et poliomyelitidis inactivatum, antigeni-o(-is) minutum, adsorbatum 770
Vaccinum diphtheriae, tetani, pertussis et poliomyelitidis inactivatum adsorbatum 785
Vaccinum diphtheriae, tetani, pertussis, poliomyelitidis inactivatum et haemophili stirpi b coniugatum adsorbatum 787
Vaccinum diphtheriae, tetani, pertussis sine cellulis ex elementis praeparatum cumque haemophili stirpi b coniugatum adsorbatum 771
Vaccinum diphtheriae, tetani, pertussis sine cellulis ex elementis praeparatum et hepatitidis B (ADNr) adsorbatum 774
Vaccinum diphtheriae, tetani, pertussis sine cellulis ex elementis praeparatum et poliomyelitidis inactivatum adsorbatum 775
Vaccinum diphtheriae, tetani, pertussis sine cellulis ex elementis praeparatum et poliomyelitidis inactivatum, antigeni-o(-is) minutum, adsorbatum 778
Vaccinum diphtheriae, tetani, pertussis sine cellulis ex elementis praeparatum, hepatitidis B (ADNr), poliomyelitidis inactivatum et haemophili stirpi b coniugatum adsorbatum 780
Vaccinum diphtheriae, tetani, pertussis sine cellulis ex elementis praeparatum, poliomyelitidis inactivatum et haemophili stirpi b coniugatum adsorbatum 783
Vaccinum encephalitidis ixodibus advectae inactivatum 845
Vaccinum encephalomyelitidis infectivae aviariae vivum 871
Vaccinum erysipelatis suillae inactivatum 955
Vaccinum febris flavae vivum **6.1**-3365
Vaccinum febris typhoidi 849
Vaccinum febris typhoidi cryodesiccatum 849
Vaccinum febris typhoidis polysaccharidicum 847
Vaccinum febris typhoidis vivum perorale (stirpe Ty 21a) 849
Vaccinum furunculosidis ad salmonidas inactivatum cum adiuvatione oleosa ad iniectionem 922
Vaccinum haemophili stirpi b coniugatum 792
Vaccinum hepatitidis A inactivatum adsorbatum 795
Vaccinum hepatitidis A inactivatum et hepatitidis B (ADNr) adsorbatum 794
Vaccinum hepatitidis A inactivatum virosomale 797
Vaccinum hepatitidis B (ADNr) 800
Vaccinum hepatitidis viralis anatis stirpe I vivum 902
Vaccinum herpesviris equini inactivatum 905
Vaccinum inactivatum diarrhoeae vituli coronaviro illatae 882

Vaccinum inactivatum diarrhoeae vituli rotaviro illatae 884
Vaccinum influenzae equi inactivatum 907
Vaccinum influenzae inactivatum ad suem 944
Vaccinum influenzae inactivatum ex cellulis corticisque antigeniis praeparatum 804
Vaccinum influenzae inactivatum ex cellulis virisque integris praeparatum 810
Vaccinum influenzae inactivatum ex corticis antigeniis praeparatum 803
Vaccinum influenzae inactivatum ex corticis antigeniis praeparatum virosomale 806
Vaccinum influenzae inactivatum ex viris integris praeparatum 808
Vaccinum influenzae inactivatum ex virorum fragmentis praeparatum 801
Vaccinum laryngotracheitidis infectivae aviariae vivum 872
Vaccinum leptospirosis bovinae inactivatum 876
Vaccinum leptospirosis caninae inactivatum 888
Vaccinum leucosis felinae inactivatum 914
Vaccinum mannheimiae inactivatum ad bovinas 927
Vaccinum mannheimiae inactivatum ad ovem 928
Vaccinum meningococcale classis C coniugatum 814
Vaccinum meningococcale polysaccharidicum 816
Vaccinum morbi Aujeszkyi ad suem inactivatum 859
Vaccinum morbi Aujeszkyi ad suem vivum ad usum parenteralem 861
Vaccinum morbi Carrei vivum ad canem 887
Vaccinum morbi Carrei vivum ad mustelidas 900
Vaccinum morbi haemorrhagici cuniculi inactivatum 949
Vaccinum morbillorum, parotitidis et rubellae vivum **6.1**-3347
Vaccinum morbillorum vivum **6.1**-3348
Vaccinum morbi Marek vivum 930
Vaccinum morbi partus diminutionis MCMLXXVI inactivatum ad pullum 904
Vaccinum Mycoplasmatis galliseptici inactivatum 932
Vaccinum myxomatosidis vivum ad cuniculum 933
Vaccinum panleucopeniae felinae infectivae inactivatum 912
Vaccinum panleucopeniae felinae infectivae vivum 913
Vaccinum parainfluenzae viri canini vivum 890
Vaccinum paramyxoviris 3 aviarii inactivatum 874
Vaccinum parotitidis vivum **6.1**-3349
Vaccinum parvovirosis caninae inactivatum 891
Vaccinum parvovirosis caninae vivum 892
Vaccinum parvovirosis inactivatum ad suem 946
Vaccinum pasteurellae inactivatum ad ovem 941
Vaccinum pertussis adsorbatum 824
Vaccinum pertussis sine cellulis copurificatum adsorbatum 822
Vaccinum pertussis sine cellulis ex elementis praeparatum adsorbatum 820
Vaccinum pestis anatis vivum 901
Vaccinum pestis classicae suillae vivum cryodesiccatum 956
Vaccinum pneumococcale polysaccharidicum 827
Vaccinum pneumococcale polysaccharidicum coniugatum adsorbatum 825
Vaccinum poliomyelitidis inactivatum 829
Vaccinum poliomyelitidis perorale **6.1**-3351
Vaccinum pseudopestis aviariae inactivatum 937
Vaccinum pseudopestis aviariae vivum 939
Vaccinum rabiei ex cellulis ad usum humanum **6.1**-3355
Vaccinum rabiei inactivatum ad usum veterinarium **6.1**-3375
Vaccinum rabiei perorale vivum ad vulpem 952
Vaccinum rhinitidis atrophicantis ingravescentis suillae inactivatum **6.1**-3373
Vaccinum rhinotracheitidis infectivae bovinae vivum 924
Vaccinum rhinotracheitidis viralis felinae inactivatum 916
Vaccinum rhinotracheitidis viralis felinae vivum 917
Vaccinum rubellae vivum **6.1**-3358
Vaccinum Salmonellae Enteritidis inactivatum ad pullum 953
Vaccinum Salmonellae Typhimurium inactivatum ad pullum 954
Vaccinum tenosynovitidis viralis aviariae vivum 875
Vaccinum tetani adsorbatum 844
Vaccinum tetani ad usum veterinarium 957
Vaccinum tuberculosis (BCG) cryodesiccatum 759
Vaccinum varicellae vivum **6.1**-3364
Vaccinum variolae gallinaceae vivum 921
Vaccinum variolae vivum **6.1**-3359
Vaccinum vibriosidis ad salmonidas inactivatum 960
Vaccinum vibriosidis aquae frigidae inactivatum ad salmonidas 959
Vaccinum viri parainfluenzae bovini vivum 878
Vaccinum viri syncytialis meatus spiritus bovini vivum 879
Vaginalia 751
Valerianae extractum hydroalcoholicum siccum 3173
Valerianae radix 3174
Valerianae tinctura 3175
Valinum 3176
Valnemulini hydrochloridum ad usum veterinarium 3177
Vancomycini hydrochloridum 3180
Vanillinum 3182
Vaselinum album 2614
Vaselinum flavum 2615
Vecuronii bromidum 3183
Venlafaxini hydrochloridum 3184
Verapamili hydrochloridum 3186
Verbasci flos 2454
Verbenae citriodoratae folium 2248
Verbenae herba 3188
Via praeparandi stirpes homoeopathicas et potentificandi **6.1**-3385
Vinblastini sulfas 3189
Vincristini sulfas 3190
Vindesini sulfas 3192
Vinorelbini tartras 3194
Vinpocetinum 3196
Violae herba cum flore 3217
Vitamini synthetici densati A pulvis 3201
Vitaminum A 3199
Vitaminum A syntheticum densatum oleosum 3200
Vitaminum A syntheticum, solubilisatum densatum in aqua dispergibile 3203

W

Warfarinum natricum 3207
Warfarinum natricum clathratum 3208

X

Xanthani gummi **6.1**-3569
Xenoni (^{133}Xe) solutio iniectabilis 1042
Xylazini hydrochloridum ad usum veterinarium 3234
Xylitolum 3235
Xylometazolini hydrochloridum 3237
Xylosum 3238

Y

Yohimbini hydrochloridum 3244

Z

Zidovudinum 3249
Zinci acetas dihydricus 3250
Zinci acexamas 3251
Zinci chloridum 3253
Zinci oxidum 3253
Zinci stearas 3254
Zinci sulfas heptahydricus 3254
Zinci sulfas hexahydricus 3255
Zinci sulfas monohydricus 3255
Zinci undecylenas 3256
Zingiberis rhizoma 1969
Zolpidemi tartras 3256
Zopiclonum 3257
Zuclopenthixoli decanoas 3259

KEY TO MONOGRAPHS

Version date of the text

01/2008:0884

corrected 6.1

Text reference number

Modification to be taken into account from the publication date of Supplement 6.1

CARBIMAZOLE

Carbimazolum

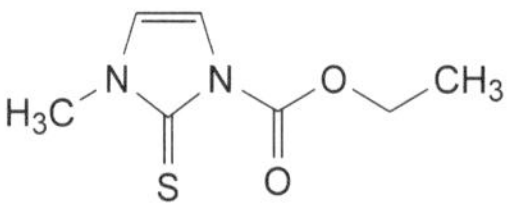

CAS number

$C_7H_{10}N_2O_2S$ [22232-54-8] M_r 186.2

DEFINITION

Chemical name in accordance with IUPAC nomenclature rules

Ethyl 3-methyl-2-thioxo-2,3-dihydro-1*H*-imidazole-1-carboxylate.

Content: 98.0 per cent to 102.0 per cent (dried substance).

CHARACTERS

Appearance: white or yellowish-white, crystalline powder.

Solubility: slightly soluble in water, soluble in acetone and in ethanol (96 per cent).

IDENTIFICATION

Application of the first and second identification is defined in the General Notices (chapter 1)

First identification: B.

Second identification: A, C.

A. Melting point (*2.2.14*): 122 °C to 125 °C.

B. Infrared absorption spectrophotometry (*2.2.24*).

Preparation: discs.

Comparison: *carbimazole CRS.*

Reference standard available from the Secretariat (see www.edqm.eu)

C. Thin-layer chromatography (*2.2.27*).

Test solution. Dissolve 10 mg of the substance to be examined in *methylene chloride R* and dilute to 10 ml with the same solvent.

Reference solution. Dissolve 10 mg of *carbimazole CRS* in *methylene chloride R* and dilute to 10 ml with the same solvent.

Plate: *TLC silica gel GF_{254} plate R.*

Mobile phase: *acetone R*, *methylene chloride R* (20:80 *V/V*).

Reagents described in chapter 4

Application: 10 µl.

Development: over a path of 15 cm.

Drying: in air for 30 min.

Further information available on www.edqm.eu (KNOWLEDGE)

Detection: examine in ultraviolet light at 254 nm.

Results: the principal spot in the chromatogram obtained with the test solution is similar in position and size to the principal spot in the chromatogram obtained with the reference solution.

TESTS

Reference to a general chapter

Related substances. Liquid chromatography (*2.2.29*).

Test solution. Dissolve 5.0 mg of the substance to be examined in 10.0 ml of a mixture of 20 volumes of *acetonitrile R* and 80 volumes of *water R*. Use this solution within 5 min of preparation.

Line in the margin indicating where part of the text has been modified (technical modification)

Reference solution (a). Dissolve 5 mg of *thiamazole R* and 0.10 g of *carbimazole CRS* in a mixture of 20 volumes of *acetonitrile R* and 80 volumes of *water R* and dilute to 100.0 ml with the same mixture of solvents. Dilute 1.0 ml of this solution to 10.0 ml with a mixture of 20 volumes of *acetonitrile R* and 80 volumes of *water R*.

Reference solution (b). Dissolve 5.0 mg of *thiamazole R* in a mixture of 20 volumes of *acetonitrile R* and 80 volumes of *water R* and dilute to 10.0 ml with the same mixture of solvents. Dilute 1.0 ml of this solution to 100.0 ml with a mixture of 20 volumes of *acetonitrile R* and 80 volumes of *water R*.

Column:

- *size*: *l* = 0.15 m, Ø = 3.9 mm,
- *stationary phase*: *octadecylsilyl silica gel for chromatography R* (5 µm).

Mobile phase: *acetonitrile R*, *water R* (10:90 *V/V*).

Flow rate: 1 ml/min.

Detection: spectrophotometer at 254 nm.

Injection: 10 µl.

Run time: 1.5 times the retention time of carbimazole.

Retention time: carbimazole = about 6 min.

System suitability: reference solution (a):

- *resolution*: minimum 5.0 between the peaks due to impurity A and carbimazole.

Limits:

- *impurity A*: not more than 0.5 times the area of the principal peak in the chromatogram obtained with reference solution (b) (0.5 per cent),
- *unspecified impurities*: for each impurity, not more than 0.1 times the area of the principal peak in the chromatogram obtained with reference solution (b) (0.10 per cent).

Loss on drying (*2.2.32*): maximum 0.5 per cent, determined on 1.000 g by drying in a desiccator over *diphosphorus pentoxide R* at a pressure not exceeding 0.7 kPa for 24 h.

Sulphated ash (*2.4.14*): maximum 0.1 per cent, determined on 1.0 g.

ASSAY

Dissolve 50.0 mg in *water R* and dilute to 500.0 ml with the same solvent. To 10.0 ml add 10 ml of *dilute hydrochloric acid R* and dilute to 100.0 ml with *water R*. Measure the absorbance (*2.2.25*) at the absorption maximum at 291 nm.

Calculate the content of $C_7H_{10}N_2O_2S$ taking the specific absorbance to be 557.

IMPURITIES

Specified impurities: A.

Other detectable impurities (the following substances would, if present at a sufficient level, be detected by one or other of the tests in the monograph. They are limited by the general acceptance criterion for other/unspecified impurities and/or by the general monograph *Substances for pharmaceutical use (2034)*. It is therefore not necessary to identify these impurities for demonstration of compliance. See also *5.10. Control of impurities in substances for pharmaceutical use): B.*

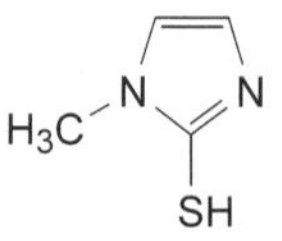

A. 1-methyl-1*H*-imidazole-2-thiol (thiamazole),